The Optics of Blood

A Handbook

Online at: https://doi.org/10.1088/978-0-7503-4806-5

IOP Series in Advances in Optics, Photonics and Optoelectronics

SERIES EDITOR

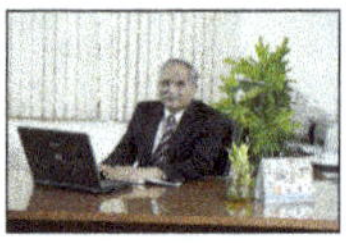

Professor Rajpal S Sirohi Consultant Scientist

About the Editor

Rajpal S Sirohi is currently working as a faculty member in the Department of Physics, Alabama A&M University, Huntsville, AL, USA. Prior to this, he was a consultant scientist at the Indian Institute of Science, Bangalore, and before that he was Chair Professor in the Department of Physics, Tezpur University, Assam. During 2000–2011, he was an academic administrator, being vice-chancellor to a couple of universities and the director of the Indian Institute of Technology, Delhi. He is the recipient of many international and national awards and the author of more than 400 papers. Dr Sirohi is involved with research concerning optical metrology, optical instrumentation, holography, and the speckle phenomena.

About the series

Optics, photonics, and optoelectronics are enabling technologies in many branches of science, engineering, medicine, and agriculture. These technologies have reshaped our outlook and our ways of interacting with each other, and have brought people closer together. They help us to understand many phenomena better and provide deeper insight into the functioning of nature. Further, these technologies themselves are evolving at a rapid rate. Their applications encompass very large spatial scales, from nanometres to the astronomical scale, and a very large temporal range, from picoseconds to billions of years. This series on advances in optics, photonics, and optoelectronics aims to cover topics that are of interest to both academia and industry. Some of the topics to be covered by the books in this series include biophotonics and medical imaging, devices, electromagnetics, fibre optics, information storage, instrumentation, light sources, charge-coupled devices (CCDs) and complementary metal oxide semiconductor (CMOS) imagers, metamaterials, optical metrology, optical networks, photovoltaics, free-form optics and its evaluation, singular optics, cryptography, and sensors.

About IOP ebooks

The authors are encouraged to take advantage of the features made possible by electronic publication to enhance the reader experience through the use of color, animation, and video and by incorporating supplementary files in their work.

A list of recent titles published in this series can be found here: https://iopscience.iop.org/bookListInfo/series-on-advances-in-optics-photonics-and-optoelectronics.

The Optics of Blood

A Handbook

Edited by
Alexandre Douplik
Head of TMU Photonics Group, Physics Department, Toronto Metropolitan University (TMU), Toronto, Canada

and

Researcher, Affiliated Scientist, Institute for Biomedical Engineering, Science and Technology (iBEST), Keenan Research Centre of the Li Ka Shing (LKS) Knowledge Institute, St. Michael Hospital, Toronto, Canada

IOP Publishing, Bristol, UK

ISBN 978-0-7503-4806-5 (ebook)
ISBN 978-0-7503-4804-1 (print)
ISBN 978-0-7503-4807-2 (myPrint)
ISBN 978-0-7503-4805-8 (mobi)

DOI 10.1088/978-0-7503-4806-5

Version: 20260301

IOP ebooks

British Library Cataloguing-in-Publication Data: A catalogue record for this book is available from the British Library.

Published by IOP Publishing, wholly owned by The Institute of Physics, London

IOP Publishing, No.2 The Distillery, Glassfields, Avon Street, Bristol, BS2 0GR, UK

US Office: IOP Publishing, Inc., 190 North Independence Mall West, Suite 601, Philadelphia, PA 19106, USA

For my spouse, Julia, and my daughter, Alice, with love and gratitude.

Dedicated to my mother, colleagues, and students; and with special thanks to Vanja Dvekar for assistance in preparing this book.

Contents

Preface

Blood is one of the most information-rich and clinically important tissues in the human body, yet it remains optically complex, dynamic, and highly context-dependent. It is simultaneously a transport medium, a diagnostic window, a therapeutic target, and an active participant in light–tissue interactions.

This handbook was conceived to bring together, in a single volume, the foundational principles, optical properties, measurement approaches, and biomedical applications that define the rapidly developing field of the optics of blood.

This book is the result of the collective efforts of a diverse and interdisciplinary group of authors and contributors whose expertise spans physics, biophotonics, biomedical engineering, chemistry, laboratory medicine, pathology, and clinical research. Their contributions reflect the inherently multidisciplinary nature of blood optics, where meaningful progress depends on close interaction between basic science, instrumentation, quantitative modeling, and clinical need.

The volume is organized to connect fundamental blood science with optical theory and practice. It moves from blood morphology, physiology, and rheology to the key optical parameters governing blood–photon interactions (including absorption, refractive index, and scattering), and then to major spectroscopic and imaging modalities, as well as therapeutic and monitoring applications in which blood is both a mediator and a measurable biomarker. This structure is intended to support readers from different backgrounds: students entering the field, researchers seeking cross-disciplinary grounding, and clinicians/engineers interested in translational optical technologies.

A central goal of this handbook is to bridge fundamental and applied perspectives. Blood optics cannot be understood adequately through isolated spectra, coefficients, or imaging examples alone; it must be interpreted in the context of cellular composition, oxygenation state, aggregation, flow, pathology, and instrumentation constraints. Another goal is to preserve methodological breadth by presenting complementary optical approaches—spectroscopic, imaging, and therapeutic—in a way that highlights both their differences and their convergence.

It is my hope that The Optics of Blood: A Handbook will serve not only as a reference, but also as a platform for dialogue across disciplines. By connecting optical physics, blood science, engineering, and medicine, this volume aims to support both current practice and future innovation.

Alexandre (Sasha) Douplik
Toronto Metropolitan University and St. Michael's Hospital
Toronto, Canada

Acknowledgements

I would like to express my sincere gratitude to all chapter authors and contributors for their scholarship, dedication, and patience throughout the development of this volume. Preparing a handbook of this scope requires not only expertise, but also sustained collaboration, flexibility, and a shared commitment to interdisciplinary knowledge-building. I am deeply appreciative of the time and care each contributor invested in this project.

I also wish to thank my colleagues, collaborators, and trainees whose discussions, feedback, and ongoing work in biophotonics and biomedical optics helped shape the vision of this handbook. Their scientific engagement and collaborative spirit have been invaluable.

I gratefully acknowledge Julia Davydova for her creative direction, iterative development of AI-assisted artwork, and preparation of the final cover design and production files.

Special thanks are extended to the editorial and production teams at IOP Publishing for their guidance, professionalism, and support during the preparation and production of this book.

Finally, I acknowledge the broader research and clinical communities working at the interface of optics, blood science, and medicine. Their continued innovation and dedication to improving diagnosis, monitoring, and therapy are the foundation on which this volume is built.

Editor biography

Alexandre Sasha Douplik

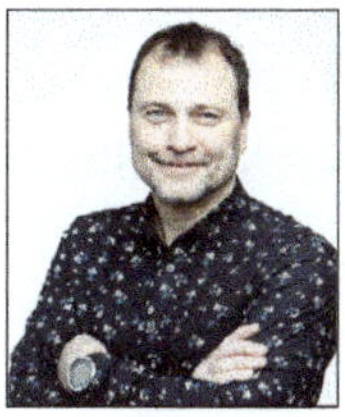

Dr. Alexandre (Sasha) Douplik is a Professor, Head of the Photonics Group in the Medical Physics Department at Toronto Metropolitan (formerly Ryerson) University since 2011, a Scientist at St. Michael's Hospital, Toronto, specializing in Biophotonics and Laser Medicine, author of more than 70 peer-reviewed papers, 55 conference papers, seven book chapters and 18 patents. He was a visiting researcher at the Okinawa Institute of Science and Technology (OIST), Japan, in 2017, 2018 and 2023. From 2007–2011, he was a contract Research Professor at Erlangen University, Germany, where he defended his Biomedical Engineering Habilitation (Dr. of Science degree) in 2011. He was a Scientific Associate at Ontario Cancer Institute, Toronto, in 2006–2007, and a Senior Researcher in Xillix Technologies, Vancouver, Canada, in 2002–2006. He is a Senior Member of SPIE and OSA.

List of contributors

Dr Jason P Acker
Department of Laboratory Medicine and Pathology, University of Albert, Edmonton, AB, Canada

Dr Mackenzie Brandon-Coatham
Department of Laboratory Medicine and Pathology, University of Albert, Edmonton, AB, Canada

Mr Timothy Burton
Department of Engineering, Toronto Metropolitan University, Toronto, ON, Canada

Miss Meiyun Cao
Department of Physics, Toronto Metropolitan University, Toronto, ON, Canada

Dr Alexandre Sasha Douplik
Department of Physics, Toronto Metropolitan University, Toronto, ON, Canada

Dr Pauline John
Laboratory of Advanced Biophotonics and Imaging in the Division of Bioengineering, New York University Abu Dhabi, Abu Dhabi, United Arab Emirates

Dr Yasuyuku Kakihana
Graduate School of Medical and Dental Sciences, Kagoshima University, Kagoshima, Japan

Dr Lothar Lige
Department of Medical Biophysics, University of Toronto, Toronto, ON, Canada

Dr Yutaro Madokoro
Department of Emergency Medicine, Kirishima Medical Center, Kirishima, Japan

Dr David M Moore
Virginia Tech Carillion School of Medicine, Blacksburg, Virginia, USA

Dr Shuhei Niiyama
Emergency and Critical Care Center, Kagoshima University Hospital, Kagoshima, Japan

Dr Susanne Pahlow
Leibniz Institute of Photonic Technologies, Jena, Germany

Celina Phan
Department of Laboratory Medicine and Pathology, University of Albert, Edmonton, AB, Canada

Dr Juergen Popp
Friedrich-Schiller-University, Institute of Physical High Technology (IPHT), Jena, Germany

Dr Scott Prahl
Department of Electrical Engineering and Renewable Energy, Oregon Institute of Technology

Dr Anika Tahsin Rahman
Department of Laboratory Medicine and Pathology, University of Albert, Edmonton, AB, Canada

Dr Anuradha Ramoji
Leibniz Institute of Photonic Technologies, Jena, Germany

Mr Faraz Sadrzadeh-Afsharazar
Department of Engineering, Toronto Metropolitan University, Toronto, ON, Canada

Dr Gennadi Saiko
Department of Physics, Toronto Metropolitan University, Toronto, ON, Canada

Dr Rajendran Soundararajan
Laboratory for Advance Bio-Photonics and Imaging, Division of Bioengineering, New York University Abu Dhabi, Abu Dhabi, United Aram Emirates

Dr Hülya Yilmaz
Leibniz Institute of Photonic Technologies, Jena, Germany

Dr Azhar Zam
Department of Bioengineering, NYU, Abu Dhabi, United Arab Emirates
Department of Biomedical engineering Department of Electrical and Computer Engineering NYU Tandon School of Engineering, Abu Dhabi, United Arab Emirates

Contributor biographies

Jason P. Acker

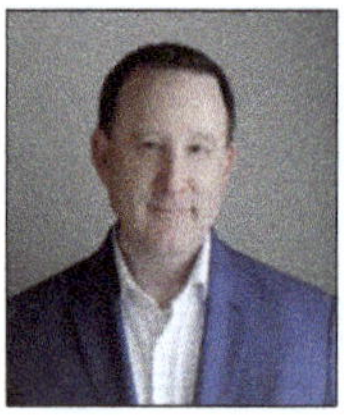

Dr. Jason P. Acker is a Senior Research Scientist with the Canadian Blood Services and a Professor in the Department of Laboratory Medicine and Pathology, Faculty of Medicine and Dentistry at the University of Alberta, Edmonton, Canada. His research program focuses on understanding the response of cells and tissues to ex vivo storage and the development of methods for their preservation and use as therapeutic products.

Faraz Sadrzadeh-Afsharazar

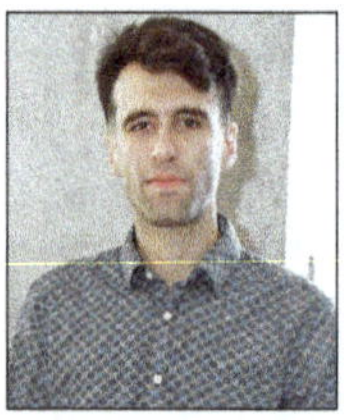

Faraz Sadrzadeh-Afsharazar is a biomedical engineer (Beng, MASc) and researcher with extensive experience in academia and the industry, including Toronto Metropolitan University, University of Toronto, Swift Medical Inc., and Oxilight Inc. Currently pursuing a PhD in Biomedical Engineering at Toronto Metropolitan University, Faraz specializes in optical, electronic, and signal processing technologies for healthcare, with a focus on wearable medical devices. He has contributed to notable projects, including the Swift Ray 1 imaging system, and co-founded EyePuck, a startup creating assistive technology for visually impaired athletes. Faraz has authored multiple peer-reviewed publications, contributed to patents in MedTech. He is passionate about advancing healthcare through innovative engineering solutions.

Timothy Burton

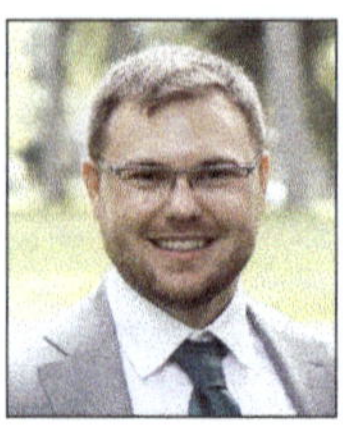

Timothy Burton is a data scientist with a strong research focus on healthcare innovation. He completed his undergraduate degree at Queen's University, earning a Bachelor of Computing (Honours) with a specialization in Biomedical Computing. He went on to complete a Master of Science (MSc) in Biomedical Engineering at Toronto Metropolitan University, where his thesis focused on contactless physiological signal acquisition and analysis. Timothy is a senior member of the IEEE. He has published extensively in peer-reviewed journals and holds numerous patents. Timothy is currently pursuing his PhD in Biomedical Engineering at Toronto Metropolitan University.

Meiyun Cao

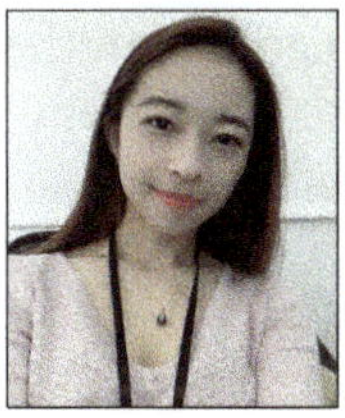

Meiyun Cao received her undergraduate degree in Co-op Medical Physics program at Toronto Metropolitan University (TMU, formerly Ryerson University), during which she completed her Co-op placement at Canadian Nuclear Laboratories in Chalk River, Ontario, where she gained experience on ex vivo and in vitro imaging. Meiyun continued to earn her Master's degree in CAMPEP credited Medical Physics from TMU. Meiyun' s master thesis project is focused on remote plethysmography (rPPG) and the signal extraction and analysis from peripheral blood flow and neck vessels. Meiyun is currently working at the Mayo Clinic Arizona as a Proton Medical Physicist Assistant, where she supports clinical and research activities in photon and proton therapy.

Dr. Mackenzie Brandon-Coatham

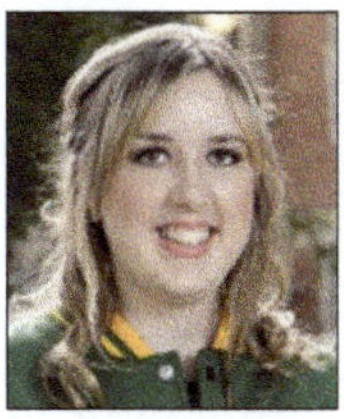

Dr. Mackenzie Brandon-Coatham was previously a Research Associate at Canadian Blood Services and is currently a Spatial Biology Specialist at the University of Alberta. Initially an enzyme kineticist and RNA biochemist specializing in molecular and synthetic biology, she transitioned into medical research becoming a cancer and red blood cell biologist. Her past and present areas of work and research all center on the molecular analysis of biomolecules or cell models.

Pauline John

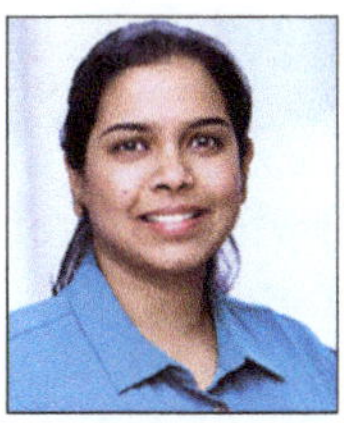

Pauline John is a Research Associate in the Laboratory for Advanced Bio-Photonics and Imaging (LAB-π) in the Division of Bioengineering at New York University Abu Dhabi (NYUAD). Before joining NYUAD, she worked as an assistant professor in the Department of Biomedical Engineering at Sri Sivasubramaniya Nadar College of Engineering (SSN), India, and as a Post-Doctoral Fellow at the School of Chemical and Biomedical Engineering, Nanyang Technological University (NTU), Singapore. She accomplished her Ph.D. in Biomedical Optics from the Indian Institute of Technology Madras (IIT Madras) and holds both Master's and Bachelor's degrees in Biomedical Engineering. Her research interests encompass the development of optical instruments and sensors for non-invasive biomedical applications, with a focus on optical coherence tomography, near-infrared spectroscopy, laser-induced breakdown spectroscopy, and flow cytometry. She has authored several peer-reviewed publications and contributed to numerous international conferences in these fields.

Dr. Yasuyuki Kakihana

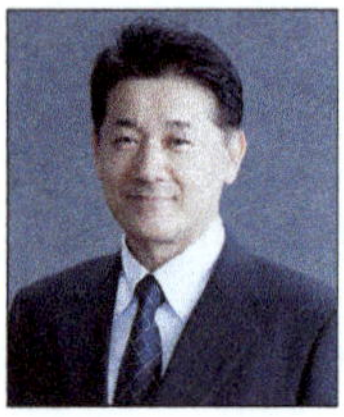

Dr. Yasuyuki Kakihana is currently Professor Emeritus at the Graduate School of Medical and Dental Sciences, Kagoshima University, and serves as Special Director of the Intensive Care Unit, Kagoshima City Hospital. From 2011 to 2025, he was Professor and Chair of the Department of Emergency and Critical Care Medicine at the Graduate School of Medical and Dental Sciences, Kagoshima University, and concurrently served as Director of the Emergency and Critical Care Center at Kagoshima University Hospital from 2014 to 2025. He is board-certified in emergency medicine, anesthesiology, and intensive care medicine, and is also a certified instructor in emergency medicine. Since 2020, he has served as Executive Director of the Japanese Society of Intensive Care Medicine and as Councilor of the Japanese Association for Acute Medicine. He was also a member of the English Journal Editorial Board from 2013 to 2018. Dr. Kakihana has authored numerous academic papers and books, and in 2023, he received the Ten-Year Most Cited Article Award from the Journal of Intensive Care.

Mr. Lilge

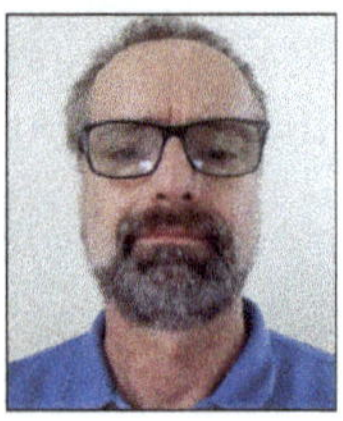

Mr. Lilge obtained his M.Sc. in Experimental Physics from the Johann Wolfgang Goethe University in Frankfurt, Germany in 1987 and his Ph.D. in biophysics from the Westfaehlische Wilhelms University in Muenster, Germany, in 1992, both with Prof. F. Hillenkamp as supervisor. His Ph.D. studies included 3 years at the Massachusetts General Hospital in Boston, USA. In 1992 he came first to McMaster University Hamilton and then the Ontario Cancer Institute for his post-doctoral training. From 1995 to 2002, he was employed by Photonics Research Ontario, a Centre of Excellence of the Province of Ontario, serving in various positions from Staff Scientist to Director of Operations for the Biophotonics User Facility. He holds a Professor appointment in the Department of Medical Biophysics at the University of Toronto. He is a Senior Scientist at the Princess Margaret Cancer Centre at University Health Network. His expertise includes photodynamic therapy, covering topics from photosensitiser evaluation to treatment planning and clinical trial support. Indications are for a range of cancers and antimicrobial infection control. Optical diagnostics for disease detection or quantification of disease prevalence, particularly for Breast Cancer. Currently, Dr. Lilge is a board member of the International Photodynamic Association (IPA) and Optics Within Life Science (OWLS).

Yutaro Madokoro

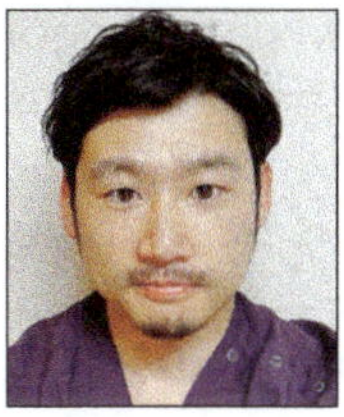

Yutaro Madokoro is a medical doctor (MD, PhD) and specialist in emergency medicine, intensive care, and disaster medicine. He is a graduate of the Faculty of Medicine at Kagoshima University. He is board-certified by the Japanese Association for Acute Medicine and the Japanese Society of Intensive Care Medicine. He currently serves as the Head of the Department of Emergency Medicine at Kirishima Medical Center in Japan and is a visiting research fellow in Emergency and Intensive Care Medicine at Kagoshima University.

He earned his doctorate through graduate research focused on sepsis, leading to a deeper understanding of its mechanisms and treatment strategies. He also conducts research on near-infrared spectroscopy and hydrogen gas inhalation therapy, seeking to advance innovative approaches in acute care and critical patient management.

David M. Moore

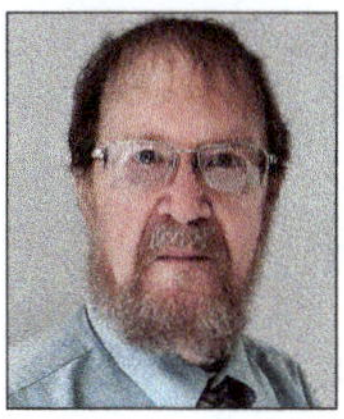

David M. Moore received a BS degree in Zoology in 1974 and an MS degree in Life Sciences in 1976 at Louisiana Tech University. He received the Doctor of Veterinary Medicine (DVM) degree from Louisiana State University in 1980. He worked in a toxicology testing facility in Louisiana, then accepted a position as Project Director for the Bionetics Corporation at the NASA Ames Research Center in California, where he also served as the veterinarian for the rats and squirrel monkeys that flew on the Space Shuttle in Spacelab 3. In late 1985, he accepted the position of University Veterinarian and Director of Animal Resources at Virginia Tech (VT). In 2000, he was appointed as the Associate Vice President for Research Compliance at VT, serving in that capacity until his retirement in late 2017. He was awarded Emeritus faculty status in 2019. He continues to provide lectures to undergraduate and graduate students in two colleges at VT. He is an Associate Professor in the Department of Biomedical Science Education at the Virginia Tech Carilion School of Medicine. He is a national and international consultant in the area of laboratory animal medicine. He is a specialty board certified lab animal veterinarian as a Diplomate of the American College of Laboratory of Laboratory Animal Medicine, and is the only US veterinarian to also be a Diplomate of the Japanese College of Laboratory Animal Medicine. He was honored as the 2021 Distinguished Alumnus by the LSU School of Veterinary Medicine.

Dr. Shuhei Niiyama

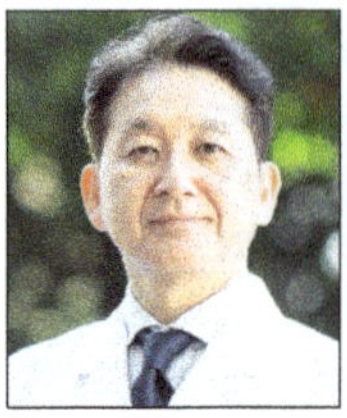

Dr. Shuhei Niiyama graduated from the Kurume University School of Medicine in 1993. He conducted research on central nervous system protection at the Graduate School of Medicine, Kurume University from 1999 to 2003. He was Postdoctoral Researcher at UMDNJ (New Jersey, USA) from 2003 to 2004. He served at the Advanced Emergency and Critical Care Center, Kurume University Hospital from 2008 to 2011, focusing primarily on research related to sepsis-associated encephalopathy. Since 2018, he has been serving at the Emergency and Critical Care Center, Kagoshima University Hospital, he was an associate Professor from 2020. He is a professor and chairman of department of Emergency and Intensive Care Medicine, Kagoshima University Graduate School of Medical and Dental Sciences from 2025. In research, he is engaged in studies on sepsis from the perspective of tetrahydrobiopterin and the development of brain resuscitation methods using near-infrared spectroscopy.

Susanne Pahlow

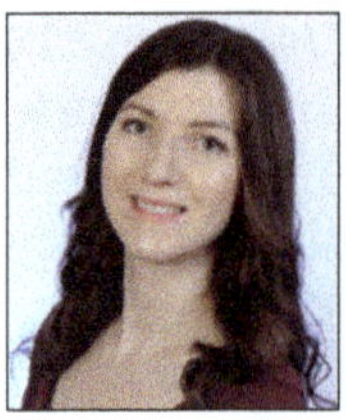

Susanne Pahlow obtained her diploma in chemistry in 2010 at the Friedrich Schiller University in Jena. Afterwards she joined the biophotonics group of Prof. Dr. Jürgen Popp at the Leibniz Institute of Photonic Technologies (Leibniz-IPHT) and worked in the field of Raman microspectroscopy, specializing in the identification of bacteria. In 2016 she defended her PhD thesis with the topic "Innovative Sample Preparation Strategies and Detection Methods for Microorganisms" and currently is leading the Applied Biospectroscopy and Bioassays group together with Dr. Anuradha Ramoji at the Leibniz-IPHT. Her main research interests are establishing Raman compatible sample preparation strategies, investigating new capture probes for microorganisms and chemical surface modification techniques.

Celina Phan

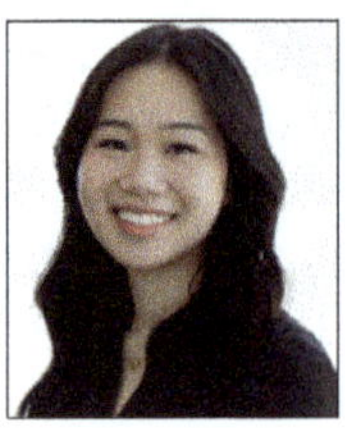

Celina Phan is the Education Program Coordinator for the Medical Laboratory Science and graduate Laboratory Medicine and Pathology program at the University of Alberta, Edmonton, Canada. After completing her Master of Science in Laboratory Medicine and Pathology, she transitioned into academic program leadership, where she now supports program development, student success, and excellence in laboratory medicine education. Her graduate research focused on blood quality, blood banking practices, and transfusion medicine, including the characterization of diabetic blood products and their performance in transfusion settings.

Juergen Popp

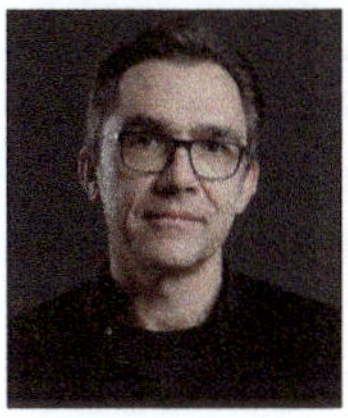

Juergen Popp studied chemistry in Erlangen and Würzburg and completed his PhD before conducting postdoctoral research at Yale University. He habilitated in Würzburg in 2002 and has since held the Chair of Physical Chemistry at Friedrich Schiller University Jena. Since 2006 he has also served as Scientific Director of the Leibniz Institute of Photonic Technology. Popp is a leading expert in biophotonics and optical health technologies, author of more than 1,140 peer-reviewed papers (>44,400 citations, h-index 88), and holds 21 patents. He has delivered over 200 invited lectures, organized major conferences, and serves as Editor-in-Chief of the Journal of Biophotonics. He is a key partner in numerous national and international research initiatives, including the Leibniz Center for Photonics in Infection Research (LPI), a German national roadmap infrastructure. Popp serves on the Photonics21 Executive Board and is frequently consulted by media and policymakers. His awards include the Pittsburgh Spectroscopy Award (2016), the Charles Mann Award (2023), an honorary doctorate from the University at Albany (2023) and the SPIE Biophotonics Technology Innovator Award 2026.

Dr. Scott A. Prahl

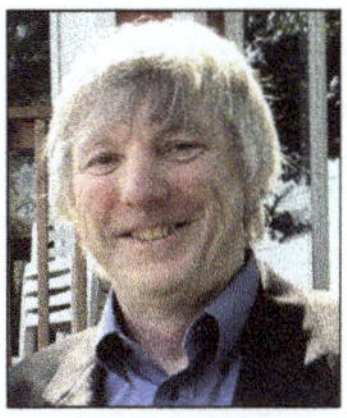

Dr. Scott A. Prahl is a Professor of Electrical Engineering & Renewable Energy at the Oregon Institute of Technology; Co-founder and Chief Technical Officer of Unfold Therapeutics; and Senior Research Scientist at Oregon Health & Science University since 2023, specializing in medical lasers and biophotonics. He has contributed to over 75 peer-reviewed papers and filed multiple patents in laser-based medical technologies. He holds a BS in Applied Physics from Caltech, a PhD in Biomedical Engineering from the University of Texas at Austin, and has completed postdoctoral training in Biomedical Optics at the Academic Medical Center, Amsterdam and the Wellman Center, Harvard Medical School.

Dr. Anika Tahsin Rahman

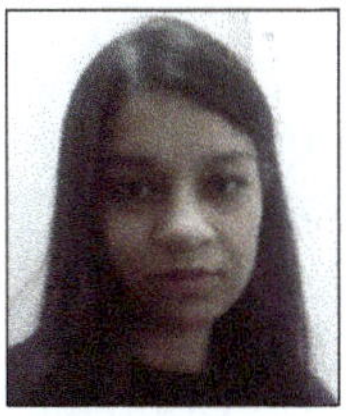

Dr. Anika Tahsin Rahman was an Alberta Innovates Postgraduate Fellowship funded postdoctoral fellow under the supervision of Dr. Jason Acker. Her research has centered on studying different types of antifreeze proteins in addition to cell preservation techniques. A trained molecular biologist, she also has experience in fluorescent protein-based assay development.

Soundararajan Rajendran

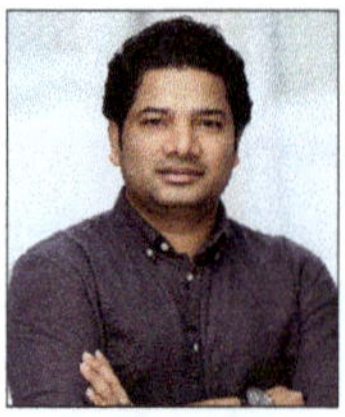

Soundararajan Rajendran, Ph.D., is a Postdoctoral Associate at the Laboratory for Advanced Bio-Photonics and Imaging (LAB-π) at New York University Abu Dhabi (NYUAD). He received his Ph.D. in Photonics and Optoelectronics from National Taiwan University (NTU), Taiwan, and holds Master's degrees in Laser and Electro-Optical Engineering and Physics. He also has extensive industrial experience in photonics and optoelectronic systems, with hands-on expertise spanning technical sales, system integration, and laser applications engineering. Prior to joining NYUAD, he served as a Postdoctoral Research Fellow at the University of California, Davis (UC Davis), where he specialized in high-resolution biomedical imaging and next-generation optical coherence tomography (OCT) platforms. His research focuses on the conception, integration, and translational advancement of multimodal optical imaging systems, including OCT (full-field, spectral-domain, and swept-source), scanning laser ophthalmoscopy, photoacoustic imaging, photodynamic therapy, and advanced spectroscopic techniques for ophthalmic, dermatological, oncological, brain organoid, and biochip-based applications. His work integrates quantitative imaging, advanced system instrumentation, and data analysis to advance high-resolution biomedical diagnostics and therapeutic applications.

Dr. Anuradha Ramoji

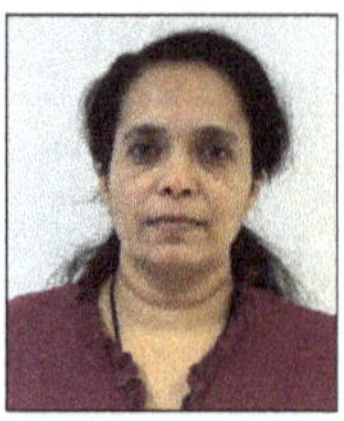

Dr. Anuradha Ramoji received her Master's degree in Physics from Karnataka University in 2002 and completed her Ph.D. in Vibrational Spectroscopy. In 2008, she joined the biophotonics group of Jürgen Popp at Friedrich Schiller University Jena as a postdoctoral researcher and later worked with Ute Neugebauer at the Center for Sepsis Control and Care, Jena University Hospital. She co-leads the Applied Biospectroscopy and Bioassays group together with Dr. Susanne Pahlow at the Leibniz Institute of Photonic Technologies and serves as Akademischer Rat at Friedrich Schiller University Jena. Her research focuses on the clinical translation of Raman spectroscopy, with key contributions demonstrating immune-cell–based Raman profiling for improved diagnosis of infection and sepsis, advancing label-free optical diagnostics toward routine clinical application.

Gennadi Saiko

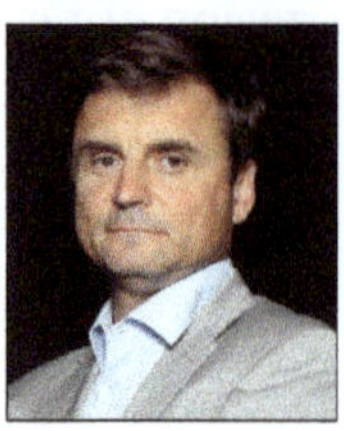

Gennadi Saiko is an accomplished scientist and entrepreneur with a successful track record in world-famous research institutes (Institute of General Physics, Moscow, Princess Margaret Hospital, Toronto), Fortune 500 companies (American Express), world-renown universities (Friedrich-Alexander-University of Erlangen-Nurnberg, Moscow Institute of Physics and Technology, Toronto Metropolitan University), and startups (Infinium Capital, Oxilight

Inc, Swift Medical Inc). Gennadi has received MSc and Ph.D. in Physics from the Moscow Institute of Physics and Technology. His primary interest is in the development of innovative optical imaging modalities for healthcare, with primary focus on wound care, cardiology, emergency and critical care. He combines both academic and industrial expertise. Gennadi has a successful experience in IP development and commercialization in MedTech. In particular, he developed a handheld multimodal imaging system primarily used in wound care, which Swift Medical Inc commercialized as Swift Ray 1. Gennadi authored more than 40 publications in peer-reviewed journals, three books, seven book chapters, and several patents. In addition, he delivered more than 30 presentations at international scientific conferences. He chaired sessions at multiple international conferences. In addition, Gennadi is a reviewer at more than 20 peer-reviewed journals and serves on boards of several scientific journals. Gennadi is an Adjunct Professor of the Department of Physics at Toronto Metropolitan University (formerly Ryerson University).

Hülya Yılmaz

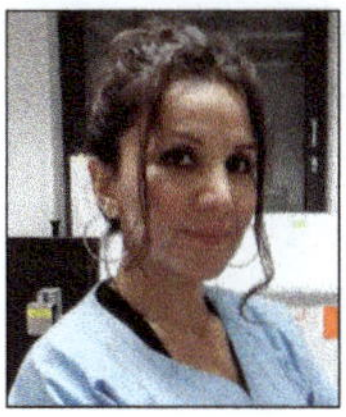

Hülya Yılmaz received her Ph.D. in chemistry from Suleyman Demirel University, Turkey, in 2018, with a research focus on the ionisation and degradation of active pharmaceutical ingredients using mass spectrometry and liquid chromatography. Following her Ph.D., she completed a postdoctoral fellowship at the Nanobiotechnology and Molecular Engineering Research Group of the Department of Genetics and Bioengineering at Yeditepe University, Istanbul, Turkey. There she worked on nanomaterials and surface-enhanced Raman scattering (SERS) for medical applications. She later joined the Nanotechnology Research and Application Centre at Sabancı University, where she contributed to EU-funded projects on safe-by-design of nanoparticles and their toxicity. She also worked at Pfizer in Turkey, where she gained valuable experience in linking academic research with industrial applications. In 2023, she moved to the Leibniz Institute of Photonic Technologies in Germany, where she continues her work in the field of biospectroscopy. Her interdisciplinary research interests span chemistry, medicine, biology, photonics, nanoscience and nanotechnology.

Azhar Zam

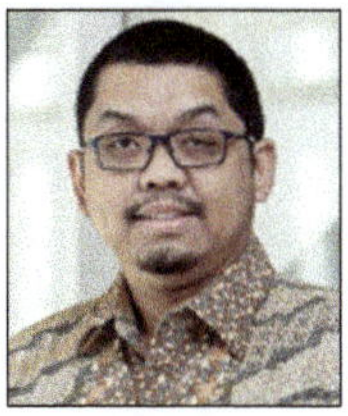

Azhar Zam is an Associate Professor of Bioengineering at NYU Abu Dhabi, where he leads the cutting-edge Laboratory for Advanced Bio-Photonics and Imaging (LAB-π). He is also an associated faculty member with the Department of Biomedical Engineering and the Department of Electrical and Computer Engineering at NYU Tandon School of Engineering in New York. Dr. Zam's impressive academic background includes a

B.S. from the University of Indonesia, an M.Sc. from the University of Luebeck, Germany, and a Ph.D. from Friedrich-Alexander-University Erlangen-Nuremberg, Germany. Before joining NYUAD, Dr. Zam was an assistant professor at the Department of Biomedical Engineering, University of Basel, Switzerland, where he founded the Biomedical Laser and Optics Group (BLOG) and co-established the MIRACLE II flagship project. He has also held research positions at prestigious institutions such as the University of Waterloo, the National University of Ireland Galway, the Toronto Metropolitan University (formerly known as Ryerson University), and the University of California at Davis. Dr. Zam's contributions include over 100 peer-reviewed articles and book chapters to his name, as well as several patents.

Dr. Alexandre (Sasha) Douplik

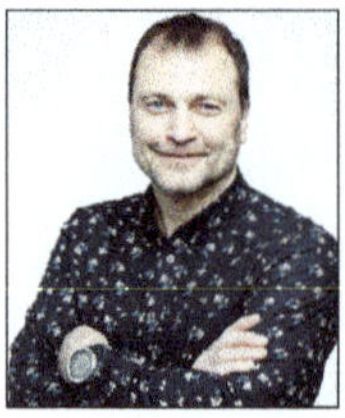

Dr. Alexandre (Sasha) Douplik is a Professor, Head of the Photonics Group in the Medical Physics Department at Toronto Metropolitan (formerly Ryerson) University since 2011, a Scientist at St. Michael's Hospital, Toronto, specializing in Biophotonics and Laser Medicine, author of more than 70 peer-reviewed papers, 55 conference papers, seven book chapters and 18 patents. He was a visiting researcher at the Okinawa Institute of Science and Technology (OIST), Japan, in 2017, 2018 and 2023. From 2007–2011, he was a contract Research Professor at Erlangen University, Germany, where he defended his Biomedical Engineering Habilitation (Dr. of Science degree) in 2011. He was a Scientific Associate at Ontario Cancer Institute, Toronto, in 2006–2007, and a Senior Researcher in Xillix Technologies, Vancouver, Canada, in 2002–2006. He is a Senior Member of SPIE and OSA.

Abbreviations

[PS]	Photosensitizer concentration
$^1O_2$	Singlet oxygen
$^1PS^*$	Electronic excited singlet state
2D	Two-dimensional
3D	Three-dimensional
$^3O_2$	Molecular oxygen
^3PS	Triplet excited state
A-Scan	Axial scan
ACS	Acute coronary syndrome
AD	Alzheimer's disease
AFM	Atomic force microscopy
aFTL	Anisotropic Fourier transform light scattering
AGES	Advanced glycation end-products
ALA	Aminolaevulinic acid
ALP	Alkaline phosphatase
ALT	Alanine aminotransferase
AMD	Age-related macular degeneration
aPDT	Antimicrobial photodynamic therapy
AR-PAF	Acoustic resolution photoacoustic flometry
AR-PAM	Acoustic resolution PAM
AST	Aminotransferases
AST	Aspartate aminotransferase
ATP	Adenosine triphosphate
BACS	Buoyancy-activated cell sorting
BGC	Blood glucose concentration
BOLD fMRI	Blood-oxygen-level-dependent functional magnetic resonance imaging
BOLD	Blood oxygen level dependent
BV	Blood volume
CA125	Cancer antigen 125
CAD	Coronary artery disease
CAM	Chick chorioallantoic membrane
CARS	Coherent anti-Stokes Raman spectroscopy
CBC	Complete/comprehensive blood count
CCD	Charge-coupled device
CCO	Cytochrome C oxidase
CD40	Cluster of differentiation 40
CEG	Clark error grid
CEP	Congenital erythropoietic porphyria
CGM	Continous glucose monitoring
CI	Cardiac index
CMP	Comprehensive metabolic panel
CNN	Convolutional neural network
CO	Cardiac output
COPD	Chronic obstructive pulmonary disease
CRDS	Cavity ring-down spectroscopy
CRID	Continuous refractive index dispersion
CRP	C-reactive protein

CTC	Circulating tumor cell
CTV	Clinical target volume
CVI	Choroidal vascularity index
DAMPs	Damage-associated molecular patterns
DAOCT	Differential absorption OCT
DAQ	Data acquistion
DCDR	Drop coating deposition Raman
DCLS	Direct classical least squares
DCS	Diffuse correlation spectroscopy
DCS	Diffuse correlation spectroscopy
DDA	Dipole discrete approximation
DEAS	Cavity-Ehnanced absorption spectroscopy
DeoxyHb	Deoxygenated hemoglobin
DHM	Digital holographic images
DIS	Double integrating sphere
DLB	Dementia with Lewy bodies
DLS-PM	Dynamic iight scattering platelet monitor
DLS	Dynamic light scattering
DNA	Deoxyribonucleic acid
DO	Oxygen delivery
DOCP	Degree of circular polarization
DOCT	Doppler optical coherence tomography
DOLP	Degree of Linear polarization
DOP	Net Degree of polarization
DOS	Diffuse Optical spectroscopy
DOT	Diffuse optical tomography
DPM	Diffraction phase microscopy
DR	Diabetic retinopathy
DRRS	Diffuse resonance Raman spectroscopy
DRS	Diffuse reflectance spectroscopy
DVT	Deep vein thrombosis
DyC-OCT	Dunamic contrast optical coherence tomography
ECDL	External cavity diode laser
EMD	Empirical mode decomposition
ESR	Erythrocyte sedimentation rate
ESS	Elastic scattering spectroscopy
FA	Fluorescein angiography
FACS	Fluorescence-activated cell sorting
FAD	Flavin adenine dinucleotide
fbMB	Frequency-band model-based
FD-OCT	Frequency-domain optical coherence tomography
FD	Fourier domain
FDTD	Finite-difference time-domain
FFR	Fractional flow reserve
FP	Fabry–Pérot
FSC	Forward scatter
FT	Fourier transform
FTIR	Fourier transform infrared
FTLS	Fourier transform light scattering
GGT	Glycoprotein gamma-glutamyltransferase

Hb A	Adult hemoglobin
Hb F	Fetal hemoglobin
Hb	Hemoglobin
HbCO	Carboxyhemoglobin
HbO2	Oxygenated hemoglobin
HbO2	Oxygenated hemoglobin
HBOC	Hemoglobin-based oxygen carrier
HbS	Sickle cell hemoglobin
HbS	Sulfhemoglobin
HCR	Hybridization chain reaction
HCT/Ht	Hematocrit
HCV	Hepatitis C virus
HDL	High density lipoprotein
He–Ne	Helium–neon
HIS	Medical hyperspectral imaging
HIV	Human immunodeficiency virus
HLS	Hyperleukocytic syndrome
Hz	Hemozoin
ICA	Intravascular coronary angiography
ICAM	Intercellular adhesion molecule
ICG	Indocyanine green
ICGA	Indocyanine green angiography
IFE	Inner filter effect
IL-4	Interleukin 4
IL-6	Interleukin 6
iMC	Inverse Monte Carlo
iRBC's	Infected erythrocytes
IS	Integrating sphere
IS/OS	Inner and outer segment
IV	Intravenous
IVUS	Intravascular ultrasound
KNN	K-nearest neighbor
LAD	Left anterior descending artery
LCI	Low coherence interferometry
LCP	Left circular polarization
LD	Laser Doppler
LDF	Laser Doppler flowmetry
LDG	Lactate dehydrogenase
LDPI	Laser per perfusion imaging
LDV	Laser Doppler velocimetry
LED	Light-emitting diode
LILT	Low-Intensity laser therapy
LLLR	Low Level laser radiation
LLLT	Low-Level laser therapy
LPS	Lipopolysaccharide
LSCI	Laser speckle contrast Imaging
LSCI	Laser speckle contrast Imaging
LSI	Laser speckle imaging
LSP	Light scattering profile/pattern
LSS	Light scattering spectroscopy

MACS	Magnetic activated cell sorting
MBP	Major basic protein
MCHC	Mean corpuscular hemoglobin concentration
MCV	Mean corpuscular volume
MetHb	Methemoglobin
METRICS OCT	Molecular imaging true-colour apectroscopic optical coherence tomography
Mfsd2a	Major facillitator auperfamily domain-containing protein 2
MPV	Mean platelet volume
MRI	Magnetic resonance imaging
MSI	Multispectral imaging
MSOT	Multispectral optoacoustic tomography
N:C	Nucleus to cytoplasm ratio
NAD+	Oxidized nicotinamide adenine dinucleotide
NADH	Reduced nicotinamide adenine dinucleotide
NDD	Neurodegenerative disease
NET	Neutrophil extracellular trap
NEU-SFL	Neutrophil side fluorescence
NEUT	Neutrophils
NIPALS	Non-linear iterative partial least squares
NIR	Near infrared
NIRS	Near infrared spectroscopy
NNLS	Non-negative least squares
NO	Nitric oxide
NRBC	Nucleated red blood cells
OAI	Optoacoustic imaging
OAT	Optoacoustic tomography
OCA	Optical clearing agent
OCM	Optical coherence microscopy
OCT-A	OCT-angiography
OCT	Optical coherence tomography
OMAG	Optical microangiography
OPO	Optical parametric oscillator
OR-PAM	Optical-resolution PAM
OxyHb	Oxygenated hemoglobin
PAE	Photoacoustic endoscope
PAF	Platelet activating factor
PAFI	Photoacoustic fluctuation Imaging
PAI	Photoacoustic imaging
PAI	Photoacoustic imaging
PAM	Photoacoustic microscopy
PAS	Photoacoustic spectroscopy
PAT	Photoaccoustic tomography
PAUS	Photoacoustic ultrasound spectroscopy
PAVT	Photoacoustic vector tomography
PBM	Photobiomodulation
PBMC	Peripheral blood mononuclear cells
PBP	Photodynamic blood purification
PBS	Periberal blood smears
PCA	Principal component analysis

PCI	Percutaneous coronary intervention
PCT	Porphyria cutanea
PCT	Procalcitonin
PCV	Packed cell volume
PDT	Photodynamic therapy
PDW	Platelet distribution width
PHA	Phytohaemagluttinin
PLS	Partial least squares
PLT's	Platelets
PMP	Platelet-derived microparticles
PMS	Phorbol-12-myristate 12-acetate
PPG	Photoplethysmography
PPIX	Free protoporphyrin
PR-OCT-A	Projection resolved OCT-A algorithm
PRP	Platelet rich plasma
PS-OCT	Polarization-sensitive optical coherence tomography
PS	Photosensitizers
PT	Photothermal
PVP	Polybinylpyrrodlidone
PVS	Polyvinyl chloride
QPA	Quantitative photoacoustic assessment
qPAT	Quantitative photoacoustic tomography
QPI	Quantitative phase imaging
RAO	Retinal artery occlusion
RBC	Red blood cells
RCP	Right circular polarization
RCS	Radar cross-section
RDG	Rayleigh-Debye–Gans
RMSE	Root mean square error
RNA-FISH	RNA fluorescence *in situ* hybridization
RNA	Ribonucleic acid
ROS	Reactive oxygen species
RPE	Retinal pigment epithelium
RVO	Retinal Vascular occlusion
S-OCM	Spectroscopic optical coherence microscopy
S-OCT	Spectroscopic optical coherence tomography
SARS-CoV-2	Severe Acute Respiratory Syndrome Coronavirus Type 2
SCD	Sickle cell diseases
SD-OCT	Spectral-domain optical coherence tomography
SERS	Surface enhanced Raman spectrocopy
SES	Synchronous emission spectra
SFC	Scanning flow cytometry
SFDI	Spatial Frequency-domain imaging
SLED	Superluminescent light-emitting diode
SMF	Spatial matched filter
SNR	Signal to noise ratio
SO2	Blood oxygenation
SOAPs	Spatially distributed optoacoustic point sources
SOCT	Speckle optical coherence tomography
SORS	Spatially offset Raman spectroscopy

SRS	Stimulated Raman scattering
SS-OCT	Swept-dource optical coherence tomography
SS	Slab subtraction
SSADA	Split-spectrum amplitude-deccorelation angiography
SSC	Side scatter
SSIM	Structured similarity Indexing
STFFT	Short-time fast Fourier transform
STS	Static light scattering
SUR	Specific uptake ratio
SVD	Singular value decomposition
SVM	Support vector machine
SXS	Synchronous excitation spectra
T2DM	Type 2 diabetes mellitus
TCR	T cell receptor
TD-OCT	Time-domain optical coherence tomography
TDF	Thermal diffusion flowmetry
TFT	Time frequency transformation
TGF	Transforming growth factor
Thal	Thalassemia
tHb	Total hemoglobin concentration
THG	Third Harmonic generation
THP1 Cells	Tohoku Hospital pediatrics-1 cells
TIR	Total impulse resonance
TLR	Toll-like receptor
TNF-alpha	Tumor necrosis factor alpha
TOC	Tissue optical clearing
TPEF	Two-photon excited fluorescence
TPM	Tomographic phase microscopy
Tregs	Regulatory T cells
TTH	Thrombotic thrombocytopenic purpura
UCB	Umbilical cord blood
US	Ultrasound
UV-VIS	Ultraviolet-visible
V/H	Vertical/horizontal
V/V	Vertical/vertical
VCAM	Vascular cell adhesion molecule
VDA	Vascular disrupting agent
vWF	von Wilebrand factor
WBC	White blood cells
ZnPP	Zinc protoporyphrin

Chapter I

Introduction to the optics of blood: a handbook

Alexandre Douplik

I.1 Blood as a multifaceted optical medium

Blood, the quintessential biological fluid, performs a vital role in systemic physiology, delivering oxygen, nutrients, and signaling molecules to tissues while removing metabolic waste. Yet beyond its well-characterized biochemical and cellular composition, blood also presents a rich and complex optical signature. This optical complexity—manifesting in absorption, scattering, fluorescence, birefringence, refractive index variation, and more—has rendered blood an important focus of biomedical optics. The capacity to interrogate blood non-invasively or minimally invasively through photonic technologies underpins diagnostic innovation across numerous clinical specialties.

The present *The Optics of Blood* volume of IOP Series in Advances in Optics, Photonics and Optoelectronics brings together a diverse collection of scholarly contributions that map the interplay between blood's structural, biochemical, and rheological properties and its optical behavior. Spanning foundational concepts to cutting-edge imaging and therapeutic modalities, this handbook seeks to establish a coherent framework for understanding how light interacts with blood and how such interactions can be harnessed to probe, monitor, explore and affect biological systems.

This introductory chapter provides a contextual overview of the themes developed in the twelve chapters that follow. We begin with the physiological, morphological and rheological review of blood, then underpinnings of blood optics, proceed through the core physical principles of light–tissue interaction as applied to blood, and focus on modern applications of optical technologies for imaging, diagnosis, and therapy. Together, these chapters elucidate the fundamental principles and emergent frontiers in the optical analysis of blood.

doi:10.1088/978-0-7503-4806-5chI

I.2 Structural, physiological and rheological foundations

I.2.1 Human blood morphology

Chapter 1 lays the physiological groundwork, providing a detailed exploration of human blood's normal composition and cellular architecture.

The chapter also addresses microscopy and quantitative hematology, laying the clinical and laboratory framework within which optical assessments can be contextualized and validated.

I.2.2 Comparative blood morphology in animal models

Chapter 2 complements the human-centric perspective with a comparative view of blood cell morphology across commonly used experimental animal species, including rodents, rabbits, pigs, and non-human primates. These models are essential in preclinical development and validation of optical techniques.

Key species-specific differences—such as the nucleation of red blood cells (RBCs) in non-mammalian models, differences in cell volume, and hematocrit levels—affect light interaction at both microscopic and macroscopic scales. These differences underscore the need for cautious interpretation when extrapolating animal-model data to human applications and justify the inclusion of a comparative morphological analysis as a reference framework for translational research.

I.2.3 Hemodynamics and rheological considerations

Chapter 3 shifts focus from static morphology to dynamic behavior—blood rheology and hemodynamics. Blood behaves also as a non-Newtonian fluid, with viscosity modulated by shear rate, hematocrit, temperature, and aggregation state of RBCs. These factors not only affect physiological perfusion but also may influence the interaction of light with blood which will be considered further in the Core optical properties of blood chapters 4–6.

Understanding these relationships is vital for optimizing sensor design, signal processing algorithms, and clinical interpretation of hemodynamic metrics.

I.3 Core optical properties of blood

Chapters 4–6 emphasize how optical phenomena—primarily light absorption, refraction and scattering—emerge from the cellular size, shape, concentration and rheology of blood components such as blood plasma, RBCs, white blood cells (WBCs), and platelets. RBCs, for instance, exhibit biconcave geometry that significantly influences scattering anisotropy, while their hemoglobin content defines key absorption peaks in the visible spectrum. Platelets and leukocytes, although less optically dominant, introduce heterogeneity in scattering patterns due to size variability and nucleated structure. Erythrocyte aggregation, particularly under low shear conditions, alters scattering cross-sections, thereby affecting signal intensity and temporal dynamics in optical modalities.

Changes in these properties across pathological states can modulate the optical profile of blood, providing a basis for diagnostic interpretation through spectroscopic and imaging modalities.

I.3.1 Absorption: hemoglobin and beyond

Chapter 4 provides an in-depth analysis of light absorption in blood, focusing on hemoglobin's complex spectral behavior. Oxyhemoglobin (HbO_2), deoxyhemoglobin (Hb), methemoglobin, and carboxyhemoglobin each exhibit distinct absorption bands, particularly in the 400–850 nm region. These spectral signatures form the basis of optical oximetry, photoacoustic tomography, and spectroscopic tissue diagnostics.

The chapter also discusses how absorption is influenced by hematocrit, oxygen saturation, chromophore heterogeneity, and blood flow. Advanced methods for measuring absorption spectra—such as integrating spheres, time-resolved spectroscopy, and spatially resolved reflectance—are surveyed, emphasizing the translation from *in vitro* studies to *in vivo* diagnostics.

I.3.2 Refractive index: integrative optical parameter

Chapter 5 explores refractometry of blood, a relatively underutilized yet insightful technique. The refractive index reflects the concentration of cellular and molecular constituents, offering a global assessment of blood composition. Variations in plasma protein levels, lipid content, and cellular volume affect the refractive index, which in turn modulates light refraction, phase delay, and scattering.

The chapter discusses techniques for measuring refractive index, highlighting their application in refractive spectroscopy.

I.3.3 Scattering and optical clearing

Chapter 6 delves into the scattering behavior of blood. Scattering arises predominantly from mismatch of the refraction index of the membrane structures such as cells and subcellular structures, at comparable levels of their contribution in the light scattering by blood within the visible range. RBCs, with size, shape, and orientation contribute to angular and spectral dependencies. Light scattering also reflects cell–cell interactions, deformability, and aggregation—making it sensitive to disease states such as sickle cell anemia and malaria.

Optical clearing techniques, which may use chemical agents or higher concentration of RBCs (hematocrit) to reduce scattering by matching refractive indices, are reviewed. These methods enhance light penetration and imaging depth, offering potential for deep-tissue visualization and therapeutic photonics.

I.4 Spectroscopic and imaging modalities

I.4.1 Fluorescence spectroscopy and autofluorescence imaging

Chapter 7 examines the intrinsic and extrinsic fluorescence properties of blood. Endogenous fluorophores—such as NADH, flavins, porphyrins, and plasma proteins—emit characteristic spectra under UV and visible excitation. These signals can be modulated by metabolic state, oxidative stress, and disease, enabling their use as biomarkers.

The chapter also reviews fluorophore-based imaging using intravenous dyes, offering insights into blood volume, flow, and vascular leakage. Applications in oncology, cardiology, and vascular surgery are reviewed.

I.4.2 Raman spectroscopy: molecular fingerprinting

Chapter 8 introduces Raman spectroscopy, a vibrational spectroscopic technique that provides molecular-specific information. Raman scattering from blood reveals chemical structures, such as hemoglobin conformation, lipid content, and protein signatures.

The chapter details spontaneous and surface-enhanced Raman spectroscopy (SERS), including fiber-based probes and confocal configurations for *in vivo* diagnostics. Case studies on cancer, diabetes, and drug monitoring demonstrate Raman's diagnostic potential and challenges in signal-to-noise ratio, tissue penetration, and spectral overlap.

I.4.3 Optoacoustics: hybrid imaging beyond scattering limits

Chapter 9 describes optoacoustic (photoacoustic) imaging, which combines optical contrast with sonic interrogation and resolution. By exploiting the strong absorption of hemoglobin, optoacoustic methods provide high-resolution maps of oxygenation and vascular architecture.

Photoacoustic tomography (PAT) and microscopy (PAM) offer multi-scale imaging from microvessels to whole organs. The chapter covers clinical applications in anemia detection, tumor angiogenesis, and real-time glucose sensing. Limitations such as acoustic distortion and light delivery to deep tissues are also considered.

I.4.4 Optical coherence and polarimetric imaging

Chapter 10 introduces optical coherence tomography (OCT) and polarimetry. OCT provides cross-sectional imaging of tissue microstructure based on light backscattering. Blood flow can be quantified through Doppler OCT, while spectroscopic OCT adds functional contrast.

Polarimetric techniques measure birefringence and depolarization, which reflect cell alignment and membrane organization. Applications in hematologic disorders and microangiopathy are presented, along with emerging multimodal systems that integrate OCT and polarimetry for comprehensive blood characterization.

I.5 Blood–photon interactions in therapeutics

I.5.1 Photodynamic therapy (PDT): blood as carrier and target

Chapter 11 explores the two-fold role of blood in photodynamic therapy. Blood acts as a carrier of photosensitizers and molecular oxygen—both critical for the generation of cytotoxic singlet oxygen upon light activation.

Additionally, PDT can target the vasculature itself, leading to vascular shutdown and tumor hypoxia. Monitoring blood flow during PDT enhances dosimetry and treatment personalization. The use of PDT for sterilizing blood products, such as in transfusion medicine, is also discussed.

I.5.2 Photobiomodulation (PBM): modulation through light

Chapter 12 presents photobiomodulation (PBM), wherein low-level light (600–1000 nm) interacts with mitochondrial chromophores, particularly cytochrome c oxidase. This interaction alters ATP production, reactive oxygen species levels, and nitric oxide release, affecting both systemic and localized physiology.

PBM influences RBC deformability, leukocyte activation, and platelet aggregation—parameters relevant in inflammation, wound healing, and vascular health. The chapter surveys experimental and clinical evidence supporting PBM's efficacy in treating circulatory and immune-mediated disorders.

I.6 Cross-cutting themes and future directions

Across the book chapters, several recurring themes emerge:

Multiscale integration: From molecular to organ-level assessments, the optical interrogation of blood spans multiple spatial and temporal scales. This integration is essential for developing comprehensive diagnostic and therapeutic platforms.

Label-free versus contrast-enhanced techniques: Intrinsic optical signatures (e.g., absorption, autofluorescence) offer non-invasive biomarkers, while contrast-enhanced modalities (e.g., dye-based fluorescence, SERS) enhance specificity. Optimal combinations depend on clinical context.

Translational relevance: Animal models, *ex vivo* studies, and preclinical trials provide pathways to human applications. However, optical properties vary with species, disease state, and environmental conditions, necessitating validation and calibration.

Technological synergy: Hybrid systems that combine imaging, spectroscopy, and flow monitoring (e.g., OCT + Raman, photoacoustics + fluorescence) promise richer datasets and more robust interpretations.

Emerging clinical applications: From glucose monitoring to oncology, cardiology, and infectious disease diagnostics, blood-based optical techniques are entering the clinical mainstream. Regulatory considerations, cost-effectiveness, and user interfaces remain areas for innovation.

I.7 Conclusion: illuminating the circulatory landscape

This volume collectively presents blood not merely as a physiological fluid but as an optically rich, diagnostically accessible, and therapeutically responsive medium. Although this volume does not address all related topics, it constitutes a foundational effort to consolidate current understanding of the morphological, physiological, and rheological properties of blood as they pertain to optics and biomedical optical applications. As biophotonics advances, blood will remain central to technological innovation—serving as both a window into systemic health and a substrate for photonic intervention.

By synthesizing physiology, optics, engineering, and clinical science, this handbook aims to equip researchers, clinicians, and developers with the foundational understanding and technical acumen required to navigate and contribute to this rapidly evolving field. The exploration of blood through light offers a unique convergence of science and medicine—an endeavor that continues to shape the future of diagnostics and therapeutics.

Chapter 1

Normal morphology and physiology of human blood including main clinical parameters and microscopy

Celina Phan, Mackenzie L Brandon-Coatham, Anika T Rahman and Jason P Acker

Human blood is composed of plasma, red blood cells (RBCs), white blood cells (WBCs), and platelets (PLTs). The physiology of these components can be characterized by their light scattering and absorption properties. Such optical properties can explain changes in the various characteristics of blood (size, shape, abundance of cells and/or molecules) throughout different conditions. This chapter will review the normal and pathological physiology of blood components from a physical and biochemical perspective that can be assessed using clinically relevant optical techniques.

Abbreviations

ALP	alkaline phosphatase
CBC	complete blood count
DAMPs	damage associated molecular patterns
GGT	glycoprotein gamma-glutamyltransferase
HCT	hematocrit
Hb	hemoglobin
HC	hormonal contraceptives
HDL	high density lipoprotein
LDL	low density lipoprotein
MBP	major basic protein
MCV	mean cell volume
MCH	mean corpuscular hemoglobin
MCHC	mean corpuscular hemoglobin concentration
MPV	mean platelet volume
PAMPs	pathogen associated molecular patterns
PBS	peripheral blood smear
PLT	platelet

doi:10.1088/978-0-7503-4806-5ch1

PCT	plateletcrit
PDW	platelet distribution width
RBC	red blood cell
RDW	red cell distribution width
WBC	white blood cell
PDW	platelet distribution width

1.1 Blood

The cells (erythrocytes, leukocytes, and thrombocytes) within blood all originate from hematopoietic stem cells. In adults, these stem cells originate from the bone marrow. Stem cells eventually become immature blasts which go on to further differentiate into either lymphoid or myeloid cell lines. Lymphoid stem cells are the precursors to lymphocytes a subset of leukocytes while the myeloid stem cells serve as the origin of all erythrocytes, thrombocytes, and remaining types of leukocytes [1, 2]. When blood is drawn in clinical settings, the whole blood sample can either be subjected to automated cell counting within light-based analyzers or upon centrifugation and sedimentation of the cellular components, the plasma can be run through analyzers that operate on similar principles but can detect the products of various biochemical reactions. Classical microscopy is often employed alongside extensive laboratory testing to ascertain the overall health of individuals.

1.2 Red blood cells

Erythrocytes, or RBCs account for 40%–54% of the total blood volume in males and 36%–48% in females, as measured by hematocrit (HCT) thereby constituting a large portion of blood [3]. With an average lifespan in circulation of $\sim$120 days, RBCs are responsible for transporting oxygen from the lungs to peripheral tissues and waste, such as carbon dioxide, from the periphery back to the lungs for exhalation [4, 5]. In all mammals, RBCs are distinctively anucleate to accommodate greater amounts of hemoglobin (Hb) while also giving rise to their flexible biconcave shape [4]. Their unique mechanical properties allow them to withstand shear forces and navigate the microcirculation, with their deformability relying on minimal alterations to their surface area-to-volume ratio [4]. The membrane of RBCs is comprised of a lipid bilayer underlaid by a network of proteins (membrane skeleton) that is 40–90 nm in thickness [6]. This lipid bilayer contains a variety of integral and peripheral proteins responsible for molecule transport (e.g., Band 3), cell adhesion (e.g., ICAM-4), membrane regulation (e.g., phosphatidylserine), and blood group specificity (e.g., Rhesus antigens) [4, 6]. The underlying membrane skeleton is composed of spectrin, actin, and other proteins capable of interacting with the lipid bilayer [6, 7]. The association between the membrane and membrane skeleton layers plays a major role in RBCs' observed flexibility. Additionally, the cytosolic viscosity of RBCs also plays a role in its deformability [4, 5]. The viscosity of the cytosol is dependent upon the concentration of Hb in the cell and the regulation of cation content (e.g. Na^+/K^-) [4, 5]. Cation levels influence RBC volume and therefore RBCs' ability to adapt in response to shear forces.

1.2.1 Normal morphology of red blood cells

Peripheral blood smears (PBS) in conjunction with various Romanowsky staining techniques can be used to assess the histology of RBCs. These approaches often use a combination of acidic and basic dyes, staining basic cell components red and acidic cell components blue [8, 9]. A PBS from a healthy individual will show well-defined RBCs with relatively uniform size as reflected by the red cell distribution width (RDW) (11.5%–14.5%) [8, 10]. In humans, RBCs can range from 6–8 μm in diameter, are 1.5–2.5 μm thick and contain a central pallor taking up approximately 1/3 of the cell size [11]. Lacking both organelles and granules, the hemoglobin located in the cell's periphery stains a pink-red hue, while the central pallor remains relatively colourless. However, artifacts of storage and handling may be present on the smear and should be carefully considered to avoid misinterpretation. Such artifacts often present as RBCs with abnormal morphology, such as echinocytes, which lack a central pallor and have a thorny appearance [12]. With artifacts considered, variations in RBC morphology often indicate a blood disorder or abnormality.

1.2.2 Normal functioning of red blood cells

Complete blood counts (CBCs) are frequently requested by healthcare providers to help assess an individual's overall health. While a CBC provides a look at all the different cellular components of blood, in the context of RBCs, some standard clinical indices that are captured include: RBC count, Hb content, HCT, mean corpuscular volume (MCV), mean corpuscular hemoglobin (MCH), and mean corpuscular hemoglobin concentration (MCHC). These indices provide insight into the functionality of RBCs by providing information regarding their size, shape, and concentration. The RBC count and Hb content can be indicative of the erythropoietic process, in which RBCs are produced [13, 14]. MCV and MCHC contribute not only to our understanding of RBC size and Hb concentration but also serve as indicators of RBC cytosolic viscosity and deformability [4, 5, 15]. In a healthy individual, while the ranges observed for these RBC parameters can be variable depending on factors such as age, ethnicity, and even testing site, typical reference intervals for both sexes are outlined in table 1.1 [10].

The RBC count reflects the number of RBCs in an individual and has been found to be influenced not only by sex, age, and ethnicity, but lifestyle choices and hormonal contraceptives (HC) as well (table 1.1) [16–19]. Normally, RBC counts decrease with age and in females using HC [16, 19]. Hb content refers to the amount of hemoglobin present in a blood sample. Males generally have higher Hb levels than females; however, their Hb levels decline with age (table 1.1) [16]. Furthermore, ethnicity and lifestyle differences can alter Hb content, with individuals identifying as Asian and Black individuals tending to possess lower Hb levels than white individuals [17, 18]. HCT, reflective of the blood volume occupied by RBCs, is influenced similarly to Hb content by the abovementioned factors [16–18]. Naturally, average cell volume (MCV), its variation (RDW), and the amount (MCH) and concentration (MCHC) of Hb in RBCs, have also been found to be

Table 1.1. RBC specific reference ranges taken from normal individuals' CBCs.

Parameter	Male range	Female range
RBC count ($10^{12}l^{-1}$)	4.5–6.1	4.0–5.4
Hb (g dl^{-1})	13.0–17.0	12.0–16.0
HCT (%)	40–52	37–47
MCV (fl)	80–98	80–98
MCH (pg)	27–33	27–33
MCHC (g dl^{-1})	31.5–37.0	31.5–37.0
RDW (%)	11.5–14.5	11.5–14.5

influenced by an array of factors specific to each individual. Cell volume increases with age, HC use and lifestyle choices such as drug use [16, 17, 19]. However, minimal variation in MCV is observed between sexes, barring use of HC (table 1.1). The deviation in RBC volumes is reported as RDW and thus follows the age and HC trends described previously for MCV [20, 21]. Despite no sex differences having been observed with MCV measurements, sex differences are reported in RDW in females until ~60 years of age [20]. Sex differences are also observed in MCH and MCHC. The amount of hemoglobin in an RBC has repeatedly been found to be greater in males and also increases with age in both sexes [16]. Alternatively, MCHC, while greater in males, remains stable in both sexes with age [16]. For those using HC however, MCH is decreased as it relies on Hb count (unaffected by HC) and RBC count (decreased in females on HC). Finally, compared to white individuals, Asians have a reduced lower limit for MCV, MCH and MCHC and increased RDW [18]. In a healthcare setting, clinicians should be aware of these normal variations to interpret and assess RBC-related CBC results accurately. Recognizing and understanding the factors influencing blood parameters helps improve the precision and context-specific interpretation of clinical data in diverse populations.

1.2.3 Abnormal morphology and functioning of red blood cells

Abnormal RBC shapes, or poikilocytes, can provide valuable information on underlying conditions. Common RBC shapes and their probable pathologies can be found in table 1.2 [22]. The abnormalities of RBC shapes are not exclusively a result of pathological conditions. Instead, various cell shapes are present in different normal physiological conditions at varying frequencies, for example during RBC aging or *ex vivo* storage. In contrast, disease can affect the morphology of the RBCs. For instance, sickle cells are the most commonly found in those homozygous for Hb S [22]. Sickle cells can be characterized by a crescent or C-like shape. However, sickle cells may be less prevalent for those heterozygous for Hb S and Hb C, and the presence of target cells or elliptocytes may be more common [22]. Target cells have an abnormal distribution of Hb such that it is concentrated centrally and peripherally, giving the appearance of a target on a PBS [12]. Alternatively, elliptocytes

Table 1.2. Variations in RBC shapes and their diagnostic significance.

Morphology	Pathology
Echinocyte	Artifact of storage or staining procedure; dehydration, renal disease, or select medication use.
Sickle cell (drepanocytes)	Sickle cell disease: homozygous Hb S (SS disease), heterozygous Hb S and Hb C (SC disease) or β-thalassemia (S/β-thalassemia)
Bite cell	Glucose-6-phosphate dehydrogenase deficiency
Elliptocyte	Hereditary elliptocytosis, iron deficiency anemia
Spherocyte	Hereditary spherocytosis, autoimmune hemolytic anemia,
Target cell (dodocytes)	Iron deficiency anemia, sickle cell disease, thalassemia's
Teardrop (dacrocyte)	Iron deficiency anemia, thalassemia's

would appear as oval/elliptical in shape due to abnormal cytoskeleton interactions [22]. Furthermore, target and teardrop cells could indicate iron deficiency anemia or, more seriously, thalassemia. In a PBS, teardrop cells, the cells take on the shape of a tear/water droplet with one end rounded and the other end pointed [12]. Identifying specific RBC shapes and their corresponding pathologies can provide valuable diagnostic information regarding both anemic conditions and hematological disorders.

RBC morphology influences routine RBC counts, thus the two methodologies are often used in conjunction for the purpose of diagnosis. Deviations from the reference ranges of the RBC clinical indices typically indicate underlying health conditions. For example, an elevated RBC count and HCT could indicate a range of conditions such as polycythemia vera, a bone marrow disease resulting in excessive RBC production, or more simply, an indicator of dehydration [23, 24]. Conversely, a low RBC count (low HCT) could suggest internal bleeding or a deficiency in vitamin B and folate [24]. Abnormalities in other blood parameters such as Hb levels, MCV, RDW, MCH and MCHC can also provide valuable information towards the ascertainment of a clinical diagnosis. In the case of anemia, a decrease in Hb levels and MCV can indicate various types of anemia, including iron deficiency anemia or vitamin B12 deficiency anemia [25]. Furthermore, an increase in RDW may aid in diagnosing macro-, normo-, or microcytic anemia based on corresponding MCV [26]. Alternatively, low Hb and MCV can also indicate thalassemia without iron deficiency [27]. In diabetic individuals, the Hb count is expected to be lower, while MCV is likely to be increased [28]. It also follows that RDW is positively correlated with glycated hemoglobin levels, a glycemic marker, and its prognosis in type 2 diabetes [10, 28]. Finally, hereditary spherocytosis, a type of hemolytic anemia characterized by an abnormal cell membrane, is associated with elevated levels of MCHC [29]. Again, though it should be noted that these conditions are not diagnosed solely based on clinical blood parameters alone, usually requiring further clinical testing, such as histological examination.

1.2.4 The current state and limitations of clinical red blood cell counting and microscopy

RBC profiling using CBC and PBS are valuable tools for healthcare providers, offering valuable insights into the state of a patient's health. Cell analyzers, while able to provide a comprehensive measure of RBC indices, are unable to account for morphological variations which may be influencing these indices [30]. Current methods rely on the manual assessment of RBC morphology, which is inherently subjective and can be time-consuming, introducing variability in results. The classification of RBC morphologies in clinical laboratories can vary across hospitals and may not consistently capture the extent of RBC abnormalities, revealing a need for more precise methodologies [30]. The manual nature of PBS assessments also prevents consistent detection of subtle changes in RBC shape abnormalities, further introducing potential diagnostic limitations. Current research has been aimed at the development of machine-learning models, capable of assessing both RBC morphology and correcting RBC indices accordingly, namely MCV, Hb content, and MCHC [30]. While not intended to replace manual assessment of PBS, these tools will be invaluable to improving the efficiency of PBS assessments as emerging studies are demonstrating their ability to discriminate various pathological conditions [30].

1.3 White blood cells

Leukocytes or WBCs are comprised of a mixture of nucleated cell types, whose circulation in the human body is responsible for defence against injury and infection. Immature WBCs released from the bone marrow, thymus, lymph nodes or spleen upon maturation have a typical lifespan of only 13–20 days prior to their destruction by the lymphatic system [31]. WBCs through recognition of pathogen- or damage-associated molecular patterns (PAMPs and DAMPs) on microbes and damaged tissue, respectively, can migrate to affected areas and enact specific roles and functions.

1.3.1 Normal morphology of white blood cells

PBS slides, stained with Giemsa or Leishman's solutions, have served for decades as the gold-standard for histologically identifying leukocytes [32]. Historically based on their microscopic appearance, WBCs are divided as either granulocytes or agranulocytes [32]. From the bone marrow of adults, granulocytes, made up of neutrophils, basophils and eosinophils, possess both lysosomes and specific granules, that under light microscopy have distinct appearances [33]. The granules within neutrophils are not well resolved under a standard microscope, while the larger granules found inside eosinophils and basophils with the aforementioned stains, appear red and blue, respectively, based on the pH of their contents (figure 1.1) [32, 34]. While not performed routinely in the clinic, granulocytes have been examined more extensively by electron microscopy which has revealed the granules of eosinophils to be both uniformly oval and full of major basic protein (MBP) [34]. Basophils' granules on

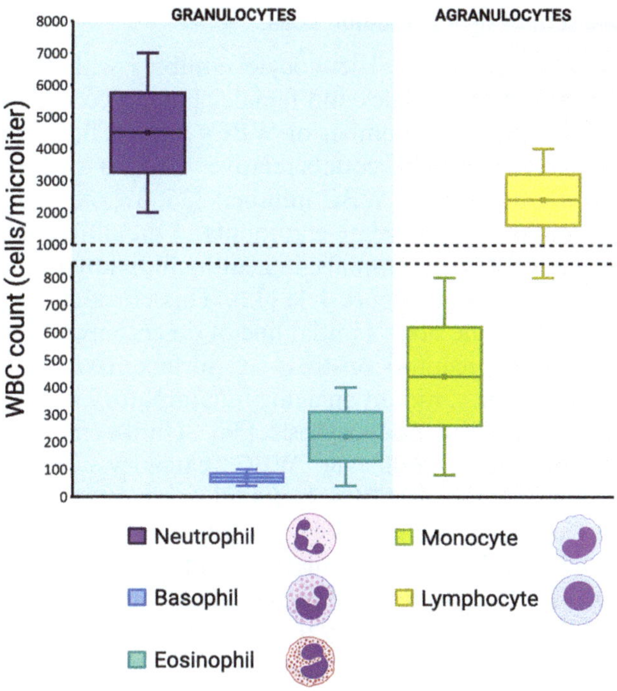

Figure 1.1. The normal morphologies and differential counts associated with all WBC types.

the other hand, under the electron microscope, are not only much larger and irregular in their shape but also found less frequently within the cell [35]. Morphologically, all granulocytes share a similar diameter, ranging in size from 12 to 15 μm but all three types exhibit distinct nuclei [32]. Eosinophils and basophils' nuclei are more bi-lobed and S-shaped, respectively, while neutrophils possess multi-lobed nuclei (figure 1.1) [32]. Made up of lymphocytes from lymphatic tissues and monocytes from reticuloendothelial tissues, the agranulocyte classification of WBCs arose since they lack any sort of specialized granules yet still contain lysosomes or azurophilic granules [32]. Examination under basic light microscopy has revealed monocytes to possess ample cytoplasm with their characteristic blue-grey color originating from the presence of lysosomes [32]. Monocytes like their granulocytic counterparts have been found to have diameters of 12–15 μm [32]. The nuclei of monocytes are on the larger side and uniquely shaped, indented into a horseshoe-like C-shape (figure 1.1) [32]. Lymphocytes can vary more in their diameter. At the lower end of 9 μm, the nuclei-to-cytoplasm ratio for these smaller lymphocytes is higher [32]. Additionally, their nuclei are spherical (figure 1.1). The larger lymphocytes with diameters nearing 18 μm, are most often in their activated state, and possess not only more lysosome-containing cytoplasm relative to their nuclei but the shape of these activated lymphocytes nuclei is less spherical and more indented [32]. Morphological changes to WBCs provide physicians with clues as to underlying conditions and diseases.

1.3.2 Normal functioning of white blood cells

In the clinic, a CBC captures total leukocyte numbers with the range of WBCs designated as normal for adult males and females having been established between 4000–11 000 cells μl^{-1} [32]. The number of WBCs though fluctuates with age with newborns possessing elevated WBC counts relative to adults while the elderly tend to experience a slight decline in their WBC numbers [36, 37]. Also measured within a CBC though is the differential or relative amounts of the different WBC types. The most abundant of the WBCs, neutrophils, in healthy individuals make up 50%–70% of the leukocytes in circulation (figure 1.1) [32]. This correlates with their cellular function which is to act as the body's initial line of defence in response to injury and infection. The membrane receptors on their cell surface, recognize the presence of debris and infectious bacteria, mount an acute inflammatory response, subsequently degrading foreign entities by phagocytosis [38]. Unlike neutrophils, basophils, another member of the granulocyte WBC category, do not phagocytize. Constituting less than 1% of all WBCs, basophil's primary role is associated with initiating the allergic response (figure 1.1) [32, 39]. The binding of antigens to the surface of basophils leads to degranulation and the release of mediators of inflammation [40, 41]. Eosinophils are found at an abundance ranging between 1% and 4%, and besides modulating the symptoms of inflammation through regulating basophils, function mainly to combat parasitic infections (figure 1.1) [32]. Their specific granules equipped with MBP, are particularly effective at killing subsets of parasites and like granulocytic neutrophils, eosinophils are capable of phagocytosis but primarily in the context of clearing allergic immune complexes [32, 42]. Monocytes from the agranulocytic class of WBCs have been established to be present at levels of approximately 2%–8% (figure 1.1) [32]. Notably these leukocytes differentiate upon leaving the bloodstream, becoming the various cells comprising the mononuclear phagocytotic system, with their function being to execute phagocytosis within tissues [43]. The most prevalent of the agranulocytes are the lymphocytes at 20%–40% of all WBCs (figure 1.1) [32]. As lymphocytes must circulate through the lymphatic system to serve as part of the adaptive immune system, their presence at higher numbers coincides with the fact that at any given time in humans, a reserve of immunocompetent WBCs needs to be readily capable of recognizing and reacting to foreign antigens [44]. In the clinical laboratory, these total WBC counts, and differentials have been captured both manually and automatically. The combined speed and accuracy of automated counters has made them superior to their predecessors, the specially designed Neubauer chambers [45]. Both high and low numbers of WBCs can serve as a signal of underlying medical conditions.

1.3.3 Abnormal morphology and functioning of white blood cells

Any deviation from the established range of 4000–11 000 cells μl^{-1} is considered either leukopenia or leukocytosis, depending on whether the counts when compared to normal are lower or higher, respectively. Leukopenia is often associated with viral infections but can occur in the context of some chronic health conditions such as lupus [32]. Leukocytosis typically presents with a higher percentage of neutrophils being evident. While higher neutrophil numbers can be witnessed with more benign patient ailments such as stress, leukocytosis is generally viewed as sign of cancer or the body's attempt to mount an inflammatory response to a serious parasitic infection [32]. Histological analysis by PBS often accompanies clinical parameter testing to provide deeper insight into cases of either leukopenia or leukocytosis [32]. WBC disorders are usually classified as either quantitative where the cellular appearance is normal, but the quantity of leukocytes is altered, or qualitative, wherein abnormal looking cells are in circulation but neither at an excess or deficit [46]. Neutrophilia often emerges because of pathologies existing outside the bone marrow, such as infectious diseases, neoplasia, metabolic disorders, hemorrhage, or stress [46]. On the other hand, neutropenia is often witnessed in response to drug treatment or radiotherapy but there are instances where congenital disorders can also decrease WBC production [46]. Notably, when granulocyte counts are below 1000 cells μl^{-1} the risk of sepsis infection increases immensely [46]. Together with corticosteroids, chemotherapeutic agents can lead to defects in the functionality of granulocytes [46]. Several genetic syndromes and anomalies though have been discovered to intrinsically impact the functioning of granulocytes too [46]. Eosinophilia while occurring in response to cancer, emerges upon parasitic infections and disorders affecting connective tissues such as rheumatoid arthritis [46]. Basophilia similar to neutrophilia is most evident with a cancer diagnosis [46]. Monocytosis which can be associated with certain malignancies and rheumatic diseases, sometimes trails chronic infections such as tuberculosis or diseases such as inflammatory bowel disease [46]. Similarly, lymphocytosis accompanies a variety of viral infections but also is evident with autoimmune diseases [46]. Lymphocytopenia, much like neutropenia, is a side effect of harsh therapeutic regimens but in other circumstances a result of congenital diseases of the immune system [46]. As WBC counts in the case of leukemias can exist across a wide spectrum, morphology and sometimes even histochemistry or cell surface marker expression is necessary to definitively classify the disease [46]. Acute leukemias will often present with large blasts, or immature WBCs with high nuclear to cytoplasmic ratios [46]. Lymphoblasts, the precursors to lymphocytes will often have coarser chromatin paired with less delineated nucleoli while the predecessors to granulocytes, myeloblasts exhibit the reverse phenomenon [46]. PBS from chronic myelogenous leukemia patients often validates their diagnosis as granulocytes appear in all stages of development [46].

1.3.4 The current state and limitations of clinical white blood cell counting and microscopy

Although the techniques employed in the medical laboratory to assess leukocytes have remained relatively consistent over time, numerous efforts are still being undertaken to improve clinical WBC testing to personalize patient treatment. As a result of the COVID-19 pandemic, it became apparent that age together with the severity of the viral infection, could significantly impacts clinical test results with some findings from the differential potentially being predicative of outcomes [47, 48]. More studies of this nature but on a larger scale and across multiple centers need to be conducted to assess whether the utility of some clinical parameters such as the WBC differential could be expanded from their current scope. While WBC counts are known to differ based on characteristics such as sex, reference intervals specific to women, particularly during pregnancy, a common and normal physiological state for a large cross-section of the population, were until very recently underdeveloped. Establishment of reference intervals for this vulnerable group would allow physicians to more accurately pinpoint causes of infection and inflammation. Furthermore, development of reference intervals for subsets of patients, needs to be done considering ethnicity and other characteristics that are often overlooked but highly influential on health-related measurements. Some of the first studies to take on this task revealed substantial changes in WBC numbers across the subtypes over the course of pregnancy and into postpartum period [49, 50]. This kind of work could have a profound impact on physicians' ability to accurately diagnose the conditions affecting expecting mothers thereby reducing the risk of maternal related morbidity and mortality. Additionally, continued improvements to analyzer technology and data analysis are constantly warranted. Clumping of WBCs, while infrequent is a source of error when specimens are counted that affects the reliability, if PBS is not performed in conjunction [51]. Improvements on automated counting of immature granulocytes is still an active area of research and technological development as improvements in their detection could lead to more confident diagnosis of infections over other abnormalities [52].

1.4 Platelets

Platelets (PLTs) are one of the smallest blood components that are disc-shaped cellular fragments. Megakaryocytes in the bone marrow will undergo membrane blebbing to produce over 5000 PLTs per cell [53]. Once produced, the PLTs are released into the vasculature with an average lifespan of 7–10 days [54]. During their lifespan, PLTs play a crucial role in homeostasis through coagulation [53]. PLTs typically remain inactive and survey the vasculature for signs of vascular damage. Like RBCs, their membrane is spectrin-based, while the cytoskeleton is made up of actin [53]. These components confer protection to the PLTs against the shear stressors in the vasculature. Once activated, PLTs undergo structural changes from a discoid shape to a spherocytic shape with pseudopodia [53, 54]. The pseudopodia, along with membrane proteins and receptors, allow adhesion to the injury site, aggregation of PLTs, and eventual release of granules. The cellular components of PLTs are involved in the clotting cascade. The complex structure and function of PLTs make them an essential component in blood, particularly in the context of hemostasis and thrombosis.

1.4.1 Normal morphology of platelets

PLTs can be visualized by PBS wherein when inactivated they are 2–3 μm in diameter and are oval disc-like in shape. When stained, mammalian PLTs can be divided into two regions: the hyalomere (protein-rich region) and the chromomere (granular region) [55]. The hyalomere stains a pale blue, while the granular region stains a darker red-purple colour [9]. Upon activation, PLTs release their granules, resulting in an agranular PLT that can also be visualized on a PBS. Three main types of granules can be secreted by PLTs: alpha granules, dense granules, and lysosomes. Of the highest abundance are the alpha granules, carrying factors influencing coagulation, inflammation, angiogenesis, and wound healing [56, 57]. These granules can range from 200–500 nm and make up approximately 10% of total PLT volume. On the other hand, dense granules, responsible for PLT aggregation, are smaller (~150 nm) and contain high concentrations of molecules such as serotonin, adenosine diphosphate, and calcium ions [56]. Lastly, lysosomes contain enzymes used to degrade cellular debris at the injury site [56]. A typical morphological finding with PLTs is the presence of clumping aggregation which leads to a false decrease in PLT count as determined by a cell analyzer [12, 58, 59]. Often this is a result of improper handling and storage of the blood sample [12, 58]. Repeating the PBS with a fresh sample is often performed to confirm PLT morphology [12].

1.4.2 Normal functioning of platelets

The normal PLT count can range from (1500–4000) $\times$ 10^9 cells per liter of blood [53]. Within a CBC, mean PLT volume (MPV), plateletcrit (PCT), and PLT distribution width (PDW) are measured alongside the PLT count. Like RBCs, these parameters can vary with sex, age, and ethnicity in addition to other factors. PLT counts have a tendency to decrease with age, and females have a naturally higher PLT count than males [60]. Furthermore, ethnicity alters PLT count, with black individuals possessing slightly higher PLT levels than white individuals [18]. PCT refers to the percentage of blood volume occupied by PLTs, and ranges from 0.22% to 0.24%. Like PLT count, PCT is higher in females than males and has been found to decrease with age in both sexes [61]. The average size of PLTs or the MPV, can range between 7–12 fl. Sex differences have also been observed with MPV, with males experiencing an increase in PLT volume with age, health conditions (hypertension and hyperglycemia), and lifestyle choices such as smoking [62]. Conversely, the MCV in females is positively correlated with menstruation and hormonal contraceptive use [62]. From the MPV, PDW can be calculated, which provides an indication of the variation and heterogeneity in PLT sizes. PDW ranges between 8.3% and 56.6% [63] and is influenced similarly to MPV. Understanding the factors that influence PLT clinical parameters helps in the interpretation and diagnosis of PLT-related disorders and diseases.

1.4.3 Abnormal morphology and functioning of platelets

Common PLT morphological abnormalities include clumping, changes to size, and granulation. These changes can indicate underlying medical conditions such as thrombocytosis or thrombopenia, myeloproliferative disorders, or medication-induced PLT dysfunction [58]. PLT morphology often helps assess the validity of CBC results. Pseudothrombocytopenia occurs when the anticoagulants used for blood collection cause PLTs to aggregate and result in falsely low PLT counts. A PBS would show aggregates of platelets, which mimics a decreased platelet count

[12]. Furthermore, hypogranulation, the lack of granules, may result from PLT activation and granular release during storage, or it could be a feature of myeloproliferative disorder [12, 58]. Lastly, PLTs can also increase or decrease in size due to several acquired and/or inherited diseases [58]. Accurate holistic assessment of PLT parameters can provide valuable diagnostic information for various pathological conditions.

In the context of PLTs, abnormalities of their indices may indicate an underlying disease or PLT-related disorder. An abnormally high platelet count would suggest thrombocythemia or thrombocytosis [64]. On the other hand, a low PLT count may indicate thrombocytopenia [65]. High levels of PLTs increase the risk of excessive clotting, while low levels of platelets can result in excessive bleeding [64, 65]. Abnormalities in PLT counts may only be transient due to acute infections, recovery from blood loss, alcohol intake, or certain medications [65, 66]. However increased PCT has also been linked to more chronic conditions such as Crohn's disease or endometrial cancer [63]. In diabetes mellitus, PLTs have increased aggregation, MPV, and PDW properties [53, 63]. This abnormal functioning of PLTs in diabetes mellitus can contribute to an increased risk of cardiovascular complications. Furthermore, increased MPV has been associated with septic shock, heart disease, and malignant tumours [63]. However, when interpreted in conjunction with decreased PDW, it could indicate threatened pre-term labour [63]. PLT parameters are influenced by several diseases such that the accurate assessment of PLT parameters can provide valuable diagnostic information for various pathological conditions.

1.4.4 The current state and limitations of clinical platelet testing

The evaluation of PLT function relies on both PLT indices and morphological assessments for insights into blood clotting and the overall vascular health of an individual. More recently, PLTs have been implicated in the pathophysiology of cancers, inflammatory diseases, and infections such as COVID-19. Despite pre-analytic influences, such as sample temperature, collection type and time between sampling and testing, PLT indices remain useful prognostic and diagnostic tools for clinicians [63]. Alongside blood analyzers, emerging techniques are being used to assess the functionality and morphology of PLTs. Current light microscopy techniques have only been able to visualize PLTs at lower resolutions. Alternatively, electron microscopy has allowed for high-resolution imaging with intra-PLT differentiation [67]. Advances in imaging can aid in the diagnosis and characterization of PLT disorders, such as identifying abnormalities in PLT size, shape, and granule content [67]. However, this technique requires specialized training, expensive equipment and is too time consuming to be clinically translated [67]. Along with electron microscopy, flow cytometry is an emerging technique, favoured for its ability to analyze numerous parameters and thus a detailed analysis of PLTs. Flow cytometry can provide insight into PLT surface marker expression, protein levels, and cellular interactions [67]. Aside from technical training and equipment, flow cytometry also requires a careful study design and is limited to antibodies currently on the market [67]. These techniques if advanced even further have the potential to enhance clinics' efficiency in evaluating PLT function and therefore have implications for not only vascular health, but management of patients afflicted with cancers, inflammatory diseases, and infections.

1.5 Plasma

Blood plasma, the solution in which erythrocytes, leukocytes, and thrombocytes are contained, originates from the water and solutes absorbed by the human digestive tract [68]. Approximately 90% water, the remaining 10% is made up of several critical components [68]. To aid in the maintenance of blood pH, electrolytes are present within plasma as well as proteins which act to preserve osmotic pressure, but other enzymes, hormones, and vitamins can also be found in small amounts [68]. Furthermore, coagulants and immunoglobins constitute plasma too and contribute to blood clotting and the fight against infections, respectively [68]. Plasma makes up the remaining total volume of whole blood besides what is constituted by RBCs. Measurements of blood volume can be conducted upon the injection of radioactive tracers into the bloodstream and are useful in tracking the proper functioning of bodily organs [69].

1.5.1 Normal appearance of plasma

Blood plasma is typically light-yellow in color [68]. Bilirubin, the product of the destruction of RBCs is the main contributor to the pigmentation of plasma [70]. Common deviations in plasmas' characteristic color can be the result of excess RBC hemolysis (red-orange), elevated ceruloplasmin from hormonal medications (green), and diet-induced lipemia (cloudy-white) [71–73].

1.5.2 Normal functioning of plasma

The numerous roles of plasma in the human body unsurprisingly overlap with many of the components it houses. Clinically, three types of chemistry tests are employed to measure the levels of various plasma constituents: basic metabolic panels, blood enzyme, and blood clotting tests. Ion selective potentiometry by clinical chemistry instrumentation is the current sensing method for electrolyte imbalances but ion selective electrodes can also be found in blood gas analyzers as well [74, 75]. The reference ranges for integral ions within healthy individuals are 135–145 mmol l^{-1} for sodium, 3.5–5 mmol l^{-1} for potassium, 95–105 mmol l^{-1} for chloride and 22–28 mmol l^{-1} for bicarbonate (figure 1.2) [76]. These ion concentrations should remain relatively consistent over time. In conjunction, employment of blood gas analysis can result in measurements of plasma pH which should be between 7.35 and 7.45 (figure 1.2) [77]. The glucose oxidase method is the most specific procedure to date performed by automated analyzers to measure blood glucose levels. It involves a series of enzymatic and biochemical conversions of glucose and its downstream products into chemical compounds that can be quantitated spectrophotometrically [78]. The concentration range for glucose upon fasting typically ranges from 3.9 to 5.6 mmol l^{-1} (figure 1.2) [79]. Similarly, the amount of lipid metabolites (total

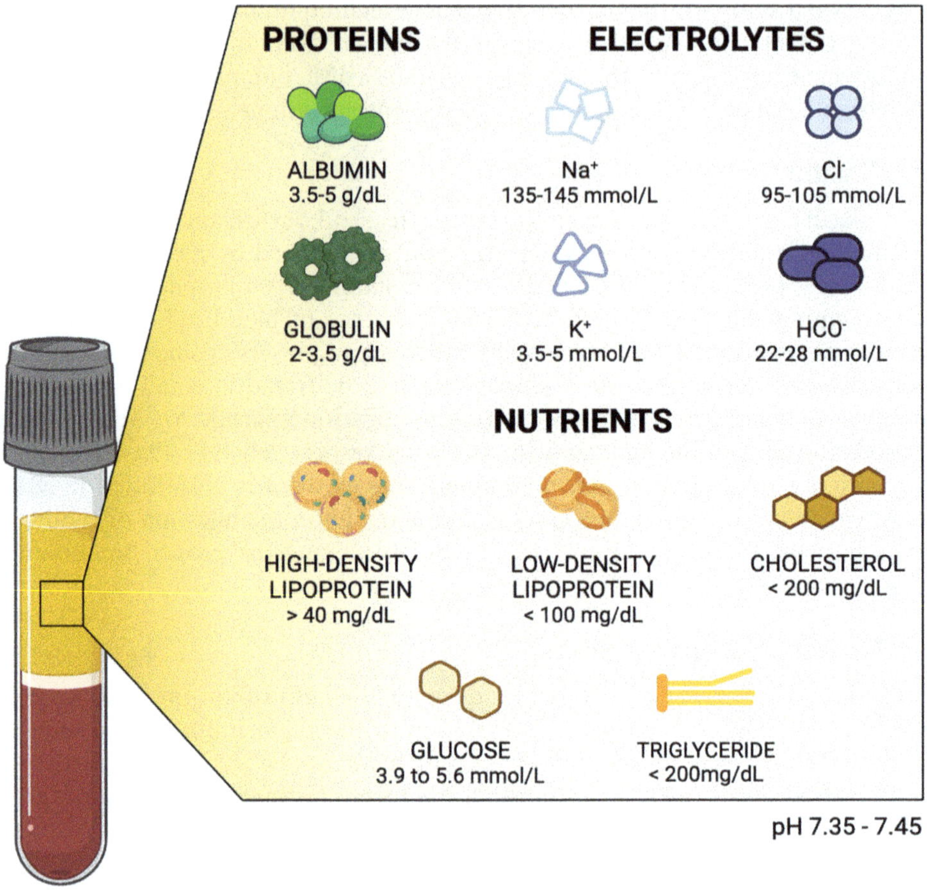

Figure 1.2. Established reference intervals for a subset of plasma constituents in healthy individuals.

cholesterol, high density lipoprotein (HDL) cholesterol, and triglycerides) in plasma is also directly determined through a series of coupled enzymatic reactions wherein colorimetric end products are measured [80]. It should be noted that low density lipoprotein (LDL) cholesterol is indirectly ascertained through calculation using directly measured values of total and HDL cholesterol [81]. Desirable total cholesterol and triglyceride levels are both less than 200 mg dl^{-1} (figure 1.2) [82]. Optimally, HDL should exceed 40 mg dl^{-1} while LDL is normally under 100 mg dl^{-1} (figure 1.2) [82].

Albumin is the most abundant protein within plasma, at 50% of the total protein content and a concentration of 3.5–5 g dl^{-1} in healthy individuals (figure 1.2) [83]. In part due to its abundance, albumin greatly impacts the osmotic pressure of plasma but additionally functions as a transporter of countless ligands such as bilirubin, ions, and fatty acids [68, 83]. Less abundant but still making up over 30% of the protein in plasma are globulins (2–3.5 g dl^{-1}) which also act as transporters of ions, hormones, and lipids (figure 1.2) [84]. Also, a subset of globulins can facilitate immune responses. Liver enzyme panels or hepatic function tests run on

Table 1.3. Broad reference intervals for liver function tests performed on normal human plasma [85].

Parameter	Range
Total Protein (g l^{-1})	60–80
ALP (IU l^{-1})	30–120
GGT (IU l^{-1})	6–50
AST (IU l^{-1})	5–30
ALT (IU l^{-1})	4–36

semi-automatic or fully automated clinical chemistry analyzers using enzymatic and colorimetric biochemical principles provide an initial indication of total protein levels (both albumin and globulin). Additional enzymes captured by this panel include alkaline phosphatase (ALP), glycoprotein gamma-glutamyltransferase (GGT), and the aminotransferases, AST and ALT [85]. Reference intervals for these photometric measurements vary not only across laboratories but are also highly variable between the sexes [85, 86]. Under normal conditions though, the results of this liver specific panel are as outlined in table 1.3 [85].

It should be noted that the preferred specimen for this clinical chemistry testing is serum rather than plasma, with the main difference between these cell-free blood solutions being that serum has undergone clotting and therefore no longer contains fibrinogen, a coagulant. While the clinical parameters discussed within this chapter are not an exhaustive list of all the testing that can be done on the plasma portion of blood, the aforementioned tests are some of the most important indicators of correctly functioning physiology and thus play a vital in the monitoring of health and disease.

1.5.3 Abnormal state of plasma

Clinical testing of plasma is often thc starting point for the diagnosis of many disease states by clinicians. While electrolyte imbalances can occur in association with more benign conditions such as dehydration or the use of certain medications, sustained severely high or low levels can disrupt multiple bodily functions and lead to life-threatening complications [76]. Hyponatremia, or low sodium can be an indication of heart failure, cirrhosis of the liver, adrenal insufficiency, among other serious disorders [76]. Higher than normal levels of potassium, or hyperkalemia, is often caused by uncontrolled diabetes, or various forms of acute and chronic kidney disease [87]. Similarly, improperly functioning kidneys underly both hypo- and hyperchlor-emia [76]. Disturbances to bicarbonate concentration, or in other words either metabolic acidosis or alkalosis are again often linked to disorders of the kidney and adrenal glands [88]. Elevated plasma glucose measurements of 5.6–6.9 $\text{mmol}\,l^{-1}$ typically coincide with a diagnosis of diabetes mellitus [89]. Hypoglycemia, most observed in type I diabetic individuals experiencing an overdose of insulin, can to a rarer extent be found in people battling such critical illnesses as sepsis, end-stage liver disease or pancreatic cancer [90]. Increased concentration of plasma lipids has been linked to various genetic disorders of both dominant and recessive inheritance patterns which ultimately give rise to hypercholesterolemia or hypertriglyceridemia [91]. Individuals with these disorders are at higher risk for developing coronary artery disease, atherosclerosis, and hypertension [91]. A few notable conditions associated with decreased serum albumin, are shock, liver disease, and Crohn's disease [92, 93]. If required for the patient's diagnosis, protein electrophoresis can also be employed on the proteins present in plasma. Within serum, separation of albumin, alpha1, alpha2, beta1, beta2, and gamma globulins can be conducted allowing for quantitative assessment of each protein fraction from its characteristic band patterning and intensity. This clinical test can reveal malignant conditions such as multiple myeloma in the case of increased gamma globulin fraction [94]. Raised alpha2 globulin concentration in plasma discovered using this methodology can be indicative of acute infections such as hepatitis or pneumonia or chronic inflammation such as lupus [95]. Unsurprisingly, elevated liver enzymes, (ALP, CGT, AST, ALT) often suggest damage or disease to the liver, either through hepatitis or cirrhosis, respectively [96]. Biochemical analysis of the bodily fluid, plasma not only can support the diagnosis of disease but also subsequent treatment.

1.5.4 The current state and limitations of clinical plasma testing

Clinical laboratory measurements are often the only means by which some late-stage organ diseases are detected. Continuous research and translation efforts will need to be focused on bringing additional identification markers for more asymptomatic conditions to standard laboratory testing panels for improved management of certain diseases [97]. Reference intervals in use for decades require reconsideration due to growing evidence suggesting variation in baseline measurements across such factors as race, ancestry, and socioeconomic status [97]. With the increased demand for personalized health monitoring by most of the general population, 'point-of-care' testing that is both rapid and accurate at assessing common analytes, has been successfully developed [97]. A bonus to these ongoing advancements has been the ability to perform testing of plasma 'near patient' allowing for health assessments to occur outside of hospital settings [97].

1.6 Conclusion

In the twenty-first century, rapid technological advances could potentially lead to further evolution of clinical blood testing approaches. From smaller volumes of blood components, more biological indicators of conditions will likely be examined as next generation -omics approaches contribute substantially to our molecular and cellular understanding of healthy and diseased states. With this anticipated influx of blood-related data though, considerations will need to be made for how this multitude of personalized information can be linked to beneficial clinical action.

References

[1] Chapman J and Zhang Y 2024 *Histology, Hematopoiesis* (Treasure Island, FL: StatPearls)

[2] Zhang Y, Gao S, Xia J and Liu F 2018 Hematopoietic hierarchy–an updated roadmap *Trends Cell Biol.* **28** 976–86

[3] Billett H H 1990 Hemoglobin and hematocrit *Clinical Methods: The History, Physical, and Laboratory Examinations* 3rd edn ed H K Walker, W D Hall and J W Hurst (Boston, MA: Butterworth)
[4] Mohandas N and Gallagher P G 2008 Red cell membrane: past, present, and future *Blood* **112** 3939–48
[5] Huisjes R, Bogdanova A, van Solinge W W, Schiffelers R M, Kaestner L and van Wijk R 2018 Squeezing for life–properties of red blood cell deformability *Front Physiol* **9** 656
[6] Lux S E 2016 Anatomy of the red cell membrane skeleton: unanswered questions *Blood* **127** 187–99
[7] Li H and Lykotrafitis G 2014 Erythrocyte membrane model with explicit description of the lipid bilayer and the spectrin network *Biophys. J.* **107** 642–53
[8] Adewoyin A S and Nwogoh B 2014 Peripheral blood film—a review *Ann Ib Postgrad Med.* **12** 71–9
[9] Horobin R W and Walter K J 1987 Understanding Romanowsky staining. I: the Romanowsky–Giemsa effect in blood smears *Histochemistry* **86** 331–6
[10] Seo I H and Lee Y J 2022 Usefulness of complete blood count (CBC) to assess cardiovascular and metabolic diseases in clinical settings: a comprehensive literature review *Biomedicines* **10** 2697
[11] Ward J, Cherrian S and Linden M A 2018 Hematopoietic and lymphoid tissues *Comparative Anatomy and Histology* 2nd edn. ed P Treuting, S M Dintzis and K S Montine (Academic) ch 19 pp 365–401
[12] Lynch E C 1990 Peripheral blood smear *Clinical Methods: The History, Physical, and Laboratory Examinations* 3rd edn ed H K Walker, W D Hall and J W Hurst (Boston, MA: Butterworth)
[13] Bhoopalan S V, Huang L J and Weiss M J 2020 Erythropoietin regulation of red blood cell production: from bench to bedside and back *F1000 Res.* **9** 1153
[14] Moras M, Lefevre S D and Ostuni M A 2017 From erythroblasts to mature red blood cells: organelle clearance in mammals *Front. Physiol.* **8** 1076
[15] Patel K V, Mohanty J G, Kanapuru B, Hesdorffer C, Ershler W B and Rifkind J M 2013 Association of the red cell distribution width with red blood cell deformability *Adv. Exp. Med. Biol.* **765** 211–6
[16] Zierk J, Krebs A, Rauh M, Metzler M, Loscher A, Strasser E *et al* 2020 Blood counts in adult and elderly individuals: defining the norms over eight decades of life *Br. J. Haematol.* **189** 777–89
[17] Feriel J, Tchipeva D and Depasse F 2021 Effects of circadian variation, lifestyle and environment on hematological parameters: a narrative review *Int. J. Lab. Hematol.* **43** 917–26
[18] Lim E, Miyamura J and Chen J J 2015 Racial/ethnic-specific reference intervals for common laboratory tests: a comparison among Asians, Blacks, Hispanics, and White *Hawaii J. Med. Public Health* **74** 302–10
[19] Grau M, Cremer J M, Schmeichel S, Kunkel M and Bloch W 2018 Comparisons of blood parameters, red blood cell deformability and circulating nitric oxide between males and females considering hormonal contraception: a longitudinal gender study *Front Physiol* **9** 1835
[20] Phillips R, Wood H, Weaving G and Chevassut T 2021 Changes in full blood count parameters with age and sex: results of a survey of almost 900000 patient samples from primary care *BJHaem* **192** e102–e5

[21] Tekle E, Gelaw Y and Asrie F 2022 Hematological profile changes among oral contraceptive users: a narrative review *J. Blood Med.* **13** 525–36
[22] Gao J and Monaghan S A 2018 Red blood cell/hemoglobin disorders *Foundations in Diagnostic Pathology, Hematopathology* 3rd edn ed E Hsi (Amsterdam: Elsevier) pp 3–56
[23] Pillai A A, Fazal S, Mukkamalla S K R and Babiker H M 2024 *Polycythemia* (Treasure Island, FL: StatPearls)
[24] George-Gay B and Parker K 2003 Understanding the complete blood count with differential *J. Perianesth Nurs.* **18** 96–114
[25] Brugnara C 2003 Iron deficiency and erythropoiesis: new diagnostic approaches *Clin. Chem.* **49** 1573–8
[26] Maner B S and Moosavi L 2024 *Mean Corpuscular Volume* (Treasure Island, FL: StatPearls)
[27] Bajwa H and Basit H 2024 *Thalassemia* (Treasure Island, FL: StatPearls)
[28] Wang Y, Yang P, Yan Z, Liu Z, Ma Q, Zhang Z, Wang Y and Su Y 2021 The relationship between erythrocytes and diabetes mellitus *J Diabetes Res.* **2021** 6656062
[29] Zamora E A and Schaefer C A 2024 *Hereditary Spherocytosis* (Treasure Island, FL: StatPearls)
[30] Foy B H, Stefely J A, Bendapudi P K, Hasserjian R P, Al-Samkari H, Louissaint A *et al* 2023 Computer vision quantitation of erythrocyte shape abnormalities provides diagnostic, prognostic, and mechanistic insight *Blood Adv.* **7** 4621–30
[31] Kline D L and Cliffton E E 1952 Lifespan of leucocytes in man *J. Appl. Physiol.* **5** 79–84
[32] Tigner A, Ibrahim S A and Murray I V 2024 *Histology, White Blood Cell* (Treasure Island, FL: StatPearls)
[33] Prinyakupt J and Pluempitiwiriyawej C 2015 Segmentation of white blood cells and comparison of cell morphology by linear and naive Bayes classifiers *Biomed. Eng. Online* **14** 63
[34] Melo R C, Dvorak A M and Weller P F 2010 Contributions of electron microscopy to understand secretion of immune mediators by human eosinophils *Microsc. Microanal.* **16** 653–60
[35] Woessner S 2005 Transmission electron microscopy in hematological diagnosis *Ultrastruct. Pathol.* **29** 237–68
[36] Sushanth , Avabratha K S, Tauro K J and Shwethadri G K 2010 Hyperleukocytosis in a neonate: a diagnostic dilemma *Indian J. Med. Paediatr. Oncol.* **31** 86–8
[37] Aminzadeh Z and Parsa E 2011 Relationship between age and peripheral white blood cell count in patients with sepsis *Int. J. Prev. Med.* **2** 238–42
[38] Malech H L, Deleo F R and Quinn M T 2014 The role of neutrophils in the immune system: an overview *Methods Mol. Biol.* **1124** 3–10
[39] Chirumbolo S, Bjorklund G, Sboarina A and Vella A 2018 The role of basophils as innate immune regulatory cells in allergy and immunotherapy *Hum. Vaccin. Immunother.* **14** 815–31
[40] Karasuyama H, Obata K, Wada T, Tsujimura Y and Mukai K 2011 Newly appreciated roles for basophils in allergy and protective immunity *Allergy* **66** 1133–41
[41] Borriello F, Iannone R and Marone G 2017 Histamine release from mast cells and basophils *Handb. Exp. Pharmacol.* **241** 121–39
[42] Kita H 2011 Eosinophils: multifaceted biological properties and roles in health and disease *Immunol. Rev.* **242** 161–77

[43] Chiu S and Bharat A 2016 Role of monocytes and macrophages in regulating immune response following lung transplantation *Curr. Opin. Organ. Transplant* **21** 239–45
[44] Larosa D F and Orange J S 2008 Lymphocytes *J. Allergy Clin. Immunol.* **121** S364–9 quiz S412
[45] Zhang M, Gu L, Zheng P, Chen Z, Dou X, Qin Q *et al* 2020 Improvement of cell counting method for Neubauer counting chamber *J. Clin. Lab. Anal.* **34** e23024
[46] Blumenreich M S 1990 The white blood cell and differential count *Clinical Methods: The History, Physical, and Laboratory Examinations* 3rd edn. ed H K Walker, W D Hall and J W Hurst (Boston, MA: Butterworth)
[47] Palladino M 2021 Complete blood count alterations in COVID-19 patients: a narrative review *Biochem. Med. (Zagreb.)* **31** 030501
[48] Anurag A, Jha P K and Kumar A 2020 Differential white blood cell count in the COVID-19: a cross-sectional study of 148 patients *Diabetes Metab. Syndr.* **14** 2099–102
[49] Dockree S, Shine B, Pavord S, Impey L and Vatish M 2021 White blood cells in pregnancy: reference intervals for before and after delivery *EBioMedicine* **74** 103715
[50] Zhu J, Li Z, Deng Y, Lan L and Yang J 2024 Comprehensive reference intervals for white blood cell counts during pregnancy *BMC Pregnancy Childbirth* **24** 35
[51] Gulati G, Uppal G and Gong J 2022 Unreliable automated complete blood count results: causes, recognition, and resolution *Ann. Lab. Med.* **42** 515–30
[52] Briggs C 2009 Quality counts: new parameters in blood cell counting *Int. J. Lab. Hematol.* **31** 277–97
[53] Ghoshal K and Bhattacharyya M 2014 Overview of platelet physiology: its hemostatic and nonhemostatic role in disease pathogenesis *Sci. World J.* **2014** 781857
[54] Williams O and Sergent S R 2024 *Histology, Platelets* (Treasure Island, FL: StatPearls)
[55] Bos-Mikich A, Ferreira M O, de Oliveira R and Frantz N 2019 Platelet-rich plasma or blood-derived products to improve endometrial receptivity ? *J. Assist. Reprod. Genet.* **36** 613–20
[56] Sharda A and Flaumenhaft R 2018 The life cycle of platelet granules *F1000Res* **7** 236
[57] Blair P and Flaumenhaft R 2009 Platelet alpha-granules: basic biology and clinical correlates *Blood Rev.* **23** 177–89
[58] Robier C 2020 Platelet morphology *J. Lab. Med.* **44** 231–9
[59] Schrezenmeier H, Muller H, Gunsilius E, Heimpel H and Seifried E 1995 Anticoagulant-induced pseudothrombocytopenia and pseudoleucocytosis *Thromb. Haemost.* **73** 506–13
[60] Balduini C L and Noris P 2014 Platelet count and aging *Haematologica* **99** 953–5
[61] Santimone I, Di Castelnuovo A, De Curtis A, Spinelli M, Cugino D, Gianfagna F *et al* 2011 White blood cell count, sex and age are major determinants of heterogeneity of platelet indices in an adult general population: results from the MOLI-SANI project *Haematologica* **96** 1180–8
[62] Panova-Noeva M, Schulz A, Hermanns M I, Grossmann V, Pefani E, Spronk H M *et al* 2016 Sex-specific differences in genetic and nongenetic determinants of mean platelet volume: results from the Gutenberg Health Study *Blood* **127** 251–9
[63] Pogorzelska K, Krętowska A, Krawczuk-Rybak M and Sawicka-Żukowska M 2020 Characteristics of platelet indices and their prognostic significance in selected medical condition—a systematic review *Adv. Med. Sci.* **65** 310–5
[64] Ashorobi D and Gohari P 2024 *Essential Thrombocytosis* (Treasure Island, FL: StatPearls)
[65] Jinna S and Khandhar P B 2024 *Thrombocytopenia* (Treasure Island, FL: StatPearls)

[66] Rokkam V R, Killeen R B and Kotagiri R 2024 *Secondary Thrombocytosis* (Treasure Island, FL: StatPearls)

[67] Tyagi T, Jain K, Gu S X, Qiu M, Gu V W, Melchinger H *et al* 2022 A guide to molecular and functional investigations of platelets to bridge basic and clinical sciences *Nat. Cardiovasc. Res.* **1** 223–37

[68] Mathew J, Sankar P and Varacallo M 2024 *Physiology, Blood Plasma* (Treasure Island, FL: StatPearls)

[69] Manzone T A, Dam H Q, Soltis D and Sagar V V 2007 Blood volume analysis: a new technique and new clinical interest reinvigorate a classic study *J. Nucl. Med. Technol.* **35** 55–63

[70] Elkassabany N M, Meny G M, Doria R R and Marcucci C 2008 Green plasma-revisited *Anesthesiology* **108** 764–5

[71] Agnihotri N and Kumar L 2014 Turbid plasma donations: need for quantification *Asian J. Transfus. Sci.* **8** 78–9

[72] Mani A, Poornima A P and Gupta D 2019 Greenish discoloration of plasma: is it really a matter of concern ? *Asian J. Transfus. Sci.* **13** 1–2

[73] Tesfazghi M T, McGill M R and Yarbrough M L 2019 What's causing this dark brown plasma? *J. Appl. Lab. Med.* **4** 125–9

[74] Burnett R W, Covington A K, Fogh-Andersen N, Kulpmann W R, Lewenstam A, Maas A H *et al* 2000 Recommendations for measurement of and conventions for reporting sodium and potassium by ion-selective electrodes in undiluted serum, plasma or whole blood. International Federation of Clinical Chemistry and Laboratory Medicine (IFCC). IFCC Scientific Division Working Group on Selective Electrodes *Clin. Chem. Lab. Med.* **38** 1065–71

[75] Yan R, Qiu S, Tong L and Qian Y 2016 Review of progresses on clinical applications of ion selective electrodes for electrolytic ion tests: from conventional ISEs to graphene-based ISEs *Chem. Speciat. Bioavailab.* **28** 72–7

[76] Shrimanker I and Bhattarai S 2024 *Electrolytes* (Treasure Island, FL: StatPearls)

[77] Singh V, Khatana S and Gupta P 2013 Blood gas analysis for bedside diagnosis *Natl. J. Maxillofac. Surg.* **4** 136–41

[78] Shaker G and Swift C J 2024 *Peroxidase-Coupled Glucose Method* (Treasure Island, FL: StatPearls)

[79] Mathew T K, Zubair M and Tadi P 2024 *Blood Glucose Monitoring* (Treasure Island, FL: StatPearls)

[80] Sharma A, Artiss J D and Zak B 1987 A method for the sequential colorimetric determination of serum triglycerides and cholesterol *Clin. Biochem.* **20** 167–72

[81] Lee Y and Siddiqui W J 2024 *Cholesterol Levels* (Treasure Island, FL: StatPearls)

[82] Expert Panel on Detection E, Treatment of High Blood Cholesterol in A 2001 Executive summary of the third report of the national cholesterol education program (NCEP) expert panel on detection, evaluation, and treatment of high blood cholesterol in adults (adult treatment panel III) *JAMA* **285** 2486–97

[83] Moman R N, Gupta N and Varacallo M 2024 *Physiology, Albumin* (Treasure Island, FL: StatPearls)

[84] Busher J T 1990 Serum albumin and globulin *Clinical Methods: The History, Physical, and Laboratory Examinations* 3rd edn ed H K Walker, W D Hall and J W Hurst (Boston, MA: Butterworth)

[85] Lala V, Zubair M and Minter D A 2024 *Liver Function Tests* (Treasure Island, FL: StatPearls)

[86] Gowda S, Desai P B, Hull V V, Math A A, Vernekar S N and Kulkarni S S 2009 A review on laboratory liver function tests *Pan. Afr. Med. J.* **3** 17

[87] Simon L V, Hashmi M F, Farrell M W and Chapagain R 2024 *Hyperkalemia (Nursing)* (Treasure Island, FL: StatPearls)

[88] Sur M and Hashmi M F 2024 *Alkalosis* (Treasure Island, FL: StatPearls)

[89] Mouri M and Badireddy M 2024 *Hyperglycemia* (Treasure Island, FL: StatPearls)

[90] Mathew P and Thoppil D 2024 *Hypoglycemia* (Treasure Island, FL: StatPearls)

[91] Cox R A and Garcia-Palmieri M R 1990 Cholesterol, triglycerides, and associated lipoproteins *Clinical Methods: The History, Physical, and Laboratory Examinations* 3rd edn ed H K Walker, W D Hall and J W Hurst (Boston, MA: Butterworth)

[92] Jensen K and Jarnum S 1976 Albumin and IgG turnover in ulcerative colitis and Crohn's disease *Plasma Protein Turnover* (London: Palgrave Macmillan)

[93] Gounden V, Vashisht R and Jialal I 2024 *Hypoalbuminemia* (Treasure Island, FL: StatPearls)

[94] O'Connell T X, Horita T J and Kasravi B 2005 Understanding and interpreting serum protein electrophoresis *Am. Fam. Physician* **71** 105–12

[95] Vandooren J and Itoh Y 2021 Alpha-2-macroglobulin in inflammation, immunity and infections *Front. Immunol.* **12** 803244

[96] Kalas M A, Chavez L, Leon M, Taweesedt P T and Surani S 2021 Abnormal liver enzymes: a review for clinicians *World J. Hepatol.* **13** 1688–98

[97] Plebani M, Laposata M and Lippi G 2019 A manifesto for the future of laboratory medicine professionals *Clin. Chim. Acta* **489** 49–52

Chapter 2

Normal and pathological morphology of blood cells of experimental animals

David Moore

To better understand the presence and function of blood cells and their role in normal physiology and in disease conditions, the use of animal models facilitates initial basic research. This chapter provides information about blood cells from commonly used experimental animals, and their properties that may affect blood optics (e.g., sizes, shapes, presence of nucleus), that will be of use in the research and development of new technologies and procedures for *in vivo* and *ex vivo* imaging of blood cells in humans and animals for research and diagnostic purposes.

2.1 Introduction

2.1.1 Milestones in the history of hematology and blood cell morphological identification [1]

2.1.1.1 17th Century

Red Blood Cells (RBCs)—Antoni van Leeuwenhoek (1632–1723), a City Hall custodian in Delft, Holland, whose hobby was the grinding of lenses, was one of the first three individuals to observe erythrocytes in blood, but his 31 letters, over 39 years, to the Royal Society in London, cemented his place in history for his microscope-based technology and study of blood cells [2]. He was the first to study and describe the structures in the blood of a variety of mammals, fish, birds, amphibians, and arthropods.

2.1.1.2 19th Century

Platelets—in 1842, Alfred Donné, a French public health physician, discovered/identified platelets in blood.

White Blood Cells (WBCs)—In 1843 Gabriel Andral, a French professor of medicine, and William Addison, an English country practitioner, reported simultaneously the first descriptions of leukocytes, noting that both RBCs and WBCs were altered by the presence of disease [3].

Between 1852 and 1876, multiple investigators developed procedures for counting RBCs and WBCs using a hemocytometer [1]. In 1878, Paul Ehrlich, a German physician, developed blood cell staining techniques to facilitate morphological identification of the cells, and subsequently identified three types of granulocytes, mast cells, and megaloblasts [4].

2.1.1.3 20th Century

Maxwell Wintrobe, MD (1901–86), near the end of the 1920s, recognized the absence of published, reliable, normal blood values to use in assessing clinical patients, and became the first to document statistically normal values in adults and children [5]. In 1942, he was the principal editor for the first edition of the textbook *Clinical Hematology*. Through his research, publications, and mentorship, he established hematology as a subspecialty.

In 1948, Wallace H Coulter developed a method to count and obtain volumetric data of blood cells, and using this 'Coulter Principle', produced the initial commercial Coulter Counter for automated blood-cell counting in 1956 [6].

Leeuwenhoek's examination of multiple vertebrate species laid the foundation for comparative hematology, and the discoveries made by the others described above led to the implementation of hematological analyses as a key tool in veterinary clinical medicine, as well as an additional source of data when assessing experimental treatments and physiological processes in laboratory animal models used in research. The recognition of optical properties of biological cells facilitates interpretation of their interaction with light, as well as deriving morphological information. In a study of tissues other than blood, it was observed that animal tissue optical properties were comparable to human counterpart tissues in the same spectral range [7]. In addition to *ex vivo* examination of blood cell optics, *in vivo* technologies have been developed to identify blood cells within the circulatory system and in tissues *in situ*; however, a majority of studies on the optical properties of blood cells has involved human blood [8–15]. In contrast, there are relatively few current published studies related to optical imaging of blood cells in experimental animals. Providing researchers with information about the morphology and optics of experimental animal blood cells will facilitate development or adaptation of technology to expand the use of animal models prior to assessing the technology in humans.

2.2 Morphology of human and laboratory animal blood cells

As can be observed in figures 2.1 and 2.2, the basic morphology/appearance of RBCs and WBCs of humans and the common laboratory animals (or better said, the majority of mammalian species) is quite similar. This similarity may allow adaptation of existing human blood cell imaging technology to the next generation imaging methodologies, using experimental animal models in research and development (R&D) prior to testing in humans. The following subsections provide descriptions of the cell types found in the peripheral blood circulation.

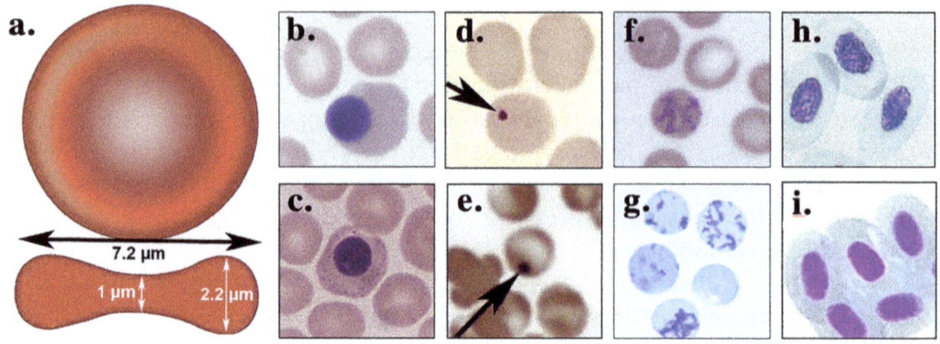

Figure 2.1. Morphology of the erythrocyte (RBC). (a) Illustration of a human erythrocyte. (b) Photomicrograph of a human nucleated RBC (NRBC). (c) Photomicrograph of a rabbit NRBC. (d) Photomicrograph of human Howell–Jolly body. (e) Photomicrograph of mouse Howell–Jolly body. (f) Photomicrograph of human reticulocytes. (g) Photomicrograph of dog reticulocytes. (h) Photomicrograph of a *Xenopus laevis* RBC. (i) Photomicrograph of a Zebrafish RBC.

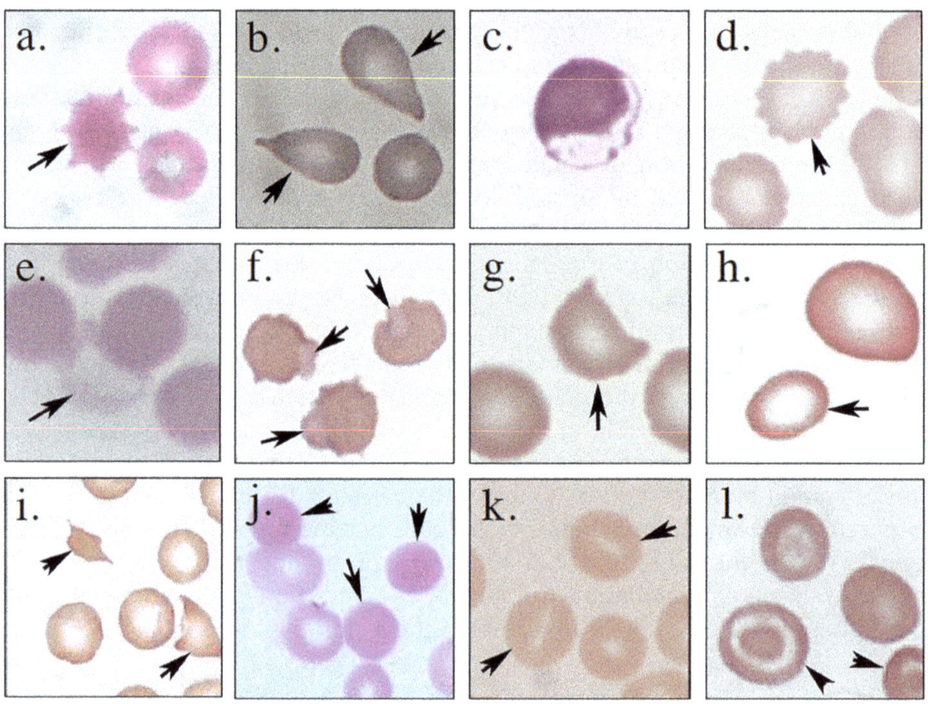

Figure 2.2. Photomicrographs of common RBC anomalies. (a) Acanthocyte. (b) Dacryocyte. (c) Eccentrocyte. (d) Echinocyte. (e) Ghost cell. (f). Heinz body. (g) Keratocyte. (h) Microcyte. (i) Schistocyte. (j) Spherocyte. (k) Stomatocyte. (l) Target cell.

2.2.1 Erythrocytes (red blood cells)

An approach to interpreting RBC morphological parameters has been previously described [16]. The morphology of the RBC (e.g., shape, volume, hemoglobin mass, and membrane stiffness) influences its ability to circulate through the body and transport oxygen to tissues [17]. RBCs contain an iron-containing pigment, hemoglobin, that gives the cell its color. Normal mammalian red blood cells are non-nucleated, biconcaved disc-shaped, with central pallor (see figure 2.1), with one exception—the RBCs of the camel are oval-shaped and nucleated in their mature form. The central pallor of RBCs in dogs is much greater than that observed in laboratory rodent species (gerbil, guinea pig, hamster, mouse, rat). The RBCs of fish, amphibians, reptiles, and birds are oval in shape, and contain a central oval nucleus, and are thus dissimilar to and inappropriate to use as models for human RBCs.

The morphology/shape of the RBC of all mammals (except camels), including humans, is virtually the same, with the primary difference between species being the average diameter of the RBC, as noted in table 2.1. Under normal conditions, human RBCs are malleable cells, approximately 7.2 μm in diameter and 2.2 μm in thickness, and have a spatially uniform refractive index because they lack nuclei and most organelles, with the refractive index mainly determined by the amount of hemoglobin in the cell [18]. RBCs can readily deform in response to circulatory shear stress, allowing them to efficiently pass through 3–5 μm diameter capillaries, smaller than the average diameter of an RBC [19]. Across vertebrate species (e.g., amphibians, snakes, birds, and rats as the representative model for mammals), it was observed that RBC diameters are about 25% larger than capillary diameters [20]. The elongation index, a measurement of RBC deformability, was determined for RBCs of humans, cats, dogs, mice, pigs, rats, and sheep, and the greatest to lowest

Table 2.1. Average values of erythrocyte diameter, mean corpuscular volume (MCV), and volume-to-diameter ratio (VDR), by species.

Species	Diameter (μm)	MCV (fl)	VDR
Human	7.2	90 [80–100]	12.5
Bovine (cattle)	5.5	44.5 [38–51]	8.1
Cat	5.0	46 [40–52]	9.2
Dog	6.3	70 [64–76]	11.1
Ferret	6.2	49.5 [45–54]	8.0
Gerbil	5.5	53 [46–60]	9.6
Goat	3.2	19 [16–22]	5.9
Guinea pig	7.1	86.5 [78–95]	12.2
Hamster	6.6	71 [64–78]	10.8
Horse	6.0	49 [43–55]	8.2
Mouse	5.8	50 [45–55]	8.6
NHP	7.2	70 [64–75]	9.7
Rabbit	6.1	62 [52–72]	10.2
Rat	6.0	58 [50–66]	9.7
Sheep	4.8	31.5 [28–35]	6.6
Swine (pig)	5.8	54.5 [44–65]	9.4

RBC deformability was found to be: humans, dogs, mice, rabbits > rats > cats, pigs > sheep [21].

Another RBC parameter is the mean corpuscular volume (MCV), indicating the average size and volume of an RBC. Table 2.1 provides a representative reference range for normal MCV values. An MCV value below the reference interval, e.g., smaller than normal cell size (normocytic), is termed microcytosis (microcytic RBCs). An MCV value above the reference interval, e.g., larger than normal cell size, is termed macrocytosis (macrocytic RBCs). Microcytosis may be caused by: iron deficient anemia; anemia of chronic diseases; Thalassemia trait; pregnancy; lead toxicity; and, sideroblastic anemia. Macrocytosis may be caused by: vitamin B_{12} deficiency; folate deficiency; HIV medications; hemolysis or hemorrhage; alcohol abuse; bone marrow disfunction; prescription medications; hypothyroidism; liver and kidney disease; and, chronic obstructive pulmonary disease (COPD).

In mammals, nucleated RBCs (NRBCs) occur in normal development as precursors to mature RBCs, with the nucleus ejected, as a normal part of cellular differentiation, prior to the cell's release into the bloodstream. The human NRBC, illustrated in figure 2.1, has a distinctive round nucleus, representative of NRBCs in other mammalian species. The presence of circulating NRBCs is associated with hematopoietic stress such as severe infection, massive hemorrhage, marrow infiltration, or extramedullary hematopoiesis [22]. Low numbers of NRBCs and Howell–Jolly bodies (shown in figure 2.1(e)) are common in normal mice and rats. In humans, Howell–Jolly bodies, DNA inclusions, remnants of the RBC nucleus, are associated with a number of pathological conditions: deficient spleen function; post-splenectomy; sepsis; congenital disorders; sickle cell hemoglobinopathies; alcoholism; lupus and other autoimmune disorders; post-bone marrow transplantation; gastrointestinal diseases (celiac and Inflammatory Bowel Diseases); neoplastic disorders; splenic vascular thrombosis; amyloidosis; geriatric patients; post-methyldopa treatment; and post-high-dose corticosteroid treatment [23].

Specific descriptions of erythrocytes of laboratory rodents and rabbits have been published previously [24–26]. Ferrets, guinea pigs, hamsters, mice, nonhuman primates (NHPs), rats, and rabbits often demonstrate moderate anisocytosis, e.g., RBCs of varying diameters, with the diameter of some cells being only one-quarter to one-third that of the standard sized RBC [24–26]. Anisocytosis may be seen in normal cats and cattle. Young gerbils, mice, and rats, in contrast to adults, have higher levels of circulating reticulocytes (non-nucleated immature RBCs). Reticulocytes have multiple particles or granules of varying size scattered throughout the cytoplasm, as illustrated in figure 2.1. Elevated or decreased reticulocyte counts may be associated with anemias and bone marrow dysfunction. One hematology analyzer, the Sysmex XT-2000iV, provides an indication of reticulocyte maturity by dividing the reticulocytes into three counting regions based on fluorescent intensity or absorbance, and has been used to assess reticulocyte counts in blood samples from dogs, mice, and rats [27]. Decreased reticulocyte counts may be caused by iron deficiency anemia, aplastic anemia, Vitamin B_{12} and folate deficiencies, hemolytic anemias associated with certain viral and bacterial infections, and myelodysplasia. Increased reticulocyte counts may be caused by hemolytic anemias (a result of RBC destruction), and acute or chronic blood loss. In stained blood smear samples, basophilic stippling is commonly observed in young and adult gerbils.

Variability in RBC shape/morphology, referred to as poikilocytosis, can be caused by a variety of diseases and nutritional deficiencies. Photomicrographs of RBCs exhibiting morphological changes are provided in figure 2.2, and descriptions of those cells are provided below.

Acanthocytes—These cells, also known as spur cells, exhibit spicules (spiny projections) of varying sizes, few in number, and at irregular intervals, projecting from the surface of the RBC. Because of their spiny surface, they can be trapped and destroyed in the spleen, leading to anemia. They are associated with diseases including abetalipoproteinemia, liver disease, chorea acanthocytosis, McLeod syndrome, neuroacanthocytosis, anorexia nervosa, infantile pyknocytosis, hypothyroidism, idiopathic neonatal hepatitis, alcoholism, congestive splenomegaly, Zieve syndrome, chronic granulomatous disease, and Bassen-Kornzweig syndrome.

Dacryocytes—These cells are teardrop-shaped, and are associated with diseases that cause bone marrow fibrosis, e.g., primary myelofibrosis, myelodysplastic syndromes, acute leukemias, and, myelophthisis; and more rarely post-irradiation, toxins, autoimmune diseases, metabolic conditions, inborn hemolytic anemias, iron-deficiency anemia or β-thalassemia.

Eccentrocytes—Eccentrocytes, associated with oxidative injury of the cell, have a crescent-shaped clear area close to the edge of the cell.

Echinocytes—Also known as burr cells, they have many small, evenly spaced thorny projections on the surface of the RBC, and more distinct central pallor. These cells are distinguished from acanthocytes by the shape of the projections, which are smaller and more numerous than in acanthocytes, and the projections are evenly spaced. They are associated with liver dysfunction, uremia, chronic kidney disease, Vitamin E deficiency, pyruvate kinase deficiency, hypomagnesemia, hypophosphatemia, hyperlipidemia, phosphoglycerate kinase deficiency, disseminated malignancy, myeloproliferative disorders, and early posttransfusion of RBCs.

Ghost cells—Ghost cells are comprised of the hollow remnant membrane of an RBC following intravascular lysis, a result of immune or nonimmune-mediated processes.

Heinz body—Oxidation or denaturation of hemoglobin in RBCs, a result of disease or treatment with certain drugs, will result in the development of a protuberance from the RBC membrane. They are associated with chronic liver disease, NADPH deficiency, glucose-6-phosphate dehydrogenase deficiency, Alpha thalassemia, and post-splenectomy.

Keratocytes—Keratocytes are fragments of RBCs with varying shapes such as half-moons or helmets. They are associated with iron deficiency anemia, disseminated intravascular coagulation, hemolytic uremic syndrome

Microcytes—These are abnormally small RBCs because the contain an insufficient amount of hemoglobin. The cells have a lower than normal mean corpuscular volume (MCV). They are associated with iron deficiency anemia, thalassemias, sideroblastic anemia, anemia of chronic disease, and chronic lead poisoning.

Schistocytes—These cells are often small in size, with no central pallor, and may be triangular, helmet shaped, or comma shaped with pointed ends. They are associated with hemolytic anemia, hemolytic uremic syndrome, thrombotic thrombocytopenic purpura, disseminated intravascular coagulation (DIC), and in individuals with mechanical heart valves.

Spherocytes—Spherocytes are created by an immune-mediated attack on RBCs, when macrophages strip off the outer membrane of the RBC, causing the loss of the discoid shape and producing a cell with a spherical shape, with the loss of the central pallor. Small numbers of spherocytes created from non-immune-mediated damage may also be observed.

Stomatocyte—These cells have a slit-like (mouth-like) area of central pallor. In these cells, there is an alteration in RBC wall permeability, leading to an increase in red cell volume. They are associated with hereditary stomatocytosis, dilantin toxicity, and alcoholism.

Target cells—Also known as codocytes or leptocytes, these cells appear bell-shaped within the circulation, but in blood smears examined microscopically, they have a characteristic target appearance. They have a dark central hemoglobinized area, surrounded by a ring of pallor, and then a dark peripheral ring of hemoglobin. These cells exhibit an increase in the ratio of surface membrane area to volume. They are associated with liver disease, thalassemia, Hemoglobin C disease, iron deficiency anemia, and post-splenectomy.

Sickle (crescent)-shaped RBCs in humans are observed in sickle cell disease, an inherited disease, associated with a genetic mutation. While it occurs primarily in individuals of African ethnicity, it can also be seen in individuals with Hispanic, Southern European, Middle Eastern, or Asian Indian backgrounds. These ‘C’-shaped cells tend to stick together, and do not move easily through blood vessels. Sickling of RBCs can be seen in goats and sheep, but has not been described as a genetic mutation.

Examples of studies involving *in vivo* imaging of RBCs in mice are provided in the references [28, 29].

2.2.1.1 Hemoglobin

Hemoglobin (Hb) is an iron-containing protein found in erythrocytes (RBCs) of mammals, including humans, comprising 96% of an RBCs dry weight (excluding water), and 35% of an RBCs total weight (including water) [30]. This protein is composed of four globular subunits, each containing one polypeptide chain, and a non-protein heme group containing iron, necessary for the binding of oxygen in the RBC. Heme is synthesized in the bone marrow and the liver of mammals. The four subunits of hemoglobin can each bind one molecule of oxygen. Hemoglobin can also bind with carbon dioxide, transporting the gas to the lungs for removal during exhalation. Hemoglobin manifests two biochemical properties—oxygen biding affinity, and cooperativity. Oxygen biding affinity denotes how tightly the hemoglobin protein binds with oxygen. The Bohr effect demonstrates that hemoglobin's oxygen binding affinity (e.g., oxygen–hemoglobin dissociation curve) is inversely related both to acidity and to the concentration of carbon dioxide. Cooperativity involves the interaction of the four Hb subunits such that the affinity of each binding site is increased. While the structure of hemoglobin is virtually the same across all mammals, including humans, from an evolutionary standpoint, hemoglobin proteins in various mammalian species have adapted oxygen biding affinity and cooperativity to meet their specific oxygen needs based on their body size, shape, physiology, and environment [31]. Mice, and by extension other small laboratory rodents, have a higher metabolic rate than humans, and in contrast to humans, they have a lower oxygen binding affinity in their Hb, facilitating dissociation of oxygen to support the higher metabolic rate [32].

Measuring hemoglobin—While a number of methods can be used to determine hemoglobin (Hb) concentration, the most accurate method for its determination is the cyanmethemoglobin (hemoglobincyanide) method, a colorimetric/spectrophotometric method [33]. In automated cell counters, the quantity of hemoglobin is determined by its absorption characteristics, and abnormal conditions such as 'hyperlipidemia, hyperbilirubinemia, very high WBC count, and high serum protein can interfere with this measurement and result in falsely elevated hemoglobin values.' [34]

One hematology assessment, mean corpuscular hemoglobin (MCH), quantifies the amount of hemoglobin per RBC. MCH values are expressed in picograms (pg) per cell. Another assessment, mean corpuscular hemoglobin concentration (MCHC), quantifies the amount of hemoglobin per unit volume, correlating the hemoglobin content with the volume of the cell. MCHC values are expressed in grams per deciliter (g dl^{-1}).

$$\text{MCH}\ (pg/cell) = \frac{\text{Hemoglobin in grams per 1000 ml of blood}}{\text{RBC count in millions per ml of blood}}$$

$$\text{MCHC}\ (g/dl) = \frac{\text{Hemoglobin in grams per 100 ml of blood} \times 100}{\text{Volume of packed cells per 100 ml of blood}}$$

Across the vertebrate species, Hb and MCHC concentrations increase from Agnatha to birds and mammals, however, the changes in Hb and MCHC concentrations do not parallel changes in RBC size [20].

The absorption spectra of hemoglobin in cattle, dogs, horses, humans, pigs, rats, and sheep have been previously described [35].

Table 2.2 provides the ranges of normal hemoglobin indices in humans and common laboratory animals.

Deficiency of hemoglobin occurs with anemia (reduced numbers of RBCs due to hemolysis or hemorrhage), bone marrow problems, chemotherapy (affecting bone marrow), nutritional deficiency of iron, kidney failure, or sickle cell disease.

A review article describes the use of blood optical properties, e.g., blood oxygenation, to assess clinical and physiological conditions including: monitoring of brain function during surgery; assessment of exercise effects on muscle for the diagnosis of peripheral vascular disease; scanning of the body for the location of

Table 2.2. Hemoglobin indices and their normal ranges in humans and lab animals.

Species	Hemoglobin (g dl^{-1})	MCH (pg/cell)	MCHC (g dl^{-1})
Human	12–18	27–31	32–36
Bovine (cattle)	8–15	11–17	30–36
Cat	9.8–15.4	13–17	30–36
Dog	11.9–18.9	21.0–26.2	32.0–36.3
Ferret	12.0–18.2	16.4–19.7	
Gerbil	12.1–16.9	16.1–19.4	30.6–33.3
Goat	8–12	5.2–8.0	30–36
Guinea pig	11.4–17.2	23.1–27.2	28.2–38.9
Hamster	13.1–19.2	19.9–25.8	27.5–37.4
Horse	10.1–16.1	13.7–18.2	35.3–39.3
Mouse	10.7–11.5	11.1–12.7	22.3–31.2
NHP	11.2–15.2	21.3–27.1	27.4–42.8
Rabbit	8–15	17.1–23.5	29–37
Rat	11.5–16.1	14.3–19.0	26.2–36.1
Sheep	9–15	8–12	31–34
Swine (pig)	10–16	17–21	30–34
Xenopus	6.06–15.19	6.9–22.1	19.3–32.3
Zebrafish	11.2–15.0	—	—

vascular occlusions; monitoring the effects of pharmaceutical and anesthetic substances and gas mixtures on tissues (especially brain); and cancer diagnostics by monitoring the level of oxygenation and total hemoglobin in the angiogenesis network of tumors [36]. In a study of Hb saturation with oxygen, it was observed that pigs, rabbits and sheep show similar trends in optical properties as a function of oxygen saturation [36].

2.2.2 Thrombocytes (platelets)

The optical properties of human platelets have been previously described [37], as well as a review of methodologies for *in vitro* and *in vivo* imaging of platelets [38].

Human platelets lack a nucleus, and are disc-shaped, as can be seen in figure 2.3. Thrombocytes of all mammalian species, including laboratory animals, are anuclear. Thrombocyte cell size ranges for humans and the common laboratory animals are provided in table 2.3.

Mouse and rat thrombocytes are round to oval to elongated in shape, as can be seen in figure 2.3. Guinea pig thrombocytes have an irregular, oval, or spindle shape, with concentric dark inner and lighter outer staining regions, as can be seen in figure 2.3. Rabbit thrombocytes may be oblong, oval, or rounded. Dog thrombocytes are oval to round, usually one-fourth to one-half the size of an RBC, though some platelets can be larger than an RBC. Cat thrombocytes are usually larger and have greater size variation than other domestic species [39]. Ferret platelets have a

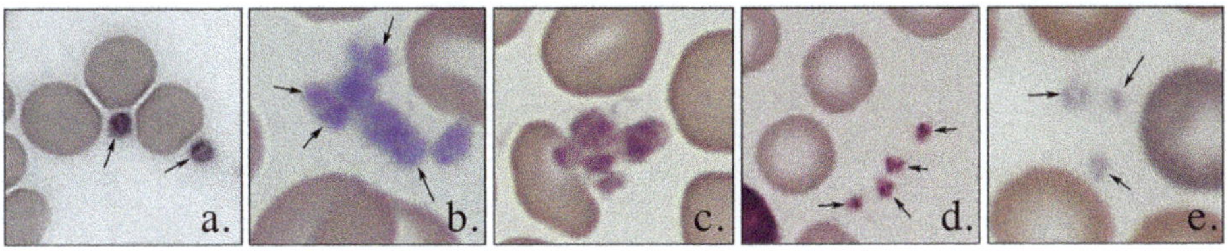

Figure 2.3. Photomicrograph images of platelets. (a) Human. (b) Guinea pig. (c) Hamster. (d) Mouse. (e) Rat.

Table 2.3. Blood cell diameter ranges for humans and common laboratory animals.

	Cell diameter (μm)						
Species	Eryth	Thromb	Basoph	Eosino	Lympho	Monocyt	Neutroph
Human	6–8	1–2	10–15	10–18	6–9	12–20	12–15
Bovine (cattle)	5–6	1–2	11.5	12	8–15	13–19	12–15
Cat	5–6	4–6	12–20	12–20	9–12	15–20	10–15
Dog	6–8	2–4	12–20	12–20	9–15	15–20	12–15
Ferret	4.6–7.7	1.5–2.3	13–14	12.7	6–13	12–18	9–13
Gerbil	5–6	1–3	10–14	10–14	10–15	10–15	10–12
Goat	3.2–3.4	2.2	8–10	10–15	6–9	13–19	10–15
Guinea pig	7.1–8.3	2–3	10–14	10–15	7–14	13–17	10–12
Hamster	4.0–7.5	1–3	10–14	10–14	9–12	10–16	10–12
Horse	5–7	2.5–3.5	13.8	13.4	6.0–9.5	15–20	12.25
Mouse	4–7	1–4	10–15	9–12	10–15	12–16	12–15
NHP	4–8	2.5–3.0	10.5–13.0	10.7–13.3	9.5–12.5	12.5–15.5	10.7–13.3
Rabbit	5.0–7.8	1–3	10–15	12–16	7–15	15–18	10–15
Rat	5–7	1–4	10–15	10–14	10–15		11
Sheep	4.4–4.5	2.6	8–10	10–15	6–9	13–19	10–15
Swine (pig)	4–8	1–3	10–12	12–15	7–15	14–18	12–15
Xenopus	12 × 16	6.7–15.6	7–16	12.5–17.0	5–11	11.5–15.0	11–19
Zebrafish	7 × 10	3–4	8–10	8–9	5–8	12–18	9–11

round to oval shape, but may be slightly irregular in size and shape. Equine thrombocytes are round, oval, or elongate. Platelets in cattle are usually round, but also are observed in varying sizes and shapes. Sheep and goats have platelets of similar shape to those found in other domestic species, but their platelets are smaller in comparison to the other species. Pig thrombocytes vary in shape and size. Nonhuman primate platelet morphology is similar to that of other lab animal species. Thrombocytes in Zebrafish (*Danio rerio*) are oval-shaped, smaller in size than RBCs, and have a centrally located elongated nucleus. Thrombocytes in the African clawed frog (*Xenopus laevis*) are either round, oval, or spindle-shaped, with a centrally located elongated nucleus

The range of cell numbers of RBCs and WBCs in humans and typical laboratory animals, found during hematology assessments, are provided in table 2.4.

Table 2.4. Blood cell count ranges for humans and common laboratory animals.

Species	Total RBC count ($\times10^6$ μl^{-1})	Total platelets ($\times10^3$ μl^{-1})	Total WBC count ($\times10^3$ μl^{-1})	Basoph # $\times10^3$ μl^{-1} (% of total)	Eosino # $\times10^3$ μl^{-1} (% of total)	Lympho # $\times10^3$ μl^{-1} (% of total)	Monocyt # $\times10^3$ μl^{-1} (% of total)	Neutroph # $\times10^3$ μl^{-1} (% of total)
Human	3.8–5.9	150–450	4.5–11.0	0.25–1.00 (0.5%–1.0%)	0.5–5.0 (1%–4%)	1–4 (20%–40%)	0.1–0.7 (2%–8%)	2.5–8.0 (55%–70%)
Bovine (cattle)	5.0–13.5	160–800	7.4–12.5	0.0–0.2 (0%–1%)	0.0–1.5 (3%–7%)	1.6–8.1 (56%–68%)	0.0–0.8 (3%–6%)	1.8–6.3 (28%–39%)
Cat	6.6–10.9	206–465	4.8–15.3	0.0–0.1 (0%–2%)	0.1–1.2 (1%–15%)	1.2–10.2 (9%–56%)	0.1–0.6 (0%–6%)	1.7–8.8 (27%–82%)
Dog	5.9–8.4	220–480	6.0–14.3	0.01–0.08 (0%–1%)	0.2–1.4 (1%–18%)	1.5–4.7 (9%–47%)	0.1–0.7 (2%–12%)	3.1–9.4 (42%–84%)
Ferret	6.5–13.2	297–910	2.2–18.2	0.0–0.1 (0.0%–3.0%)	0.0–0.7 (0.0%–8.5%)	0.6–10.5 (12%–67%)	0.0–0.5 (0.0%–8.3%)	0.7–7.4 (24%–78%)
Gerbil	7.1–9.4	432–710	4.3–12.8	0.0–0.01 (0.0%–0.8%)	0.0–0.22 (0.0%–2.3%)	1.96–9.47 (58.9%–78.1%)	0.0–1.11 (0.0%–6.5%)	1.31–5.01 (9.3%–25.8%)
Goat	8–16	300–600	2–19	0–1 (0%–3%)	0–2 (0%–6%)	1–12 (35%–80%)	0–1 (0%–6%)	1–9 (18%–57%)
Guinea pig	3.3–6.8	260–740	5.2–17.5	0.0–0.2 (0.0%–1.7%)	0.0–0.9 (0.0%–7.0%)	2.56–5.68 (40.0%–80.4%)	0.0–0.1 (1.0%–5.3%)	1.6–3.1 (20.3%–56.0%)
Hamster	3.9–10.3	300–573	5.0–10.6	0.0–0.23 (0%–5%)	0.17–2.25 (0.2%–1.5%)	20.18–51.63 (50.9%–92.3%)	6.19–16.95 (0.4%–4.4%)	1.36–5.63 (17.1%–35.2%)

(Continued)

Table 2.4. (*Continued*)

Species	Total RBC count ($\times 10^6\ \mu l^{-1}$)	Total platelets ($\times 10^3\ \mu l^{-1}$)	Total WBC count ($\times 10^3\ \mu l^{-1}$)	Basoph # $\times 10^3\ \mu l^{-1}$ (% of total)	Eosino # $\times 10^3\ \mu l^{-1}$ (% of total)	Lympho # $\times 10^3\ \mu l^{-1}$ (% of total)	Monocyt # $\times 10^3\ \mu l^{-1}$ (% of total)	Neutroph # $\times 10^3\ \mu l^{-1}$ (% of total)
Horse	6.2–10.2	100–250	5.5–12.5	Rare (0%–3%)	0.0–0.4 (0%–16%)	1.5–5.5 (18%–55%)	0.2–0.4 (0%–7%)	2.5–8.0 (36%–79%)
Mouse	6.9–11.7	157–412	12.1–15.9	0.0–0.13 (0.01%–1.24%)	0.0–2.03 (1.3%–2.8%)	0.12–23.46 (62.4%–82.8%)	0.0–5.08 (0.9%–2.4%)	0.03–32.03 (13.2%–21.6%)
NHP	5.3–5.4	410–437	5.3–10.5	0.0–0.2 (0.0%–0.2%)	0.1–0.3 (1.9%–4.6%)	1.3–4.4 (19.2%–52.7%)	0.08–0.30 (1.4%–3.5%)	2.5–6.5 (39.7%–68.1%)
Rabbit	5.1–7.9	270–656	5.2–12.5	0.0–0.7 (2.4%–7.5%)	0.0–0.3 (0.5%–3.5%)	0.8–7.6 (28.0%–52.1%)	0.0–0.8 (4.0%–13.4%)	0.8–8.0 36.4%–54.0%)
Rat	6.7–9.7	150–460	6.6–12.6	0.0–0.02 (0.0%–0.6%)	0.03–0.21 (0.1%–1.9%)	2.09–7.66 (50.2%–84.5%)	0.08–0.76 (0.0%–1.8%)	0.19–1.43 (4.4%–49.2%)
Sheep	9.2–13.0	426–1142	5.1–15.9	0.0–0.2 (0.0%–0.01%)	0.0–0.2 (4.0%–5.4%)	0.8–6.3 (43.6%–49.6%)	0.1–0.8 (1.9%–3.7%)	5.1–15.9 (41.9%–48.1%)
Swine (pig)	5–8	200–500	11–22	0.0–0.2 (0%–2%)	0.2–1.1 (0.5%–11.0%)	5.5–18.7 (39%–62%)	03–1.32 (2%–10%)	4.5–10.0 (28%–47%)
Xenopus	0.80–1.48	12–24	2.92–9.56	0.0–1.9 (22.9%–65.6%)	0.0–1.4 (0.0%–5.5%)	3.2–11.4 (15.4%–44.7%)	0.2–3.9 (0.0%–3.2%)	1.9–28.1 (10.6%–40.0%)
Zebrafish	2.9–3.2			(0%–2%)	(0%–2%)	(64%–92%)	(5%–15%)	(2%–18%)

2.2.3 Leukocytes (white blood cells)

In general, leukocytes are relatively similar in appearance across mammalian species. Descriptions of those cells are provided below, and comparative photomicrographic images of human and experimental animal blood cells are provided in figure 2.4. There are five basic types of leukocytes (WBCs) in mammalian and non-mammalian vertebrate species—basophils, eosinophils, lymphocytes, monocytes, and neutrophils. Leucocyte cell shapes are dynamic, allowing them to pass through capillaries and into tissues. Generally, in pathological states in lab animals, there is an alteration in numbers of cells rather than an alteration in morphology.

Examples of studies involving *in vivo* imaging of WBCs in humans are provided in the references [40–42].

2.2.3.1 Basophils

Basophils are rarely seen in the peripheral circulation in the majority of domestic mammals, but may be found in the blood of horses. Basophils are present in the peripheral circulation for only a few hours before migrating into tissues [43]. Increased numbers of basophils in circulation (basophilia) is usually rare, but

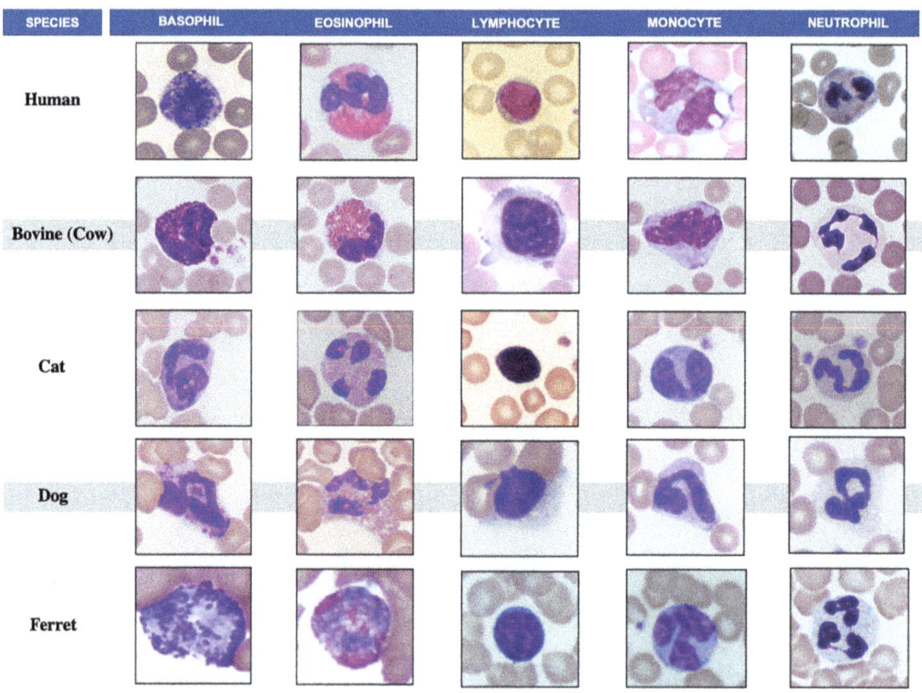

Figure 2.4. (a) Comparative photomicrograph images of human and common lab animal blood cells. (b) Comparative photomicrograph images of human and common lab animal blood cells. (c) Comparative photomicrograph images of human and common lab animal blood cells. (d) Comparative photomicrograph images of human and common lab animal blood cells.

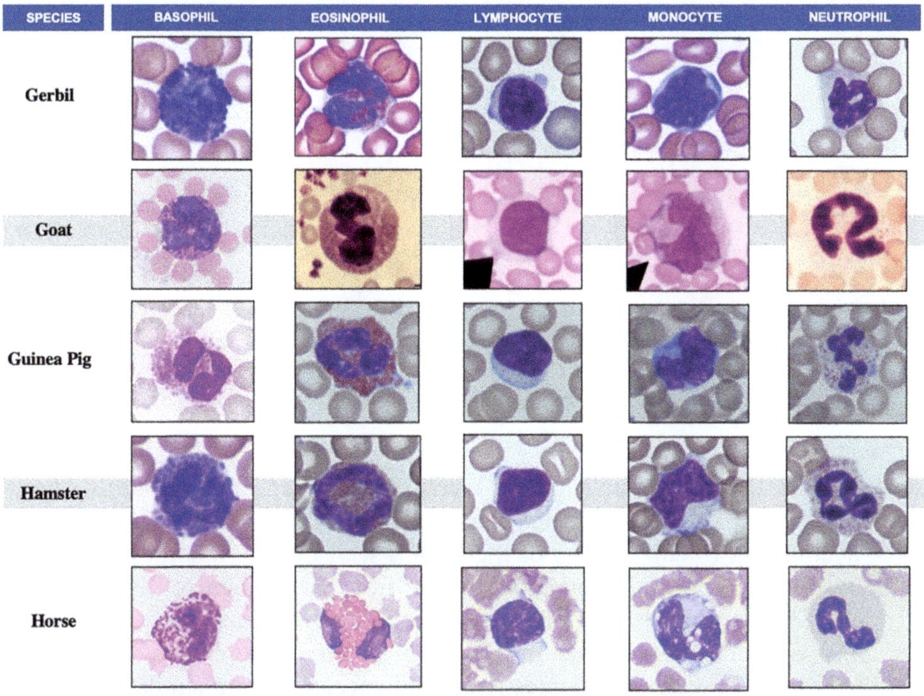

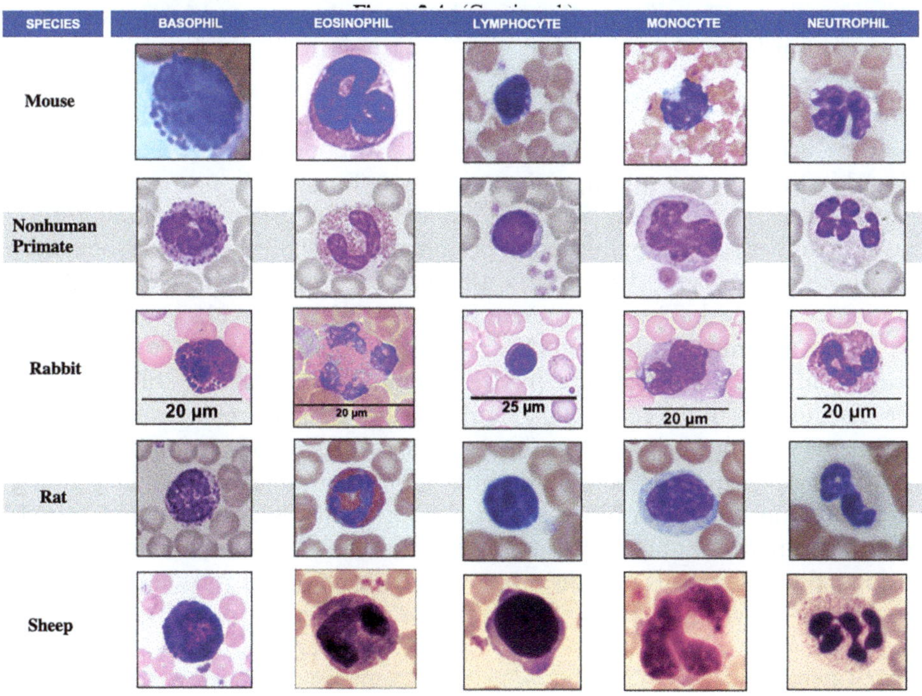

Figure 2.4. (Continued.)

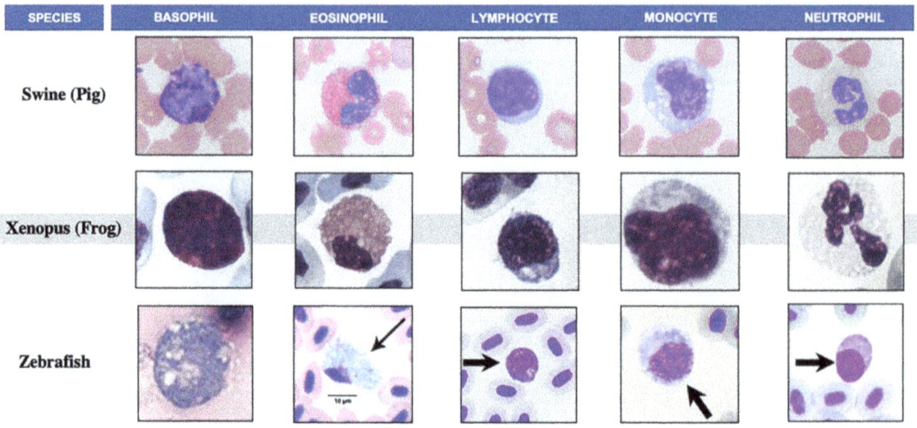

Figure 2.4. (Continued.)

when it occurs there may also be an increased number of eosinophils observed (eosinophilia). Unlike other mammalian species, basophils are commonly seen in rabbits, accounting for up to 30% of the WBCs seen in a peripheral blood smear.

The basophil nucleus is segmented, but not as segmented as the mature neutrophil. The cytoplasm contains a small number of scattered round granules, which may obscure the nucleus in some cells. The basophils of the common laboratory rodent species and domestic animal species have a similar appearance. Photomicrographs of representative basophils from the common laboratory animals are provided in figure 2.5.

2.2.3.2 Eosinophils

While the majority of eosinophils are produced in bone marrow, they may also be produced in the thymus, spleen, and cervical lymph nodes. In normal animals, they are either absent or present in low numbers in the peripheral circulation. An increased number of eosinophils in the peripheral circulation can be associated with the presence of parasitic disease and allergic reactions, when antigens are being continuously released. They are present in the peripheral circulation for only a few hours before moving into tissues [43].

Eosinophils are usually similar in size to neutrophils, but may often be slightly larger. The nucleus of the eosinophil, similar to that of neutrophils, is segmented, but the segments may not be as well defined. The cytoplasm contains multiple granules of varying shapes and numbers depending upon the animal species. Depending on the type of stain used with blood smears, the granules may appear red to reddish pink. In contrast to mice, rats, and gerbils, whose eosinophils have rounded inclusions, the eosinophils of guinea pigs and hamsters have rod-shaped inclusions. The inclusions in eosinophils in rabbits appear needle-shaped.

2.2.3.3 Lymphocytes

Lymphocytes are the most common WBC found in the peripheral blood of rodents (e.g., gerbils, guinea pigs, hamsters, mice, and rats) and ruminants (e.g., cattle,

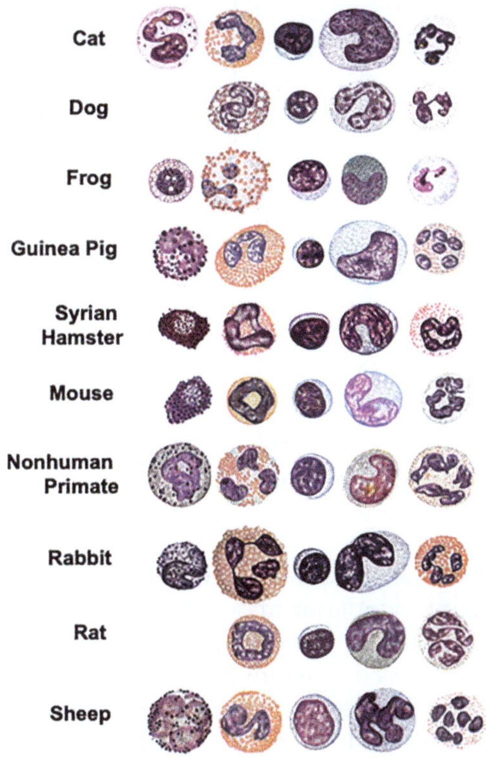

Figure 2.5. Drawings of WBCs of the common laboratory animals. (columns L to R: basophils, eosinophils, lymphocytes, monocytes, neutrophils).

sheep, goats), and the second most common WBC in other mammals. Lymphocytes are the dominant WBC in amphibians. Lymphocytes are usually round in shape, with a round-to-oval nucleus. The nucleus may be central or slightly eccentric within the cell. The variation in appearance of mammalian lymphocytes can be attributed to the amount of nuclear chromatin condensation, staining characteristics of the cytoplasm, and size. Photomicrographs of representative lymphocytes from the common laboratory animals are provided in figure 2.5. 'Small' lymphocytes are more commonly seen in the peripheral circulation, with a high nucleus-to-cytoplasm (N:C) ratio, e.g., there is a scant amount of cytoplasm surrounding the nucleus. 'Medium' to 'large' lymphocytes may also be seen, observed more frequently in ruminants, with a lower N:C ratio, e.g., there is a greater amount of cytoplasm surrounding the nucleus. Examples of small and large lymphocytes are provided in figure 2.6.

2.2.3.4 Monocytes

Monocytes are either absent or found in very low numbers in peripheral blood circulation. The numbers of monocytes are usually higher in juveniles than in adult mammals. The nucleus may present with a variety of shapes, such as round to oval

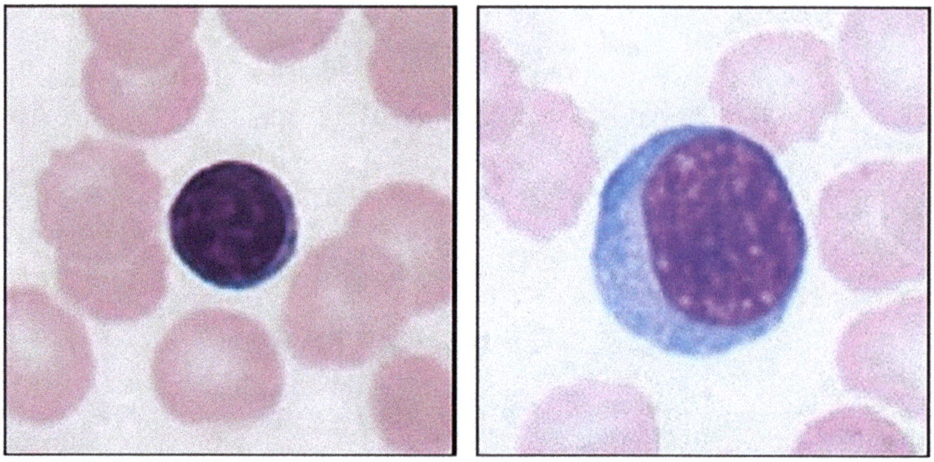

Figure 2.6. Photomicrographic images of small and large lymphocytes. (a). Small lymphocyte. (b). Large lymphocyte.

with a single indentation (kidney bean-shaped), or multiple indentations/lobulations. The moderately abundant cytoplasm may contain a number of clear vacuoles of varying sizes. Photomicrographs of representative monocytes from the common laboratory animals are provided in figure 2.5.

Increased numbers of monocytes in the peripheral circulation (monocytosis) may be seen with certain bacterial infections (e.g., brucellosis and tuberculosis), during recovery from acute infections, neoplasia, and collagen diseases.

2.2.3.5 Neutrophils

Mature neutrophils, containing segmented nuclei, are the most common WBCs found in the peripheral blood of mammals, however, in rodents (e.g., gerbils, guinea pigs, hamsters, mice, and rats) and ruminants (e.g., cattle, sheep, goats), the lymphocyte is the most common cell type seen in peripheral blood.

The neutrophils in guinea pigs, hamsters, and rabbits are referred to as heterophils. The cytoplasm of heterophils contains rounded or rod-shaped granules which stain pink to red, making the cell appear similar to an eosinophil, thus heterophils are sometimes referred to as pseudoeosinophils. The nucleus of the heterophil is dense, and has five or more segments. The granules in the cytoplasm are round, as compared to the elongated inclusions of eosinophils.

Band neutrophils (see figure 2.7) are immature neutrophils that lack the nuclear segmentation seen in more mature cells. The nucleus is U-shaped, resembling a horseshoe, and the width (side-to-side) of the nucleus is constant along its length. As the cell matures, indentations begin to form, resulting in the final segmented appearance. The N:C ratio is approximately 1:2. Release of band neutrophils into circulation indicates that the bone marrow is responding to a severe inflammatory/infectious stimulus.

Guinea pigs have mononuclear leukocytes in their peripheral circulation, known as Kurloff cells, that contain an inclusion body composed of glycoprotein. These cells, unique to guinea pigs, have natural killer (NK) and natural cytotoxic activity.

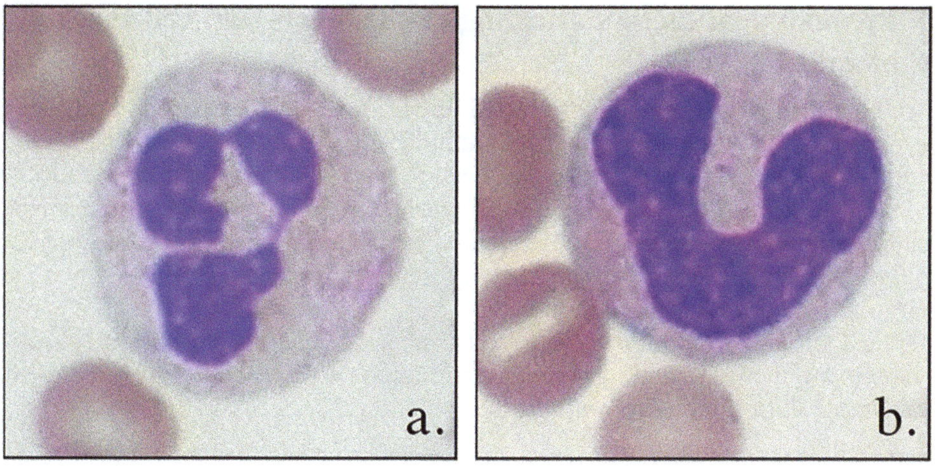

Figure 2.7. Photomicrographic images of mature and immature neutrophils. (a) Mature segmented nucleus. (b) Immature band nucleus.

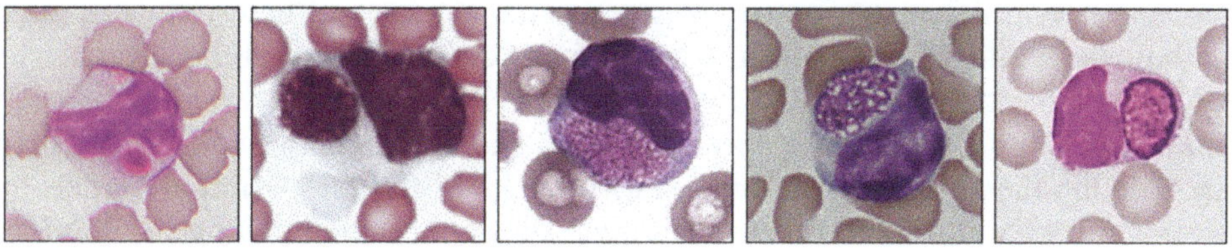

Figure 2.8. Photomicrographic images of guinea pig Kurloff cells.

Table 2.5. Nucleus to cytoplasm ratios for mature human leucocytes.

	Basoph	Eosino	Lympho	Monocyt	Neutroph
N:C ratio	1:3	1:3	5:1 to 2:1	3:1 to 2:1	1:3

They are seen more often in females than in males, and are seen in increased numbers in pregnant females. Representative examples of Kurloff cells are provided in figure 2.8.

2.2.3.6 Nucleus-to-cytoplasm ratio of leucocytes

The N:C ratio is a ratio of the size (volume) of the nucleus of a cell to the size of the cytoplasm of that cell. In normal leucocytes, the N:C ratio indicates the maturity of a cell. Immature WBCs, referred to as blasts, are released from the bone marrow into the general circulation. As the blast cell matures, the size of its nucleus generally decreases. Table 2.5 provides N:C ratios for mature human leucocytes, which would be comparable to their counterparts in animals. In body tissues other than blood cells, an increased N:C ratio is observed in precancerous dysplasia and in malignant cells.

2.3 Preanalytical factors affecting cell numbers and cell types observed

When conducting *in vivo* or *ex vivo* blood optics analyses, the quantity and types of cells observed may be affected by a number of intrinsic and extrinsic factors including, but not limited to: blood collection site; frequency of blood collection; age; sex; strain; animal vendor; diet; environment; handling/restraint; transport; circadian rhythms; anesthesia/analgesia; and euthanasia [44]. A knowledge of those variables will help in assessing the likely presence or absence of WBCs when using *in vivo* or *ex vivo* imaging of blood cells.

Optical property assessment of blood can be affected by sample preparation, measurement method, and assessment conditions (e.g. blood flow), as there is considerable light attenuation in undiluted blood [13].

2.4 Establishing experimental animal blood cell datasets for AI machine learning

As mentioned earlier, mammalian blood cell morphology is similar across the various species, differing primarily in size, and in the case of heterophils in guinea pigs, hamsters, and rabbits, with the inclusion of cytoplasmic granules. Researchers might select the animal model and its blood cells for a variety of reasons (e.g., animal size, cost of procurement and housing, and commercial availability), rather than selecting the animal based on the morphology of the cells. Animal models may be selected based on the need for developing species-specific imaging of blood cells for that species in support of biomedical research or veterinary clinical care.

A number of papers have been published describing the use of artificial intelligence (AI) for identification of human blood cells for diagnostic and research purposes [45–53]. Development of AI for recognition of experimental animal blood cells will facilitate development of the next generation of *in vivo* and *ex vivo* imaging technology. Technology requiring US Food and Drug Administration (FDA) review and approval may require initial testing in animal models prior to use in humans.

Datasets of images of human WBCs [54–60] and RBCs [61–63] are available for use in machine learning in support of new imaging technologies. At the present time, similar datasets for blood cells of the common laboratory animal species are not readily available. In the absence of 'off the shelf' datasets, acquiring cell images for animal blood cells can be accomplished in two ways—collecting whole blood from live animals, or purchasing blood or specific blood cells from commercial sources.

2.5 Acquiring and collecting blood from animals

Prior to acquiring and using live animals as the source of blood samples, permission/approval must be sought from the researcher's institution's Animal Care and Use Committee, Animal Ethics Committee, or applicable regulatory committee as required in that individual's country. After approval is granted, animals may be purchased and housed in accordance with the institution's policies and requirements, or blood samples from agricultural and domestic species may be sought from local veterinarians. Guidance on blood collection techniques for the various species should be sought from the institution's laboratory animal veterinarian. Agricultural animals (cow, goat, horse, pig, sheep) and 'pet' species (cat, dog, ferret, guinea pig, rabbit) do not typically require the use of anesthesia prior to blood collection. Laboratory rodent species (gerbil, mouse, rat) and aquatic species (*Xenopus* frog, Zebrafish) are usually anesthetized prior to blood collection. The institution's laboratory animal veterinarian should be consulted for guidance in the dosing and administration of anesthetic agents. Blood samples should be collected in an EDTA blood tube, and then a blood smear made on a microscope slide prior to staining. Descriptions and illustrations of the process involved in making blood smears are available on the internet [64, 65]. Staining of the blood smear is accomplished by standard procedures [66]. Once the smear is stained, no coverslip is required, a drop of immersion oil is placed in the feathered edge of the smear, and the slide examined under a microscope using the 1000x objective lens. Digital photographs of individual cells are taken, and the images included in an appropriate dataset.

Individual cell types can be isolated from peripheral blood samples prior to making blood smears, facilitating imaging of larger numbers of the same cell type in the absence of other cells. Procedures for isolating ***basophils*** have been described for guinea pigs [67, 68] and mice [69]. Procedures for isolating ***eosinophils*** have been described for cattle [70], guinea pigs [71, 72], horses [73], mice [74–76], nonhuman primates [77], and rats [78, 79]. Procedures for isolating ***lymphocytes*** have been described for goats [80], guinea pigs [81], horses [82], mice [83–85], pigs [86, 87], and rats [88, 89]. Procedures for isolating ***macrophages*** have been described for ferrets [90], guinea pigs [91, 92], hamsters [93], horses [94], pigs [95], rats [96], and sheep [97]. Procedures for isolating ***monocytes*** have been described for goats [98], guinea pigs [99], horses [100], mice [101–103], nonhuman primates [104], pigs [105, 106], and rats [107, 108]. Procedures for isolating ***neutrophils*** have been described for cattle [70], dogs [109], ferrets [110], goats [109], horses [109, 111], mouse [109, 112–116], nonhuman primates [109], pigs [109, 117, 118], rabbits [109], rats [109, 119, 120], and sheep [109, 121].

2.5.1 Purchasing whole blood or specific blood cells from experimental animal species

2.5.1.1 Whole blood vendors

BioChemed, Winchester, VA USA

Bovine (cattle), Cat, Dog, Ferret, Guinea Pig, Hamster, Mouse, Nonhuman Primate, Pig, Rabbit, Rat, Sheep

BIOIVT, Westbury, NY USA

Swine (Gottingen minipig)

Charles River Laboratories, Wilmington, MA USA

Mouse, Rat

HemoStat Laboratories, Dixon, CA USA
Bovine, Goat, Guinea Pig, Horse, Pig, Rabbit, Sheep

HumanCells Biosciences, Milpitas, CA USA
Nonhuman Primate (Cynomologus; Rhesus)

Innovative Research, Novi, MI USA
Guinea Pig, Swine (pig)

2.5.1.2 Commercial sources of individual blood cells

Erythrocytes (Red Blood Cells—RBCs)

AcceGen Biotechnology, Fairfield, NJ USA
Guinea Pig, Hamster

Biocompare, South San Francisco, CA USA
Dog, Mouse, Nonhuman Primate, Rabbit, Rat

BIOIVT, Westbury, NY USA
Bird, Bovine (cattle), Mouse, Nonhuman Primate, Rat, Sheep

Fisher Scientific, Waltham, MA USA
Bovine, Horse, Nonhuman Primate, Rabbit, Rat, Sheep

Innovative Research, Novi, MI USA
Guinea Pig, Rat, Swine (pig)

Rockland Immunochemicals, Pottstown, PA USA
Guinea Pig

TCS Biosciences, Buckingham, UK
Guinea Pig, Horse, Rabbit, Sheep

Lymphocytes

SBS Genetech Co., Beijing, China
Rat

Macrophages

AcceGen Biotechnology, Fairfield, NJ USA
Mouse

Cell Biologics, Chicago, IL USA
Canine, Hamster, Mouse, Nonhuman Primate, Porcine (pig), Rabbit, Rat

ScienCell Research Laboratories, Carlsbad, CA USA
Mouse, Rat

Monocytes

AcceGen Biotechnology, Fairfield, NJ USA
Mouse

BIOIVT, Westbury, NY USA
Nonhuman Primate

Cell Biologics, Chicago, IL USA
Mouse, Rat

Neutrophils
AcceGen Biotechnology, Fairfield, NJ USA
Mouse
BIOIVT, Westbury, NY USA
Mouse, Nonhuman Primate
Cell Biologics, Chicago, IL USA
Mouse, Rat

PERIPHERAL BLOOD MONONUCLEAR CELLS (PBMCs)—(Lymphocytes, Monocytes, Macrophages)
BIOIVT, Westbury, NY USA
Canine (dog), Minipig, Mouse, Nonhuman Primate, Rat
Fisher Scientific, Waltham, MA USA
Rabbit
3H Biomedical, Uppsala, Sweden
Mouse, Rat
iQ Biosciences. Alameda, CA USA
Canine, Guinea Pig, Mouse, Nonhuman Primate, Rabbit, Rat
iXCells Biotechnologies, San Diego, CA USA
Bovine, Mouse, Rat
HumanCells Biosciences, Milpitas, CA USA
Nonhuman Primate (Cynomologus; Rhesus)

References

[1] Coller B S 2015 Blood at 70: its roots in the history of hematology and its birth *Blood* **126** 2548–60

[2] Davis I M 2022 Round, red globules floating in a crystalline fluid'—Antoni van Leeuwenhoek's observations of red blood cells and hemocytes *Micron* **157** 103249

[3] Hajdu S I 2003 The discovery of blood cells *Ann Clin Lab Sci.* **33** 237–8

[4] Tifford M 2010 Paul Ehrlich: histological staining, immunology, chemotherapy *Lab. Med.* **41** 497–8

[5] Kushner J P 2007 Maxwell Myer Wintrobe: influential teacher in the field of hematology *Hematologist* **4** 1306

[6] Graham M D 2022 The coulter principle: a history *Cytometry* **101** 8–11

[7] Frabasile L *et al* 2023 Non-invasive estimation of *in vivo* optical properties and hemodynamic parameters of domestic animals: a preliminary study on horses, dogs, and sheep *Front. Vet. Sci.* **18** 1243325

[8] Lindberg L and Oberg P A 1993 Optical properties of blood in motion *Opt. Eng.* **32** 253–7

[9] Sardar D K and Levy L B 1998 Optical properties of whole blood *Lasers Med. Sci.* **13** 106–11

[10] Roggan A *et al* 1999 Optical properties of circulating human blood in the wavelength range 400–2500 NM *J. Biomed. Opt.* **4** 36–46

[11] Semyanov K *et al* 2007 Optics of leucocytes *Optics of Biological Particles* NATO Science Series **vol 238** ed A Hoekstra, V Maltsev and G Videen (Dordrecht: Springer) pp 253–64
[12] Maltsev V P, Hoekstra A G and Yurkin M A 2011 Optics of white blood cells: optical models, simulations, and experiments *Advanced Optical Flow Cytometry: Methods and Disease Diagnoses* ed V V Tuchin (New York: Wiley-VCH) pp 63–93
[13] Meinke M C, Freibel M and Helfman J 2011 Optical properties of flowing blood cells *Advanced Optical Flow Cytometry: Methods and Disease Diagnoses* ed V V Tuchin (New York: Wiley-VCH) pp 95–132
[14] Bosschaart N *et al* 2014 A literature review and novel theoretical approach on the optical properties of whole blood *Lasers Med Sci.* **29** 453–79
[15] Yaroslavsky A N and Yaroslavsky I V 2016 Optics of blood *Handbook of Optical Biomedical Diagnostics, Volume 1: Light-Tissue Interaction* 2nd edn ed V V Tuchin (SPIE Press) pp 161–219
[16] Doig K and Zhang B 2017 A methodical approach to interpreting the red blood cell parameters of the complete blood count *Clin. Lab. Sci.* **30** 173–85
[17] Paul R *et al* 2020 Quantitative absorption imaging of red blood cells to determine physical and mechanical properties *RSC Adv.* **10** 38923–36
[18] Gautam R *et al* 2019 Optical force-induced nonlinearity and self-guiding of light in human red blood cell suspensions *Light: Sci. Appl.* **8** 31
[19] McMahon T J 2019 Red blood cell deformability, vasoactive mediators, and adhesion *Front. Physiol.* **10** 1417
[20] Snyder G K and Sheafor B A 1999 Red blood cells: centerpiece in the evolution of the vertebrate circulatory system *Am. Zool.* **39** 189–98
[21] Varga A *et al* 2022 Interspecies diversity of osmotic gradient deformability of red blood cells in human and seven vertebrate animal species *Cells* **11** 1351
[22] Pikora K *et al* 2023 Diagnostic value and prognostic significance of nucleated red blood cells (NRBCs) in selected medical conditions *Cells* **12** 1817
[23] Scafidi J M *et al* 2023 Histology, Howell Jolly bodies *StatPearls* (Treasure Island, FL: StatPearls Publishing) https://ncbi.nlm.nih.gov/books/NBK557489/
[24] Lindstrom N M *et al* 2015 Hematologic assessment in pet rats, mice, hamsters, and gerbils—blood sample collection and blood cell identification *Vet. Clin. Exot. Anim.* **18** 21–32
[25] Zimmerman K *et al* 2015 Hematological assessment in pet guinea pigs (*Cavia porcellus*)—blood sample collection and blood cell identification *Vet. Clin. Exot. Anim.* **18** 33–40
[26] Moore D M *et al* 2015 Hematological assessment in pet rabbits—blood sample collection and blood cell identification *Vet. Clin. Exot. Anim.* **18** 21–32
[27] Mathers A *et al* 2012 Reticulocyte measurements in rat, dog and mouse whole blood samples using the Sysmex XT-2000iV *Comp. Clin. Pathol.* **21** 631–7
[28] Avsievich T *et al* 2020 The advancement of blood cell research by optical tweezers *Rev. Phys.* **5** 100043
[29] Jeon J *et al* 2021 Intravital imaging of circulating red blood cells in the retinal vasculature of growing mice *Transl. Vis. Sci. Technol.* **10** 31
[30] Weed R I *et al* 1963 Is hemoglobin an essential structural component of human erythrocyte membranes? *J. Clin. Invest.* **42** 581–88
[31] Rapp O and Yifrach O 2019 Evolutionary and functional insights into the mechanism underlying body-size-related adaptation of mammalian hemoglobin *eLife* **8** e47640

[32] Perlman R L 2016 Mouse models of human disease: an evolutionary perspective *Evol., Med. Public Health* **2016** 170–6
[33] https://laboratorytests.org/cyanmethemoglobin-method/
[34] Sarma P R 1990 Red cell indices *Clinical Methods: The History, Physical, and Laboratory Examinations* **Chapter 152** 3rd edn ed H K Walker *et al* (Boston: Butterworths)
[35] Zijlstra W G *et al* 2019 *Visible and Near Infrared Absorption Spectra of Human and Animal Haemoglobin—Determination and Application* (Boca Raton, FL: CRC Press) pp 55–188
[36] Savateeva E V *et al* 2002 Optical properties of blood at various levels of oxygenation studied by time-resolved detection of laser-induced pressure profiles *Proc. SPIE* **4618**
[37] Meinke M *et al* 2007 Optical properties of platelets and blood plasma and their influence on the optical behavior of whole blood in the visible to near infrared wavelength range *J. Biomed. Opt.* **12** 014024
[38] Montague S J *et al* 2020 Imaging platelet processes and function—current and emerging approaches for imaging *in vitro* and *in vivo Front. Immunol.* **11** 00078
[39] Schaefer D M 2022 Hematology of cats *Schalm's Veterinary Hematology* 7th edn ed M B Brooks *et al* (New York: Wiley) pp 984–6
[40] Fanous M J *et al* 2017 White blood cell detection, classification and analysis using phase imaging with computational specificity (PICS) *Sci. Rep.* **12** 20043
[41] Yoon J *et al* 2015 Label-free characterization of white blood cells by measuring 3D refractive index maps *Biomed. Opt. Express* **6** 3865–75
[42] Yoon J *et al* 2022 Identification of non-activated lymphocytes using three-dimensional refractive index tomography and machine learning *Sci. Rep.* **7** 6654
[43] Whalen J E 2015 *A Toxicologist's Guide to Clinical Pathology in Animals* (New York: Springer) p 20
[44] Enos K E and Moore D M 2022 Hematology of laboratory animals *Schalm's Veterinary Hematology* 7th edn ed M B Brooks *et al* (New York: Wiley) pp 1061–7
[45] Alam M M and Islam M T 2019 Machine learning approach of automatic identification and counting of blood cells *Healthc. Technol. Lett.* **6** 103–8
[46] Radakovich N, Nagy M and Nazha A 2020 Artificial intelligence in hematology: current challenges and opportunities *Curr. Hematol. Malig. Rep.* **15** 203–10
[47] Diaz-Del-Pino S *et al* 2023 Artificial intelligence to assist specialists in the detection of haematological diseases *Heliyon* **9** e15940
[48] Hu Y *et al* 2022 Artificial intelligence and its applications in digital hematopathology *Blood Sci.* **4** 136–42
[49] Tayebi R M *et al* 2022 Automated bone marrow cytology using deep learning to generate a histogram of cell types *Commun. Med. (Lond)* **2** 45
[50] Yonfei H *et al* 2022 Artificial intelligence and its applications in digital hematopathology *Blood Sci.* **4** 136–42
[51] Gedefaw L *et al* 2023 Artificial intelligence-assisted diagnostic cytology and genomic testing for hematologic disorders *Cells* **12** 1755
[52] Lewis J E and Pozdnyakova O 2023 Digital assessment of peripheral blood and bone marrow aspirate smears *Int. J. Lab. Hematol.* **45** 50–8
[53] Lewis J E *et al* 2023 An automated pipeline for differential cell counts on whole-slide bone marrow aspirate smears *Mod. Pathol.* **36** 100003
[54] Acevedo A *et al* 2020 A dataset of microscopic peripheral blood cell images for development of automatic recognition systems *Data Brief* **30** 105474

[55] Kouzehkanan Z M *et al* 2022 A large dataset of white blood cells containing cell locations and types, along with segmented nuclei and cytoplasm *Sci. Rep.* **12** 1123
[56] Bodzas A, Kodytek P and Zidek J 2023 A high-resolution large-scale dataset of pathological and normal white blood cells *Sci. Data* **10** 466
[57] https://doi.org/10.1101/2021.05.02.442287
[58] https://github.com/Shenggan/BCCD_Dataset
[59] https://github.com/MrAnayDongre/BloodCell-Detection-Datatset
[60] https://bbbc.broadinstitute.org/BBBC045
[61] Cimrák I *et al* 2023 Curated dataset for red blood cell tracking from video sequences of flow in microfluidic devices *Data* **8** 106
[62] https://data.mendeley.com/datasets/rg7f6bwvb7/1
[63] https://zenodo.org/records/5656057
[64] https://agric.wa.gov.au/livestock-biosecurity/blood-smear-technique-veterinarians
[65] https://uvm.edu/~jschall/pdfs/techniques/bloodsmears.pdf
[66] https://statlab.com/pdfs/ifu/svw001.pdf
[67] Graziano F M *et al* 1984 Isolation of guinea pig basophils using anti-leukocyte antibody and density gradient centrifugation on Percoll *J. Immunol. Methods* **67** 157–65
[68] MacGlashan D W *et al* 1982 Purification of basophilic leukocytes from guinea pig and human blood and from guinea pig bone marrow *Cell Separation* ed T G Pretlow and T P Pretlow (New York: Academic) pp 301–20
[69] Yoshimoto T and Nakanishi K 2012 Generation and characterization of mouse basophils from bone marrow and purification of basophils from spleen *Curr. Protoc. Immunol.* **98** 3.24.1–16
[70] Roth J A and Kaeberle M L 1981 Isolation of neutrophils and eosinophils from the peripheral blood of cattle and comparison of their functional activities *J. Immunol. Methods* **45** 153–64
[71] Tsuda S *et al* 1986 Isolation of peritoneal eosinophils from Polymyxin B-treated guinea pigs on density gradients of Nycodenz, a new non-ioniciodinated gradient medium *Biomed. Res.* **7** 389–97
[72] Gleich G J and Loegering D 1973 Selective stimulation and purification of eosinophils and neutrophils from guinea pig peritoneal fluids *Transl. Res.* **82** 522–8
[73] Jörg A *et al* 1978 A rapid and simple method for the isolation of pure eosinophilic leukocytes from horse blood *Experientia* **34** 1654–56
[74] Geslewitz W E, Percopo C M and Rosenberg H F 2018 FACS isolation of live mouse eosinophils at high purity via a protocol that does not target Siglec F *J. Immunol. Methods* **454** 27–31
[75] Percopo C M *et al* 2021 Detection of mouse eosinophils in tissue by flow cytometry and isolation by Fluorescence-Activated Cell Sorting (FACS) ed G M Walsh *Eosinophils. Methods in Molecular Biology* **vol. 2241** (New York: Humana) pp 49–58
[76] Reichman H, Rozenberg P and Munitz A 2017 Mouse eosinophils: identification, isolation, and functional analysis *Curr. Protoc. Immunol.* **119** 14.43.1–22
[77] Legrand F 2021 Eosinophil purification from peripheral blood of rhesus monkeys *Methods Mol. Biol.* **2241** 27–35
[78] Cypcar D *et al* 1996 Rat eosinophils: isolation and characterization of superoxide production *J. Leukoc. Biol.* **60** 101–5

[79] James S L, Leid R W Jr and Sher A 1979 Purification of rodent eosinophils on discontinuous metrizamide gradients *J. Immunol. Methods* **27** 373–82
[80] Banks K L and Greenlee A 1982 Lymphocyte subpopulations of the goat: isolation and identification *Am. J. Vet. Res.* **43** 314–7
[81] Pollack V A, Brandhorst J S and Hanna M G J 1981 Separation of guinea pig peripheral blood lymphocytes by discontinuous density gradient centrifugation using Ficoll-metrizoate *J. Immunol. Methods* **41** 29–41
[82] Banks K L and Greenlee A 1981 Isolation and identification of equine lymphocytes and monocytes *Am. J. Vet. Res.* **42** 1651–54
[83] Lim J F, Berger H and Su I H 2016 Isolation and activation of murine lymphocytes *J. Vis. Exp.* **30** 54596
[84] Qiu Z and Sheridan B S 2018 Isolating lymphocytes from the mouse small intestinal immune system *J. Vis. Exp.* **132** 57281
[85] Polakova A *et al* 2023 Isolation of lymphocytes from human skin and murine tissues: a rapid and epitope—preserving approach *JID Innov.* **3** 100155
[86] Solano-Aguilar G I *et al* 2000 Isolation and purification of lymphocyte subsets from gut-associated lymphoid tissue in neonatal swine *J. Immunol. Methods* **241** 185–99
[87] Parkes A B and Bradley D M 1974 Isolation and fractionation of porcine peripheral lymphocytes *Biochim. Biophys. Acta (BBA)—Gen. Sub.* **362** 527–33
[88] Hewitt C W *et al* 1980 A simple method for the isolation of platelet-free lymphocyte suspensions from rat whole blood *J. Immunol. Methods* **36** 227–34
[89] Lee J *et al* 2009 Improved isolation methods for mucosal leukocytes from small and large intestines in rats *Biosci., Biotechnol., Biochem.* **73** 1732–40
[90] Lee J S *et al* 2021 Single-cell transcriptome of bronchoalveolar lavage fluid reveals sequential change of macrophages during SARS-CoV-2 infection in ferrets *Nat. Commun.* **12** 4567
[91] Knowles M and Hughes D A 1970 A technique for rapid isolation of macrophages from guinea-pig peritoneal exudates *J. Clin. Pathol.* **23** 824–5
[92] Winter H S *et al* 1983 Isolation and characterization of resident macrophages from guinea pig and human intestine *Gastroenterology* **85** 358–63
[93] Kobzik L *et al* 1988 Isolation and antigenic identification of hamster lung interstitial macrophages *Am. Rev. Respir. Dis.* **138** 908–14
[94] Werners A H *et al* 2004 Generation and characterization of an equine macrophage cell line (e-CAS cells) derived from equine bone marrow cells *Vet. Immunol. Immunopathol.* **97** 65–76
[95] Meli V S *et al* 2021 Isolation and characterization of porcine macrophages and their inflammatory and fusion responses in different stiffness environments *Biomater. Sci.* **9** 7851–61
[96] Jin X *et al* 2022 Isolation of monocyte-macrophage lineage cells from rat bones by secondary adherence method *J. Vis. Exp.* **185** e64053
[97] Liu Y *et al* 2018 Isolation and characterization of ovine monocyte-derived macrophages from peripheral blood *Vet. Immunol. Immunopathol.* **205** 83–92
[98] Liggitt H D 1983 Characterization of short- and long-term cultured goat peripheral blood monocytes *Am. J. Vet. Res.* **44** 919–24
[99] Noga S J, Normann S J and Weiner R S 1984 Methods in laboratory investigation. Isolation of guinea pig monocytes and Kurloff cells: characterization of monocyte subsets by morphology, cytochemistry, and adherence *Lab. Invest.* **51** 244–52

[100] Bruyninckx W J and Blancquaert A M 1983 Isolation of horse mononuclear cells, especially of monocytes, on Isopaque-Ficoll neutral density gradient *Vet. Immunol. Immunopathol.* **4** 493–504

[101] Francke A *et al* 2011 Generation of mature murine monocytes from heterogeneous bone marrow and description of their properties *J. Histochem. Cytochem.* **59** 813–25

[102] Houthuys E *et al* 2010 A method for the isolation and purification of mouse peripheral blood monocytes *J. Immunol. Methods* **359** 1–10

[103] Oliva-Martin M J *et al* 2015 Evaluation of a method for murine monocyte isolation by bone marrow depletion *Anal. Biochem.* **480** 42–28

[104] Nielsen M C, Andersen M N and Møller H J 2020 Monocyte isolation techniques significantly impact the phenotype of both isolated monocytes and derived macrophages *in vitro Immunology* **159** 63–74

[105] de Gruijter M *et al* 1990 Isolation of human and porcine monocytes and lymphocytes by three parameter flow sorting *Zentralbl. Veterinarmed.* A **37** 585–91

[106] Berg C *et al* 2013 Isolation of porcine monocyte population: a simple and efficient method *Vet. Res. Commun.* **37** 239–41

[107] Scriba A, Luciano L and Steiniger B 1996 High-yield purification of rat monocytes by combined density gradient and immunomagnetic separation *J. Immunol. Methods* **189** 203–16

[108] Wagner M *et al* 2014 Isolation and intravenous injection of murine bone marrow derived monocytes *J. Vis. Exp.* **94** e52347

[109] Reifenberg K, Stahl M and Lösch U 1989 Granulocyte isolation from whole blood of goat, sheep, cattle, horse, dog, pig, and man *Zentralbl. Veterinarmed.* B **36** 191–8

[110] Nakata M, Itou T and Sakai T 2007 Isolation and chemiluminescent properties of ferret (*Mustela putorius furo*) polymorphonuclear cells *J. Vet. Med. Sci.* **69** 1321–4

[111] Pycock J F, Allen W E and Morris T H 1987 Rapid, single-step isolation of equine neutrophils on a discontinuous Percoll density gradient *Res. Vet. Sci.* **42** 411–2

[112] An Y *et al* 2017 An optimized method for purification and functional evaluation of neutrophils from living mouse *J. Clin. Exp. Med.* **10** 4618–28

[113] Marchi L F *et al* 2014 Comparison of four methods for the isolation of murine blood neutrophils with respect to the release of reactive oxygen and nitrogen species and the expression of immunological receptors *Comp. Clin. Pathol.* **23** 1469–76

[114] Swamydas M *et al* 2015 Isolation of mouse neutrophils *Curr. Protoc. Immunol.* **110** 3.20.1–15

[115] Swamydas M and Lionakis M S 2013 Isolation, purification and labeling of mouse bone marrow neutrophils for functional studies and adoptive transfer experiments *J. Vis. Exp.* **77** e50586

[116] Ubags N D J and Suratt B T 2018 Isolation and characterization of mouse neutrophils *Lung Innate Immunity and Inflammation. Methods in Molecular Biology* **vol 1809** ed S Alper and W Janssen (New York: Humana Press) pp 45–57

[117] Roberts R L *et al* 1987 Purification and properties of porcine polymorphonuclear cells *J. Immunol. Methods* **103** 27–32

[118] Dodek P M, Ohgami M and Minshall D K 1988 One step isolation of porcine neutrophils using an elutriator *Clin. Invest. Med.* **11** C7

[119] He L *et al* 2022 Bone marrow is the preferred source for isolation of rat neutrophils and the subsequent acquisition of neutrophil extracellular traps *Ann. Transl. Med.* **10** 823

[120] Russo-Carbolante E *et al* 2002 Comparative study of four isolation procedures to obtain rat neutrophils *Comp. Clin. Path.* **11** 71–6

[121] Rezapour A and Majidi J 2009 An improved method of neutrophil isolation in peripheral blood of sheep *J. Anim. Vet. Adv.* **8** 11–5

IOP Publishing

The Optics of Blood
A Handbook
Alexandre Douplik

Chapter 3

Blood rheology and hemodynamics at health and pathology: aggregation, viscosity, fluid mechanics

Yasuyuki Kakihana, Yutaro Madokoro and Shuhei Niiyama

3.1 Introduction

Rheology is a field of study broadly concerned with the deformation and flow of materials, named by the American chemist E C Bingham in 1929. The term 'rheo-' originates from the Greek word 'rheos,' meaning 'to flow.' This is linked to the famous saying of the Greek philosopher Heraclitus, 'panta rei' (everything flows), where 'rei' is related to 'rheos.' With the advancement of rheology, the area of biorheology, which focuses on biological aspects, has rapidly developed. The physiological significance of blood circulation lies in the transport of substances, including oxygen, which maintains the internal environment and ensures the normal function of the body. Since William Harvey's discovery of blood circulation, blood and its circulation have continued to attract new interest from physicians, physicists, and fluid dynamics engineers. Poiseuille experimentally established the relationship between flow rate, pressure drop, and viscosity in a tube, laying the foundation for rheology and fluid dynamics [1, 2] (Poiseuille 1844). The driving force of blood circulation is the pressure generated by the heart's contraction. However, the flow of blood is significantly influenced by its fluid dynamic properties, even when subjected to the same driving pressure. The study of the fluid dynamic properties of blood and its flow behaviour is known as blood rheology or hemorheology. Recently, these issues have become subjects of various experimental, theoretical, and numerical studies. Accompanying technical and conceptual advancements (such as imaging, flow rate measurement, flowmetry, numerical methods, and microfluidics), there is ongoing integration of various foundational research studies related to model systems, clinical studies, and biomedical interests. The scope of this research spans from the cellular level to the organ level, with progress being made in analyzing the

doi:10.1088/978-0-7503-4806-5ch3

rheological properties of cells, including molecular-level analysis and the incorporation of nanotechnology.

3.2 Poiseuille's law and its physiological significance

Poiseuille's law is a fundamental principle for understanding the flow of blood within blood vessels. It states that when a fluid flows through a rigid cylindrical tube at a flow rate Q, there is a relationship between the pressure difference ΔP at both ends of the cylinder, the radius r of the cylinder, its length l, and the viscosity η of the fluid, given by:

$$Q = [(\pi r^4)/8\eta] \cdot [\Delta P/l] \tag{3.1}$$

While it is difficult to apply this law to the entire circulatory system, it is essential for understanding the general overview of blood circulation and local blood flow conditions. Rewriting Poiseuille's law, it becomes

$$\Delta P = Q \cdot [8\eta l/(\pi r^4)] \tag{3.2}$$

indicating that blood pressure (ΔP) depends on cardiac output (Q) and peripheral resistance ($R = \eta/r^4$) [3].

Peripheral resistance is influenced by the constriction state of the blood vessels (r) and the viscosity of the blood (η) (figure 3.1). Since red blood cells (RBCs) account for about half of the total blood volume, the viscosity and flow properties of blood largely depend on the behaviour of RBCs [4]. Particularly, the behaviour of RBCs in the microcirculation is significant for maintaining bodily functions, as it dramatically affects the exchange of oxygen and carbon dioxide between tissues [5].

Arterial blood pressure is expressed as the product of cardiac output (Q) and peripheral resistance (R). Peripheral resistance (R) is directly proportional to the

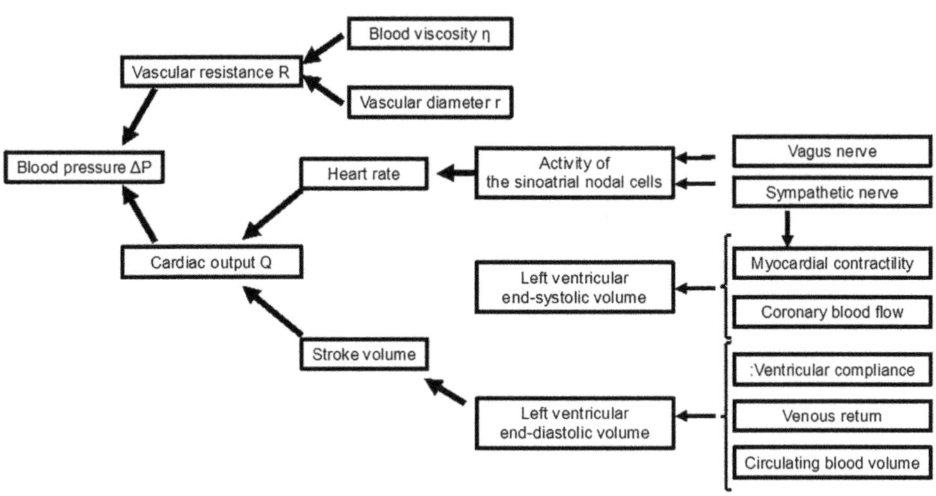

Figure 3.1. Factors governing arterial blood pressure.

viscosity of blood (η) and inversely proportional to the fourth power of the radius of the blood vessels (r) [3].

3.3 Blood flow in blood vessels

In living organisms, the flow of blood within blood vessels is a critical consideration. To understand how blood viscosity is related to blood circulation within the body, it's essential to explain the basic principles of fluid flow within blood vessels.

3.3.1 Laminar and turbulent flow

Figure 3.2 illustrates the velocity profile of the fluid in a cylindrical tube, as well as the relationship between the flow rate Q (or average velocity v(av)) and the pressure gradient $\Delta P/l$. At low flow rates, a laminar flow state is maintained, but as the flow rate increases, it transitions to a turbulent state [6].

If a Newtonian fluid flows through a cylindrical tube, forming numerous thin concentric cylindrical layers, then, similar to the case of two flat plates, each minute part of the fluid moves parallel to the axis of the tube. The layer in contact with the tube wall remains stationary, while layers closer to the tube axis move faster. These layers slide over each other without mixing. Such a flow is referred to as laminar flow [7]. In this state, if ink is carefully injected into the cylindrical tube, it flows straight and stably without disturbance. The velocity profile is parabolic, and since Poiseuille's law is applicable, the flow rate Q is proportional to the pressure gradient $\Delta P/l$. Turbulent flow, on the other hand, refers to a state where the fluid moves irregularly, not only in the direction of the tube axis but also in the perpendicular direction. In this state, even if ink is carefully injected, it quickly becomes disturbed

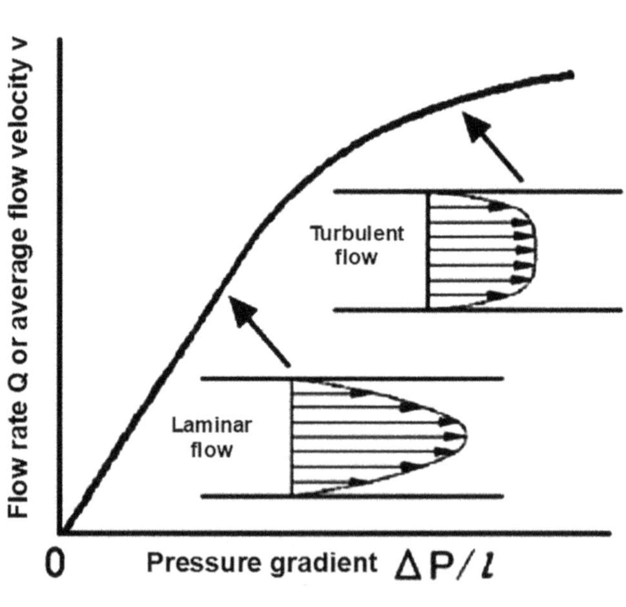

Figure 3.2. Laminar and turbulent flow in a cylindrical tube.

Table 3.1. Typical values of flow parameters in different levels of the vascular network [9]. John Wiley & Sons © 2020.

	Diameter (mm)	Average velocity (mm s^{-1})	Reynolds, Re	Womersley α	Wall shear rate (1 s^{-1})
Aorta	25	400	3000	17	130
Arteries	4	450	550	3	900
Arteriole	0.05	50	0.75	0.03	8000
Capillary	0.008	1	0.002	0.006	1000
Venule	0.02	2	0.01	0.01	800
Veins	5	100	150	3	160
Vena cava	30	380	3500	20	100

and spreads throughout the tube. In turbulent flow, the velocity profile near the tube center axis becomes flattened, and the velocity gradient near the tube wall is steep [8].

During the contraction phase of the heart, the pressure reaches about 120 mmHg (16 kPa) in the aorta and about 25 mmHg (3.3 kPa) in the pulmonary artery, and then drops sharply during the heart's relaxation phase. These blood flows are characterized by two key numbers: the Reynolds number, $\mathrm{Re} = \rho UD/\eta$ (where ρ is the blood density, around 1060 $\mathrm{kg\,m^{-3}}$, U is the typical flow speed, D is the vessel diameter, and η is the dynamic viscosity, about 3–4 mPa.s) and the Womersley number, $\alpha = R(\omega\rho/\eta)^{1/2}$ (where R is the vessel radius, and ω represents pulsation, around 20 rad s^{-1} for a heart rate of 60 beats per minute). In large vessels, such as arteries and veins, the flow becomes turbulent and inertial forces become significant ($\mathrm{Re} >> 1$), leading to a constant turbulent state in the large aorta, where noise can be heard during auscultation. In anemia, blood viscosity decreases, increasing Re and the tendency towards turbulence. Conversely, beyond the end of the aorta, the vessel diameter and flow speed decrease, leading to a smaller Reynolds number (Re) and a laminar flow, where viscous forces become more significant. Therefore, Poiseuille's law applies to blood circulation in the vessel region beyond the aorta. Meanwhile, the Womersley number is used to characterize pulsatile flow (flow caused by the heart's pulsation) and primarily affects large vessels ($\alpha > 10$) (table 3.1).

3.3.2 Blood viscosity

The viscosity of blood is influenced by various factors: the physicochemical properties and quantity of different cellular components, the composition and concentration of plasma constituents, the interaction between cellular and plasma components, and the physicochemical environment in which the blood is situated [10].

3.3.2.1 Newton's law of viscosity

In steady flow, if the moving velocity at a point P in a fluid is V (cm s^{-1}) and the perpendicular distance from point P to a fixed flat plate A is Y (cm), then V/Y is constant at any point in the fluid (figure 3.3). The velocity gradient of this flow is

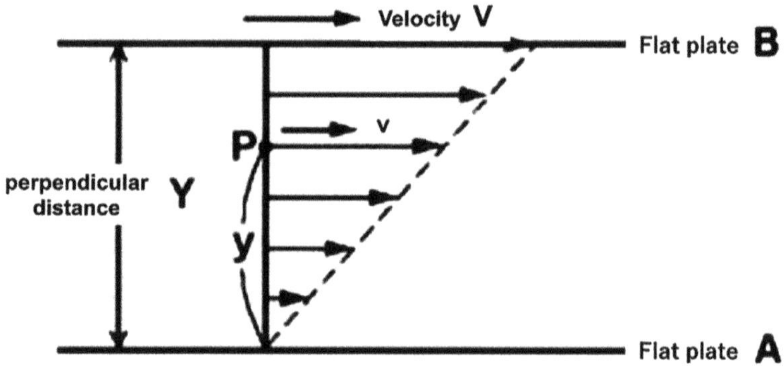

Figure 3.3. Steady flow.

referred to as the shear rate (dv/dy), which indicates how rapidly the layers of the fluid are moving relative to one another. The dimension of the shear rate is (cm s^{-1}/cm). The shear rate dv/dy is related to the force per unit area applied to the moving flat plate B, which is the shear stress (τ), measured in dyn cm^{-2} (or Pascal, Pa). If η represents the viscosity of the fluid (or the coefficient of viscosity), indicating the 'stickiness' of the fluid, then according to Newton's law of viscosity [11]:

$$\eta = \tau/(dv/dy) \tag{3.3}$$

In the above situation, the faster a thin layer of fluid near plate B tends to accelerate, the slower the thin layer of fluid near plate A, while the slower part of the fluid tries to decelerate the faster part of the fluid next to it, creating a tangential force. The magnitude of this internal friction, which attempts to minimize the velocity difference between these adjacent thin layers, corresponds to the viscosity. The dimension of viscosity is expressed in CGS units as dyn s cm^{-2}. This unit is called poise (P), after Poiseuille (1 P = 100 centipoise (cP)). When converted to the International System of Units (SI system), the pascal (1 Pa = 1 N m^{-2}; 1 N = 1 kg m s^{-2}) is used as the pressure (stress) unit, so 1 cP = 1 mPa s [12].

3.3.2.2 Apparent viscosity

In simple liquids like water, Newton's law of viscosity applies, and such fluids are called Newtonian fluids. The viscosity of a Newtonian fluid is a material constant determined only by the type of fluid at a certain constant temperature. On the other hand, fluids like blood, which do not follow Newton's law of viscosity, are called non-Newtonian fluids. In this case, the shear rate dv/dy is expressed as a function of the shear stress τ, $(dv/dy) = f(\tau)$. Therefore, in the relationship between dv/dy (s^{-1}) and τ(dyn cm^{-2}), for Newtonian fluids, it forms a straight line passing through the origin, and the reciprocal of the slope $\tau/(dv/dy)$ represents the viscosity η(mPa · s). However, for non-Newtonian fluids, it becomes a curve [13]. But even in non-Newtonian fluids, if we consider $\eta_a = \tau/(dv/dy)$, η_a is called the 'apparent viscosity.' Apparent viscosity has the same dimension as the viscosity of a Newtonian fluid. Still, it depends not only on temperature but also on dv/dy (and therefore τ), making it not a material constant (see figure 3.4).

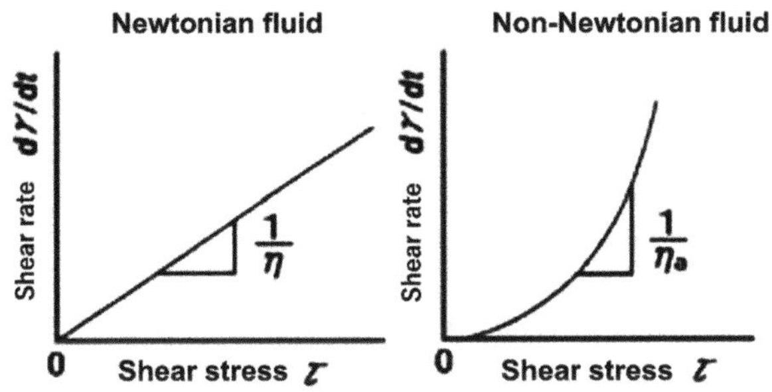

Figure 3.4. Flow curves of Newtonian and non-Newtonian fluids.

The viscosity can be determined from the slope of the line or curve that represents the relationship between the shear rate and shear stress.

3.3.2.3 Factors governing the viscosity of blood

When blood serum, a Newtonian fluid, is flowed through a capillary, the flow rate Q is directly proportional to the pressure difference ΔP, resulting in a linear relationship, regardless of the flow condition (shear rate). However, with blood, this relationship is nonlinear, and as ΔP increases, the rate of increase in Q becomes greater. This indicates that as ΔP increases in Poiseuille's equation, the viscosity μ decreases. The factors governing blood viscosity are (1) to (4), with (3) and (4) mainly showing dependence on the shear rate.

(1) RBC volume (or Ht): As the Ht increases, the viscosity of blood increases, but it increases exponentially when it exceeds about 50% [14–16].
(2) Plasma viscosity: Depends on the type and concentration of plasma proteins. Plasma is generally considered a Newtonian fluid, but it can exhibit non-Newtonian properties under certain conditions [17, 18].
(3) Erythrocyte deformation: This phenomenon occurs at high shear rates where RBCs passively deform. By deforming, they reduce the disruption in flow lines, decrease the effective hydrodynamic volume, reduce flow resistance, and thus lower blood viscosity. Therefore, when RBCs become stiffer, they disrupt flow lines more, increasing viscosity [19, 20].
(4) Erythrocyte aggregation: a condition in which erythrocytes adhere to each other due to interactions between erythrocytes and high-molecular-weight plasma proteins in the low shear rate region. When aggregation occurs, the viscosity of the blood increases because the hydrodynamic effective volume increases, greatly disturbing the streamlines and increasing flow resistance. The phenomenon of erythrocyte deformation is dependent on displacement stress, whereas erythrocyte aggregation is a phenomenon that occurs over time under slow flow conditions. In the body, blood viscosity varies significantly across different vascular regions, including arteries, capillaries, and veins, due to varying shear rates [15].

RBC aggregates are often formed pathologically (for example, due to an increase in fibrinogen concentration caused by an acute phase reaction, or due to diabetes, ischemia/reperfusion injury, etc). In the relatively large arteriole region, RBC aggregates form a pathologically flowing cord at the central axis due to the Fåhraeus effect [21]. They are eliminated at the branching points of the microvessels. In the capillary region, RBCs adhere to each other and become congested like a string of beads. This phenomenon is called sludge. Sometimes, the aggregates are fragmented, and the flow becomes heterogeneous and discontinuous due to the exclusion effect at the branching points of the blood vessels. In the venule region where the flow velocity decreases, RBC aggregates settle at the bottom of the blood vessels running horizontally due to gravity, increasing the flow resistance. Since the state of RBC aggregates depends on the time they are exposed to low shear rates, it is essential to physically improve circulation by utilizing muscle pumping actions, such as exercise [21, 22].

3.3.2.4 Pathophysiological significance of blood viscosity

Below Ht of 30%, the viscosity varies almost linearly with Ht; however, when Ht exceeds this value, the viscosity increases exponentially (figure 3.5). At the same Ht, the blood viscosity varies slightly because the hydrodynamic effective volume varies with erythrocyte morphology and erythrocyte index. In general, the relationship between Ht (%) and blood viscosity ηs is expressed as [23]:

$$\eta s/\eta p = 1/(1 - \alpha \cdot Ht/100) \tag{3.4}$$

(ηs is the total viscosity of blood, ηp is the viscosity of plasma, α is the correction factor, and Ht is the hematocrit value) and, as the Ht value increases, the overall

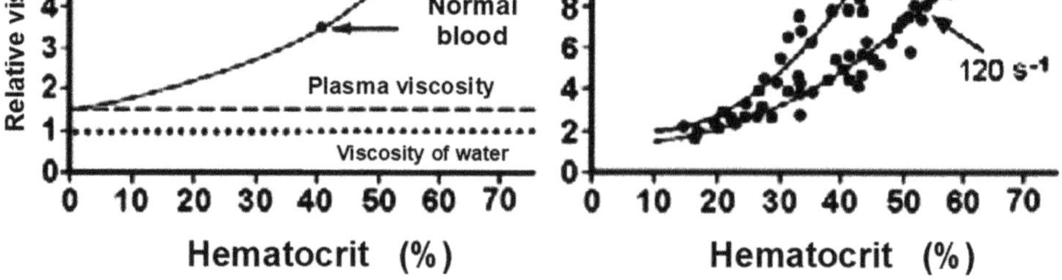

Figure 3.5. Relationship between Ht and blood viscosity. (Left) Ht dependence of blood viscosity taken from Guyton's textbook. Reprinted from [24], copyright (1991), with permission from Elsevier. The displacement velocity is not specified in this figure. (Right) Viscosity of whole blood at 12 and 120 s^{-1} measured at 37 °C using a conical plate viscometer. Reproduced with permission from [25], copyright 1962 The American Society for Clinical Investigation. Viscosity values of the 43 studies were plotted against per cent Ht at the lowest shear rate of 12 s^{-1} and the highest shear rate of 120 s^{-1}.

ratio $\eta s/\eta p$ has been shown to increase. However, this equation is a simplified model that assumes blood is a non-Newtonian fluid. In actual clinical practice, blood viscosity is influenced by numerous factors, making this equation an approximate measure.

Blood viscosity is a risk factor for cardiovascular disease. In the arterial system, as blood viscosity increases, blood pressure rises to maintain blood flow to the tissues. Conversely, in the venous system, as blood flow decreases, the displacement velocity decreases, which in turn increases blood viscosity and further reduces blood flow. These conditions, when morbidly progressive, are sometimes fatal. Circulatory disorders caused by increased blood viscosity are referred to as hyperviscosity syndrome. Epidemiological studies have shown that (i) adult men have higher Ht and therefore higher blood viscosity than adult women. (ii) Smokers have an increase in plasma viscosity and blood viscosity dependent on the amount of smoking, which returns to normal when smoking is stopped. (iii) Increased relaxation phase blood pressure is associated with increased blood viscosity. (iv) Increased plasma cholesterol is associated with increased blood viscosity [26–29].

3.4 Components involved in the rheology of blood

Blood, a dense suspension of generally deformable objects (blood cells) in plasma, is a complex fluid in terms of its composition and rheology. RBCs account for 40%–45% Ht of the total blood volume, while white blood cells (WBCs) and platelets are negligibly small in volume.

3.4.1 Rheology of erythrocytes

Erythrocytes are heterogeneous cell populations with a life span of 120 days in circulating blood, are nucleusless and have a characteristic biconcave disk with a mean diameter of 7.7 ± 0.7 μm, approximately 2.8 ± 0.5 μm at its thickest part and 1.4 ± 0.5 μm in the center. The mean erythrocyte volume (MCV), a critical hematological parameter, averages 82–98 μm^3, and its surface area (120–140 μm^2) is 30%–40% larger than that of a sphere of the same volume (85–105 μm^3) as the erythrocyte. The large surface area of erythrocytes to their volume ratio enables effective oxygen transport to tissues. The primary oxygen carrier is the high concentration of hemoglobin (32–36 $g\,dl^{-1}$) contained in the cytoplasm of the erythrocyte. Conditions causing increased Ht include relative increases due to dehydration (or decreased plasma volume) and absolute increases, as in true erythrocyte hyperplasia. Living at high altitudes, chronic hypoxia, inappropriate use of recombinant erythropoietin, smoking, etc, can cause erythrocyte hyperplasia secondarily. Even in anemias with a reduced erythrocyte mass, such as pernicious anemia and iron deficiency anemia, the viscosities differ despite having the same Ht.

3.4.1.1 The phenomenon of erythrocyte deformation

One of the physiological significances of the unique shape of erythrocytes, the biconcave disc, is that it can deform and pass through capillaries thinner than its size with minimal energy and can flow with reduced flow resistance in large vessels. When homogeneous displacement stress is applied to RBCs, they deform into elongated ellipsoid plates (bodies) and move in the direction of flow, resulting in less turbulence in the streamlines and less flow resistance. In this state, the RBC membrane rotates like the caterpillar tread of a tank. This phenomenon is called tank-tread motion. However, hard erythrocytes and erythrocytes with irregular shapes rotate almost in their original state (tumbling), increasing the effective hydrodynamic volume and disrupting the flow line, thus increasing the viscosity of the blood. This impaired erythrocyte deformation results in higher blood pressure and reduced blood flow to the tissues due to increased circulatory resistance [30].

3.4.1.2 Viscoelasticity of erythrocyte membranes

Changes in the quantitative and qualitative properties of erythrocyte membrane components, as well as changes in the state of organization, can alter the 'hardness' of the membrane. Structural changes in membrane backbone proteins have a significant effect. The erythrocyte membrane is composed of a lipid bilayer and proteins. The lipid bilayer is composed of approximately equal molar amounts of phospholipids and cholesterol. The outer layer of the bilayer is rich in choline phospholipids, and the inner layer is rich in aminophospholipids. A tetrameric structure consisting of two each of the α and β chains of spectrin among the membrane proteins constitutes the membrane backbone. This basic structure maintains a dynamic conformation that can be freely deformed by external forces [31]. Young erythrocytes immediately after neogenesis in the bone marrow are relatively large in diameter, and the medium hollow is well maintained. Aging erythrocytes, however, are less hollow and show a tendency to thicken and become more spherical. As RBCs age, (a) their surface area decreases and they become small, (b) MCHC (mean corpuscular hemoglobin concentration) increases due to impairment of the calcium pump mechanism, and (c) the viscosity of the RBC membrane increases and its deformability decreases [32]. Erythrocytes of the elderly are generally less deformable than those of the young. Abnormalities in the membrane skeleton structure, such as those caused by hereditary diseases, and abnormal interactions between the membrane skeleton and cytoplasmic components destabilize the membrane structure, impairing erythrocyte deformation. Injury to skeletal proteins by various oxidants or peroxides is also a problem. The accumulation of Ca^{2+} in erythrocytes and the resulting changes in membrane–protein interactions contribute to the reduced deformability observed in essential hypertension. Mechanical stimulation of erythrocytes or contact with heterogeneous surfaces alters membrane permeability, increasing permeability to Ca ions and decreasing deformability. In diabetes mellitus, the glycation status of hemoglobin and membrane skeletal proteins correlates well with reduced erythrocyte deformability. Erythrocyte deformability can be quantified by monitoring cell shape changes resulting from applied fluid forces, either through direct microscopic visualization or by analyzing laser-diffraction patterns generated by the deformed cells [33].

3.4.1.3 Abnormal hemoglobin in red blood cells
Several pathologies, whether congenital, infectious, or metabolic in origin, can significantly alter cytosol or membrane properties, as well as erythrocyte morphology, and consequently impact blood rheology. Sickle cell disease (SCD), which affects approximately 300 000 births per year worldwide [34], causes the production of hemoglobin S (HbS), an abnormal hemoglobin due to a genetic mutation, and is associated with stressors such as hypoxia, dehydration, cold, and infection, resulting in the characteristic stiff sickle-like shape related to the polymerization of fibrous HbS (figure 3.6). Sickle-shaped erythrocytes tend to clog as they pass through blood vessels, thereby reducing oxygen supply to tissues and organs and causing pain and dysfunction. Thalassemia (a or b), depending on the type of hemoglobin subunit affected) is another family of hereditary hemoglobinopathies [35], characterized by microcytic hemolytic anemia.

3.4.1.4 Aggregation and sedimentation phenomena in red blood cells
Increased blood viscosity due to erythrocyte aggregation is a problem in the vessels immediately after passing through the capillaries, i.e. in the region of small veins and

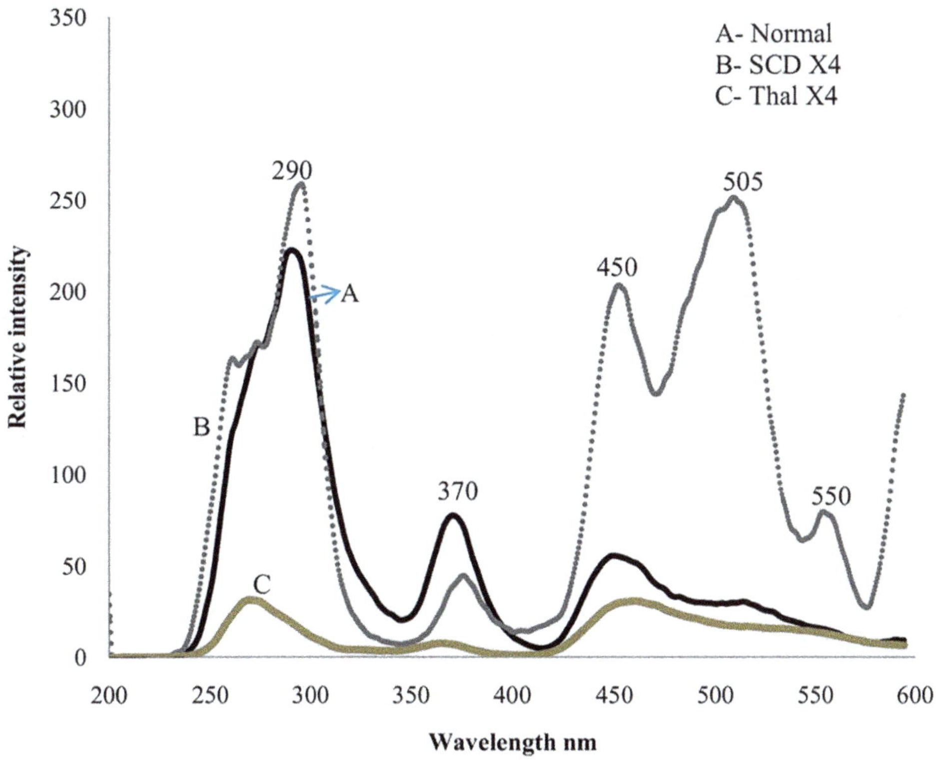

Figure 3.6. Synchronous excitation spectra (SXS), (with $\Delta\lambda = 70$ nm) of blood plasma of (a) normal, (b) SCD, (c) thalassemia (Thal). Reprinted from [56], copyright 2013, with permission from Elsevier B.V. All rights reserved. It is important to note that the intensities of all bands for SCD and Thal are significantly low. They have been multiplied by a factor of four to become noticeable.

small venules. Erythrocyte aggregation is a reversible adhesion phenomenon between erythrocytes that occurs in the presence of polymeric compounds in the low shear rate region, whereby the adherent erythrocytes fall apart when shear stress is applied. One-dimensional erythrocyte aggregates, such as a stack of coins, are particularly referred to as Renqian rouleaux [36]. When erythrocytes or branches of other coins attach to the sides of the coins, they grow into three-dimensional aggregates. Another essential feature of this phenomenon is the vicious circle in which the pathological formation of aggregates and stagnation of flow lead to an increased tendency to form aggregates. When erythrocytes form aggregates, the blood, as a fluid of suspended erythrocytes, becomes extremely unstable and prone to sedimentation. Erythrocyte aggregate formation occurs *in vivo*, primarily in smaller blood vessels, particularly within the microcirculation. These aggregates can form in capillaries and small veins and are influenced by various factors, including blood flow, the presence of specific proteins, and the overall health of the blood. In a healthy state, RBCs typically move smoothly through the blood vessels. Still, under certain conditions—like high viscosity, low shear stress, or the presence of specific proteins like fibrinogen—RBCs can start to clump together, forming aggregates. These aggregates can affect blood flow and are often observed in conditions such as inflammation, diabetes, and certain types of anemia. The mechanism of this phenomenon was first proposed by R Fåhraeus (1917) [37]. Working in the maternity ward of a hospital in Stockholm during World War I, Fåhraeus noticed that the blood of pregnant women was unstable and that the erythrocytes settled rapidly and showed that the leading cause of this was the aggregation of the erythrocytes. The Westergren method [38] was used to measure the erythrocyte sedimentation rate (ESR). As the erythrocytes begin to settle, a layer of plasma increases in the upper part of the settling tube and a layer of settling erythrocytes separates in the lower part. During the settling process of erythrocyte aggregates, a downward movement of the aggregates and an upward flow of plasma replacing the descending aggregates are observed; A E Boycott (1920) discovered a phenomenon whereby the settling of erythrocytes becomes faster when the settling tube is tilted. This phenomenon is due to an upward flow of plasma along the upper tube wall of the inclined tube, causing the aggregates formed along the lower tube wall to settle faster, a phenomenon known as the Boycott effect. Careful attention should be paid when measuring ESR. RBC aggregation, including the Boycott effect, can indeed alter the optical properties of blood. Various optical methods, such as laser Doppler flowmetry, dynamic light scattering, and spectrophotometry, can be employed to assess these changes and provide valuable information about blood flow and aggregation dynamics [39].

3.4.1.5 Factors affecting the aggregation of red blood cells

Various physicochemical conditions influence RBC aggregation. (1) As the shear rate (blood flow velocity) increases, the formed aggregates disperse. (2) RBC deformability is an essential cellular property for aggregation [40]. RBC flattening (alkaline pH, high osmotic pressure) promotes the formation of aggregates, while spherization (acidic pH, low osmotic pressure, low temperature) inhibits it. However, exposure to temperatures below 15 °C significantly promotes aggregation. (3) Even in conditions that form three-dimensional aggregates on the ground, only rouleaux are formed under zero-gravity conditions. Conversely, increased hydrostatic pressure promotes the aggregation of RBCs. In smokers, factors such as increased fibrinogen levels promote aggregation compared to non-smokers. A high-fat diet can increase plasma triglyceride levels within 2–3 h, which in turn stimulates the aggregation of RBCs.

For characterizing aggregation at the suspension scale and its structural impacts, techniques such as image analysis [41, 42], aggregometry and ektacytometry [43, 44], light scattering [45], and acoustic backscatter [46, 47] are employed. These techniques enable the establishment of a correlation between aggregate size statistics and rheology; however, more localized techniques are also used. These include the study of aggregation and disaggregation mechanisms at the microscopic scale, the derivation of information on fundamental mechanisms, and the characterization of interaction forces at the cellular scale. Techniques such as micropipette aspiration [48] and AFM (atomic force microscopy) measurements are employed, which determine the interaction energy between two RBCs in double aggregation experiments [49]. Currently, the measurement of interaction forces in aggregation or disaggregation situations is being performed using multiple optical tweezers, allowing for better control of the interaction surfaces [50].

3.4.1.6 Microcirculation of red blood cells

In blood vessels, RBCs near the vessel wall move towards the center of the vessel due to differences in shear rate, undergoing a rotational 'tank-tread' motion. This phenomenon is known as axial accumulation of RBCs. As a result, a thin layer of plasma, several micrometres thick, where only plasma flows, forms along the slower-moving vessel wall. This layer is referred to as the plasma (cell-free) layer. This plasma layer reduces friction (circulatory resistance) between RBCs and the endothelial cells lining the blood vessels, thus facilitating blood flow.

When the Ht decreases, the collision between RBCs reduces, promoting axial accumulation and thickening the plasma layer, which in turn lowers the flow resistance. If the deformability of RBCs decreases, their membranes' rotational movement becomes less likely, hindering axial accumulation. Additionally, the RBCs collide with each other and fail to adapt to the flow, resulting in a poor formation of the plasma layer and increased flow resistance. When RBC aggregation is promoted, the axial accumulation of RBCs in the central part of the vessel accelerates, thickening the plasma layer. This increase in the plasma layer at least locally alleviates the increase in circulatory resistance. In microvessels with diameters less than 10 μm, such as capillaries, the flow of RBCs becomes either laminar or single-layered, making the formation of the plasma layer independent of Ht. Thus, the deformability of RBCs becomes more significant—the plasma layer forms between the deforming RBCs and the vessel wall. As the flow rate increases, RBC deformation is promoted, and the plasma layer thickens. Therefore, when RBC deformability decreases, the plasma layer becomes thinner, increasing flow resistance.

On the other hand, the endothelial cells lining blood vessels have a layer of glycoproteins (glycocalyx) about 0.5 μm thick on their surface. It is said that this increases the flow resistance about threefold compared to smooth vessels. However, the glycocalyx also plays a role in reducing flow resistance by preventing direct contact between RBCs and the vessel wall. The glycocalyx layer not only protects RBCs from external forces but also plays a crucial role in cell interactions, protection, substance transport, and cellular response. Damage or reduction of the glycocalyx in blood vessels can lead to disturbances in blood flow and the development of pathological conditions [51]. Therefore, the flow resistance of blood within microvessels is complexly constituted, influenced not only by the flow behaviour of RBCs but also by the intricate structure of the endothelial lining.

As a result of the axial concentration phenomenon of RBCs, the cells flowing near the center of the vessel move faster compared to the plasma flowing near the vessel wall [23]. This difference in flow rate between the RBCs and plasma results in a lower Ht inside microvessels compared to larger vessels (figure 3.7, left). This phenomenon is known as the Fåhraeus effect [52]. As shown in figure 3.7 (left), if we assume that HT is the Ht in the blood flowing through a thin tube and HD is the Ht in the blood after it is discharged from the thin tube, in the Fåhraeus effect, HT (tube Ht) is lower than HD (discharge Ht), so the HT/HD ratio is HT $<$ HD (or HT/HD $<$ 1). This occurs because RBCs concentrate in the middle of the tube, while the area near the vessel wall is filled with plasma that has fewer RBCs, making the proportion of RBCs in the tube appear lower than it is. This phenomenon is especially pronounced in vessels with small diameters, which enhances the fluidity of blood and thereby optimizes oxygen supply to tissues. The effect starts in microvessels with an inner diameter of less than 300 μm and is most pronounced in diameters of 10–20 μm.

On the other hand, the Ht (HD) of blood discharged from a thin tube can be considered as the Ht of venous blood. For example, even if the same amount of RBCs and plasma enter the thin tube, the amount of RBCs discharged will be greater than the amount of plasma because the RBCs pass through the thin tube faster than the plasma. In other words, the Fåhraeus effect causes the venous Ht to be higher than the body Ht. Factors influencing the Fåhraeus effect are the same as those affecting the formation of the plasma layer; as the diameter decreases, HT/HD

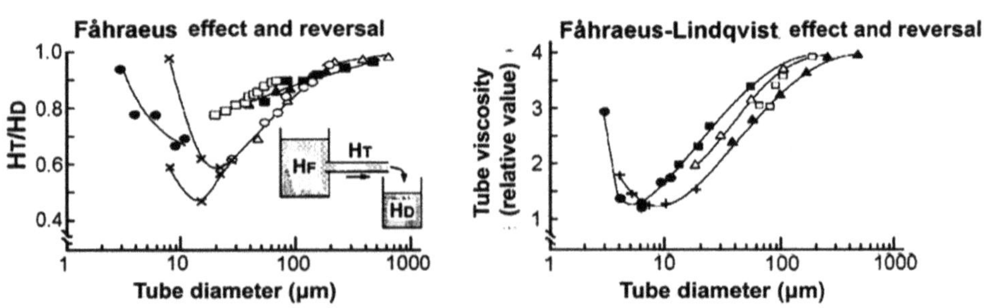

Figure 3.7. The Fåhraeus effect (left) and the Fåhraeus–Lindqvist effect (right), Along with the reversal phenomena [58] HF (feeding Ht): Ht in the storage tank of blood (RBC suspension); HT (tube Ht): Ht of blood flowing inside a tube; HD (discharge Ht): Ht after exiting the tube.

decreases, but it increases when the flow rate decreases [53]. When the vessel diameter is less than 15–20 μm, the flow of RBCs changes to a two-layer or single-layer flow, eliminating the difference in flow rate between RBCs and plasma. This increases the proportion of RBCs in the vessel, thereby increasing the Ht again. This phenomenon is called the reversal of the Fåhraeus effect. When the diameter becomes less than 6 μm, the deformation of RBCs reaches its maximum, and HT/HD becomes independent of the flow rate or Ht [54].

As the Ht in microvessels decreases due to the Fåhraeus effect, the blood viscosity also decreases (figure 3.7, right). This phenomenon is known as the Fåhraeus–Lindqvist effect [55]. The reversal of the Fåhraeus effect occurs in microvessels with diameters of approximately 20 μm figure 3.7, right. Still, since RBCs exhibit complex behaviour in microvessels, the Fåhraeus–Lindqvist effect reverses in vessels with diameters of 5–7 μm or less, where the viscosity increases again (figure 3.7, right).

In the microvascular network, vessels branch repeatedly, and RBCs and plasma are distributed into each branching vessel. Even if the diameter of these branches is the same, RBCs tend to flow into the faster-flowing microvessels. As a result, the Ht becomes higher on the side of the faster-flowing vessels, while it becomes even lower on the side of the slower-flowing vessels. This phenomenon is known as the network Fåhraeus effect [59]. This effect becomes more pronounced as blood moves towards the periphery while passing through the branching points. This phenomenon is closely related to the deformability of RBCs. As the flow rate increases, the deformation of RBCs is promoted, weakening their screening. Conversely, when the flow rate decreases, RBCs are more easily screened [60].

3.4.1.7 Red blood cell screening and plasma separation

As the diameter of capillaries decreases to approximately 30 μm or smaller, RBCs begin to have difficulty entering these narrow tubes smoothly. This phenomenon is known as RBC exclusion, also referred to as cell screening. It occurs at sites where thick microvessels branch into thinner ones. As shown in figure 3.7 (left), if we assume that HF is the Ht in the storage tank of blood (RBC suspension), HT is the Ht in the blood flowing through a thin tube, and HD is the Ht in the blood after it is discharged from the thin tube, it is necessary to distinguish between the Fåhraeus effect (HT $<$ HD) and the phenomenon of RBC screening (HD $<$ HF). Due to the RBC screening effect, the distribution of RBCs and plasma in the microvascular network becomes even more heterogeneous. Since plasma flows along the vessel walls, at the branching points of the tubes, plasma preferentially flows into the smaller branches. This phenomenon is known as plasma skimming [61]. Especially when the diameter of the vessel approaches the size of RBCs, the cells are more likely to be excluded from the plasma flow. However, these phenomena are not fixed in the living body's microvascular network. Changes in the flow state due to vasomotion, or alterations in the spatial relationships of vessels resulting from movements of surrounding tissues, can cause RBCs to flow through vessels that previously did not carry them. From the perspective of oxygen supply to tissues, vessels with flowing RBCs are called functional capillaries, while those carrying only plasma are referred to as non-functional capillaries [62].

3.4.1.8 Red blood cell rheology and oxygen transport

The rheological properties of RBCs are closely related to the transfer of oxygen from RBCs to tissues during the microcirculatory process [63].

3.4.1.8.1 Regulation of blood flow to tissues

The circulation of RBCs in the microvascular network of tissues is well-regulated according to the state of tissue metabolic activity. It adapts efficiently to changes in the internal environment. For example, (1) if the oxygen partial pressure decreases, erythropoietin is secreted from the kidneys to stimulate RBC production in the bone marrow [64]. (2) An increase in stress on the vascular walls or a decrease in oxygen partial pressure causes vasodilation, increasing blood flow. (3) When RBCs are mechanically stimulated or their oxygen content decreases, they release ATP, which promotes NO synthesis in endothelial cells, leading to vasodilation and increased blood flow [65]. Conversely, in conditions such as advanced atheromatous arteriosclerosis in diabetes, synergistic adverse effects on blood circulation can occur due to changes in the elasticity of the vessel walls, decreased deformability of RBCs, and increased formation of RBC aggregates [66].

3.4.1.8.2 Red blood cell volume and oxygen transport to tissues

The amount of oxygen transported to tissues per unit time ($Q(O_2)$) can be expressed as the product of blood flow (Q) and the oxygen content in arterial blood (CaO_2), so:

$$Q(O_2) = Ca\ O_2 \times Q \tag{3.5}$$

In this equation, CaO_2 is proportional to the Ht (or RBC volume). In the formula for CaO_2 used in clinical practice, the oxygen-binding capacity of hemoglobin is 1.34 ml l^{-1} g^{-1} of Hb; however, this is not entirely accurate. This is because there are metHb and HbCO in our blood that cannot bind oxygen. One mole of hemoglobin will bind four moles of oxygen; the weight of Hb is 64,458.5g/mol^{-1}, and thus 1/64 458.5th of Hb (i.e., 1 g). If we assume that oxygen is an ideal gas, one mole of it will occupy 22.4 l of volume at standard temperature and pressure; thus, the ideal oxygen-binding capacity of hemoglobin must be $(4 \times 22.4) \div 64\,458.5$, or around 1.39 ml g^{-1}. The amount of oxygen dissolved in blood is 0.0031 ml per 1 mmHg, so CaO_2 is expressed as [67]:

$$CaO_2\ (ml/dl) = 1.39 \times SaO_2 \times Hb + 0.0031 \times PaO_2 \tag{3.6}$$

However, considering that metHb and HbCO levels cannot be measured directly in clinical practice in many cases, it may be better to calculate the oxygen-binding capacity of hemoglobin as 1.34 ml g^{-1} of Hb [68]).

Meanwhile, Q is inversely proportional to blood viscosity (η) according to Poiseuille's law, so $Q(O_2)$ is expressed as:

$$Q(O_2) = k \times Ht \times (1/\eta) \tag{3.7}$$

(where k is a constant).

This equation shows that as Ht increases, $Q(O_2)$ does not necessarily increase because η increases. In normal blood, oxygen transport is maximized at an Ht of

30%–50%, but even with a normal Ht, $Q(O_2)$ decreases if there is a pathological decrease in erythrocyte deformability or an increase in blood viscosity due to accelerated erythrocyte aggregation. Therefore, blood transfusions and RBC volume expansion for anemia can also be counterproductive if not performed appropriately [30, 69].

3.4.1.8.3 Red blood cell dynamics

Numerous theoretical approaches have been proposed for modelling blood cells, extending to models of elastic capsules [70] and vesicles [71, 72]. These models, in their simpler versions (two-dimensional, incompressible fluid with bending elasticity for vesicles and extensional and shear elasticity for quasi-two-dimensional solids), are capable of qualitatively describing the behaviour of RBCs. However, recent models tend to incorporate as many mechanical parameters as possible (extensibility, bending and shear elasticity, membrane viscosity). Much of the recent research has focused on the dynamics of simple shear in RBCs [73–76]. Experimentally, numerous studies have been conducted to confirm or identify various dynamic regimes [77, 78]. These are performed to create a diagram of the transitions between different motions, such as tank-treading, tumbling, rolling, and other more complex motions that combine rotations, oscillations, or deformations.

3.4.2 White blood cell rheology

In their inactive state, WBCs are spherical and have fine wrinkled surfaces. The diameter of WBCs (9–12 μm) is larger than that of RBCs. Among WBCs, lymphocytes (approximately 25% of the total) are smaller than granulocytes (approximately 70%), which in turn are smaller than monocytes (approximately 5%). While WBCs have a minimal impact on blood viscosity when their numbers are normal, an increase in WBC count (greater than 100 000 μl^{-1}) raises blood viscosity, leading to circulatory disturbances due to adherence to vessel walls. This condition is known as hyperleukocytic syndrome (HLS). HLS WBCs exhibit significantly reduced deformability compared to normal WBCs, which contributes to circulatory disturbances. Lymphocytes and monocytes, which have a larger nucleus-to-cytoplasm volume ratio compared to granulocytes, exhibit reduced deformability and higher viscosity due to restricted cytoplasmic fluidity. Intracellular and extracellular Ca^{2+} concentrations influence the deformability of granulocytes; reducing the physiological extracellular free Ca^{2+} concentration (1.25 mM) to approximately 0.1 mM improves deformability by lowering the intracellular Ca^{2+} concentration [79].

3.4.2.1 Microcirculation of white blood cells

WBCs slowly flowing along the vessel walls (WBC rolling) eventually stop and adhere to the surface of endothelial cells. Such WBCs resist blood flow. Furthermore, when physical or chemical stimuli activate WBCs, the phenomena of rolling and adherence on the surface of endothelial cells are enhanced, significantly affecting local blood circulation. Such adhesion of WBCs primarily occurs in the post-capillary venule region and involves interactions between WBC adhesion molecules and receptors on endothelial cells [80]. In atherosclerosis, diabetes, and inflammatory diseases, the adhesion molecule VCAM-1 (vascular cell adhesion molecule-1) is abnormally expressed on endothelial cells. In conditions such as rheumatoid arthritis and infections, the intercellular soluble adhesion molecule ICAM-1 (intercellular adhesion molecule-1) or VCAM is increased. When WBCs are activated, the release of free radicals and proteolytic enzymes can impair the deformability of RBCs and damage endothelial cells, thereby affecting blood microcirculation in a complex manner.

3.4.3 Platelet rheology

Platelets are the smallest cellular components, with a diameter of 2–3 μm. Inside platelets, there are complex organelles and contractile proteins, and when activated by stimulation, their mechanical properties change.

Platelets are smaller and have a more complex internal structure than RBCs. Additionally, when platelets are activated by stimulation, the state of the microtubule coils on the inner surface of the platelet membrane changes, promoting membrane extension or, conversely, exhibiting resistance, thereby displaying complex behaviour [81].

3.4.3.1 Platelet microcirculation

Since platelets are extremely small compared to RBCs, they do not cause significant rheological problems as long as they flow normally. A characteristic phenomenon in the flow of platelets within capillaries is that larger RBCs flow near the central axis of the vessel due to axial concentration. In contrast, smaller platelets flow along the vessel walls. Observing the distribution of platelets in arterioles, the number of platelets near the wall is the highest, nearly twice that in the central axis region. Such a flow of platelets is incredibly purposeful, maximizing their characteristic of adhering immediately to the vessel wall when it is damaged.

Regarding the function of platelets, issues related to bleeding and thrombosis arise. Bleeding and thrombosis arise from the disturbance of the complex interaction balance of three fundamental elements: blood, vessels, and blood flow, known as Virchow's triad. When a vessel is damaged, platelets adhere to the subendothelial tissue surface to form a thrombus, which stops the bleeding. However, in capillaries, the formed thrombi can obstruct blood flow and sometimes occlude the vessel [82].

3.4.3.2 Arterial and venous thrombosis

In venous thrombosis, which forms in low shear rate areas (low shear aggregation), von Willebrand factor (vWF) and fibrinogen bridge between the damaged vessel wall and platelets. Venous thrombi are relatively platelet-poor red thrombi, and as Ht increases, ADP is released from RBCs as an aggregating agent, chemically promoting thrombus formation. Therefore, anticoagulants (e.g., warfarin, heparin) are used in the treatment of fibrin-dependent thrombi, such as deep vein thrombosis (DVT). On the other hand, in arterial thrombosis, which forms in high-shear-rate areas (high-shear aggregation), vWF primarily provides a stable bridge between platelets and the subendothelial tissue. Arterial thrombi are white thrombi formed solely from platelets, and as Ht increases, physical shear stress increases, promoting thrombus formation. Therefore, in cases of arterial thrombosis in the heart or brain, which are primarily caused by platelet aggregation, antiplatelet drugs (e.g., aspirin, clopidogrel) are used rather than anticoagulants for treating conditions such as stroke or myocardial infarction [83].

3.4.3.3 Platelet aggregation under high shear stress

With arterial thrombus formation, the relationship between shear stress and platelet aggregation is essential. When shear stress (= plasma viscosity × shear rate) is applied [83] to platelet-rich plasma of healthy individuals, platelet aggregation begins at around 10–20 dynes cm^{-2}. Further increasing the shear stress initially dissociates the platelet aggregates, but at approximately 90–100 dyn cm^{-2}, extremely dense aggregates are formed. Shear stress plays a crucial role in signalling for platelet aggregation, involving calcium ions. When shear stress is applied, the intraplatelet calcium ions increase approximately tenfold, coinciding with platelet aggregation. When extracellular calcium ions are chelated and removed by EDTA, the increase in intraplatelet calcium ions mediated by vWF and aggregation is completely suppressed [84].

In atherosclerosis, atherosclerotic lesions (especially at sites of plaque rupture) emit signals similar to those of vessel injury, promoting platelet adhesion and aggregation, and pathologically narrowing vessels. However, as the vessel narrows, the wall shear rate at the stenotic site further increases, accelerating thrombus formation. Clinically, treatments are performed to stop bleeding or dissolve formed thrombi. Conversely, diseases in which platelet aggregation is weakened due to high shear stress include platelet disorders with abnormalities in membrane proteins, such as thrombasthenia and Bernard–Soulier syndrome, as well as von Willebrand disease [85].

3.4.4 Rheology of plasma components

Plasma proteins in blood plasma, such as albumin (4–5 g dl^{-1}), various globulins (3–6 g dl^{-1}), fibrinogen (0.2–0.4 g dl^{-1}), as well as glucose and various lipids (triglycerides, cholesterol, fatty acids, etc), are closely related to the rheology of blood. A pathological increase in high-molecular-weight plasma proteins leads to significantly increased plasma viscosity, a condition known as plasma hyperviscosity syndrome. Lipids in plasma are closely related to the development of arterial vascular lesions. An increase in plasma triglycerides, even if temporary, raises plasma viscosity and promotes RBC aggregation. Generally, as the molecular weight and the length of fibrous molecules increase, plasma viscosity rises, making RBC aggregation more likely. The tendency to form aggregates is in the order of IgM (pentamer) > IgA (dimer) > IgG (monomer), but fibrinogen forms aggregates more readily than IgG, and an increase in fibrinogen is known as a risk factor for cardiovascular diseases. Albumin inhibits aggregate formation, making the albumin/globulin (A/G) ratio an important indicator in considering RBC aggregation.

Pathological proteins, such as those found in myeloma proteins in multiple myeloma and macroglobulin in Waldenström's macroglobulinemia, cause a significant increase in plasma viscosity. Increased plasma viscosity can lead to symptoms of circulatory disorders, including bleeding, retinopathy, and neurological symptoms such as headaches, dizziness, and convulsions. Symptoms improve when pathological proteins are removed by plasma pheresis, reducing plasma viscosity [86].

3.5 Conclusion

The rheological properties of blood, including its viscosity and the intravascular flow behaviour of individual blood components, greatly influence blood circulation, which in turn is directly linked to organ dysfunction, especially concerning the supply of oxygen to organs. To understand the essence of hypoxia caused by circulatory disorders, it is necessary to comprehensively examine blood components, blood viscosity, blood flow, the state of the vascular system, the status of oxygen release, and physiological regulatory mechanisms. The study of blood rheology, an ancient field of research, remains a new discipline due to its physiological importance and its foundational relevance to all areas of clinical medicine.

References

[1] Beris A N and Giacomin A J 2014 Everything flows *Appl. Rheol.* **24** 52918

[2] Pfitzner J 1976 Poiseuille and his law *Anaesthesia* **31** 273–5

[3] Delong C and Sharma S 2025 *Physiology, Peripheral Vascular Resistance* (Treasure Island (FL): StatPearls Publishing)

[4] Baskurt O K and Meiselman H J 2024 Blood rheology and hemodynamics *Semin. Thromb. Hemost.* **50** 902–15

[5] Kwon O, Krishnamoorthy M, Cho Y I, Sankovic J M and Banerjee R K 2008 Effect of blood viscosity on oxygen transport in residual stenosed artery following angioplasty *J. Biomech. Eng.* **130** 011003

[6] Stigler J 2014 Analytical velocity profile. in tube for laminar and turbulent flow *Eng. Mech.* **21** 371–9

[7] Lowe G D O and Barbenel J C 1988 *Plasma and Blood Viscosity Clinical Blood Rheology* **Vol 1** ed G D O Lowe (Boca Raton, FL: CRC Press) pp 11–44

[8] Gurovich A N and Braith R W 2013 Enhanced external counterpulsation creates acute blood flow patterns responsible for improved flow-mediated dilation in humans *Hypertens. Res.* **36** 297–305

[9] Podgorski T 2022 *Hemodynamics and Hemorheology: Biological Flow in Large Vessels* ed V Deplano, J M Fullana and C Verdier (ISTE: WILEY) pp 1–41

[10] Alexy T, Detterich J, Connes P, Toth K, Nader E, Kenyeres P, Arriola-Montenegro J, Ulker P and Simmonds M J 2022 Physical properties of blood and their relationship to clinical conditions *Front. Physiol.* **13** 906768

[11] Gooch J W 2011 Viscosity coefficient ed J W Gooch *Encyclopedic Dictionary of Polymers* (New York: Springer)

[12] Roux E, Bougaran P, Dufourcq P and Couffinhal T 2020 Fluid shear stress sensing by the endothelial layer *Front. Physiol.* **11** 861

[13] Martínez-Padilla L P 2023 Rheology of liquid foods under shear flow conditions: recently used models *J. Texture Stud.* **55** e12802

[14] Rampling M W 1988 *Red Cell Aggregation and Yield Stress: Clinical Blood Rheology* ed G D O Lowe (Boca Raton, FL: CRC Press) pp 11–44

[15] Baskurt O K and Meiselman H J 2003 Blood rheology and hemodynamics *Semin. Thromb. Hemost.* **29** 435–50

[16] Lenz C, Rebel A, Waschke K F, Koehler R C and Frietsch T 2008 Blood viscosity modulates tissue perfusion: sometimes and somewhere *Transfus. Altern. Transfus. Med.* **9** 265–72

[17] Somer T and Meiselman H J 1993 Disorders of blood viscosity *Ann. Med.* **25** 31–9

[18] Késmárky G, Kenyeres P, Rábai M and Tóth K 2008 Plasma viscosity: a forgotten variable *Clin. Hemorheol. Microcirc.* **39** 243–6

[19] Evans E A and La Celle P L 1975 Intrinsic material properties of the erythrocyte membrane indicated by mechanical analysis of deformation *Blood* **45** 29–43

[20] Mohandas N and Shohet S B 1981 The role of membrane-associated enzymes in regulation of erythrocyte shape and deformability *Clin. Haematol.* **10** 223–37

[21] Popel A S and Johnson P C 2005 Microcirculation and hemorheology *Annu. Rev. Fluid Mech.* **37** 43–69

[22] Tschakovsky M E and Sheriff D D 2004 Immediate exercise hyperemia: contributions of the muscle pump vs. rapid vasodilation *J. Appl. Physiol.* **97** 739–47

[23] Pries A, Neuhaus D and Gaehtgens P 1992 Blood viscosity in tube flow: Dependence on diameter and hematocrit *Am. J. Physiol.* **263** H1770–8

[24] Guyton A C 1991 *Guyton's Textbook: Textbook of Medical Physiology* 8th edn ed M J Wonsiewicz and R Hallowell (Philadelphia, PA: Saunders) p 157

[25] Wells R E J and Merrill E W 1962 Influence of flow properties of blood upon viscosity-hematocrit relationships *J. Clin. Invest.* **41** 1591–8

[26] Grau M, Cremer J M, Schmeichel S, Kunkel M and Bloch W 2018 Comparisons of blood parameters, red blood cell deformability and circulating nitric oxide between males and females considering hormonal contraception: a longitudinal gender study *Front. Physiol.* **9** 1835

[27] Ilkkilic K, Karadogan D, Telatar T G, Cure O and Klisic A 2025 Effect of smoking and smoking cessation on hematological parameters in polycythemic patients *Open Med.* **20** 20251181

[28] Tripolino C, Gnasso A, Carallo C *et al* 2016 Hemorheological profiles of subjects with prehypertension *Hypertens. Res.* **39** 519–23

[29] Irace C, Carallo C, Scavelli F *et al* 2014 Influence of blood lipids on plasma and blood viscosity *Clin. Hemorheol. Microcirc.* **57** 267–74

[30] Nader E *et al* 2019 Blood rheology: key parameters, impact on blood flow, role in sickle cell disease and effects of exercise *Front. Physiol.* **10** 1329

[31] Evans E and Fung Y C 1972 Improved measurements of the erythrocyte geometry *Microvasc. Res.* **4** 335–47

[32] Rendell M, Luu T, Quinlan E, Knox S, Fox M, Kelly S and Kahler K 1992 Red cell filterability determined using the cell transit time analyzer (CTTA): effects of ATP depletion and changes in calcium concentration *Biochim. Biophys. Acta* **1133** 293–300

[33] Hardeman M R, Goedhart P T, Dobbe J G G and Lettinga K P 1994 Laser assisted optical rotational cell analyzer (LORCA): a new instrument for measurement of various structural hemorheological parameters *Clin. Hemorheol. Microcirc.* **14** 605–18

[34] Rees D C, Williams T N and Gladwin M T 2010 Sickle-cell disease *Lancet* **376** 2018–31
[35] Higgs D R, Engel J D and Stamatoyannopoulos G 2012 Thalassaemia *Lancet* **379** 373–83
[36] Eisenberg R 2009 Thickening of small bowel folds *AJR Am. J. Roentgenol.* **193** W1–6
[37] Fåhraeus R 1921 The suspension stability of the blood *Phys. Rev.* **IX** 241
[38] Westergren A 1921 Studies of the suspension stability of the blood in pulmonary tuberculosis *Acta Med. Scand.* **54** 247–82
[39] Semenov A, Lugovtsov A, Ermolinskiy P, Lee K and Priezzhev A 2022 Problems of red blood cell aggregation and deformation assessed by laser tweezers, diffuse light scattering and laser diffractometry *Photonics* **9** 238
[40] Baskurt O K and Meiselman H J 1997 Cellular determinants of low-shear blood viscosity *Biorheology* **34** 235–47
[41] Jan K M and Chien S 1973 Role of surface electric charge in red blood cell interactions *J. Gen. Physiol.* **61** 638–54
[42] Chen S, Gavish B, Zhang S, Mahler Y and Yedgar S 1995 Monitoring of erythrocyte aggregate morphology under flow by computerized image analysis *Biorheology* **32** 487–96
[43] Başkurt O K and Mat F 2000 Importance of measurement temperature in detecting the alterations of red blood cell aggregation and deformability studied by ektacytometry: a study on experimental sepsis in rats *Clin. Hemorheol. Microcirc.* **23** 43–9
[44] Baskurt O K, Uyuklu M, Ulker P, Cengiz M, Nemeth N, Alexy T, Shin S, Hardeman M R and Meiselman H J 2009 Comparison of three instruments for measuring red blood cell aggregation *Clin. Hemorheol. Microcirc.* **43** 283–98
[45] Shin S, Ku Y, Park M S and Suh J S 2005 Slit-flow ektacytometry: laser diffraction in a slit rheometer *Cytometry B Clin. Cytom.* **65** 6–13
[46] Boynard M and Lelievre J C 1990 Size determination of red blood cell aggregates induced by dextran using ultrasound backscattering phenomenon *Biorheology* **27** 39–46
[47] Franceschini E, Yu F T, Destrempes F and Cloutier G 2010 Ultrasound characterization of red blood cell aggregation with intervening attenuating tissue-mimicking phantoms *J. Acoust. Soc. Am.* **127** 1104–15
[48] Buxbaum K, Evans E and Brooks D E 1982 Quantitation of surface affinities of red blood cells in dextran solutions and plasma *Biochemistry* **21** 3235–9
[49] Steffen P, Verdier C and Wagner C 2013 Quantification of depletion-induced adhesion of red blood cells *Phys. Rev. Lett.* **110** 018102
[50] Yaya F 2021 Physical properties of red blood cells in aggregation *PhD thesis* Universität des Saarlandes, Saarbücken and Université Grenoble Alpes, Grenoble
[51] Weinbaum S, Tarbell J M and Damiano E R 2007 The structure and function of the endothelial glycocalyx layer *Annu. Rev. Biomed. Eng.* **9** 121–67
[52] Goldsmith H L, Cokelet G R and Gaehtgens P 1989 Robin Fåhraeus: evolution of his concepts in cardiovascular physiology *Am. J. Physiol.* **257** H1005–15
[53] Pries A R, Secomb T W, Gaehtgens P and Gross J F 1990 Blood flow in microvascular networks. Experiments and simulation *Circ. Res.* **67** 826–34
[54] Dintenfass L 1967 Inversion of the Fahraeus–Lindqvist phenomenon in blood flow through capillaries of diminishing radius *Nature* **215** 1099–100
[55] Farina A, Rosso F and Fasano A 2021 A continuum mechanics model for the Fåhræus-Lindqvist effect *J. Biol. Phys.* **47** 253–70

[56] Masilamani V, Al Salhi M S, Devanesan S, Algahtani F H, Abu-Salah K M, Ahamad I and Agastian P 2013 Spectral detection of sickle cell anemia and thalassemia *Photodiagnosis Photodyn. Ther.* **10** 429–33

[57] Soutani M, Suzuki Y, Tateishi N and Maeda N 1995 Quantitative evaluation of flow dynamics of erythrocytes in microvessels: influence of erythrocyte aggregation *Am. J. Physiol.* **268** H1959–65

[58] Chien S, Usami S and Skalak R 1984 Microcirculation *Blood Flow in Small Tubes: Handbook of Physiology, Section 2: The Cardiovascular System* **Vol IV** ed E M Renkin and C C Michel (Bethesda, MD: American Physiological Society) pp 217–49

[59] Reinhart W H, Piety N Z and Shevkoplyas S S 2017 Influence of feeding hematocrit and perfusion pressure on hematocrit reduction (Fåhraeus effect) in an artificial microvascular network *Microcirculation* **24**

[60] Maeda N 1996 Erythrocyte rheology in microcirculation *Jpn. J. Physiol.* **46** 1–14

[61] Possenti L, di Gregorio S, Gerosa F M, Raimondi G, Casagrande G, Costantino M L and Zunino P 2019 A computational model for microcirculation including Fahraeus-Lindqvist effect, plasma skimming and fluid exchange with the tissue interstitium *Int. J. Numer. Method Biomed. Eng.* **35** e3165

[62] Poole D C, Copp S W, Ferguson S K and Musch T I 2013 Skeletal muscle capillary function: contemporary observations and novel hypotheses *Exp. Physiol.* **98** 1645–58

[63] Maeda N and Shiga T 1994 Velocity of oxygen transfer and erythrocyte rheology *Physiology* **9** 22–7

[64] Jelkmann W 1992 Erythropoietin: structure, control of production, and function *Physiol. Rev.* **72** 449–89

[65] Helms C C, Gladwin M T and Kim-Shapiro D B 2018 Erythrocytes and vascular function: oxygen and nitric oxide *Front. Physiol.* **9** 125

[66] Williams A, Bissinger R, Shamaa H, Patel S, Bourne L, Artunc F and Qadri S M 2023 Pathophysiology of red blood cell dysfunction in diabetes and its complications *Pathophysiology* **30** 327–45

[67] McLellan S A and Walsh T S 2004 Oxygen delivery and haemoglobin *Contin. Educ. Anesth. Crit. Care Pain* **4** 123–6

[68] Dijkhuizen P, Buursma A, Fongers T M, Gerding A M, Oeseburg B and Zijlstra W G 1977 The oxygen binding capacity of human haemoglobin. Hüfner's factor redetermined *Pflugers Arch.* **369** 223–31

[69] Pasipoularides A 2012 Optimal hematocrit: a Procrustean bed for maximum oxygen transport rate? *J. Appl. Physiol.* **113** 353–4

[70] Lac E and Barthès-Biesel D 2005 Deformation of a capsule in simple shear flow: effect of membrane prestress *Phys. Fluids* **17** 072105

[71] Vlahovska P M, Podgorski T and Misbah C 2009 Vesicles and red blood cells in flow: from individual dynamics to rheology *C R Physique* **10** 775–89

[72] Biben T, Farutin A and Misbah C 2011 Three-dimensional vesicles under shear flow: numerical study of dynamics and phase diagram *Phys. Rev. E Stat. Nonlin. Soft Matter Phys.* **83** 031921

[73] Cordasco D and Bagchi P 2014 Intermittency and synchronized motion of red blood cell dynamics in shear flow *J. Fluid Mech.* **759** 472–88

[74] Peng Z, Mashayekh A and Zhu Q 2014 Erythrocyte responses in low-shear- rate flows: effects of non-biconcave stress-free state in the cytoskeleton *J. Fluid Mech.* **742** 96–118

[75] Sinha K and Graham M D 2015 Dynamics of a single red blood cell in simple shear flow *Phys. Rev. E Stat. Nonlin. Soft Matter Phys.* **92** 042710
[76] Lanotte L, Mauer J, Mendez S, Fedosov D A, Fromental J M, Claveria V, Nicoud F, Gompper G and Abkarian M 2016 Red cells' dynamic morphologies govern blood shear thinning under microcirculatory flow conditions *Proc. Natl. Acad. Sci. USA* **113** 13289–94
[77] Levant M and Steinberg V 2016 Intermediate regime and a phase diagram of red blood cell dynamics in a linear flow *Phys. Rev.* E **94** 062412
[78] Mauer J, Mendez S, Lanotte L, Nicoud F, Abkarian M, Gompper G and Fedosov D A 2018 Flow-induced transitions of red blood cell shapes under shear *Phys. Rev. Lett.* **121** 118103
[79] Zaiss S 1990 The influence of calcium on the deformability of human granulocytes *Biorheology* **27** 701–9
[80] Isfahani A H and Freund J B 2012 Forces on a wall-bound leukocyte in a small vessel due to red cells in the blood stream *Biophys. J.* **103** 1604–15
[81] Sadoul K 2015 New explanations for old observations: marginal band coiling during platelet activation *J. Thromb. Haemost.* **13** 333–46
[82] Ruggeri Z M 2009 Platelet adhesion under flow *Microcirculation* **16** 58–83
[83] Yazdani A, Li H, Humphrey J D and Karniadakis G E 2017 A general shear-dependent model for thrombus formation *PLoS Comput. Biol.* **13** e1005291
[84] Chow T W, Hellums J D, Moake J L and Kroll M H 1992 Shear stress-induced von Willebrand factor binding to platelet glycoprotein Ib initiates calcium influx associated with aggregation *Blood* **80** 113–20
[85] Peterson D M, Stathopoulos N A, Giorgio T D, Hellums J D and Moake J L 1987 Shear-induced platelet aggregation requires von Willebrand factor and platelet membrane glycoproteins Ib and IIb–IIIa *Blood* **69** 625–8
[86] Weaver A, Rubinstein S and Cornell R F 2020 Hyperviscosity syndrome in paraprotein secreting conditions including waldenstrom macroglobulinemia *Front. Oncol.* **10** 815

Chapter 4

Light absorption of blood

Gennadi Saiko, Faraz Sadrzadeh-Afsharazar, Scott Prahl and Alexandre Douplik

4.1 Introduction

Blood is a critically important biofluid responsible for transporting oxygen and nutrients to all body tissues and removing waste from them. Blood has distinct spectral features in the visible spectrum range, enabling multiple biomedical optical methods.

Blood consists of four essential components: red blood cells (RBCs), white blood cells (WBCs), platelets, and plasma.

Blood plasma is a light amber-colored liquid component of blood, which contains proteins (e.g., albumin) and other constituents of whole blood in suspension. It makes up about 55% of the body's total blood volume.

Cellular components comprise another 45% of the body's total blood volume. RBCs (or erythrocytes) dominate among cell components ($\sim$4500 × 10^3 μl^{-1} blood). Other types of cells are WBCs (leukocytes, $\sim$8 × 10^3 μl^{-1} blood) and platelets (thrombocytes, $\sim$300 × 10^3 μl^{-1} blood).

The study of optical and particularly absorption properties of blood has a long history. Van Assendelft [1] wrote in the introduction to his book 'Since the introduction of spectrophotometry, the technique has been applied in the study of haemoglobin and its derivatives. Among those who have contributed to the early spectrophotometric studies of haemoglobin derivatives mention should be made of the following. Angstrom was the first to describe spectral characteristics of blood in 1855 [2]. Hoppe–Seyler [3] in 1862 described the light absorption bands of oxy-haemoglobin and haemoglobin in the visible part of the spectrum. First mention of spectral characteristics of haemoglobin in the ultraviolet is made by Soret [4] in 1878. His work was improved upon by Gamgee [5] in 1897 using a quartz spectroscope with the sun as light source. Vierordt [6] again described spectral characteristics of haemoglobin and oxyhaemoglobin, also supplied a method to determine the haemoglobin content of blood samples using spectrophotometry. Calculation of the relative and total concentration of different haemoglobin

doi:10.1088/978-0-7503-4806-5ch4

derivatives was introduced by Hüfner [7] … Also in the nineteen thirties a great deal of work on the spectral characteristics of haemoglobin derivatives was published by Drabkin and co-workers [8].' The first comprehensive monograph on this topic appeared in 1933 [9].

Light absorption by blood is a key phenomenon with distinct features that has found multiple applications in biooptics.

4.2 Primary absorbers in blood

The primary absorbers of the blood are hemoglobins and water. Blood absorption can be described as a mixture of these two chromophores in different spectral ranges. However, other chromophores are also present.

4.2.1 Water

Water is the most abundant component of biological tissues. It accounts for 60%–80% of overall body weight.

While being a simple molecule, water has surprisingly complex absorption spectra, with strong absorption in the infrared and terahertz spectrum ranges. These peculiarities have profound implications. One particular implication for biomedical optics is a small (on a scale of hundred microns or less) penetration depth in tissues in the broad spectral range from mid-IR to terahertz.

In the visible range, minimal water absorption can be ignored for practical purposes. However, the water spectrum in NIR has multiple features which can be used in diagnostics and therapy. In particular, water has overtone bands of the O–H bonds with peak absorption at 760, 970 nm (the second overtone of the O–H stretching band), 1190 nm (the combination of the first overtone of the O–H stretching and the O–H bending band), 1450 nm (the first overtone of the OH-stretching band and a combination band), and 1940 nm (combination of the O–H stretching band and the O–H bending band) [10].

The absorption coefficients of water at 970, 1190, 1450, and 1940 nm wavelengths are 0.45, 1.04, 28.6, and 119.83 cm^{-1}, respectively [10].

4.2.2 Hemoglobins

In most vertebrates, the hemoglobin molecule is an assembly of four globular protein subunits (globins). As such, a hemoglobin molecule is a tetramer, where four subunits are roughly arranged as a tetrahedron. Each globin subunit contains a heme moiety of an organic protoporphyrin ring and a central iron ion in the ferrous state (Fe^{2+}).

The hemoglobin molecule is called oxyhemoglobin or HbO_2 if bound to oxygen. If the hemoglobin molecule is bound to carbon monoxide, it is called carboxyhemoglobin or HbCO. If the hemoglobin molecule is bound to nothing, it is called deoxyhemoglobin or Hb. Methemoglobin (sometimes called ferrihemoglobin) is a hemoglobin in which the iron in the heme group is in the Fe^{3+} (ferric) state, not the Fe^{2+} (ferrous) of normal hemoglobin. All these hemoglobin states have different absorption spectra.

4.2.2.1 Oxy- and deoxyhemoglobins

The two primary blood chromophores are deoxygenated and oxygenated hemoglobin (Hb and HbO_2). These chromophores are of great clinical interest as they define clinically significant total hemoglobin concentration ($tHb = Hb + HbO_2$) and blood oxygenation ($sO_2 = HbO_2/(HbO_2 + Hb)$).

Arterial and venous blood are oxygenated by approximately 97.5% and 75%, respectively [11].

When arterial blood is 95% saturated, some hemoglobin molecules have four oxygens bound, some have three, and a few have one or two. The statistical average of all oxygen bound to hemoglobin molecules relative to the total amount that can be bound is its oxygen saturation.

Deoxyhemoglobin has absorption peaks at 272, 433, 556, and 758 nm [12].

Oxyhemoglobin has absorption peaks at 274, 344, 414 (Soret band), 542, and 576 nm (Q bands) and a broad peak around 940 nm [12].

4.2.2.2 Methemoglobin

Methemoglobin (metHb) is a biomolecule formed when the iron in hemoglobin is oxidized to its ferric state. In healthy individuals, only 1% of hemoglobin is methemoglobin; anything above this is called methemoglobinemia. The hemoglobin-methemoglobin couple acts as an oxygen tension sensor by reacting with nitric oxide (NO). NO dilates vessels and increases perfusion to areas with poor oxygenation. Studies have shown that inadequate wound healing in diabetics is linked to reduced NO production in the wound [13].

Most of the daily reduction of methemoglobin in healthy people is due to the NADH cytochrome b5/cytochrome b5 reductase system, an efficient antioxidant found in RBCs [14]. On average, methemoglobin is reconverted at a rate of $15\% \, h^{-1}$.

4.2.2.3 Other hemoglobins

In addition to Hb, HbO_2, and metHb, other hemoglobins, such as sulfhemoglobin (HbS) and carboxyhemoglobin (HbCO), may also be present in the blood, though typically in much smaller quantities.

Fetal hemoglobin (Hb F) is the major hemoglobin in fetal RBCs during gestation, constituting 60%–80% of total hemoglobin in the full-term newborn. By approximately 6–12 months of age, Hb F is almost entirely replaced by adult hemoglobin (Hb A) [15].

4.2.3 Other blood chromophores

4.2.3.1 β-Carotene

β-Carotene is a precursor of vitamin A in the human diet, which turns into vitamin A in the liver. β-carotene belongs to the family of carotenoids, which are found in many fruits and vegetables, as well as some animal products such as egg yolks. Vitamin A is essential for proper production of RBCs in the bone marrow.

Along with lycopene, β-carotene is among the most frequently consumed dietary carotenoids in human subjects, ranking among the highest in blood/plasma concentrations [16]. Carotenoids are primarily stored in fatty tissue which holds around 80%–85% of the β-carotene available in the organism; the rest stays in the liver (8%–12%) and muscles (2%–3%) [17].The normal range of β-carotene in serum is 50 to 300 μg dl^{-1} or 0.93 to 5.59 μmol l^{-1} [18].

The long chain of alternating double bonds (conjugated) is responsible for the orange color of beta-carotene as they absorb in the green/blue part of the spectrum.

4.2.3.2 Bilirubin

Bilirubin is a red-orange compound produced in the normal catabolic pathway of heme breaking down. It is mainly found in the spleen and liver. Excess bilirubin secretion in the liver can no longer be stored in bile and, therefore, flows into the bloodstream and leaks into the tissue, causing the skin to appear yellow. This chromophore has its central absorption peak around 467 nm. The absorption peak's location and width depend on the solute in which it was diluted. Approximately 60% of term and 80% of pre-term newborns develop clinical jaundice in the first week after birth [19].

4.3 Experimental techniques

Traditionally, the most common way to measure the absorption of solutions is to use optical density measurements in a cuvette of the known path length. In early studies, this method was used in blood optics as well.

However, blood is an optically dense solution, particularly in the visible spectrum range. Thus, very thin layers (0.1 mm or less) or low hematocrits are used in such measurements.

The integrating sphere (IS) method has emerged as a de facto gold standard [20] in measuring optical parameters of materials that scatter and absorb light, including blood.

4.3.1 Transmission spectrophotometry

In the absence of scattering, the transmitted light intensity through a cuvette is described by the Beer–Lambert law:

$$I(L) = I_0 e^{-\mu_a L} \tag{4.1}$$

Here, L is the path length [cm] and μ_a is the absorption coefficient of the medium in the cuvette [cm^{-1}]. Thus, it is possible to extract the absorption coefficient by measuring the degradation of light through a cuvette of the known path length.

However, blood strongly scatters light which is unaccounted for in the Beer–Lambert law. The scattering coefficient μ_s can be included in a modified Beer–Lambert law.

$$\ln\left(\frac{I(L)}{I_0}\right) = -\mu_a L - \mu_s L \tag{4.2}$$

However, the way in which the scattering coefficient μ_s maybe decoupled from the absorption coefficient μ_a depends on the geometry of the experiment and making certain assumptions.

Transmission spectrophotometric measurements in blood differ from typical analytical methods that measure the absorption of liquids and gases. For liquids and gasses with low light absorption, like water in the visible range of the spectrum, different versions of optical cavity-based techniques are used, including cavity ring-down spectroscopy (CRDS) [21] and cavity-enhanced absorption spectroscopy (CEAS) [22].

4.3.2 Integrating sphere technique

The integrating sphere (IS) technique uses a thin sample placed at the entrance of an integrating sphere. The scattered reflection R_d, the total transmission T_t, and the unscattered transmission T_c of the sample are measured. Then, the optical properties, including absorption coefficient μ_a, scattering coefficient μ_s, and anisotropy factor g, can be extracted using several techniques, inverse Monte Carlo (iMC) simulations [23], inverse adding-doubling [24], or lookup tables. For example, the iMC uses forward Monte Carlo simulations iteratively to calculate the optical parameters μ_a, μ, and g based on a given phase function and the experimentally measured values for reflection and transmission R_d, T_t, and T_c.

The thickness of the sample is typically quite small. For example, Meinke *et al* [25] used a sample thickness of 2.6 mm for measuring plasma and platelets; leukocytes were measured using a sample thickness of 0.52 mm. For RBCs, the thickness was set to 0.116 mm.

The integrating sphere technique can be enhanced by adding one more integrating sphere [26]. Since the double integrating sphere (DIS) system facilitates simultaneous measurement of reflectance and transmittance from a sample without repositioning, it is a preferred approach for measuring fresh tissue samples [27]. In the double integrating sphere technique, a thin sample is placed between two integrating spheres, and the same measurements above are made. The optical properties, including absorption coefficient μ_a, scattering coefficient μ_s, and anisotropy factor g, can be extracted using several techniques, including inverse Monte Carlo simulations [23], inverse adding-doubling [24], or lookup tables.

4.4 Absorption-based techniques (techniques for biomedical research that are absorption-based)

Multiple biomedical modalities are based on light absorption by blood components (hemoglobins).

4.4.1 Pulse oximetry

Pulse oximetry is ubiquitous and is undoubtedly the most common technology among medical optical devices. Pulse oximetry probes the blood volume changes caused by pulse propagation using optical means. The pulse oximetry is based on the observation that pressure changes caused by pulse wave propagation are confined to the arterial compartment. Thus, blood volume changes during the cardiac cycle (linked to blood pressure changes via compliance) are also localized to the arterial compartment. A typical pulse oximeter contains a spatially resolved light source and detector applied to a body prominence (e.g., finger or ear lobe). A typical scenario uses both red light (660 nm) and infrared light (880 or 940 nm). The average change in each channel across the cardiac cycle (AC component) is normalized on the slow-moving DC component to obtain the AC/DC ratio for each channel (red and IR). Then, the 'ratio of ratios' R is calculated: $R = \frac{\frac{AC_R}{DC_R}}{\frac{AC_{IR}}{DC_{IR}}}$. The tissue oxygenation is calculated from R using the empirical relationship.

$$sO_2 = \frac{k_1 - k_2 R}{k_3 - k_4 R} \tag{4.2}$$

Coefficients k_1, k_2, k_3, and k_4 are determined experimentally for each specific pulse oximeter by best-fit analysis of the measured parameters in the calibration process [28].

4.4.2 NIRS

Diffuse reflectance spectroscopy (DRS), diffuse optical spectroscopy (DOS), and near-infrared spectroscopy (NIRS) refer to a broad range of technologies that use diffuse photons to extract functional and morphological information about underlying tissue. As scattering and absorption of light by tissues are lower in the NIR range of the spectrum, NIR light sources are often used. Thus, this group of technologies is commonly known as NIRS, particularly in neuroscience.

The utility of NIRS has been explored in many medical applications. For example, in wound care, using DRS, considerable differences in Hb and HbO_2 were observed for ulcerated areas compared to control sites in clinical studies. In addition, the total hemoglobin (tHb) concentration was higher in foot ulcers [29].

Photoplethysmography (PPG) is a NIRS subclass that exploits the volumetric changes caused by pulse propagation. A pulse oximeter is the best-known PPG device.

The utility of NIRs is well-established in several medical fields, including patient monitoring (pulse oximeter) and sports medicine (muscle oximetry [30]).

Fundamentals of diffuse optics have been reviewed by Durduran *et al* [31]. NIRS technology aims to extract the coefficient of absorption and reduced scattering coefficient of the media. The concentrations (absolute or relative) of chromophores (oxy-, deoxyhemoglobin, water, lipids) can be extracted from them.

NIRS methodology comes in three flavors: time-domain, frequency-domain, and continuous-wave (CW) [32].

In time-domain imaging, the tissue is irradiated with short (typically picoseconds) light pulses. Then, the shape of the received signal is analyzed to extract optical parameters.

In the frequency-domain schema, the light source is modulated at high frequency (typically 100 MHz), and the tissue response (in particular, amplitude and phase delay) is measured to extract tissue optical parameters. Some tools use modulation at several frequencies up to 1 GHz [32].

Continuous-wave spectroscopy typically explores several source-to-detector distances.

DRS, DOS, and NIRS typically refer to contact modalities that provide single-point measurements. NIRS modalities are usually based on the principle of spatially resolved spectroscopy [32].

Diffuse optical tomography (DOT) is an extension of the NIRS or DOS to several sources and detectors. The technology relies heavily on image reconstruction. So, it is not true imaging technology but a synthetic imaging modality. DOT can be used to reconstruct 2D (topographic) and 3D (tomographic). DOT has been studied intensively across various medical domains [33]. It is widely used as functional NIRS (fNIRS) imaging in neuroscience. It was also tried as optical mammography in breast cancer [32].

4.4.3 Multispectral/hyperspectral imaging

Medical hyperspectral and multispectral imaging (HSI/MSI) refer to a broad group of non-contact spectroscopy-based technologies that extract information about underlying tissues from relatively large areas.

HSI/MSI is an extension of traditional RGB imaging, where concentrations of tissue chromophores are deconvoluted from reflectance spectra sampled at several (MSI) or multiple equally-spaced (HSI) wavelengths. In a typical scenario, HSI/MSI uses reflectance geometry. Existing systems use either the visible range of spectrum or NIR.

In biomedical applications, hyperspectral or multispectral imaging is used primarily to extract data about components of the blood, which are chromophores in the visible and NIR spectrum [34]. The primary outcome of HSI/MSI methods is tissue sO_2 maps, which indicate abnormalities in blood circulation. Occasionally, oxyhemoglobin (HbO_2), deoxyhemoglobin (Hb), and total hemoglobin (tHb) or their proxies are also reported.

The primary clinical utility of HSI/MSI techniques is to determine blood circulation abnormalities in tissues (perfusion). It might indicate insufficient (e.g., hypoxia) or abnormally high blood supply (e.g., angiogenesis).

For example, Khaodhiar *et al* [35] measured Hb and HbO_2 in non-diabetic controls ($n = 14$) as well as diabetic patients with ($n = 10$) and without diabetic foot ulcer ($n = 13$) four times over six months using HSI. HbO_2 and Hb measurements in the peri-wound of non-healing ulcers were lower than in healing ulcers ($p<0.01$) and contralateral foot ($p<0.001$).

4.4.4 Photoacoustics

If the absorbed light energy is not re-emitted as luminescence, it will be transferred to other processes, which may give rise to the local temperature. This rise in temperature can lead to multiple phenomena, from sound wave generation to tissue destruction.

Photoacoustic imaging is based on sound wave generation caused by the rapid tissue expansion due to local heating by the pulsed laser light. It is a hybrid technology that uses optical excitation and ultrasonic detection. The ultrasound (US) waves are captured using US transducers and converted to images with conventional medical ultrasound procedures.

Photoacoustic imaging (PAI), photoacoustic tomography (PAT), or optoacoustic (OA) tomography uses pulsed laser light to irradiate tissues. As a result, pressure waves are produced due to the increased temperature and volume [36]. The process of photoacoustic signal generation can be described in three steps: (1) an object absorbs light, (2) the absorbed optical energy is converted into heat and generates a temperature rise, and (3) thermoelastic expansion takes place, resulting in the emission of acoustic waves [37]. For effective PAT signal generation, the laser pulse duration should be less than the thermal and stress confinement times [38]. Thus, the typical laser pulse duration used in PAT is on scales of several nanoseconds or less.

High-frequency ultrasound transducers monitor these generated pressure waves and a 3D reconstruction is performed. Visible and near-infrared light is used to perform PAT. The contrast in PAT images depends mainly upon the absorption properties of tissues [39]. The optical absorption is specific to tissue chromophores, and by changing the wavelength of light, one can tune the images to obtain enhanced contrast for particular chromophores.

While PA can be based on exogenous or endogenous chromophores, most PA applications are based on blood chromophores (hemoglobins). By projecting light at hemoglobin's peak absorption, inflamed hyperemic tissue appears dark (hypoechoic) on PAT, while surrounding tissues reflecting such light waves appear bright (hyperechoic).

In a typical scenario, multispectral PA imaging systems are used to allow spectral unmixing and the detection of chromophores of interest. Typical outputs of these multispectral PA systems are oxyhemoglobin, deoxyhemoglobin, total hemoglobin, and oxygen saturation. For example, Yang *et al* [40] used PAI to characterize circulatory and metabolic functions by monitoring hemodynamic changes in the skeletal muscle (forearm) during cuff occlusion. They found a similar trend to that of conventional NIRS.

Photoacoustic imaging will be covered in more detail in chapter 9.

4.4.5 Other techniques

Several other techniques have emerged in biomedical research and clinical practice. Here, we present several examples of such techniques.

4.4.5.1 Photothermal imaging

Photothermal (PT) imaging is similar to photoacoustic imaging in that both are mediated by heating. PT is an all-optical technology. The PT signal arises from slight changes in the index of refraction in a sample caused by sample heating due to absorption of the (heating) beam. Then, the refractive index changes are measured with a second (probing) beam, usually of a different wavelength.

PT imaging is a microscopic technique. Typically, two different strategies are used for the PT imaging of single nanoparticles: (i) photothermal interference contrast imaging [41] and (ii) photothermal heterodyne imaging [42]. This method has reached the sensitivity of single particles and single molecules. As such, it has multiple applications in biology and material science. The status of PT and its applications have been reviewed by Adhikari *et al* [43]. Pertinent to blood, Lu *et al* [44] applied two-photon PT to image heme proteins with 3D sectioning in live cells.

4.4.5.2 Deep UV microscopy

Deep UV microscopy is a technique that allows high-resolution molecular imaging and absorption-based label-free mass mapping. Deep UV microscopy measures optical density in transmission geometry. Knowing the extinction coefficients and molar weights of its components, the dry mass per unit area (σ) is calculated from these measurements. Kaza *et al* [45] proposed using deep UV microscopy to extract RBCs' morphological properties and hemoglobin (Hb) content. They imaged whole blood smears with a multispectral UV microscopy system at four wavelengths (220, 260, 280, and 300 nm) and calculated the dry mass of RBCs. They found consistent Hb mass and mean corpuscular Hb (MCH) values at all wavelengths, with the precision of the single-cell mass measurements being nearly identical at 220, 260, and 280 nm but slightly lower at 300 nm. They also compared their technique to quantitative phase imaging (QPI)-based mass mapping (see section 5.3.2) and found excellent agreement on average between the two methods.

4.5 Absorption properties of blood and its components

4.5.1 Absorption and extinction coefficients

Light propagation in a non-scattering medium is described by the Beer–Lambert law (equation (4.1)), where the distance is measured in [cm] and μ_a is measured in [cm^{-1}].

However, different sets of units are used in laboratory optical measurements. Historically, the base 10 is used instead of *e*. When the concentration of chromophore, C [mol l^{-1}] or [M] is included in equation (4.1) can be written

$$I(L) = I_0 10^{-\varepsilon CL} \tag{4.3}$$

Here, ε is the extinction coefficient [cm^{-1} M^{-1}] or [l cm^{-1} mol^{-1}]. The extinction coefficients are typically reported in the spectroscopic literature.

Also, it should be noted that as the hemoglobin is a tetramer, different authors report extinction differently, either per globin (e.g., Zijlstra [46]) or per the whole molecule (e.g., Prahl [47]). This results in a correction factor of 4, which may need to be included.

The absorption coefficient μ_a of a tissue is the sum of contributions from all absorbing chromophores within the tissue. Using equation (4.1) and equation (4.3) the absorption coefficient of the medium can be expressed through extinction coefficients and concentrations of its chromophores

$$\mu_a = \ln\,(10)\sum_i \varepsilon_i C_i \tag{4.4}$$

However, molar concentrations are not always known. In this case, volume fractions f_i of chromophores are used:

$$\mu_a = \sum_i \mu_{a,i} f_i \tag{4.5}$$

Absorption can also be derived from the complex refractive index of the sample. In particular, the complex refractive index $m(\omega)$ can be split into the sum of real and imaginary parts $m(\omega) = n(\omega) + i\kappa(\omega)$, where the imaginary part refers to dissipation, which can be linked to the absorption coefficient [48]

$$\kappa(\omega) = \frac{c\mu_a}{2\omega} \tag{4.6}$$

Here, c is the speed of light and ω is the angular frequency of light.

Using this formalism, the imaginary part (absorption) can be linked with the real part of the refractive index using Kramers–Kronig equations (See chapter 5 for further details). As it is usually easier to measure absorption than refractive index, these relationships are typically used in one direction—to determine the imaginary refractive index using absorption measurements.

4.5.2 Absorption of blood and its components

Blood primarily consists of plasma (55% of blood by volume) and RBCs (45% of blood by volume), the primary cell components of blood. Other cell types can be broadly grouped into leucocytes (WBCs) and thrombocytes (platelets).

4.5.2.1 Serum and plasma

Cell-free plasma consists of 90% water and 10% proteins [49]. Thus, the optical properties of blood in most spectral regions are dominated by the optical properties of water. The absorption spectrum of serum compiled from two sources is depicted in figure 4.1. For comparison, the absorption spectrum of the water is included.

4.5.2.1.1 Water

Optical constants of water were measured and reviewed on multiple occasions (see, for example, Querry *et al* [53]). Prahl [54] reviewed the optical properties of water, including absorption. He found that data to be consistent between different authors.

The water absorption coefficient in the 200–200 μm range is depicted in figure 4.2.

4.5.2.1.2 Proteins

The absorption of plasma in the IR is dominated by water absorption. However, for UV and visible wavelengths, plasma has significant absorption due to the proteins and other molecules (see figure 4.1). Moreover, the absorption is subject to individual variability and sample preparation techniques; plasma from different individuals can vary from yellow to green to orange to brown.

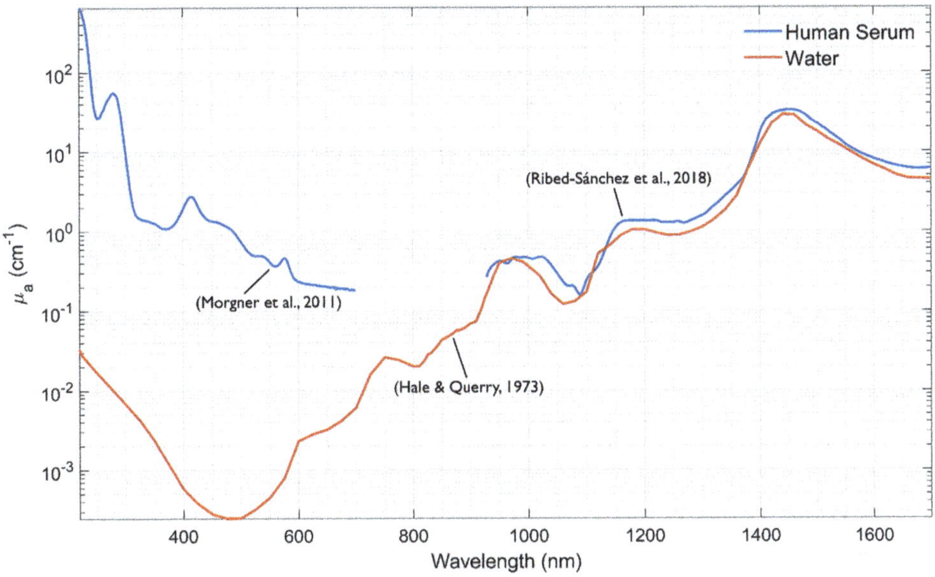

Figure 4.1. Compilation of the absorption spectra of human serum [50, 51] in the 200–1700 nm range. Water spectra compiled by Hale and Querry [52] added as reference.

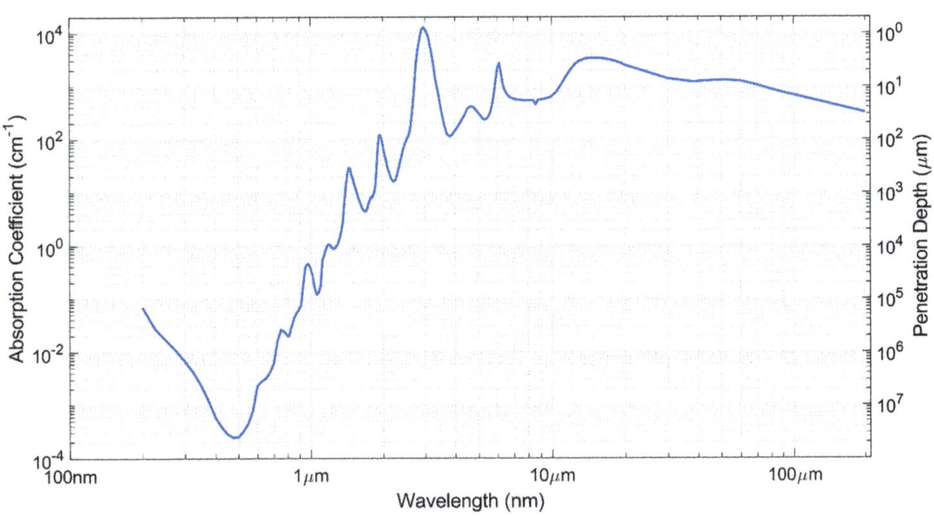

Figure 4.2. Absorption coefficient of water in 200–200 μm range based on data by Hale and Querry [52].

Meinke *et al* [25] found that plasma absorption deviates from water absorption in some spectral regions and depends on the preparation. For example, plasma centrifuged at 62 000 g for 1 h showed an absorption peak at 460 nm (attributed to bilirubin), reaching a value of 0.08 mm^{-1}. Plasma centrifuged at 1600 g for 30 min showed an absorption peak of 0.37 mm^{-1}at 415 nm and 0.02 mm^{-1} at 580 nm.

These peaks are most likely attributed to free hemoglobin. They also found that plasma absorption above 750 nm generally follows that of water.

4.5.2.2 Hemoglobin

There have been several studies on the absorption coefficients of hemoglobins. For example, using transmission spectrophotometry, Zijlstra *et al* [55] measured the absorption of hemolysed hemoglobin in the 450–800 nm range.

A widely-used hemoglobin absorption dataset has been compiled by Prahl [47] for molar extinction coefficients of oxy- and deoxyhemoglobins in water in the range of 250–1000 nm, citing data from van Assendelft [1], Gratzer and Kollias [56], Moaveni [57], Schmitt [58], and Takatani and Graham [59].

As mentioned in section 4.5.1, extinction coefficients can be turned into absorption coefficients for any particular hemoglobin content, x, measured in [g l^{-1}]

$$\mu_a = \frac{2.303\varepsilon x}{64\,500\ \mathrm{g\ mol^{-1}}} \tag{4.7}$$

The absorption coefficients for human oxy- and deoxyhemoglobin at normal hematocrit (150 g l^{-1}) are provided in table 4.1 and depicted in figure 4.3. They were calculated from the extinction coefficients provided by Prahl [47].

The absorption spectra of oxy, deoxy-, carboxy-, and methemoglobins in the visible and near-infrared spectral range (450–1000 nm) were measured by Zijlstra *et al* [60]. In addition, they found that the small differences between fetal and adult hemoglobin absorption were significant enough to be considered in multicomponent analysis of hemoglobin derivatives.

The absorption coefficients for human carboxy-and methemoglobin at normal hematocrit (150 g l^{-1}) are provided in table 4.2 and depicted in figure 4.4. They were calculated from the extinction coefficients provided by Zijlstra and Buursma [46].

4.5.2.3 Other blood components

Meinke *et al* [25] found that the existence of physiological concentrations of leucocytes has no measurable influence on the optical properties of plasma and, therefore, on the optical parameters of whole blood.

Platelets absorb light similarly to pure plasma [25]. Even when platelets are highly concentrated the plasma absorption maximum at 410 nm is shifted to 420 nm at 0.79 cm^{-1}.

4.5.2.4 Whole blood

Whole blood consists of blood plasma and blood cells (primarily RBCs). Whole blood is a densely packed solution of RBCs, where neighboring RBCs are often in contact with one other. The concentration of RBCs in whole blood is characterized by hematocrit (hct), the cell volume fraction within the whole blood volume. A typical range for hematocrit is from 39%–55% in men and 36%–48% in women [61]. The hemoglobin concentration ranges from 139–163 g l^{-1} (men) and 120–150 (women) for whole blood or 299 to 357 g l^{-1} for packed RBCs [62].

Table 4.1. The absorption coefficient μ_α [cm^{-1}] of oxy-and deoxyhemoglobin was calculated at 150 g l^{-1} of Hb (normal hematocrit). Calculated from the extinction coefficients provided by Prahl [47].

Wavelength, nm	HbO_2, cm^{-1}	Hb, cm^{-1}	Wavelength, nm	HbO_2, cm^{-1}	Hb, cm^{-1}	Wavelength, nm	HbO_2, cm^{-1}	Hb, cm^{-1}
250	573.00	608.77	500	113.04	112.65	750	2.80	7.59
252	569.98	608.77	502	111.22	117.90	752	2.88	8.18
254	581.36	608.77	504	110.26	123.14	754	2.96	8.33
256	592.86	614.65	506	107.71	128.38	756	3.03	8.43
258	609.90	621.22	508	107.98	133.62	758	3.10	8.43
260	628.43	628.00	510	108.19	139.18	760	3.16	8.36
262	649.02	634.85	512	108.81	145.46	762	3.23	8.15
264	671.82	641.93	514	110.32	151.74	764	3.29	7.88
266	694.96	649.12	516	113.41	158.02	766	3.36	7.62
268	718.55	656.34	518	121.55	164.30	768	3.44	7.35
270	734.77	663.55	520	130.69	170.58	770	3.51	7.08
272	741.05	664.72	522	142.83	177.40	772	3.58	6.82
274	747.40	658.54	524	158.05	185.75	774	3.66	6.55
276	742.09	652.36	526	175.48	194.10	776	3.72	6.28
278	733.43	647.14	528	194.35	202.45	778	3.78	6.02
280	712.45	641.91	530	215.77	210.80	780	3.83	5.81
282	689.69	635.19	532	236.93	219.15	782	3.89	5.59
284	660.31	620.03	534	253.39	227.28	784	3.95	5.38
286	629.14	604.84	536	268.66	235.40	786	4.00	5.17
288	585.81	578.56	538	279.24	243.50	788	4.04	4.98
290	565.66	531.17	540	287.47	251.60	790	4.08	4.81
292	534.25	494.83	542	287.78	260.00	792	4.13	4.64
294	475.93	463.43	544	281.32	268.42	794	4.17	4.48
296	428.31	416.34	546	269.29	276.85	796	4.25	4.34
298	382.77	375.00	548	251.96	283.48	798	4.36	4.22

(Continued)

Table 4.1. *(Continued)*

Wavelength, nm	HbO_2, cm^{-1}	Hb, cm^{-1}	Wavelength, nm	HbO_2, cm^{-1}	Hb, cm^{-1}	Wavelength, nm	HbO_2, cm^{-1}	Hb, cm^{-1}
300	356.25	347.98	550	232.29	288.42	800	4.41	4.11
302	341.32	331.02	552	214.25	292.03	802	4.47	4.02
304	334.54	317.67	554	198.80	294.41	804	4.51	3.98
306	336.70	307.30	556	186.17	294.52	806	4.56	3.94
308	339.42	311.15	558	180.66	292.49	808	4.62	3.91
310	342.10	319.44	560	176.11	290.46	810	4.67	3.87
312	356.25	336.14	562	176.15	282.29	812	4.71	3.84
314	372.69	352.86	564	183.14	273.09	814	4.75	3.82
316	390.98	368.88	566	197.07	263.67	816	4.79	3.79
318	407.89	384.52	568	216.93	253.52	818	4.87	3.76
320	425.26	402.34	570	240.28	243.39	820	4.95	3.75
322	444.18	422.73	572	265.53	234.04	822	5.02	3.75
324	464.25	443.12	574	287.86	225.27	824	5.10	3.74
326	484.90	462.20	576	299.92	216.50	826	5.16	3.74
328	506.35	477.99	578	295.53	207.73	828	5.21	3.74
330	526.56	490.62	580	270.56	199.91	830	5.26	3.74
332	545.21	503.24	582	233.84	192.65	832	5.31	3.74
334	558.92	515.87	584	187.05	185.40	834	5.35	3.74
336	566.83	538.88	586	143.64	177.40	836	5.41	3.74
338	574.84	564.17	588	106.72	167.81	838	5.46	3.74
340	582.57	585.75	590	77.76	152.95	840	5.52	3.74
342	588.92	599.38	592	56.53	137.54	842	5.57	3.74
344	594.50	613.03	594	41.47	121.90	844	5.63	3.74
346	588.77	626.68	596	30.69	106.92	846	5.67	3.74
348	583.11	641.26	598	24.32	92.12	848	5.69	3.73
350	575.51	659.30	600	17.28	79.26	850	5.71	3.73
352	567.22	677.35	602	14.39	73.56	852	5.73	3.73
354	559.96	695.39	604	11.49	67.87	854	5.76	3.73

356	548.47	713.45	606	9.66	62.17	856	5.79	3.73
358	528.27	721.61	608	8.90	56.58	858	5.84	3.74
360	511.62	728.68	610	8.13	51.00	860	5.90	3.75
362	498.14	734.64	612	7.37	46.39	862	5.95	3.76
364	485.11	739.65	614	6.60	41.91	864	6.00	3.77
366	477.81	744.66	616	5.99	39.66	866	6.04	3.78
368	472.56	749.82	618	5.54	37.41	868	6.07	3.79
370	476.15	755.83	620	5.09	35.15	870	6.09	3.81
372	494.60	761.85	622	4.63	33.44	872	6.12	3.83
374	513.76	767.86	624	4.18	31.90	874	6.14	3.86
376	534.25	773.88	626	3.82	30.35	876	6.17	3.88
378	558.53	779.89	628	3.56	28.98	878	6.20	3.90
380	591.65	784.25	630	3.29	27.80	880	6.23	3.92
382	631.63	784.25	632	3.03	26.63	882	6.26	3.94
384	677.27	802.81	634	2.77	25.55	884	6.29	3.96
386	729.71	831.10	636	2.59	24.85	886	6.32	3.98
388	799.74	861.54	638	2.49	24.16	888	6.34	4.00
390	905.84	906.01	640	2.39	23.46	890	6.36	4.02
392	1024.60	972.02	642	2.29	22.77	892	6.38	4.04
394	1145.12	1034.32	644	2.19	22.08	894	6.40	4.05
396	1250.70	1091.47	646	2.11	21.41	896	6.43	4.07
398	1341.38	1148.64	648	2.05	20.83	898	6.45	4.09
400	1437.65	1205.80	650	1.99	20.25	900	6.47	4.11
402	1534.81	1275.42	652	1.93	19.67	902	6.49	4.13
404	1667.07	1368.19	654	1.87	19.09	904	6.51	4.14
406	1912.72	1460.96	656	1.81	18.51	906	6.53	4.16
408	2280.53	1551.72	658	1.76	17.93	908	6.54	4.17
410	2520.94	1641.36	660	1.73	17.42	910	6.56	4.18
412	2701.08	1735.26	662	1.70	16.96	912	6.57	4.20

(*Continued*)

Table 4.1. (*Continued*)

Wavelength, nm	HbO_2, cm^{-1}	Hb, cm^{-1}	Wavelength, nm	HbO_2, cm^{-1}	Hb, cm^{-1}	Wavelength, nm	HbO_2, cm^{-1}	Hb, cm^{-1}
414	2831.11	1850.02	664	1.67	16.49	914	6.58	4.20
416	2818.15	1964.78	666	1.64	16.03	916	6.59	4.20
418	2783.81	2082.67	668	1.61	15.56	918	6.60	4.20
420	2593.94	2200.82	670	1.59	15.09	920	6.61	4.20
422	2332.15	2321.35	672	1.57	14.63	922	6.62	4.20
424	2031.67	2490.48	674	1.54	14.19	924	6.63	4.19
426	1760.57	2601.94	676	1.52	13.79	926	6.62	4.17
428	1528.80	2704.54	678	1.51	13.40	928	6.61	4.15
430	1328.79	2854.44	680	1.50	13.00	930	6.60	4.12
432	1156.25	2981.66	682	1.49	12.61	932	6.59	4.06
434	892.79	2981.66	684	1.48	12.21	934	6.57	3.98
436	717.23	2954.02	686	1.47	11.82	936	6.56	3.90
438	643.36	2708.42	688	1.48	11.42	938	6.56	3.82
440	553.93	2231.71	690	1.49	11.08	940	6.56	3.74
442	501.01	1961.50	692	1.50	10.80	942	6.55	3.67
444	439.80	1526.71	694	1.51	10.52	944	6.55	3.57
446	412.15	1281.01	696	1.52	10.25	946	6.54	3.46
448	362.04	935.93	698	1.54	9.97	948	6.52	3.36
450	339.21	557.78	700	1.57	9.69	950	6.50	3.25
452	317.87	338.26	702	1.59	9.40	952	6.48	3.15
454	289.18	195.32	704	1.61	9.11	954	6.47	3.07
456	267.28	165.77	706	1.64	8.83	956	6.45	2.99
458	256.48	139.79	708	1.67	8.55	958	6.43	2.92
460	240.19	126.30	710	1.70	8.32	960	6.40	2.84
462	223.13	112.81	712	1.73	8.09	962	6.38	2.76
464	214.96	104.01	714	1.76	7.85	964	6.36	2.67
466	200.20	97.97	716	1.79	7.62	966	6.34	2.56
468	188.30	91.94	718	1.84	7.39	968	6.31	2.44

470	179.33	87.24	720	1.88	7.16	970	6.27	2.32
472	170.75	82.67	722	1.92	6.94	972	6.24	2.24
474	162.61	81.26	724	1.97	6.72	974	6.21	2.17
476	155.79	79.88	726	2.01	6.50	976	6.18	2.10
478	149.68	79.15	728	2.06	6.23	978	6.13	2.02
480	143.80	78.57	730	2.11	5.95	980	6.09	1.94
482	138.79	80.36	732	2.15	5.95	982	6.05	1.86
484	135.97	82.15	734	2.20	5.95	984	6.00	1.78
486	133.22	83.94	736	2.26	5.95	986	5.95	1.69
488	130.54	85.85	738	2.33	5.94	988	5.89	1.61
490	127.90	90.09	740	2.41	6.03	990	5.83	1.53
492	124.67	94.34	742	2.48	6.27	992	5.77	1.45
494	121.27	98.58	744	2.56	6.52	994	5.71	1.36
496	117.99	102.82	746	2.63	6.84	996	5.65	1.28
498	114.80	107.41	748	2.72	7.20	998	5.59	1.20
						1000	5.53	1.12

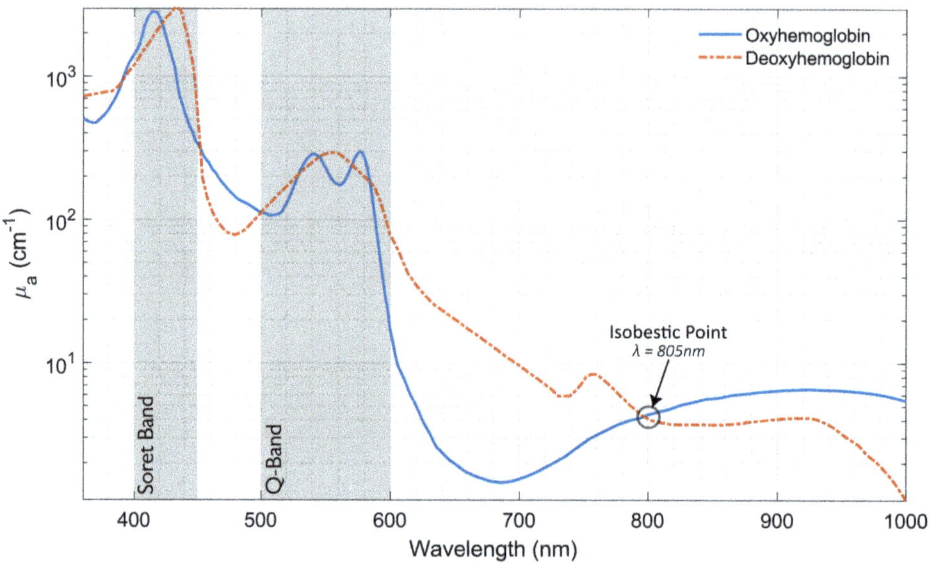

Figure 4.3. Absorption coefficient of various forms of oxy- and deoxyhemoglobin at normal hematocrit (150 g l^{-1}). Calculated from the extinction coefficients provided by Prahl [47].

Table 4.2. Absorption coefficient μ_α [cm^{-1}] of carboxy-and methemoglobin, calculated at 150 g l^{-1} of Hb (normal hematocrit). Calculated from the extinction coefficients provided by Zijlstra and Buursma [46]

Wavelength, nm	HbCO	metHb	Wavelength, nm	HbCO	metHb
450	217.51	211.68	590	62.42	76.90
480	121.39	174.31	600	23.76	69.77
500	114.05	196.78	630	4.10	84.02
510	128.30	187.27	660	1.30	17.71
520	179.28	166.97	680	0.65	5.62
530	265.46	149.90	700	0.43	4.32
538	308.88	140.40	750	0.22	5.40
540	308.23	136.94	775		6.91
542	303.26	133.27	800		8.64
550	261.58	111.46	805		8.96
554	251.21	100.66	840		11.23
560	264.60	90.29	880		13.18
568	311.69	86.62	904		14.26
570	312.34	86.62	920		15.12
576	254.02	86.40	940		15.77
578	221.83	86.18	960		16.20
580	186.62	85.32	1000		16.42

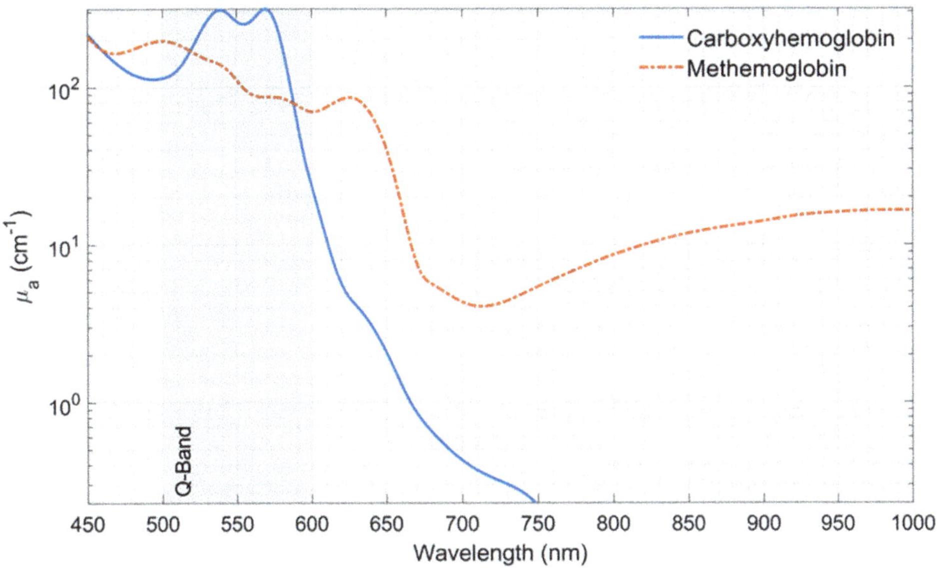

Figure 4.4. Absorption coefficient of carboxy- and methemoglobin at normal hematocrit (150 g l^{-1}). Calculated from the extinction coefficients provided by Zijlstra and Buursma [46]

The absorption of whole blood has been investigated on several occasions. Most recently, they were reviewed by Bosschaart *et al* [63].

Schmitt [58] measured hct and blood sO_2 using an implantable oximeter.

Roggan *et al* [62] investigated the optical properties of circulating human blood at 633 nm using a double integrating sphere technique and Monte Carlo simulations. Pertinent to absorption, they found that (a) scattering and absorption increased linearly with hematocrit if hct $< 50\%$, (b) absorption and scattering decreased slightly with increasing shear rate, (c) the deformation of erythrocytes had no significant impact on the optical properties if volume and hemoglobin content was kept constant, (d) increasing osmolarity leads to an increase of absorption while scattering and anisotropy decreased, (e) increasing hemolysis led to a reduction in absorption and scattering and (f) hemoglobin solutions had a smaller absorption coefficient than whole blood at the same hemoglobin concentration.

Probably the most surprising finding by Roggan *et al* [62] was that the absorption coefficient μ_a significantly decreased with increasing hemolysis. In particular, when blood was completely hemolyzed, μ_a amounted to 0.11 ± 0.03 mm^{-1} which was only 55% of the value for intact blood (0.20 ± 0.05 mm^{-1}).

Roggan *et al* [62] also measured the absorption coefficients of water and solutions of oxy- and deoxyhemoglobin in water in the 400–2500 nm range (figure 4.5). The absorption of hemoglobin solutions closely follows the spectral dependence of water in the 1350–2500 nm range (figure 4.5).

The position of the absorption peaks of the blood depends on numerous factors. In particular, the position of Q-band peaks (535, 555, 576 nm) depends on oxygenation. The peak in the Soret band (400–450 nm) depends on numerous

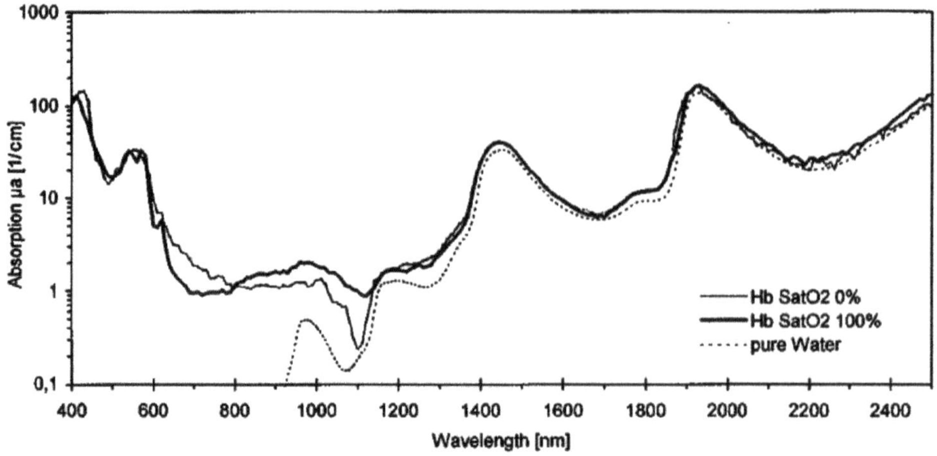

Figure 4.5. Absorption coefficients of water and solutions oxy- and deoxyhemoglobin in water at hct = 5% and a shear rate of 500 s^{-1}. Reproduced with permission from [62], copyright (1998) Society of Photo-Optical Instrumentation Engineers (SPIE).

factors. For example, it depends on the age of the bloodstain [64], which can be used in criminology. Hanson and Ballantyne [64] found a blue shift in the visible absorption spectrum of the Hb Soret band (from 414 to 408 nm) that strongly correlates with the age of the bloodstain. In addition to the age, the magnitude of the shift (0–7 nm) also depends upon the ambient temperature and relative humidity. The molecular basis for the observed Soret band blue shift is likely based upon oxidation, dehydration, and hemichrome formation, followed by the eventual loss of coordinated heme and release of free iron.

The absorption of the whole blood is affected by multiple factors. Below are the primary factors that may impact measurements.

4.5.2.4.1 Hematocrit

Blood absorption is affected by hematocrit. As mentioned, Roggan *et al* [62] found that scattering and absorption increased linearly with hematocrit if hct < 50%. Several other effects may affect light absorption by blood, including so-called *detour* and *sieve effects.*

Pigments are typically found to be concentrated in cells (hemoglobins) or organelles (melanin); thus, the distribution of hemoglobin in the blood is not uniform. As a result, when light traverses the turbid media, refractive index mismatches between cell walls and intercellular medium cause multiple internal scatterings that increase the light optical path length, increasing the probability of light absorption. This lengthening of the optical path length is referred to as the *detour effect* [65].

The distribution of absorbers within a target media can also have an opposite effect on light absorption. For example, light may traverse a turbid media, such as blood, without encountering any pigment-containing structures, effectively passing through a sieve. The *sieve effect* in blood can decrease absorption at strongly absorbed wavelengths.

Detour and sieve effects have opposite impacts on absorption. Moreover, they are dominant in different spectral ranges. While the detour effect is more noticeable in bands of absorption minima [66], the sieve effect is more noticeable in bands of absorption maxima [67]. Because of this, absorption spectra with strong sieve effects show flattened absorption peaks, hence the alternative term *flattening effect*.

Northam and Baranoski [68] investigated the sieve factor in blood samples and its dependence on hct and blood sample thickness using *in silico* modeling, namely ray-casting techniques to compute the probability of a light ray intersecting these cells as it traverses a blood sample. In addition to a strong dependence on hct, they found a strong dependence on the blood sample thickness (see figure 4.7). However, the effect is noticeable only for low hct (below 10%) and thin sample thicknesses (below 1 mm).

4.5.2.4.2 Oxygenation

The absorption of whole blood depends on the oxygenation. The isosbestic point, where absorption is independent of the oxygenation level, is at 805 nm.

The difference in absorption between Hb and HbO_2 is used to determine blood oxygenation by optical means. In a typical scenario, two wavelengths are used, one with dominant Hb absorption (e.g., 660 nm) and one with dominant HbO_2 absorption (e.g., 880 nm).

4.5.2.4.3 Shear rate

RBC movement in blood vessels affects many things including optical interactions. Overall, absorption and scattering decrease slightly with increasing shear rate [62]. High shear rates deform the RBCs and their orientation in the flow (see figure 4.6 for illustration).

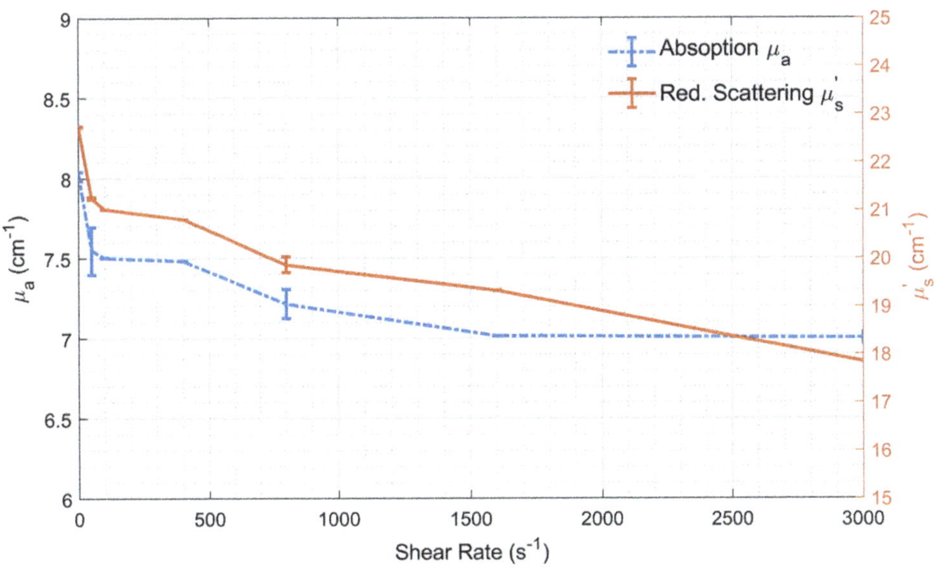

Figure 4.6. Mean values for μ_a and $\mu_{s'}$ versus shear rate. Modified with permission from [62], copyright (1998) Society of Photo-Optical Instrumentation Engineers (SPIE)..

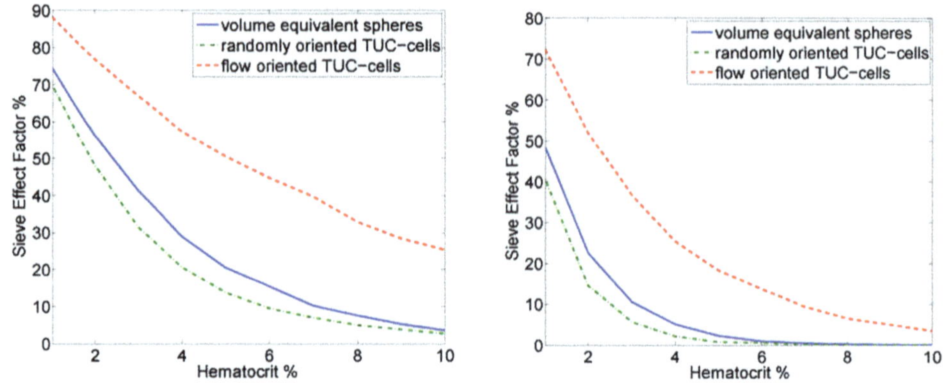

Figure 4.7. Plots of sieve effect factors (comparison with uniformly distributed hemoglobin from lysed blood cells) computed for blood samples with thickness equal to 0.1 mm (left panel) and 0.5 mm (right panel). Three representations for the erythrocytes were considered in these experiments: volume equivalent spheres, randomly oriented torus with a cylinder or TUC-cells, and flow-oriented TUC-cells. Reprinted with permission from[68], copyright Optica Publishing Group.

The optical impact of deformation is most likely relatively minimal, as Roggan *et al* [62] found that the deformation of erythrocytes had no significant impact on the optical properties when volume and hemoglobin content are kept constant.

However, flow-induced orientation (alignment) changes of RBCs may substantially influence optical properties through the sieve effect. In figure 4.7, the absorption depends significantly on the orientation of RBCs (randomly oriented versus flow-oriented). This effect is most likely noticeable only in solutions with low hematocrits (less than 10%) and thin thicknesses (less than 1 mm).

4.5.2.4.4 Osmolarity

A fluid's osmotic concentration or osmolality measures the total number of solute particles (measured in osmoles or Osm) per kilogram of solvent. Osmolarity is a very similar concept, which measures the total number of solute particles (measured in osmoles or Osm) per liter of solvent. Blood osmolality or osmolarity characterizes the body's electrolyte–water balance. The normal osmolality range is between 285 and 295 mOsm kg^{-1} for adults and 275 and 290 mOsm kg^{-1} for children [69]. Blood osmolarity is primarily regulated by vasopressin, also known as antidiuretic hormone (ADH), which controls the body's water balance.

Changes in the plasma osmolarity lead to significant changes in the shape of the erythrocytes. In hyper-osmotic plasma, RBCs shrink, often taking on a crenated appearance. In hypo-osmotic plasma, RBCs swell and may become spherical.

The shape of the RBCs affects the optical properties of blood. As mentioned, Roggan *et al* [62] found that increasing osmolarity leads to increased absorption while scattering and anisotropy decrease. Specifically, the absorption coefficient μ_a increases with osmolarity, i.e., with cell shrinkage. At 225 mOsm l^{-1}, μ_a amounted to 60% of the value measured under isotonic conditions (300 mOsm l^{-1}), while μ_a was 150% of the isotonic value at 450 mOsm l^{-1} [62].

4.5.2.4.5 Absorption heterogeneity

The blood distribution in tissues is highly heterogeneous. In healthy tissues, hemoglobin molecules are confined in the RBCs, and RBCs are confined within blood vessels. When hemoglobin strongly absorbs light, the light intensity in the center of the RBC or vessel will be less than at its periphery. As inner layers contribute less to absorption, it results in smaller apparent (or measured) absorption than theoretical absorption.

This mechanism is occasionally called *self-shielding* (see, for example, Moço *et al* [70]), and it causes spectral flattening. The self-shielding mechanism is similar for RBCs and blood vessels. However, they have different geometries: spherical or ellipsoidal in the case of RBCs and cylindrical in the case of blood vessels.

4.5.2.4.5.1 Red blood cells

Duysens [71] examined the absorption differences between particles in suspension and in solution, identifying this as a factor causing the absorption spectrum of a particle suspension to appear flattened compared to that of a solution. Building on Duysens' approach, Bosschaart *et al* [63] derived an absorption correction for blood

$$\mu_{a,\mathrm{bl}} = \frac{1 - \exp\left(-\mu_{a,\mathrm{RBC}} d_{\mathrm{RBC}}\right)}{\mu_{a,\mathrm{RBC}} d_{\mathrm{RBC}}} \mu_{a,\mathrm{Hb}} \tag{4.8}$$

where, $\mu_{a,\mathrm{bl}}$, and $\mu_{a,\mathrm{Hb}}$ are the absorption coefficient of a blood sample and hemoglobin solution, respectively. Here, d_{RBC} and $\mu_{a,\mathrm{RBC}}$ are the diameter of RBC and the absorption coefficient inside the RBC.

4.5.2.4.5.2 Blood vessel diameter

Similarly, due to strong light absorption by blood, the fluence rate near the center of the larger vessel is much lower than at the periphery. Thus, RBCs near the vessel's center absorb less light than those at the periphery. However, unlike RBCs, which have similar volumes, blood vessels have different diameters, which may impact light propagation. Thus, in the case of blood vessels, the correction factor depends on its diameter instead of a generic correction factor.

Verkruysse *et al* [72] investigated the effect of inhomogeneous blood distribution in tissues by calculating a single blood vessel's cross-sectional average fluence rate. They numerically estimated a scaling factor and found that diffuse and collimated light depends on the product of the blood vessel radius R and blood absorption coefficient, $\mu_{a,\mathrm{bl}}$. They observed that the use of a homogeneous distribution of blood to represent the influence of blood vessels on light distributions in skin tissue overestimates the influence of absorption of light by the blood when the absorption length ($1/\mu_{a,\mathrm{bl}}$) is equal to or less than the vessel radius R.

The scaling factor f connects the actual blood volume (C_{bl}) with the apparent blood volume ($C_{\mathrm{bl,app}}$):

$$C_{\mathrm{bl,app}} = f\left(\mu_{a,\mathrm{bl}} R\right) C_{\mathrm{bl}} \tag{4.9}$$

Several approaches have been proposed to approximate the scaling factor. For example, Moço *et al* [70] used the following scaling function for collimated light

$$f(\mu_{a,\text{bl}}R) = \frac{1}{1 + 1.007(\mu_{a,\text{bl}}R)^{1.228}} \tag{4.10}$$

4.5.3 Pathologies

The primary clinical utility of blood absorption-based techniques is to provide information about tissue perfusion[1]. While it is difficult to measure perfusion non-invasively, it can be done indirectly through its proxies, i.e., blood oxygen saturation or skin temperature. For example, blood oxygen saturation in microvasculature is the balance between blood supply (perfusion) and demand (consumption). Thus, one can indirectly assess the blood perfusion by determining blood oxygen saturation in the microvasculature. Blood absorption-based techniques do not provide direct information about perfusion. Instead, they typically provide information on the concentration of oxy- and deoxyhemoglobins. Other metrics, such as blood sO_2 and total hemoglobin (tHb), can be derived from this information.

As such, blood absorption techniques are helpful in the identification of abnormalities of circulation, including insufficiently low blood supply associated with hypoxia and abnormally high blood supply, which are typical for angiogenesis.

4.5.3.1 Hypoxia

Insufficient blood supply is characterized by the reduced sO_2.For example, Greenman *et al* [73] used hyperspectral imaging to measure blood oxygen saturation in healthy, diabetic, and diabetic neuropathic individuals. They found that in the foot at resting, sO_2 was lower in the neuropathic group (30±12; $p = 0.027$) than in the control (38±22) and non-neuropathic groups (37±12).

4.5.3.2 Angiogenesis

Optical imaging of cancers often finds elevated total hemoglobin (tHb), typically attributed to angiogenesis. For example, multiple studies found that breast carcinomas have an increased hemoglobin content compared to host tissue. Average values of this increase range from about 15% [74] to 200%. [75, 76]

4.6 Conclusions

Blood is a critically important biofluid responsible for transporting oxygen and nutrients to all body tissues and removing waste from them. Blood has distinct spectral features in the visible spectrum range, enabling multiple biomedical optical methods.

---

[1] Perfusion refers to fluid movement through the circulatory or lymphatic system towards a particular organ or tissue, typically in reference to the blood supply to capillary beds within tissues. The measurement of perfusion is based on the amount of blood delivered to the tissue per unit time per unit tissue mass ([ml/ml/s] or [ml/100 g min^{-1}]).

Blood absorption is dominated by the absorption of water and hemoglobins. Hemoglobins dominate in the 400–1100 nm range. Above 1350 nm, the blood absorption closely follows water absorption.

Among blood components, the optical properties of blood (including absorption) are dominated by RBCs, whose absorption and scattering are two to three orders of magnitude larger than those of the other blood components [25].

Several techniques are used for blood absorption measurements. The integrating sphere (IS) technique became the de facto gold standard in tissue optical measurements. A double integrating sphere (DIS) system is preferred for measuring fresh tissue samples as it allows simultaneous measurement of reflectance and transmittance from a sample.

Absorption of whole blood is affected by multiple factors, including hct, oxygenation, shear rate, and osmolarity. Due to the high heterogeneity of chromophore distribution in the blood (hemoglobins are concentrated in RBCs), optical measurements may be impacted by several effects, including the detour and sieve effects. As blood is a strong absorber for visible light, optical measurements are affected by the diameter of the blood vessels (a self-shielding effect). Thus, careful experimental planning is required.

Multiple blood absorption-based techniques have emerged for clinical use. Most newer modalities involve imaging. The primary clinical utility of blood absorption-based techniques is to provide information about tissue perfusion. They do it indirectly by providing total hemoglobin and blood oxygen saturation information. Thus, microcirculation abnormalities like insufficient blood supply (e.g., hypoxia) or abnormally high blood supply (e.g., angiogenesis) can be visualized.

References

[1] van Assendelft W 1970 *Spectrophotometry of Haemoglobin Derivatives* (Charles C Thomas)

[2] Ångström A J 1855 Optische Untersuchungen *Ann. PhysAnnal. Physik* **170** 141–65

[3] Hoppe–Seyler F 1862 Ueber das Verhalten des Blutfarbstoffes im Spectrum des Sonnenlichtes *Patholog. Anat. Physiol. Klin. Med.* **24** 441–9

[4] Soret J L 1878 Analyse spectrale: Sur le spectre d'absorption du sang dans la partie violette et ultra-violette *C. R. Acad. Sci.* **86** 1269

[5] Gamgee A and Hill A C 1902–1903 On the optical activity of haemoglobin and globin *Proc. Royal Soc. London* **71** 376–85

[6] Vierordt K 1873 *Die Anwendung des Spectralapparates zur Photometrie der Absorptionsspectren und zur quantitativen chemischen Analyse* (Tübingen: Verlag der H. Laupp'schen Buchhandlung)

[7] Hüfner G 1899 *Über den Ursprung und die Berechtigung besonderer Lehrstühle für physiologische Chemie* (Germany: F. Pietzcker)

[8] Drabkin D L and Austin J H 1935 Spectrophotometric studies: preparations from washed blood cells; nitric oxide hemoglobin and sulfhemoglobin *J. Biol. Chem.* **110** 51–65

[9] Heilmeyer L 1933 *Medizinische Spektrophotometrie* (Jena: Fischer)

[10] Hale G M and Querry M R 1973 Optical constants of water in the 200 nm to 200 micron wavelength region *Appl. Opt.* **12** 555–63

[11] Boulpaep E L 2009 'Blood' (chapter 18) *Medical Physiology* 2nd edn ed F Boron and E L Boulpaep (Philadelphia: Saunders) pp 448–81

[12] Prahl S 2001 https://omlc.org/spectra/

[13] Schaffer M R, Tantry U, Efron P A, Ahrendt G M, Thornton F J and Barbul A 1997 Diabetes-impaired healing and reduced wound nitric oxide synthesis: a possible pathophysiologic correlation *Surgery* **121** 513–9

[14] Minetti M and Malorni W 2006 Redox control of red blood cell biology: the red blood cell as a target and source of prooxidant species *Antioxid Redox Signal* **8** 1165–9

[15] Steinberg M H and Thein S L 2024 Fetal hemoglobin (Hb F) in health and disease https://uptodate.com/contents/fetal-hemoglobin-hb-f-in-health-and-disease (accessed 3 February 2024)

[16] Wawrzyniak A, Hamulka J, Friberg E *et al* 2013 Dietary, anthropometric, and lifestyle correlates of serum carotenoids in postmenopausal women *Eur. J. Nutr.* **52** 1919–26

[17] Grune T, Lietz G, Palou A *et al* 2010 β-carotene is an important vitamin A source for humans *J. Nutr.* **140** 2268S–85S

[18] Markell M and Siddiqi H A 2022 Vitamins and trace elements *Henry's Clinical Diagnosis and Management by Laboratory Methods* 24th edn. ed R A McPherson and M R Pincus (Philadelphia, PA: Elsevier) ch 27

[19] Mitra S and Rennie J 2017 Neonatal jaundice: aetiology, diagnosis and treatment *Br. J. Hosp. Med. (Lond.)* **78** 699–704

[20] Aernouts B, Zamora-Rojas E, Van Beers R *et al* 2013 Supercontinuum laser based optical characterization of Intralipid® phantoms in the 500–2250 nm range *Opt. Express* **21** 32450–67

[21] O'Keefe A and Deacon D A G 1988 Cavity ring-down optical spectrometer for absorption measurements using pulsed laser sources *Rev. Sci. Instrum.* **59** 2544

[22] Fiedler S E, Hese A and Ruth A A 2003 Incoherent broad-band cavity-enhanced absorption spectroscopy *Chem. Phys. Lett.* **371** 284–94

[23] Roggan A, Albrecht H J, Doerschel K *et al* 1995 Experimental set-up and Monte-Carlo model for the determination of optical tissue properties in the wavelength range 330 to 1100 nm *Laser Interaction with Hard and Soft Tissue II* **vol 2323** (SPIE) pp 21–36

[24] Prahl S A, van Gemert M J C and Welch A J 1993 Determining the optical properties of turbid media by using the adding-doubling method *Appl. Opt.* **32** 559–68

[25] Meinke M, Müller G, Helfmann J and Friebel M 2007 Optical properties of platelets and blood plasma and their influence on the optical behavior of whole blood in the visible to near infrared wavelength range *J. Biomed. Opt.* **12** 014024

[26] Pickering J W, Prahl S A, van Wieringen N *et al* 1993 Double-integrating-sphere system for measuring the optical properties of tissue *Appl. Opt.* **32** 399–410

[27] Lemaillet P, Bouchard J-P, Hwang J and Allen D W 2015 Double-integrating-sphere system at the National Institute of Standards and Technology in support of measurement standards for the determination of optical properties of tissue-mimicking phantoms *J. Biomed. Opt.* **20** 121310

[28] Nitzan M, Romem A and Koppel R 2014 Pulse oximetry: fundamentals and technology update *Med Devices (Auckl).* **7** 231–9

[29] Anand S, Sujatha N, Narayanamurthy V B *et al* 2014 Diffuse reflectance spectroscopy for monitoring diabetic foot ulcer—a pilot study *Optics Lasers Eng* **53** 1–5

[30] Perrey S and Ferrari M 2018 Muscle oximetry in sports science: a systematic review *Sports Med* **48** 597–616

[31] Durduran T, Choe R, Baker W B and Yodh A G 2010 Diffuse optics for tissue monitoring and tomography *Rep. Prog. Phys.* **73** 076701
[32] Ferrari M and Quaresima V 2012 A brief review on the history of human functional near-infrared spectroscopy (fNIRS) development and fields of application *NeuroImage* **63** 921–35
[33] Hoshi Y and Yamada Y 2016 Overview of diffuse optical tomography and its clinical applications *J. Biomed. Opt.* **21** 091312
[34] Lu G and Fei B 2014 Medical hyperspectral imaging: a review *J. Biomed. Opt.* **19** 010901
[35] Khaodhiar L, Dinh T, Schomacker K T *et al* 2007 The use of medical hyperspectral technology to evaluate microcirculatory changesin diabetic foot ulcers and to predict clinical outcomes *Diabetes Care* **30** 903–10
[36] Leahy M J, Enfield J G, Clancy N T *et al* 2007 Biophotonic methods in microcirculation imaging *Med. Laser Appl.;* **22** 105–26
[37] Xia J, Yao J and Wang L V 2014 Photoacoustic tomography: principles and advances *Electromagn. Waves (Camb)* **147** 1–22
[38] Wang L V 2008 Tutorial on photoacoustic microscopy and computed tomography' selected topics in quantum electronics *IEEE J.* **14** 171–9
[39] Beard P 2011 Biomedical photoacoustic imaging *Interface Focus* **1** 602–31
[40] Yang J, Zhang G, Chang W *et al* 2020 Photoacoustic imaging of hemodynamic changes in forearm skeletal muscle during cuff occlusion *Biomed. Opt. Express* **11** 4560–70
[41] Boyer D, Tamarat P, Maali A *et al* 2002 Photothermal imaging of nanometer-sized metal particles among scatterers *Science* **297** 1160–3
[42] Berciaud S, Lasne D, Blab G A *et al* 2006 Photothermal heterodyne imaging of individual metallic nanoparticles: theory versus experiment *Phys. Rev. B: Condens. Matter Mater. Phys.* **73** 045424
[43] Adhikari S, Spaeth P, Kar A *et al* 2020 Photothermal microscopy: imaging the optical absorption of single nanoparticles and single molecules *ACS Nano* **14** 16414–45
[44] Lu S, Min W, Chong S *et al* 2010 Label-free imaging of heme proteins with two-photon excited photothermal lens microscopy *Appl. Phys. Lett.* **96** 113701
[45] Kaza N, Ojaghi A and Robles F E 2021 Hemoglobin quantification in red blood cells via dry mass mapping based on UV absorption *J. Biomed. Opt.* **26** 086501
[46] Zijlstra W G and Buursma A 1997 Spectrophotometry of hemoglobin: absorption spectra of bovine oxyhemoglobin, deoxyhemoglobin, carboxyhemoglobin, and methemoglobin *Compar. Biochem. Physiol. B: Biochem. Mol. Biol.* **118** 743–9
[47] Prahl S https://omlc.org/spectra/hemoglobin/summary.html
[48] Faber D J, Aalders M C G, Mik E G *et al* 2004 Oxygen saturation-dependent absorption and scattering of blood *Phys. Rev. Lett.* **93** 028102
[49] 2006 InformedHealth.org *What Does Blood Do?* (Cologne, Germany: Institute for Quality and Efficiency in Health Care (IQWiG)) https://ncbi.nlm.nih.gov/books/NBK279392/
[50] Morgner F, Stufler S, Geissler D *et al* 2011 Terbium to quantum dot FRET bioconjugates for clinical diagnostics: influence of human plasma on optical and assembly properties *Sensors (Basel, Switzerland)* **11** 9667–84
[51] Ribed-Sánchez B, González-Gaya C, Varea-Díaz S *et al* 2018 Economic analysis of the reduction of blood transfusions during surgical procedures while continuous hemoglobin monitoring is used *Sensors (Basel, Switzerland)* **18** 1367
[52] Hale G M and Querry M R 1973 Optical constants of water in the 200 nm to 200 μm wavelength region *Appl. Opt.* **12** 555–63

[53] Querry M R, Wieliczka D M and Segelstein D J 1991 Water (H_2O) *Handbook of Optical Constants of Solids II* (Academic) pp 1059–77
[54] Prahl S https://omlc.org/spectra/water/abs/index.html
[55] Zijlstra W G, Buursma A and van Assendelft O W 2000 *Visible and Near Infrared Absorption Spectra of Human and animal Haemoglobin* (Utrecht: VSP)
[56] Gratzer W B and Kollias N 1999 Personal communication from Gratzer *Medical Research Council Labs* (Holly Hill, London, and N Kollias: Wellman Laboratories, Harvard Medical School, Boston)
[57] Moaveni M K 1970 A multiple scattering field theory applied to whole blood *PhD Dissertation* Department of Electrical Engineering, University of Washington
[58] Schmitt J M 1986 *Optical measurement of blood oxygenation by implantable telemetry* Technical Report G558-15
[59] Takatani S and Graham M D 1987 Theoretical analysis of diffuse reflectance from a two-layer tissue model *IEEE Trans. Biomed. Eng., BME* **26** 656–64
[60] Zijlstra W G, Buursma A and Meeuwsen-van der Roest W P 1991 Absorption spectra of human fetal and adult oxyhemoglobin, de-oxyhemoglobin, carboxyhemoglobin, and methemoglobin *Clin. Chem.* **37** 1633–8
[61] Miale J B 1982 *Laboratory Medicine: Hematology* (C.V. Mosby Company)
[62] Roggan A, Friebel M, Dorschel K *et al* 1999 Optical properties of circulating human blood in the wavelength range 400–2500 nm *J. Biomed. Optics* **4** 36–46
[63] Bosschaart N, Edelman G J, Aalders M C, van Leeuwen T G and Faber D J 2014 A literature review and novel theoretical approach on the optical properties of whole blood *Lasers Med. Sci.* **29** 453–79
Erratum in:Bosschaart N, Edelman G J, Aalders M C G, van Leeuwen T G and Faber D J 2022 Correction to: A literature review and novel theoretical approach on the optical properties of whole blood *Lasers Med. Sci.* **37** 691
[64] Hanson E K and Ballantyne J 2010 A blue spectral shift of the hemoglobin soret band correlates with the age (time since deposition) of dried bloodstains *PLoS One* **5** e12830
[65] Butler W L 1964 Absorption spectroscopy *in vivo*: theory and applications *Ann. Rev. Plant Physiol.* **15** 451–70
[66] Garlaschi F, Zucchelli G and Jennings R 1989 Studies on light absorption and photochemical activity changes in chloroplast suspensions and leaves due to light scattering and light filtartion across chloroplasts and vegetation layers *Photosynth. Res.* **20** 207–20
[67] Rabinowitch E I 1951 *Light Absorption by Pigments in the Living Cell* **vol II** (New York: Interscience Publishers) ch 22
[68] Northam L and Baranoski G V G 2010 A novel first principles approach for the estimation of the sieve factor of blood samples *Opt. Express* **18** 7456–69
[69] https://webmd.com/a-to-z-guides/serum-osmolality-test
[70] Moço A V, Stuijk S and de Haan G 2018 New insights into the origin of remote PPG signals in visible light and infrared *Sci. Rep.* **8** 8501
[71] Duyens L N M 1956 The flattening of the absorption spectrum of suspensions, as compared to that of solutions *Biochim. Biophys. Acta* **19** 1–12
[72] Verkruysse W, Lucassen G W, de Boer J F *et al* 1997 Modelling light distributions of homogeneous versus discrete absorbers in light irradiated turbid media *Phys. Med. Biol.* **42** 51–65

[73] Greenman R L, Panasyuk S, Wang X *et al* 2005 Early changes in the skin microcirculation and muscle metabolism of the diabetic foot *Lancet* **366** 1711–7
[74] Choe R, Konecky S D, Corlu A *et al* 2009 Differentiation of benign and malignant breast tumors by in-vivo three-dimensional parallel-plate diffuse optical tomography *J. Biomed. Optics* **14** 024020–0
[75] Grosenick D, Wabnitz H, Moesta K T *et al* 2005 Time-domain scanning optical mammography: II. Optical properties and tissue parameters of 87 carcinomas *Phys. Med. Biol.* **50** 2451
[76] Spinelli L, Torricelli A, Pifferi A *et al* 2005 Characterization of female breast lesions from multi-wavelength time-resolved optical mammography *Phys. Med. Biol.* **50** 2489

IOP Publishing

The Optics of Blood
A Handbook
Alexandre Douplik

Chapter 5

Refractometry of blood

Gennadi Saiko, Timothy Burton and Alexandre Douplik

5.1 Introduction

Refraction is a fundamental property of light on the interface between two media. It gives rise to the whole range of physical phenomena, including scattering, reflection, and total internal reflection.

The optical properties of biofluids (including refractive index) contain important information about health. Different diseases may cause local or integral changes of the refractive index, making refractive index a potential marker to differentiate between healthy and pathological conditions [1]. For example, refractive index measurements were proposed to monitor blood protein glycation [2].

In addition to new and promising applications, knowledge of refractive index is important for a wide group of existing applications. For example, knowledge of the refractive index of red blood cells (RBCs) can be used to derive their hemoglobin (Hb) content and corresponding cell volume from light scattering measurements in flow cytometry [3].

In this chapter we will explore optical properties of the blood and blood components with particular focus on their refractive index. We will start with discussing methods how the refractive index of blood and its components is determined. Then, we will consider experimental results obtained for blood and its components.

5.1.1 Group versus phase velocity

Phase velocity and group velocity are two important concepts in wave mechanics. Phase velocity is the speed at which a point of constant phase travels as the wave propagates. Group velocity is the velocity with which the overall envelope shape of the wave's amplitudes—known as the modulation or envelope of the wave—propagates

doi:10.1088/978-0-7503-4806-5ch5

through space. It is defined as $v_g = \frac{\partial \omega}{\partial k}$, where ω is the angular frequency of the wave, and k is the wavenumber[1].

If the angular velocity ω is directly proportional to wavenumber k, then the group velocity is exactly equal to the phase velocity. However, it is not true in many cases. Thus, as refractive index describes the relative speed of the electromagnetic wave in media compared to the speed of light in vacuum, then two types of refractive indices are possible: related to phase velocity, n, and related to the group velocity n_g.

In this chapter, by refractive index we will refer to the refractive index associated with the phase velocity. The group refractive index, n_g, can be found from the phase refractive index, n, using dispersion equation:

$$n_g(\omega) = n(\omega) + \omega \frac{\partial n}{\partial \omega} \tag{5.1}$$

5.2 Experimental techniques

Experimental techniques, which are used to determine the refractive index of blood and blood components, can be roughly split into two large groups: refractometry and synthetic methods that are based on absorption measurements and consequent application of the Kramers–Kronig (KK) transformation.

As absorption measurement techniques were discussed in chapter 4 of this book, we will limit our discussion of this group of techniques to Kramers–Kronig transformation.

5.2.1 Synthetic methods based on Kramers–Kronig transformation

The refractive index can be considered as a complex function, which gives an ability to use the powerful mathematical apparatus of complex analysis.

In particular, the complex refractive index $m(\omega)$ can be split into the sum of real and imaginary parts $m(\omega) = n(\omega) + i\kappa(\omega)$, where the imaginary part refers to dissipation, which can be linked to the absorption coefficient [4]

$$\kappa(\omega) = \frac{c\mu_a}{2\omega} \tag{5.2}$$

Here, c is the speed of light, and ω is the angular frequency of light.

For realistic physical systems, the response $\chi(t-t')$ to an initial action at the moment t' must be zero for $t < t'$, since a system cannot respond to a force before it is applied. It can be shown (see, for example [5]) that this causality implies that the Fourier transform $\chi(\omega)$ of the response function $\chi(t-t')$ is analytic in the upper-half plane of the complex plane.

[1] By convention in spectroscopy, the wavenumbers (measured in [cm^{-1}]) are used instead of wavelengths. Wavelength can be converted in wavenumber using ν [cm^{-1}] = 10 000/λ [μm].

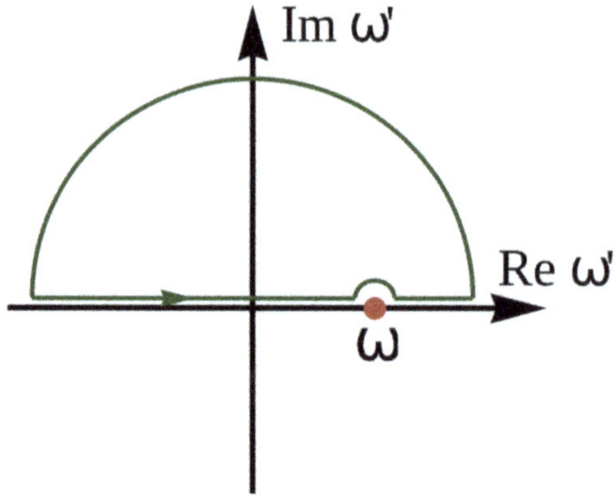

Figure 5.1. Integral contour for deriving Kramers–Kronig equations. This image has been obtained by the author(s) from the Wikimedia website [https://commons.wikimedia.org/w/index.php?curid=5553863], where it is stated to have been released into the public domain. It is included within this article on that basis.

For a complex function $\chi(\omega)$, which is analytic in the closed upper-half of the complex plane ω, and diminishes faster than $1/|\omega|$ for $\omega\to\infty$, the Cauchy's residue theorem can be applied (see figure 5.1), which gives the following expression:

$$\chi(\omega) = \frac{1}{i\pi} PV \int_{-\infty}^{\infty} \frac{\chi(\omega')}{\omega' - \omega} d\omega' \tag{5.3}$$

Here, PV denotes the Cauchy principal value of the integral (figure 5.1).

Thus, for the complex refractive index $m(\omega)$: $m(\omega) = n(\omega) + i\kappa(\omega)$, the following equations can be derived, which link real and imaginary parts:

$$n(\omega) = \frac{1}{\pi} PV \int_{-\infty}^{\infty} \frac{\kappa(\omega')}{\omega' - \omega} d\omega' \tag{5.4}$$

and

$$\kappa(\omega) = -\frac{1}{\pi} PV \int_{-\infty}^{\infty} \frac{n(\omega')}{\omega' - \omega} d\omega' \tag{5.5}$$

These equations are known as Kramers–Kronig (KK) equations or KK transformation.

However, for practical purposes, further simplifications can be done for realistic physical systems. In particular, we can realistically assume that $\chi(-\omega) = \chi^*(\omega)$, which means that its real part is an even function and imaginary part is an odd function. Thus, by multiplying the numerator and denominator of the integrand in equation (5.3) by $\omega + \omega'$, after some simple transformations we can reduce integration to the physically meaningful $[0, \infty)$ interval:

$$n(\omega) = \frac{2}{\pi} PV \int_{0}^{\infty} \frac{\omega' \kappa(\omega')}{\omega'^2 - \omega^2} d\omega' \tag{5.6}$$

and

$$\kappa(\omega) = -\frac{2\omega}{\pi} PV \int_0^\infty \frac{n(\omega')}{\omega'^2 - \omega^2} d\omega' \tag{5.7}$$

Further improvements have been proposed. For example, a subtractive KK equation [6] offers greater convergence than the conventional expression (equation (5.6)) when reflectance data are available over a limited spectral range:

$$n(\omega) = n(\omega_0) + \frac{1}{2\pi}(\omega^2 - \omega_0^2) PV \int_0^\infty \frac{\omega' \kappa(\omega')}{(\omega^2 - \omega'^2)(\omega_0^2 - \omega'^2)} d\omega' \tag{5.8}$$

where $n(\omega_0)$ is the refractive index measured at a reference frequency ω_0 to provide scaling of the calculated curves.

5.2.2 Explicit refractive index measurements

A myriad of techniques exist to use light for determining the refractive index in general, and of blood specifically, including those based on scattering, transmission/absorption, interference, and diffraction.

5.2.2.1 Abbé refractometry

The Abbé refractometer was the first commercially available device to measure refractive index, designed by Ernst Abbé in 1869 and commercialized by Carl Zeiss in 1881. Abbé refractometry measures refractive index using an instrument designed to leverage Snell's Law, where n_1 and n_2 are the refractive indices of the first and second mediums, respectively, and i and r are the angles of incidence and refraction, respectively:

$$n_1 \sin(i) = n_2 \sin(r) \tag{5.9}$$

The Abbé refractometer measures the refractive index of a sample placed between two prisms—an illuminating prism and a refracting prism. Light (of any wavelength) from a source enters the illuminating prism and passes through a matted surface that contacts the sample. This allows light to enter the sample at various angles. The refracting prism then refracts the light, and if the angle is suitable, it passes through; otherwise, it undergoes total internal reflection. The refracted light creates a distinct boundary or shadow line, and the user observes this boundary to determine the critical angle, which is used to calculate the refractive index of the sample according to the following rearrangement of Snell's law:

$$n_2 = n_1 \frac{\sin(i)}{\sin(r)} \tag{5.10}$$

The disadvantage of using Abbé refractometry to study blood is that, due to the high absorption of blood, the sample must be very thin to get an accurate refractive index (~10 μm) [7]. However, since blood cells have an approximate thickness of 1.2–2.2 μm [8], it is only possible to have a few layers of blood cells in the samples, significantly impacting the realism of the sample.

5.2.2.2 *Current measurement techniques*

Beyond Abbé refractometry, over the last decades, various techniques to determine refractive index of biological tissues were developed, including: confocal microscopy [9, 10], optical fiber cladding method [11], minimum deviation angle method [12, 13], optical coherence tomography [14] with multiple modifications, total internal reflection method [15–17], measurement of the intensity profile of diffuse light refracted into the prism around the critical angle [18], various modifications of nonlinear phase microscopy [19–21], and quantitative phase imaging techniques.

5.2.2.2.1 Confocal microscopy

Confocal microscopy enhances traditional optical stage microscopy through the rejection of out of focus light, enabling high resolution imaging of deep tissues [9, 10]. Confocal microscopy functions by focusing both the point light source and detection optics on a single, diffraction-limited, spot. Anything outside of that spot is rejected as out of focus noise. The spot is moved across the full sample to build a complete image. The wavelength of the light source may vary, from UV to visible light, to IR, depending on what may achieve maximum fluorescence of the sample.

Confocal microscopy may be used to measure the refractive index of a biological sample using the axial scaling factor. Specifically, changes at the interface between the immersion medium and sample causes axial scaling, introducing differences between the optical and physical thicknesses of the sample. By accounting for the point spread function, refractive index can be derived from axial scaling factor.

5.2.2.2.2 Optical fiber cladding

Optical fiber cladding is material that surrounds an optical fiber to confine the light within the fiber core, possible through a lower refractive index than the fiber core, causing total internal reflection, thus enabling light propagation. Further, the angle at which the light emerges from the optical fiber is determined by the refractive indices of the cladding material, along with the optical fiber and the air. Since the refractive indices of the optical fiber and air are known, the refractive index of the cladding material may be determined given the known refractive indices and the angle of the emergent light. This principle may be utilized to determine the refractive index of biological samples by removing any existing cladding material from the optical fiber, and creating an experimental design that involves routing the fiber through the sample [11].

5.2.2.2.3 Minimum deviation angle method

The minimum deviation angle is determined experimentally by varying the angle of incidence and measuring the corresponding angle of deviation to find the minimum value, which occurs when the incident ray and the refracted ray are symmetrical with respect to the prism's base. The refractive index can then be measured using Snell's law.

To measure the refractive index of a sample (liquid, in this case) using the minimum deviation angle method, a hollow prism can be filled with the sample, and an appropriate wavelength of laser selected (e.g., to minimize scattering and absorption) [13].

However, while this method is a fundamental technique, it has limitations. Firstly, angle measurements, including the prism angle, must be precise to prevent propagating error in the refractive index measurement. Secondly, the laser beam must penetrate the sample with minimal scattering and absorption, to ensure that the emergent beam is measurable, and therefore this technique is not well-suited to solid sample types.

5.2.2.2.4 Optical coherence tomography

Optical coherence tomography (OCT) uses interferometry, with short coherence length light, to interrogate the sample. OCT instrumentation is composed of an interferometer, with a split beam that is directed to both the sample, and a reference mirror. OCT can be used to assess refractive index using multiple techniques [14]. For instance, OCT measurement of optical path length may be used to derive the refractive index, though this is more suited to physically thin samples (e.g., *ex vivo* tissue). However, thicker samples (e.g., noninvasive measurement of *in vivo* tissue) may be assessed through movement of the sample stage towards the objective of a specific distance, and then movement of the reference until maximum signal is detected—based on the two distances, Snell's law can be used to derive the refractive index.

5.2.2.2.5 Total internal reflection

The principle of measurement of refractive index using total internal reflection is similar to the basis of Abbé refractometry; however, only one prism is required, and light is reflected from the interface of this prism and the sample. The reflected light is captured for assessment of refractive index, thus enabling the study of samples with higher optical thickness.

The fundamental concept of such a device is the use of a triangular prism upon which the sample is placed, as well as a laser emitter and detector. For instance, an experimental design used a triangular prism with a refractive index of 1.515 at a wavelength of 632.8 nm, which was provided by a He–Ne laser emitter [15]. A detector captures the reflected light from the prism. The emitter and detector are rotated in a synchronized manner around the stationary prism and sample, and the light recorded at each angle, to ensure comprehensive measurement across the spectrum of incident light angles. Snell's law is used to calculate the refractive index based on the angle of the reflected light.

The investigators determined that the described device is capable of measuring refractive indices from 1.0 to 1.51. Should the refractive index of the sample be projected to be in a higher range, then the prism can be substituted for an alternative with a higher refractive index (for example, a refractive index of 1.62 can cover 1.33–1.61).

5.2.2.2.6 Diffuse light intensity profile

Diffuse light is an underutilized light–tissue interaction in the assessment of refractive index. A device has been proposed to isolate diffuse light for this purpose: a semi-cylindrical prism is positioned atop the sample, with a laser providing the emitted light that traverses the prism and interacts with the sample [17]. A plano-concave lens, followed by a thin convex lens, is used to direct the light into a CCD camera. The diffuse light that is emitted by the sample into the prism is limited to a cone, with the angle of the cone dictated by the refractive indices of both the sample and prism. The camera then registers the angle. Calibration of the device is performed using water as the sample.

5.2.2.2.7 ***Nonlinear phase microscopy***

Absorption, scattering, refraction, and fluorescence are light–tissue interactions that can be used through conventional (linear) microscopy to derive refractive index. In contrast, nonlinear phase microscopy utilizes interactions such as second harmonic generation, which is the interaction of two photons of the same frequency with a material, resulting in the generation of a photon with twice the energy of the original photons [21]. Second harmonic generation only occurs in non-centrosymmetric media (i.e., does not have inversion symmetry). Many biological materials are non-centrosymmetric (e.g., muscle, collagen) and therefore exhibit second harmonic generation.

Experimentally, second harmonic generation can be exploited to determine refractive index through phase extraction from holographic second harmonic generation microscopy, though the refractive index derivation is complex.

5.2.2.2.8 Other methods

Wang *et al* [22] proposed a new method for measuring continuous refractive index dispersion (CRID). They used a homemade symmetrical arm-linked apparatus to measure refractive index of solutions. The method is based on the measurement of reflection coefficient on sample/air interface measured at different incident angles in a continuous wavelength range. Then using Fresnel equations, the refractive index is derived. They alluded that the developed method is superior to the Fresnel reflectance measurement, for avoiding the problem of light saturation in highly concentrated Hb solutions.

5.2.2.3 IR range

Interferometry is a common method to extract refractive index of samples. In particular, Michelson interferometric schema is commonly used. In this schema, the interferogram of a sample is acquired. The phase shift is calculated from the interferogram. Then, for the known path length, the refractive index can be easily extracted. Interferometric schema is the basis of several quantitative phase imaging (QPI) techniques (see section 5.3.2).

However, interferometric techniques are more commonly used in infrared range of the spectrum. In particular, it is the core technology in Fourier transform infrared (FTIR) spectroscopy [23]. FTIR is a method of obtaining infrared spectra, which includes initially the collection of an interferogram of a sample signal using an interferometer and then performance of a Fourier transform (FT) on the interferogram to obtain the spectrum.

As a spectroscopic technique in the infrared range of spectrum FTIR is preferred to the traditional dispersion optics. In particular, it allows faster acquisition time.

FTIR can be performed in three modes: transmission, attenuated total reflectance (ATR), and reflectance.

In transmission mode as light passes through the sample, typically it requires sample preparation (e.g. dilution).

ATR is the most common sampling method in FTIR, as it does not require sample preparation. ATR technique (see, for example, [24]) measures the changes that occur to an internally reflected IR beam when the beam comes into contact with a sample. An IR beam is directed through an optically dense crystal with a high refractive index on the interface with the sample at the angle larger than the critical angle. The total internal reflectance creates an evanescent wave that extends beyond the surface of the crystal into the sample held in contact with the crystal. The probing depth is several micrometers.

Reflectance mode (specular reflection and diffuse reflectance or DRIFTS) is typically used for analysis of solid samples, where transmission mode or ATR are impossible or impractical.

The refractive index can be obtained from FTIR system in several ways. Firstly, it can be done from absorption spectra using the Kramers–Kronig transformation (see section 5.2.1). Secondly, it can be assessed by measuring the total internal reflection angle in ATR mode (as the ATR prism has high refractive index).

Bonnal *et al* [25] proposed a new approach to determine the complex refractive index in the IR range, which uses a classical setup to control the incident angle, without the need for a polarizer. They found that the refractive index can be measured with a relative uncertainty close to 10^{-3} over a wide range of wavelengths.

5.3 Methods based on refractive index

Multiple methods exploit refractive index of blood explicitly or implicitly. Here, we present several common refractive index-based approaches used in life sciences.

5.3.1 Qualitative assessment of compounds

The use of transmitted light is also an effective mechanism to measure the refractive index of blood. In one application, Ali *et al* [26] sought to use red laser light (650 nm) to non-invasively measure blood glucose concentration, which is a key unmet clinical need, as diabetic patients currently need to prick their fingers to monitor glucose. Integral to the working principle of their proposed technique is that glucose molecules modify the refractive index of blood proportionally to their concentration (see section 5.4.1), and therefore changes in measured refractive index likely correspond to changes in blood glucose—increasing concentration yielding decreasing refractive angle. Specifically, emitted laser light is transmitted through the tissue and is refracted proportional to the glucose concentration, then striking a photodetector that registers the angle of the beam. Given the calculated calibration, the glucose concentration can then be determined. The refractive index device was validated on a cohort of ten healthy subjects using a standard finger prick glucose instrument as the gold standard, exhibiting a relative error of 3%–8%, with variations due to sources such as shape and thickness of the finger and swelling caused by the laser light.

5.3.2 Quantitative phase imaging

Quantitative phase imaging (QPI) has emerged in recent years as a valuable method for investigating cells and tissues. As the images represent quantitative maps of optical path-length delays introduced by the specimen, QPI provides an objective measure of morphology and dynamics, free of variability due to contrast agents [27]. Several approaches to QPI have emerged.

Diffraction phase microscopy, DPM is a common-path QPI method, capable to accurately monitor the dynamics of various nanoscale phenomena in a wide variety of environments [28], including *in situ*. The method combines the principles of common-path interferometry and single-shot phase imaging and is characterized by subnanometer path-length stability and millisecond-scale acquisition time [29].

Tomographic phase microscopy (TPM) uses digital holographic measurements of complex scattered fields to reconstruct three-dimensional refractive index maps of cells with diffraction-limited resolution by solving inverse scattering problems [30].

Ojaghi *et al* [31] developed ultraviolet hyperspectral interferometric (UHI) microscopy. A key element of this technology is the use of a 4 *f* interferometric setup that permits coherent detection using an incoherent, broadband light source. The system consists of a modified Mach-Zehnder interferometer with a series of lenses in a 4 *f* configuration to limit the number of modes illuminating each detected region of the sample, where each light-mode to be given by the square of the transverse coherence length of the light source. With Fourier domain (FD) detection, this configuration yields an interferometric signal with high fringe visibility, and access to the complex optical fields across a large spectral region (e.g., 240–450 nm). The method can recover quantitative phase images with sensitivity to optical path lengths in the order of 1 nm.

5.4 Experimental results

5.4.1 Blood and component refractive indices

Blood represents a complex mixture of components dominated by water. If we know the refractive index of these components, there are several analytical approaches, which can be used to calculate the refractive index of the media.

In particular, the law of Gladstone and Dale states that resulting value of refractive index of a mixed substance is represented as the average of the refractive indices of the components related to their volume fraction, i.e.,

$$n = \sum_{i=1}^{N} n_i f_i \tag{5.11}$$

where n_i and f_i are the refractive index and volume fraction of the individual components, respectively, and N is the number of the components [32].

Modeling of the behavior of refractive index of tissues, blood, and their components, can be based on a remarkable property of proteins: that equal concentrations of aqueous solutions of different proteins all have approximately the same refractive index, n_{pw} [33]. Moreover, the refractive index varies almost linearly with concentration, c_p:

$$n_{pw}(\lambda) = n_w(\lambda) + \alpha_p(\lambda)\, c_p \tag{5.12}$$

where n_w is refractive index of water and α_p is the specific refractive increment; c_p is measured in grams per 100 ml (g dl^{-1}). For example, the refractive index of human erythrocyte cytoplasm, defined by the cell-bounded Hb solution, can be found from this equation at $\alpha_p = 0.001\,942$ valid for a wavelength of 589 nm; i.e., for normal Hb concentration in cytoplasm of 300–360 g l^{-1}, the RBC refractive index $n_{RBC} = 1.393$–1.406 [34]. Values of specific refractive increment α_p for total serum (human) and total albumin measured by Abbé refractometer at a wavelength 589 nm were found to be 0.00179 and 0.00181, respectively [12].

The refractive indices of water over a broad wavelength range from 200 nm to 200 μm have been reported by Hale and Querry [35] and can be approximated by the following expression:

$$\begin{aligned} n_w = {} & 1.58 - 8.45 \times 10^{-4}\lambda + 1.1 \times 10^{-6}\lambda^2 - 7.19 \times 10^{-10}\lambda^3 \\ & + 2.32 \times 10^{-13}\lambda^4 - 2.98 \times 10^{-17}\lambda^5 \end{aligned} \tag{5.13}$$

Here, the wavelength λ is measured in [nm]. As the refractive index of the water depends on the wavelength, the blood's refractive index depends on the wavelength too. Thus, blood can be considered as a dispersive medium[2].

Dispersion curves of the blood and its components are typically characterized by several standard fitting functions (e.g. the Cauchy equation for plasma).

It should be noted that typically the optical properties of blood and its components are measured at several wavelengths. Just several works have measured the refractive index across whole spectral regions. For example, Liu *et al* [36] using an internal reflection technique measured the refractive indexes of whole blood and its components, such as serum, plasma, and Hb in the spectral range of 400–750 nm with spectral resolution of about 0.263 nm.

Below, we will summarize experimental results for various blood components.

5.4.1.1 Serum and plasma

Meinke *et al* [37] using an Abbé refractometer found that the refractive index of plasma is 1.3577 at 400 nm, 1.3506 at 500 nm, 1.3473 at 600 nm, and 1.3438 at 700 nm.

Jin *et al* [16] measured the refractive indexes of serum and plasma and reported only a marginal difference between them.

[2] In optics, dispersion (or chromatic dispersion) is the phenomenon in which the phase velocity of a wave depends on its frequency. A medium having this property is termed a dispersive medium.

Table 5.1. Estimations for empirical coefficients of the Cauchy equation (CRID—complex refractive index dispersion).

Sample	A	B	C	Method, range, and source
Serum	1.3350	4.6513×10^3	-1.3069×10^8	Continuous CRID, 400–750 nm [36]
Plasma	1.3353	4.4048×10^3	-9.1925×10^7	Continuous CRID, 400–750 nm [36]
Human whole blood	1.3587	1.4744×10^3	1.7103×10^9	488, 632.8, 1079.5 and 1341.4 nm [39]
Human whole plasma	1.3194	1.4578×10^4	-1.7383×10^9	488, 632.8, 1079.5 and 1341.4 nm [39]

The refractive indexes of serum and plasma in the visible range of spectrum decrease while the wavelength increases. The most common approach to characterize dispersion of serum and plasma is to use the so-called Cauchy equation:

$$n_r = A + \frac{B}{\lambda^2} + \frac{C}{\lambda^4} \tag{5.14}$$

Here, the empirical coefficients A, B, and C are calculated by a fitting program, and λ is the wavelength [nm]. Estimations for empirical coefficients of the Cauchy equation reported by several groups are presented in table 5.1.

Tuchin *et al* [38] obtained another approximation for refractive index of blood plasma in the 400–1000 nm spectral range, which include an extra term

$$n_{bp} = 1.3254 + 8.4052 \times 10^3\lambda^{-2} - 3.9572 \times 10^8\lambda^{-4} - 2.3617 \times 10^{13}\lambda^{-6} \tag{5.15}$$

Another approximation, which is commonly used in blood optics is the so-called Sellmeier formula:

$$n^2(\lambda) = 1 + \frac{A_1\lambda^2}{\lambda^2 - B_1} + \frac{A_2\lambda^2}{\lambda^2 - B_2} \tag{5.16}$$

For example, Liu *et al* [36] used it to approximate the dispersion of the whole blood.

5.4.1.2 Hemoglobin

Faber *et al* [4] determined the complex refractive index of oxygenated and deoxygenated Hb in the wavelength range 250–1000 nm using a Kramers–Kronig analysis from tabulated data[3]. The calculated values were calibrated with optical path at 800 nm explicitly measured using OCT. They found that the refractive index depends on oxygenation.

[3] Tabulated data from various sources compiled by S Prahl at http://omlc.ogi.edu/spectra.

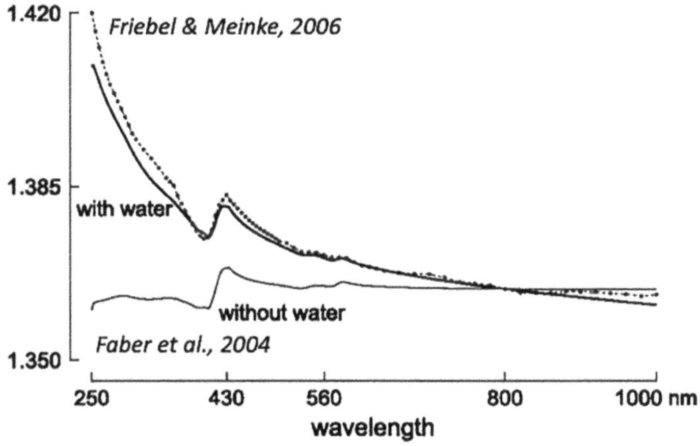

Figure 5.2. Real part of the complex refractive index of HbO2 obtained from a subtractive KK analysis with (upper solid curve) and without (lower solid curve) inclusion of water RI dispersion. Modified with permission from [43], copyright 2012 Society of Photo-Optical Instrumentation Engineers (SPIE).

The Hb solution demonstrates anomalous dispersion at 420 nm (the Soret band) and slight anomalies in the range of 500–600 nm (Q bands) (see figure 5.2).

Friebel and Meinke [40] used Fresnel reflectance to measure the real part of the complex refractive index of oxygenated native Hb solutions in the wavelength range 250–1100 nm. They measured several concentrations, including 0, 4.6, 10.4, 16.5, and 28.7 g dl^{-1}. As a result, instead of Barer's formula (equation (5.12)) they proposed a modified model function:

$$n_{Hb}(\lambda) = n_w(\lambda)(1 + \beta_{Hb}(\lambda)c_{Hb}) \tag{5.17}$$

They found that in the wavelength ranges 310–355 nm and 500–1100 nm (normal dispersion) a mean specific refractive increment $\beta = (0.001\,99 \pm 0.000\,036)$dl g^{-1} can be used without increasing the error significantly. They also found that the specific refractive increment of their model function gives a 44% higher value at 589 nm compared to Barer's formula (equation (5.12)).

Park *et al* [41] measured the dispersion of Hb solutions, prepared from Hb protein powder, at 440, 546, 560, 580, 600, 655, and 700 nm using spectroscopic phase microscopy.

Zhernovaya *et al* [42] measured the refractive index of human deoxygenated and oxygenated Hb for nine wavelengths between 400 and 700 nm for various Hb concentrations (up to 140 g l^{-1}). They found that the refractive indices are well described by linear dependence on concentration (see equation (5.12)). They also found specific refraction increments for each wavelength (see table 5.2). They also used a modified Barer's equation (equation (5.12)), where instead of refractive index of water they used empirically found the effective refractive indices at zero concentration, n_0 (see table 5.2).

Table 5.2. The effective refractive indices at zero concentration and the specific refraction increments for the deoxygenated and oxygenated Hb (HbO_2). Reproduced from [20] with permission.

	Wavelength (nm)								
	401.5	435.8	486.1	546.1	587.6	589.3	632.8	656.3	706.6
n_0	1.345	1.343	1.340	1.337	1.336	1.336	1.334	1.334	1.330
α, Hb (ml g^{-1})	0.146	0.177	0.154	0.148	0.147	0.147	0.144	0.146	0.140
α, HbO_2 (ml g^{-1})	0.170	0.163	0.150	0.150	0.147	0.148	0.144	0.145	0.143

Sydoruk *et al* [43] demonstrated that in calculation of refractive index of Hb solution using KK transformation, the dispersion of the refractive index of the nonabsorbing solvent (water) needs to be taken into account in addition to the absorption of Hb (imaginary part). In particular, they obtained a practical equation for calculation of refractive index of Hb solutions:

$$n(\omega) = n_{H_20}(\omega) + n(\omega_0) - n_{H_20}(\omega_0) + \frac{1}{2\pi}(\omega^2 - \omega_0^2)PV\int_0^{\infty} \frac{\omega' \kappa_{Hb}(\omega')}{(\omega^2 - \omega'^2)(\omega_0^2 - \omega'^2)}d\omega' \tag{5.18}$$

Here, k_{Hb} is the imaginary part of the Hb refractive index.

By accounting for water refractive index dispersion, Sydoruk *et al* [43] obtained good agreement with the experimental results of Friebel and Meinke [40] in the range 250–1000 nm and Zhernovaya *et al* [42] in the range 440–700 nm.

Figure 5.2 demonstrates the importance of explicit inclusion of the refractive index of water. Calculations by Faber *et al* [4] (bottom curve) do not agree with experimental data by Friebel and Meinke [40] (dotted curve). However, explicit inclusion of refractive index of water (equation (5.18)) provides a much better fit of experimental data.

Wang *et al* [22] measured CRID of oxygenated and deoxygenated Hb solutions in continuous wavelength range of 400–750 nm with spectral resolution of about 0.259 nm. They also compared results with those obtained using KK transformation, and they found a good match. For example, the Soret band appeared almost at the same location for the two methods and the CRID results gave fair agreement, with a shift of no more than 0.002.

Lazareva and Tuchin [44] using a multiwavelength Abbé refractometer measured the refractive index of Hb solutions in the visible/near-infrared (NIR) spectral range at room temperature for characteristic laser wavelengths: 480, 486, 546, 589, 644, 656, 680, 930, 1100, 1300, and 1550 nm. They used the Sellmeier formula (see equation (5.16)) to approximate refractive index dispersion. They found the refractive index-specific increment of Hb as 0.192 ± 0.005 ml g^{-1} for the wavelength 589 nm and temperature at 23 °C, which is quite close to Barer's result [33]. They also summarized refractive index measurements from the literature.

Jin *et al* [16] using an internal reflection technique developed in [4] measured the refractive indexes of Hb and other blood components in the spectral range of 400–750 nm. However, the Hb they used was not controlled for oxygenation.

5.4.1.3 Red blood cell

The human RBC is a unique anucleous cell that can be considered as a concentrated Hb solution encapsulated by the lipid membrane. As such, the refractive index of RBC may have different values when measured by different methods.

In light scattering measurements the primary mode of scattering will be caused by the refractive index mismatch on the membrane/plasma layer. Thus, this method will provide a surface refractive index. However, the quantitative phase imaging (e.g. tomographic phase microscopy) will sample the refractive index of the whole RBC. Thus, it can be considered as a bulk refractive index.

The concentration of Hb inside erythrocytes is 250–350 $g\,l^{-1}$ [45]. Preparation of such high Hb concentrations is challenging, with problems arising from the strong absorbance in this spectral range and from sample preparation at physiological concentrations exceeding cHb = 300 $g\,l^{-1}$, due to high viscosity or incomplete dissolution of Hb [46]. However, there are good reasons to expect that the linear relationship with concentration (equation (5.12)) holds true for these concentrations as well. In particular, Zhernovaya *et al* [42] experimentally observed a linear dependence for solutions of methemoglobin in water with the Hb concentrations up to 280 $g\,l^{-1}$. Thus, they estimated refractive indices at 320 $g\,l^{-1}$, as 1.383 for both Hbs at 589 nm.

Ojaghi *et al* [31] determined optical properties (including refractive index) of RBC in the 240–450 nm range using ultraviolet hyperspectral interferometric microscopy. They found excellent agreement between the data measured from an intact RBC and the expected results on Hb solution at 33.6 g dl^{-1}.

Gienger *et al* [47] determined refractive index of human RBCs between 290 and 1100 nm by optical extinction measurements in six volunteers. They found the refractive index increment using Barer's formula (see figure 5.3). They also found, that while there is significant interpatient variability, all six curves lie around $\alpha \approx 0.22$ ml g^{-1}, with differences of about 0.015 ml g^{-1} being present between the highest curve (A) and the lowest (D) for most wavelengths, however reaching 0.036 ml g^{-1} at the Soret band around 420 nm (figure 5.3). The comparison oexperimental data for f oxygenated human RBCs. is depicted in figure 5.4.

5.4.1.3.1 Birefringence

The normal RBCs are typically considered not birefringent [49]. However, Nagesh *et al* [50] found that a normal human RBC, when trapped with a linearly polarized laser, reorients about the electric polarization direction and then remains rotationally bound to this direction. This behavior is expected for a birefringent object. The birefringence is confined to the cell's dimple region and the slow axis is along a diameter [20]. The study reported an average retardation of 3.5 ± 1.5 nm for linearly polarized green light ($\lambda = 546$ nm) using a polarizing microscope, and also estimated a retardation of 1.87 ± 0.09 nm from the optomechanical response of the RBC in an

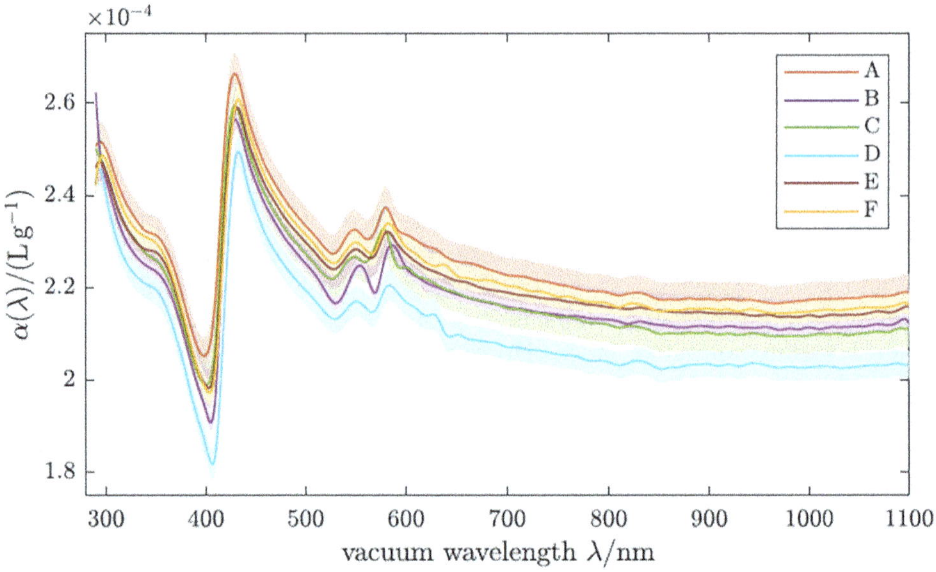

Figure 5.3. Real refractive index increment of oxygenated human RBCs. Shaded bands indicate ±1 estimated uncertainties, accounting for noise in the analysed spectra and uncertainties of complete blood count (CBC) parameters. Curves A–F stand for different volunteers. Reproduced from [47] CC BY 4.0.

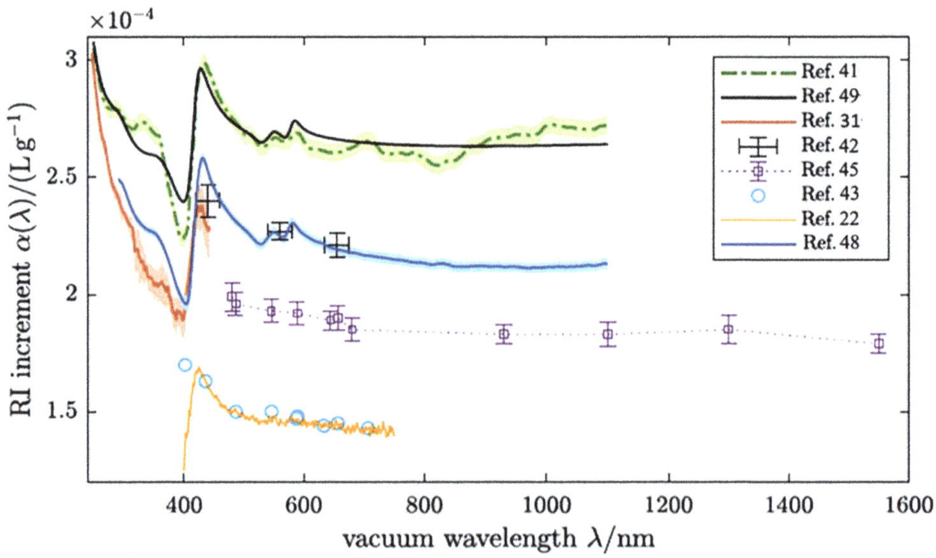

Figure 5.4. Real refractive index increment of oxygenated human RBCs. The blue line is the arithmetic mean of the individual curves in figure 5.3. Various literature values for the refractive index increment of oxygenated Hb solutions and RBCs are shown for comparison. Samples for these measurements were: (i) Hb solutions from powder [22, 41, 42], (ii) Hb solutions from freshly hemolysed RBCs [40, 44] and (iii) single native RBCs [31]. The Kramers–Kronig computation [48] matched to [40] shows the refractive index dispersion expected from the accurately known extinction spectrum $\gamma(\lambda)$. Modified from [47] CC BY 4.0.

optical trap [20]. The authors attributed birefringence to the phospholipid molecules in the lipid bilayer and the variation to the membrane curvature.

5.4.1.4 Other blood cells

5.4.1.4.1 White blood cells

White blood cells are the immune response component of blood, and contain a myriad of cell types, including neutrophils, lymphocytes and monocytes, eosinophils and basophils. Lymphocytes and monocytes are the most simple from a structural perspective, having an approximate spherical shape and containing only one nucleus [51]. Zharinov *et al* [51] validated a five-layered spherical model using light scattering data to simulate the optical properties of lymphocytes and monocytes, and found refractive indices of 1.345 ± 0.006 and 1.344 ± 0.010. These results are similar to those found by Metcalf *et al* [52] using the index matching method, which yielded a lymphocyte refraction index of 1.3572 ± 0.0002.

5.4.1.4.2 Platelets

Platelets have the thrombotic function in blood, aggregating in response to injury. Kolesnikova *et al* [53] studied the refractive index of platelets using a theoretical methodology validated with experimental data based on the light scattering approach, and found a refractive index ranging from 1.36–1.44, similar to that used in clinical optical platelet counters [54].

5.4.1.5 Whole blood

In the visible range of spectrum (400–750 nm), Liu *et al* [36] measured the refractive index of whole blood and its component based on internal reflection and used the Sellmeier formula (see equation (5.16)) to approximate the dispersion of the whole blood. They obtained 0.7960, 5.1819, 1.0772×10^4, and -7.8301×10^5 for A_1, A_2, B_1, and B_2, respectively

The optical properties of the whole blood in the 250–2500 nm range were reviewed by Bosschaart *et al* [55]. They also calculated the real part of the refractive index from absorption measurements using the subtractive KK transformation (see equation (5.7)). The results are presented in figure 5.5.

Rowe *et al* [56] analyzed the complex refractive index of the blood in the mid-IR range. They found that it closely resembles the refractive index of water. In figure 5.6, one can see the deviations of the refractive index of whole blood from the refractive index of water.

The complex refractive index of the blood in the mid-IR range can be found in the Rowe (2017) dataset [57].

5.4.2 Pathologies

The refractive index of blood samples, which reflects the physiological state and functions, appears crucial in many fields.

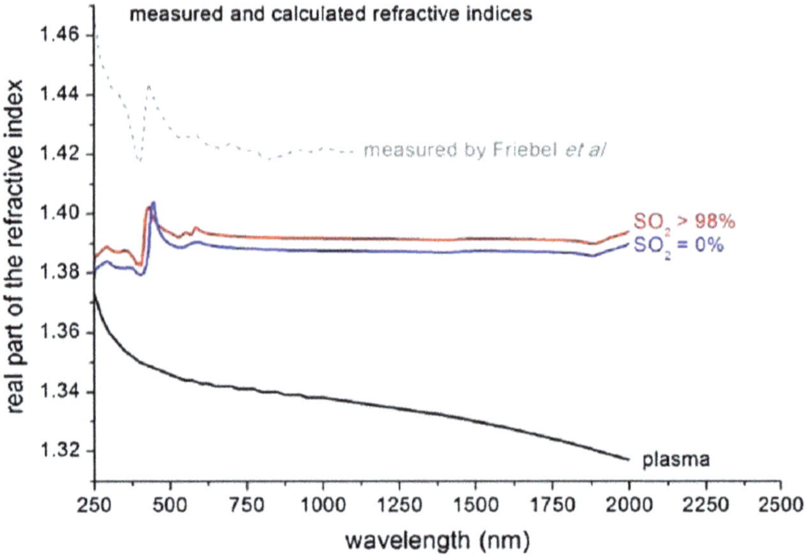

Figure 5.5. Theoretical analysis (Kramers–Kronig) of the real part of the refractive index of whole blood. Reproduced from [55] CC BY 4.0.

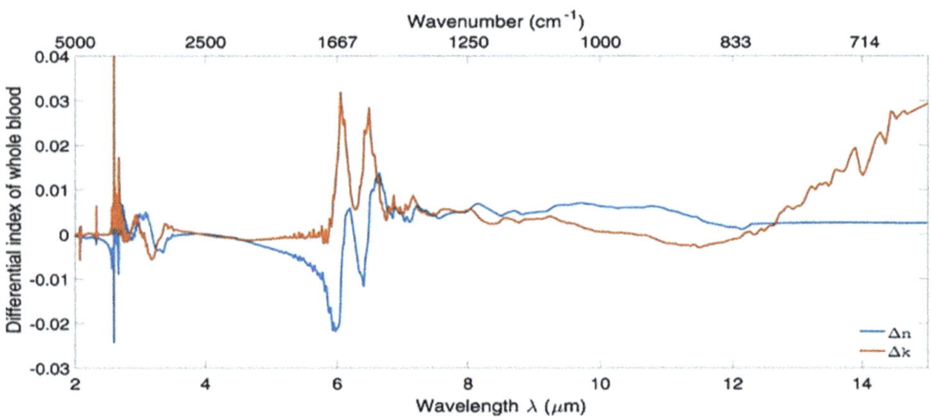

Figure 5.6. Change in the real and imaginary parts of refractive index for whole blood with respect to water in the mid-IR range. Reproduced from [56] CC BY 4.0.

Mazarevica *et al* [58] reported a qualitative relationship that the values of the refractive indices of RBCs significantly decrease for the diabetic patients compared with healthy volunteers at the same pH level.

While there are different types of blood pathologies, we will consider just several examples, including blood glucose measurements and sickle cell anemia.

5.4.2.1 Blood glucose measurements

Quantitatively the measure of diabetes complications, including retinopathy, neuropathy and cardiovascular disease, is represented by the level of glycated

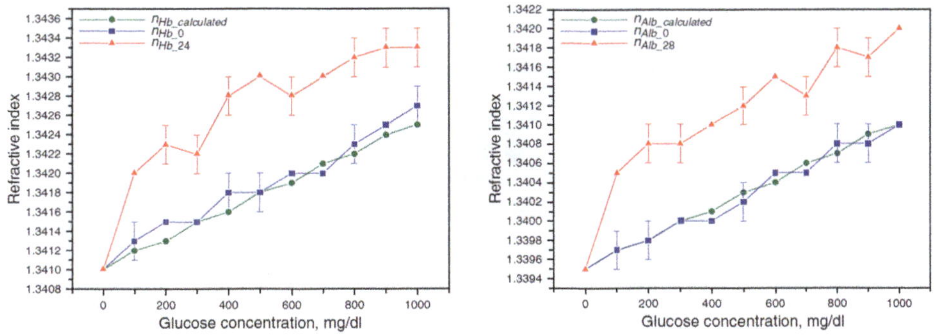

Figure 5.7. Experimental ($n_{p\ 0}$, n_{p24}) and calculated ($n_{p\ \text{calculated}}$) values of refractive indices of water solutions of proteins with glucose. Incubation time for n_{Hb24} is 24 days, $n_{Hb\ 0}$ correspond to the refractive index measurements of freshly prepared samples for Hb (left panel). Incubation time for n_{Ab28} is 28 days, $n_{Ab\ 0}$ correspond to the refractive index measurements of freshly prepared samples for albumin (right panel) [2]. John Wiley & Sons. 2008 by Astro Ltd., Published exclusively by WILEY-VCH Verlag GmbH & Co. KGaA.

(glycosylated) Hb and albumin, which are the main blood proteins that react with glucose forming glycated Hb and glycated albumin.

The percentage of glycated Hb and glycated albumin rises with increasing free glucose concentration [59], which fluctuates within a day. The rate of formation of glycated hemoglobin is proportional to free blood glucose concentration, e.g. the increase of HbA1c for 1% corresponds to enhancing of mean glucose level in plasma for 35 mg dl^{-1} (1.95 mmol l^{-1}) [60]. Inherently, less than 7% of hemoglobin and 6%–15% of total serum albumin are glycated in normal conditions [59].

Zhernovaya *et al* [2] using an Abbé refractometer measured refractive indexes of water solutions of Hb and albumin with glucose at 589 nm. They found that the refractive index of solutions incubated for 24 days (Hb) and 28 days (albumin) have considerably higher refractive index than the freshly prepared samples (see figure 5.7). They attributed this difference to glucose binding to Hb and albumin molecules.

5.4.2.2 Sickle cell anemia

Anemia is a health condition that occurs when body does not have enough RBCs or when the RBCs in the body are unable to function properly[4]. Anemia can cause symptoms such as fatigue, dizziness, and shortness of breath [30]. There are many types of anemia, each with different causes, severity, and treatment options [30].

Blood cytometry can be used to derive Hb content [3]. A common medical test called the complete blood count (CBC) measures different aspects of the blood cells. Some of these aspects are the mean corpuscular Hb concentration (MCHC), the mean corpuscular volume (MCV), and the variability of the RBC sizes, which is

[4] Types of Anemia: What Are the Most Common Types of Anemia?—Healthline. https://www.healthline.com/health/anemia/types-of-anemia.

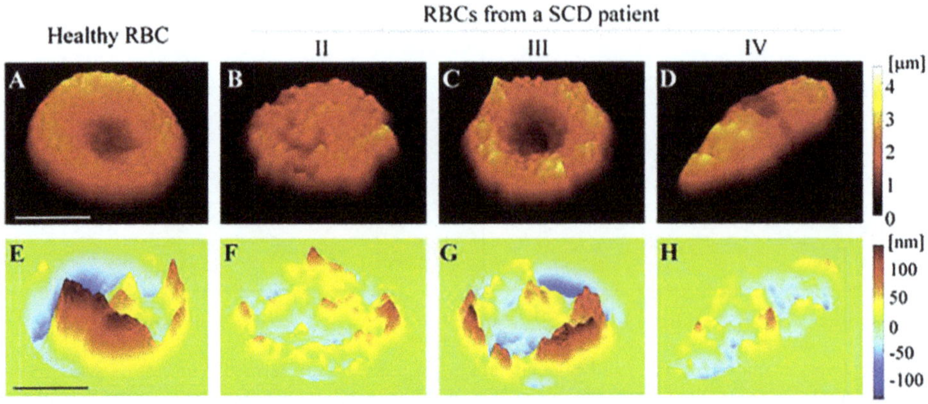

Figure 5.8. (A–D) Topographies of individual RBCs from healthy individuals (A), type II sickle cell (B), type III sickle cell (C), and type IV sickle cell (D). (E–H) Instantaneous membrane displacement maps of RBCs in (A–D). The scale bar is 5 μm. Reprinted from [61], copyright (2012), with permission from Acta Materialia Inc. Published by Elsevier Ltd. All rights reserved.

measured by red cell distribution width (RDW). These aspects allow discriminating between the healthy and patients with low blood levels, such as anemia.

Sickle cell anemia is a severe hereditary form of anemia in which a mutated form of Hb distorts the RBCs into crescent shape at low oxygen levels[5].

Byun *et al* [61] investigated biomechanical properties of sickle cells using a diffraction phase microscopy, DPM. Based on the morphological features, they classified the sickle RBCs into three groups: echinocytes (type II); discocyte (type III); and crescent-shaped irreversibly sickled cells (ISCs, type IV) (see figure 5.8).

Unlike healthy erythrocytes, the sickled cells are birefringent and the reduced Hb forms tactoids [13]. With the polarizing microscope the tactoids appear birefringent and their optical axis is perpendicular to their length. The mean retardation of each sickled red cell is 7.5 ± 0.15 nm and the birefringence is approximately 0.0037.

Ghosh *et al* [62] used scattering approach, involving a 632.8 nm (red color) He–Ne laser as the light source to generate a scattering spectra, acquired by a CCD detector, and a Fourier transform to estimate the refractive index of a normal volunteer (1.41) and a pair of anemic patients ((1.38) and (1.39)).

5.5 Conclusions

Refractive index is a key optical parameter, which determines ways how the light interacts with the media.

The refractive index of blood and blood components, which reflects the physiological state and functions, appears crucial in many medical fields. It is used in

[5] Anemia: Symptoms, types, treatment, causes, diet, and more. https://www.medicalnewstoday.com/articles/158800.

scattering calculations in blood cytometry. However, it can be used directly to assess the physiological state and functions, as in the case of blood proteins glycation.

In addition to traditional refractometry (Abbé refractometer), over the last several decades multiple techniques to determine the refractive index of blood and its components have emerged. They can be roughly split into two large groups: refractometry and synthetic methods that are based on absorption measurements and consequent application of the Kramers–Kronig transformation.

Since Barer's pioneer work in 1953, there has been a lot of understanding on the properties of refractive index of the blood and its components. The refractive index of blood and blood components has been determined in UV, visible, NIR, and mid-wave IR ranges of spectrum by multiple groups. While, traditionally, the refractive index was measured at several wavelengths and approximated by a fitting function like Cauchy or Sellmeier, with the advancement in technologies, and particularly in the automation, the possibility to perform continuous wavelength range measurements has emerged.

References

[1] Wang Z, Tangella K, Balla A and Popescu G 2011 Tissue refractive index as marker of disease *J. Biomed. Opt.* **16** 116017

[2] Zhernovaya O S, Tuchin V V and Meglinski I V 2008 Monitoring of blood proteins glycation by refractive index and spectral measurements *Laser Phys. Lett.* **5** 460–4

[3] Tycko D H, Metz M H, Epstein E A and Grinbaum A 1985 Flow-cytometric light scattering measurement of red blood cell volume and hemoglobin concentration *Appl. Opt.* **24** 1355–65

[4] Faber D J, Aalders M C G, Mik E G *et al* 2004 Oxygen saturation-dependent absorption and scattering of blood *Phys. Rev. Lett.* **93** 028102

[5] Jackson J D 1999 *Classical Electrodynamics* (Wiley) pp 332–3

[6] Ahrenkiel R K 1971 Modified Kramers–Kronig analysis of optical spectra *J. Opt. Soc. Am.* **61** 1651–5

[7] Nahmad-Rohen A, Contreras-Tello H, Morales-Luna G and García-Valenzuela A 2015 On the effective refractive index of blood *Phys. Scr.* **91** 015503

[8] Diez-Silva M, Dao M, Han J, Lim C T and Suresh S 2010 Shape and biomechanical characteristics of human red blood cells in health and disease *MRS Bull.* **35** 382–8

[9] Dirckx J J J, Kuypers L C and Decraemer W F 2005 Refractive index of tissue measured with confocal microscopy *J. Biomed. Opt.* **10** 044014

[10] Elliott A D 2020 Confocal microscopy: principles and modern practices *Curr. Protoc. Cyt.* **92** e68

[11] Bolin F P, Preuss L E, Taylor R C and Ference R J 1989 Refractive index of some mammalian tissues using a fiber optic cladding method *Appl. Opt.* **28** 2297–303

[12] Daimon M and Masumura A 2007 Measurement of the refractive index of distilled water from the near-infrared region to the ultraviolet region *Appl. Opt.* **46** 3811–20

[13] SardarD K and LevyL B 1998 Optical properties of whole blood *Lasers Med. Sci.* **13** 106–11

[14] Tearney G J, Brezinski M E, Southern J F *et al* 1995 Determination of the refractive index of highly scattering human tissue by optical coherence tomography *Opt. Lett.* **20** 2258–60

[15] Deng Z, Wang J, Ye Q *et al* 2016 Determination of continuous complex refractive index dispersion of biotissue based on internal reflection *J. Biomed. Opt.* **21** 015003

[16] Jin Y L, Chen J Y, Xu L and Wang P N 2006 Refractive index measurement for biomaterial samples by total internal reflection *Phys. Med. Biol.* **51** N371–9
[17] García-Valenzuela A and Contreras-Tello H 2013 Optical model enabling the use of Abbé-type refractometers on turbid suspensions *Opt. Lett.* **38** 775–7
[18] Contreras-Tello H and García-Valenzuela A 2014 Refractive index measurement of turbid media by transmission of backscattered light near the critical angle *Appl. Opt.* **53** 4768–78
[19] Lue N and Popescu G 2006 Live cell refractometry using microfluidic devices *Opt. Lett.* **31** 2759–61
[20] Robles F E, Satterwhite L L and Wax A 2011 Non-linear phase dispersion spectroscopy *Opt. Lett.* **36** 4665–7
[21] Shaffer E, Marquet P and Depeursinge C 2011 Second harmonic phase microscopy of collagen fibers *Multiphoton Microscopy in the Biomedical Sciences XI* **vol 7903** (SPIE) pp 63–8
[22] Wang J, Deng Z, Wang X *et al* 2015 Measurement of the refractive index of hemoglobin solutions for a continuous spectral region *Biomed. Opt. Exp.* **6** 2536–41
[23] Griffiths P R and de Haseth J A 2007 *Fourier Transform Infrared Spectrometry* (New York: Wiley)
[24] Milosevic M 2004 Internal reflection and ATR spectroscopy *Appl. Spectr. Rev.* **39** 365–84
[25] Bonnal T, Belarouc A, Orobtchouk R *et al* 2020 How to determine the complex refractive index from infrared reflectance spectroscopy? *SN Appl. Sci.* **2** 2070
[26] Ali H, Bensaali F and Jaber F 2017 Novel approach to non-invasive blood glucose monitoring based on transmittance and refraction of visible laser light *IEEE Access* **5** 9163–74
[27] Park Y, Depeursinge C and Popescu G 2018 Quantitative phase imaging in biomedicine *Nat. Photon* **12** 578–89
[28] Bhaduri B, Edwards C, Pham H *et al* 2014 Diffraction phase microscopy: principles and applications in materials and life sciences *Adv. Opt. Photon.* **6** 57–119
[29] Popescu G, Ikeda T, Dasari R R and Feld M S 2006 Diffraction phase microscopy for quantifying cell structure and dynamics *Opt. Lett.* **31** 775–7
[30] Jin D, Zhou R, Yaqoob Z and So P T C 2017 Tomographic phase microscopy: principles and applications in bioimaging *J. Opt. Soc. Am.* **B 34** B64–77
[31] Ojaghi A, Fay M E, Lam W A and Robles F E 2018 Ultraviolet hyperspectral interferometric microscopy *Sci. Rep.* **8** 9913
[32] Khlebtsov N G, Maksimova I L, Tuchin V V and Wang L V 2002 Introduction to light scattering by biological objects *Chap. 1 in Handbook of Optical Biomedical Diagnostics* **vol PM107** ed V V Tuchin (Bellingham, WA: SPIE Press) p 31167
[33] Barer R, Ross K F and Tkaczyk S 1953 Refractometry of living cells *Nature* **171** 720–4
[34] Roggan A, Friebel M, Do Rschel K, Hahn A and Mu Ller G 1999 Optical properties of circulating human blood in the wavelength range 400–2500 nm *J. Biomed. Opt.* **4** 36–46
[35] Hale G and Querry M R 1973 Optical constants of water in the 200 nm to 200 μm wavelength region *Appl. Opt.* **12** 555563
[36] Liu S, Deng Z, Li J *et al* 2019 Measurement of the refractive index of whole blood and its components for a continuous spectral region *J. Biomed. Opt.* **24** 035003
[37] Meinke M C *et al* 2007 Optical properties of platelets and blood plasma and their influence on the optical behavior of whole blood in the visible to near infrared wavelength range *J. Biomed. Opt.* **12** 014024

[38] Tuchin V V, Zhestkov D M, Bashkatov A N and Genina E A 2004 Theoretical study of immersion optical clearing of blood in vessels at local hemolysis *Opt. Express* **12** 2966–71

[39] Cheng S, Shen H Y, Zhang G, Huang C H and Huang X J 2002 Measurement of the refractive index of biotissue at four laser wavelengths *Proc. SPIE Optics in Health Care and Biomedical Optics: Diagnostics and Treatment* 4916

[40] Friebel M and Meinke M 2006 Model function to calculate the refractive index of native hemoglobin in the wavelength range of 250–1100 nm dependent on concentration *Appl. Opt.* **45** 2838–42

[41] Park Y, Yamauchi T, Choi W, Dasari R and Feld M S 2009 Spectroscopic phase microscopy for quantifying hemoglobin concentrationsin intact red blood cells *Opt. Lett.* **34** 3668–70

[42] Zhernovay O, Sydoruk O, Tuchin V V and Douplik A 2011 The refractive index of human hemoglobin in the visible range *Phys. Med. Biol.* **56** 4013–21

[43] Sydoruk O, Zhernovaya O, Tuchin V V and Douplik A 2012 Refractive index of solutions of human hemoglobin from the near-infrared to the ultraviolet range: Kramers–Kronig analysis *J. Biomed. Opt.* **17** 115002

[44] Lazareva E N and Tuchin V V 2018 Measurement of refractive index of hemoglobin in the visible/NIR spectral range *J. Biomed. Opt.* **23** 035004

[45] Meinke M C, Friebel M and Helfmann J 2011 Optical properties of flowing blood cells *Advanced Optical Flow Cytometry: Methods and Disease Diagnoses* ed V V Tuchin (Weinheim: Wiley-VCH) ch 5 pp 95–129

[46] Barer R and Joseph S 1954 Refractometry of living cells: part I. Basic principles *Quart. J. Microsc. Sci.* **s3–95** 399–423

[47] Gienger J, Smuda K, Müller R, Bär M and Neukammer J 2019 Refractive index of human red blood cells between 290nm and 1100nm determined by optical extinction measurements *Sci. Rep.* **9** 4623

[48] Gienger J, Groß H, Neukammer J and Bär M 2016 Determining the refractive index of human hemoglobin solutions by Kramers–Kronig relations with an improved absorption model *Appl. Opt.* **55** 8951–61

[49] Ascenzi A and Silvestroni E 1953 On the optical properties of the hemoglobin in microdrepanocytic disease *Blood* **8** 1061–6

[50] Nagesh B V, Yogesha , Pratibha R, Parthasarathi P *et al* 2014 Birefringence of a normal human red blood cell and related optomechanics in an optical trap *J. Biomed. Opt.* **19** 115004

[51] Zharinov A E, Tarasov P A, Shvalov A N *et al* 2006 A study of light scattering of mononuclear bloodcells with scanning flow cytometry *J. Quant. Spectrosc. Radiat. Transfer* **102** 121–8

[52] Metcalf W K, Metcalf N F and Gould R N 1978 Lymphocyte cytoplasmic refractive index (LCRI) *Laboratory Testing for Cancer* **vol 22** (Karger Publishers) pp 149–54

[53] Kolesnikova I V, Potapov S V, Yurkin M A *et al* 2006 Determination of volume, shape and refractive index of individual blood platelets *J. Quant. Spectrosc. Radiat. Transfer* **102** 37–45

[54] Marionneaux , FranciscoN S, Chan V *et al* 2013 Comparison of automated platelet counts and potential effect on transfusion decisions in cancer patients *Am. J. Clin. Pathol.* **140** 747–54

[55] Bosschaart N, Edelman G J, Aalders M C *et al* 2014 A literature review and novel theoretical approach on the optical properties of whole blood *Lasers Med. Sci.* **29** 453–79 Erratum in:Bosschaart N, Edelman G J, Aalders M C G, van Leeuwen T G and Faber D J

2021 Correction to: A literature review and novel theoretical approach on the optical properties of whole blood *Lasers Med. Sci.* **37** 691

[56] Rowe D J, Smith D and Wilkinson J S 2017 Complex refractive index spectra of whole blood and aqueous solutions of anticoagulants, analgesics and buffers in the mid-infrare *Sci. Rep.* **7** 7356

[57] Rowe D 2017 *Dataset—Complex refractive index spectra of whole blood and aqueous solutions of anticoagulants, analgesics and buffers in the mid-infrared* (University of Southampton [Dataset])

[58] Mazarevica G, Freivalds T and Jurka A 2002 Properties of erythrocyte light refraction in diabetic patients *J. Biomed. Opt.* **7** 244–7

[59] Day J F, Thorpe S R and Baynes J W 1979 *J. Biol. Chem.* **254** 595

[60] Rohlfing C L, Wiedmeyer H-M, Little R R *et al* 2002 Defining the relationship between plasma glucose and HbA(1c): analysis of glucose profiles and HbA(1c) in the diabetes control and complications trial *Diab. Care* **25** 275

[61] Byun H, Hillman T R, Higgins J M *et al* 2012 Optical measurement of biomechanical properties of individual erythrocytes from a sickle cell patient *Acta Biomater.* **8** 4130–8

[62] Ghosh N, Buddhiwant P, Uppal A *et al* 2006 Simultaneous determination of size and refractive index of red blood cells by light scattering measurements *Appl. Phys. Lett.* **88** 084101

Chapter 6

Light scattering and optical clearing of blood

Gennadi Saiko, Scott Prahl and Alexandre Douplik

6.1 Introduction

Light scattering on blood and blood components is an essential phenomenon with multiple applications in biomedical optics.

The blood consists of four essential components: red blood cells (RBCs), white blood cells (WBCs), platelets, and plasma.

Blood plasma is a light, amber-colored liquid component of blood, which contains proteins (e.g., albumin) and other constituents of whole blood in suspension. It comprises about 55% of the body's total blood volume (50%–59% in men and 56%–64% in women [1]).

Cellular components comprise another 45% of the body's total blood volume (hematocrit is 41%–50% in men and 36%–44% in women [1]).

Cellular components of the blood:

- Erythrocytes (RBCs)—anuclear cells, 7.5 μm in diameter, 2.6-μm thick at the rim, but only 0.75-μm thick in the center.
- Leucocytes (WBCs)[2]
  - o Granulocytes—2 or more lobes to nuclei
    - ■ Neutrophils—60%–70% of circulating leukocytes, 12–15 μm, 3–5 multi-lobed nuclei
    - ■ Eosinophil—2%–4% of circulating leukocytes, 12–17 μm, 2-lobed nuclei
    - ■ Basophil—less than 1% of circulating leukocytes, 12–15 μm, 2-lobed nuclei
  - o Agranulocytes—single-lobed nuclei
    - ■ Monocytes—3%–8% of circulating leukocytes, largest of circulating leukocytes (12–20 μm), large, acentric kidney-shaped nucleus
    - ■ Lymphocytes—20%–25% of circulating leukocytes, variable in size, 7–8 μm in diameter, single, round, heterochromatic nucleus
- Thrombocytes (Platelets)—2 μm in diameter (very small) and anucleate

doi:10.1088/978-0-7503-4806-5ch6

The light scattering arises from a mismatch of refractive indices. Thus, the light scattering in blood arises primarily from a mismatch of refractive indices between the plasma and cells.

The refractive index of normal blood plasma is typically modeled by the Cauchy dispersion equation (see, for example [3]). Still, in the visible range of the spectrum, it can be assessed as 1.351 [4]. Cell membranes mostly comprise lipids and proteins, with refractive indices of 1.46–1.54 [5]. Refractive indices of blood components are discussed in more detail in chapter 5 (Refractometry of blood).

Based on the sizes of cellular blood components (2–20 μm range; see cellular components above), they can be considered the Mie scatterers in the visible and near-infrared (NIR) spectrum ranges. For example, Steinke and Shepherd [6] compared Mie theory predictions with experimental results on RBCs and found that Mie theory yielded adequate values for the RBC's microscopic scattering cross-section. Since Mie's theory treats the RBCs as spheres, it did poorly predict the scattering anisotropy. Osmotically swelled RBCs matched Mie predictions better. Overall, scattering by cellular blood components is strongly forward-directed.

While the scattering on the plasma/cell interface is the most likely the primary scattering mechanism, light experiences additional scattering on large biomolecules and organelles (e.g., mitochondria and nucleus).

As blood is composed of multiple shapes and sizes of cells, scattering patterns vary significantly between different cell types. Various physical methods based on light scattering are used to characterize the blood cell sizes, shapes, velocities, and their distributions. These methods and results of their application for blood and blood component characterization are the primary focus of this chapter.

Note that in the current chapter, we will consider elastic scattering only. Inelastic (Raman) scattering will be addressed in chapter 8 of this Book (Raman scattering spectroscopy and imaging of blood).

6.2 Methods

There are several approaches for light scattering measurements. Broadly, they can be categorized into static and dynamic light scattering.

Static light scattering (SLS) measures the time-averaged intensity of the scattered light.

Dynamic light scattering (DLS) measures the time-dependent fluctuations in the scattered light intensity. DLS allows the determination of the translational diffusion coefficients (i.e., Brownian motion) and particle/molecular size.

6.2.1 Analytical and numerical approaches

6.2.1.1 Rayleigh scattering

Rayleigh scattering describes the elastic scattering of light by particles much smaller than the wavelength of light. The intensity of the scattered radiation in the Rayleigh scattering limit is given by the following equation [7]

$$I = I_0\left(\frac{1+\cos^2\theta}{2R^2}\right)\left(\frac{2\pi}{\lambda}\right)^4\left(\frac{m^2-1}{m^2+2}\right)^2\left(\frac{d}{2}\right)^6 \tag{6.1}$$

Here, I_0 is the light intensity before scattering, R is the distance between the particle and the observer, θ is the scattering angle, λ is the wavelength of the light, m is the relative refractive index (ratio of absolute refractive indices of the scatterer to its environment), and d is the diameter of the particle.

The Rayleigh scattering model breaks down when the particle size becomes larger than around 10% of the wavelength of the incident radiation.

In the context of light scattering in blood, Rayleigh scattering describes the scattering on the individual biomolecules. Thus, it can be applicable to scattering on certain blood substitutes (see section 6.4.1), like cross-linked, polymerized, and conjugated hemoglobins (Hbs).

6.2.1.2 Mie scattering

Gustav Mie found an exact solution to Maxwell's equations for scattering an electromagnetic plane wave by a homogeneous sphere [8]. This solution is known as the Lorenz–Mie solution, the Lorenz–Mie–Debye solution, or Mie scattering [9].

Even though Mie found the solution only for spheres, the current usage of the term 'Mie solution' indicates a series approximation of a solution of Maxwell's equations. There are several known objects that allow such a solution: spheres, concentric spheres, infinite cylinders, clusters of spheres, and clusters of cylinders. There are also known series solutions for scattering by ellipsoidal particles.

Mie solutions can be found for conducting and dielectric spheres (see, for example [10]).

Mie scattering refers to light scattering by relatively large particles, which are of the order of the wavelength or larger. In biooptics, in the visible range, the Mie scattering occurs on cells, the nucleus, and cellular components like mitochondria, lysosomes, etc. In blood optics, the primary scattering occurs on RBCs. As RBCs are 7.5 μm in diameter, scattering is Mie-type in the visible spectrum range and near IR.

The Mie formalism allows the calculation of the electric and magnetic fields inside and outside a spherical object. It is generally used to calculate how much light is scattered (the total optical cross-section) or where it goes (the form factor or scattering function).

6.2.1.2.1 Optical cross-section

As the radars and radiolocation are the primary use cases of reflectance of different targets, the target's (or particle) reflectance is frequently characterized in terms of the radar cross-section (RCS), which is the area that intercepts the radar's transmitted signals and reflects them back to the radar receiver.

The Mie solution for the conducting metal sphere (perfect electric conductor, or PEC) is depicted in figure 6.1 [9].

In figure 6.1, one can see two distinct regimes: Rayleigh and Mie scattering. In the left part of the chart, in agreement with equation (6.1), the RCS dependence on

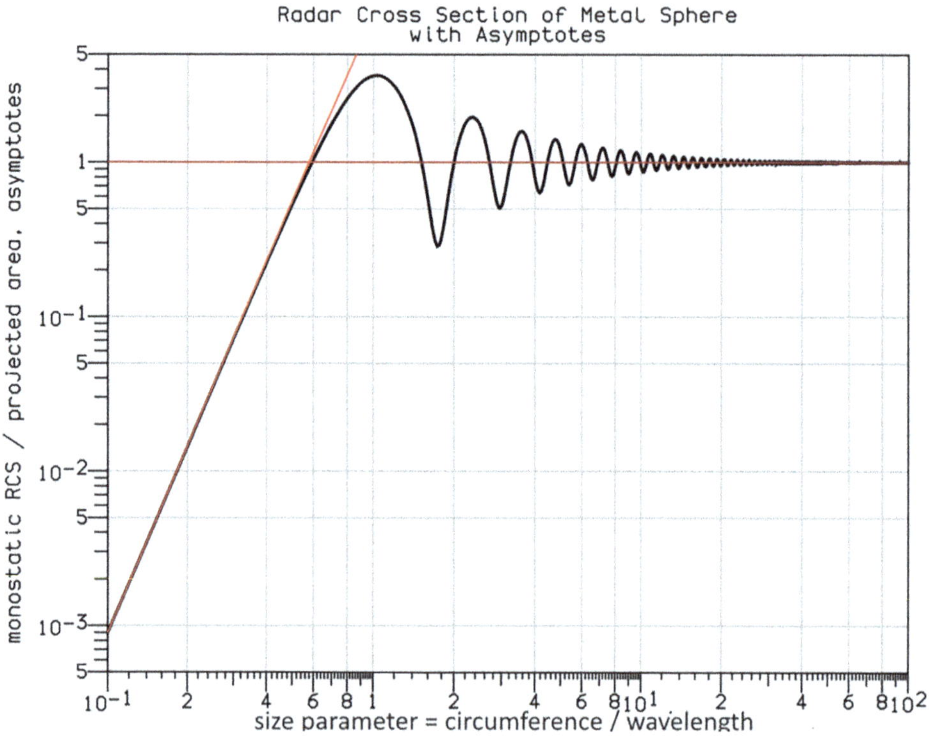

Figure 6.1. The RCS of a perfectly conducting metal sphere as a function of size parameter x, defined as $x = \pi d/\lambda$ (calculated by Mie theory). This image has been obtained by the authors from the Wikimedia website https://en.wikipedia.org/wiki/Mie_scattering, where it is stated to have been released into the public domain. It is included within this article on that basis.

the size parameter x (defined as $x = \pi d/\lambda$, here r is the diameter of the particle, λ is the wavelength) in log-log representation can be approximated by a straight line (Rayleigh regime). This relationship holds approximately to $x = 0.6$ ($d/\lambda = 0.2$). At this point, the RCS is very close to the projected area of the particle ($\pi d^2/4$). However, beyond this point, the cross-section starts oscillating around the projected area of the particle (Mie regime). Thus, the notable feature of Mie scattering is the presence of the particle size-dependent Mie resonances.

6.2.1.3 Form factor

Scattering of electromagnetic radiation is caused by the interaction of radiation with matter, resulting in the re-radiation of part of the energy. Re-radiation is caused by oscillations of electrons, which are induced by the electric field of the electromagnetic wave. If the particle size is much smaller than the wavelength, then the electric field across the particle is homogeneous. Thus, electrons oscillate synchronously as a simple antenna that emits dipole radiation (Rayleigh scattering).

As the particle size increases, the electrons in different particle parts start oscillating in different phases. Thus, oscillation configurations other than dipoles

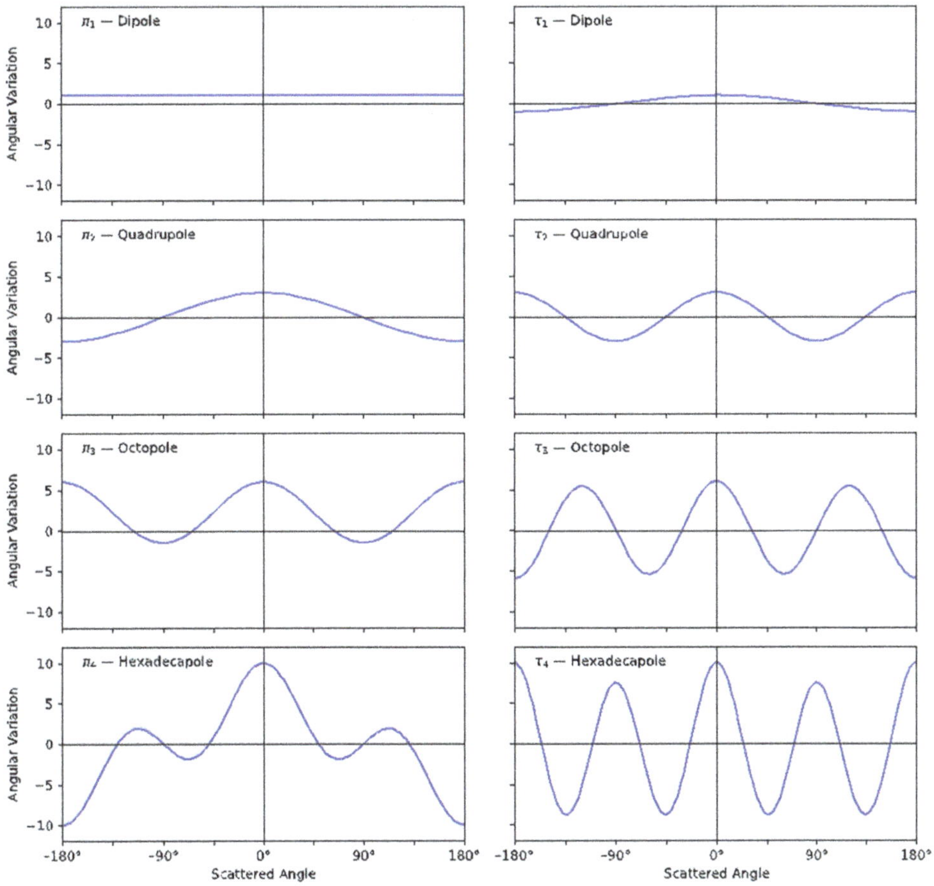

Figure 6.2. The angular dependence of scattered light arising from dipole (top row), quadrupole (2nd row), octopole (3rd row), and hexadecapole (last row) terms.

start emerging. As these oscillations interfere with each other, a complex scattering pattern emerges.

This interference of fields can be evaluated in terms of the contribution of a series of electrical and magnetic multipoles. The angular dependence of electric amplitudes of the first four multipoles (dipole, quadrupole, octopole, and hexadecapole) for light polarized perpendicularly (left column) or parallel (right column) with respect to the scattering plane is presented in figure 6.2.

In figure 6.2, it is evident that the functions $\pi_k(\theta)$ and $\tau_k(\theta)$ increase both in oscillation and magnitude with k. These functions must be multiplied by their electric and magnetic field multipole contributions to calculate the electric field amplitude of the scattered light. Figure 6.3 illustrates the scattered intensities for the first three multipoles (dipole, quadrupole, and octupole) as well as their combined effect. Note that the intensities of the individual multipoles cannot be directly summed. Instead, the field amplitudes must first be summed, and then parallel and perpendicular scattered intensities can be calculated from the results.

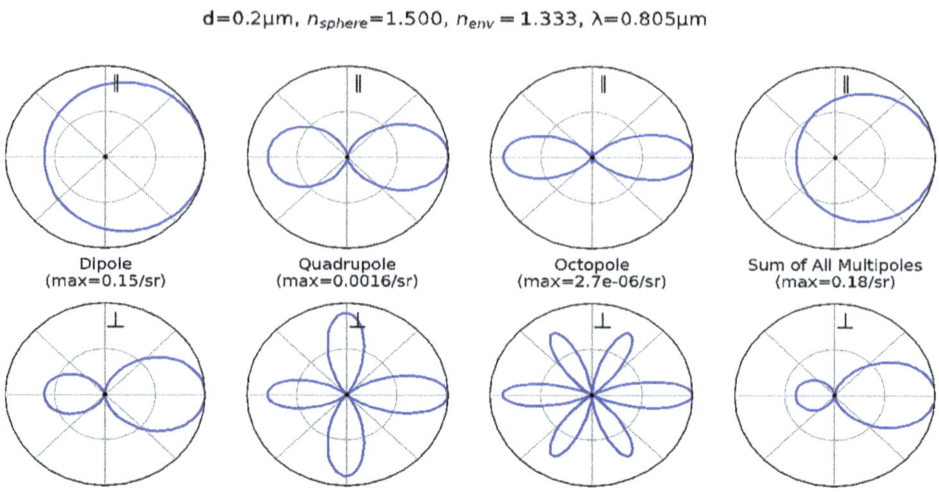

Figure 6.3. Scattering profiles (normalized intensities [1/sr]) of different multipoles: dipole, quadrupole, and octopole, and their combination (last column) for light polarized parallel (first row) or perpendicular (second row) with respect to the scattering plane. $d = 0.2$ μm, $n_{\text{sphere}} = 1.500$, $n_{\text{env}} = 1.333$, ï ¬ = 805 nm

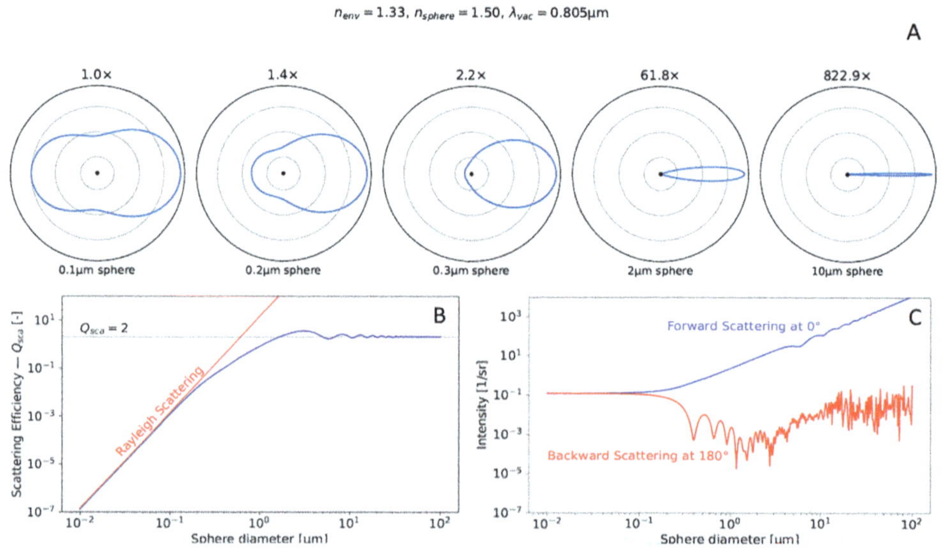

Figure 6.4. Mie angular scattering intensity patterns for spheres with different diameters (panel A). The scattering efficiency as a function of the particle diameter is depicted in panel B. Intensity of forward (blue line) and backward (red line) scattering as a function of the particle diameter is depicted in panel C. $n_{\text{sphere}} = 1.500$, $n_{\text{env}} = 1.333$, $\lambda = 805$ nm.

The angular distribution of the Mie scattering depends strongly on the particle's relative refractive index and size relative to the wavelength (the Mie-equivalent radius or size parameter)—see figure 6.4.

As the RBCs are the primary blood scatterers and their size is 7.5 μm in diameter and 2.6 μm thick at the rim, whole blood is characterized by strong forward scattering in the visible and NIR ranges of the spectrum.

There are several broadly used approximations. For example, for monodispersed dielectric spheres, the reduced scattering coefficient (which is defined as $\mu_s' = \mu_s(1-g)$, where μ_s is the scattering coefficient, and g is the anisotropy factor discussed later) can be approximated as [11]:

$$\mu_s' = 3.28\pi r^2 \rho \left(\frac{2\pi r}{\lambda}\right)^{0.37} (m - 1)^{2.08} \tag{6.2}$$

Here, r is the radius of the particles, m is the relative refractive index, and ρ is the volume density of scattering centers.

As the Mie solution contains an infinite series of spherical multipole partial waves, multiple approximations have been found and used for computational efficiency.

6.2.1.4 Rayleigh–Gans–Debye approximation

The Rayleigh–Gans–Debye approximation is an approximate solution to light scattering when the relative refractive index of the particle, n, is close to that of the environment.

$$|n - 1| \ll 1 \tag{6.3}$$

and

$$2x\,|n - 1| \ll 1 \tag{6.4}$$

Here, $x = d\pi/\lambda$ is the size parameter, and d is the particle's linear dimension (diameter). Equation (6.3) is often referred to as optically soft, and the approximation holds for particles of arbitrary shape [12]. The second condition (equation (6.4)) is a statement of the Born approximation; that is, the incident field is not significantly altered within one particle so that each volume element is considered to be illuminated by intensity and phase determined only by its position relative to the incident wave, unaffected by scattering from other volume elements [12].

The Rayleigh–Debye–Gans (RDG) approximation is often used for calculations of scattering amplitude, as it is considered appropriate for small relative refractive indices between a scatterer and the surrounding medium. In particular, RDG theory is a commonly used approximation for light scattering and absorption by nanoparticles in the visible spectrum [13]. The feasibility of RDG for monitoring biological particles in UV–visible spectrum ranges was assessed by Garcia–Lopez *et al* [14]. They found disagreement with Mie theory for refractive indices and spherical sizes representative of biological particles and suggested a correction using a hybrid model [15] by combining RDG with Mie theory.

6.2.1.5 Fraunhofer diffraction

Fraunhofer diffraction theory describes the intensity distribution in the forward direction of a uniformly illuminated opaque particle. The Fraunhofer diffraction equation is used to model the diffraction of waves when plane waves are incident on a diffracting object, and the diffraction pattern is viewed at a sufficiently long distance, L, from the object (so-called far-field region)

$$L \gg \frac{W^2}{\lambda} \tag{6.5}$$

Here, W is the largest size of a diffracting object. Equation (6.5) is called a Fraunhofer condition.

For example, this approximation is commonly used in ektacytometry to characterize small-angle light scattering by ellipsoidal RBCs.

6.2.1.6 Anomalous diffraction approximation

For large optically soft particles, van de Hulst [16] derived the expression for the efficiency factor of extinction, which is defined as the ratio of the extinction cross-section and geometrical cross-section ($\pi d^2/4$). This value is like the RCS depicted in figure 6.2.

$$Q_{\text{ext}} = 2 - \frac{4}{x}\sin(x) \quad + \frac{4}{x^2}(1 - \cos(x)) \tag{6.6}$$

where the size parameter $x = \pi d/\lambda$.

The anomalous diffraction approximation is found to have a broader range of applicability for the extinction efficiency than the Rayleigh–Debye–Gans approximation [17]. For example, Sharma and Banerjee [18] found that for biological tissues, the anomalous diffraction approximation yields reasonably good results for the tissue scattering coefficient, the phase function, and the anisotropy parameter.

Streekstra *et al* [19] found that anomalous diffraction is a better approximation than the commonly used Fraunhofer diffraction approach to describe small-angle light scattering by ellipsoidal RBCs used in ektacytometry.

6.2.1.7 Scattering phase function

The scattering distribution or scattering function of an individual scatterer like RBC can be found using Mie theory (see section 6.2.1.2).

However, as in the whole blood, the concentration of cellular components (RBCs, primarily) is very high, and the multiple scattering effects have to be considered. Thus, instead of scattering phase functions of individual scatterers, statistical approaches are more relevant, and the scattering phase functions of the ensemble of the particles can be used.

If scattering is symmetric relative to the direction of the incident wave, then the phase function depends only on the scattering angle θ: $p(\vec{s}, \vec{s'}) = p(\vartheta)$. This applies to spherical scatterers. More complex shapes (ellipsoids, cylinders, or biconcave like RBC) can be oriented randomly with respect to the incident wave in the media, which breaks this symmetry. Nevertheless, multiple scattering acts on multiple scattering centers, distributed randomly in the tissues, and 'averages' multiple individual scattering phase functions. Thus, the collective scattering phase function becomes symmetrical with respect to the incident wave direction and can be characterized by a single parameter: the scattering angle θ.

In biooptics, the most used scattering phase function for tissue is the Henyey–Greenstein function (HG), first proposed by Jacques *et al* [20]:

$$p(\vartheta) = \frac{1}{4\pi}\frac{1 - g^2}{(1 + g^2 - 2g\cos\vartheta)^{3/2}} \tag{6.7}$$

where g is the scattering an isotropy parameter defined as the average cosine of the scattering phase function $g = \langle\cos\theta\rangle$. When $g = 0$ scattering is isotropic, $g = 1$ implies total forward scattering, and $g = -1$ is for total backward scattering. Note that the HG function (equation (6.7)) works well even for single scattering events, as was demonstrated by Jacques *et al* [20] on 20 μm thick samples.

For realistic tissues, the scattering an isotropy g is 0.7 or more. Thus, it is primarily forward scattering. Blood is characterized by extremely high anisotropy ($g > 0.98$ over the visible range of the spectrum).

In addition to HG, other scattering phase functions, including the Gegenbauer [21] and Reynolds–McCormick [22, 23] scattering phase functions, have been proposed to characterize the scattering on ensembles of RBCs.

6.2.2 Experimental techniques

Many experimental techniques can be used to measure the scattering properties of blood or blood components. In addition, another large group of technologies is based on the light-scattering properties of blood components. Steelman *et al* [24] proposed the following categories: wavelength-dependent, angle-resolved, and Fourier Domain methods. We further separate scattering-based techniques used in medicine from those used in biomedical research (see section 6.2.3). This section focuses primarily on the core light scattering techniques.

6.2.2.1 Angle-resolved techniques

The scattering light intensity depends strongly on the scattering angle (see figure 6.4). Moreover, some information about the size and shape of the particle can be inferred from the scattering angle dependence (or phase function). As such, it can be considered a 'signature'.

As such, angle-resolved or goniometric techniques are the most common methods to investigate the scattering properties of cells and particles.

In the typical scenario, the particle is illuminated with a monochromatic light, and a photodetector measures the angular dependence of the scattering light intensity.

In a goniometer system, a collimated beam of light is incident on a tank filled with an index-matching solution, and the sample is located at the center of the rotation axis. A detector is rotated about the sample on the goniometer arm to collect and map the scattered light intensity as a function of angle. The size distribution of scatterers can be determined by fitting the angular scattering data to simulated scattering distributions of spherical and ellipsoidal scatterers.

6.2.2.2 Wavelength-based techniques

Strong dependence of the scattering on the wavelength (see, for example, equation (6.2) or equation (6.6)) makes it possible to analyze the scattering properties of the particle by fixing the scattering angle and scanning across various wavelengths. This observation is at the core of several light scattering techniques. In particular, light scattering spectroscopy (LSS) is based on detecting a light-scattering spectrum that depends on its size and refractive index [25].

In a typical scenario, the particle is illuminated with a broad-spectrum light source, and the spectroscopic output is analyzed to detect the particle sizes and their distribution. Originally, LSS was proposed to probe the structure of living epithelial cells *in situ* without the need for tissue removal [26]. This technology can be used in cytometry as well.

6.2.2.3 Integrating sphere

In addition to the scattering phase function measurements, total scattering also needs to be measured. For this purpose, the integrating sphere method emerged as the gold standard in biomedical optics in general and blood optics in particular.

In the integrating sphere (IS) technique, a thin sample is placed at the entrance of the integrating sphere, and the diffusely backscattered light R_d, the total transmission T_t (or diffusely transmitted light T_d), and the collimated or unscattered transmission T_c are measured. Then, the optical properties, including absorption coefficient μ_a, scattering coefficient μ_s, and anisotropy factor g, can be extracted using several techniques, including the Kubelka–Munk model [27], inverse Monte Carlo (iMC) simulations [28], inverse adding-doubling [29], or lookup tables. For example, the iMC uses forward Monte Carlo simulations iteratively to calculate the optical parameters μ_a, μ_s, and g based on a given phase function and the experimentally measured values for reflection and transmission R_d, T_t, and T_d.

The integrating sphere technique can be enhanced by adding one more integrating sphere [30]. A thin sample is placed between two integrating spheres in the double-integrating sphere (DIS) technique. Since the DIS system facilitates simultaneous measurement of reflectance and transmittance from a sample without repositioning, it is a preferred approach for measuring fresh tissue samples [31]. The typical DIS setup is depicted in figure 6.5.

The thickness of the sample should be quite small. For example, Meinke *et al* [23] used a sample thickness of 2.6 mm for measuring plasma and platelets; leukocytes were measured using a sample thickness of 0.52 mm. For RBCs, the thickness was set to 0.116 mm.

6.2.2.4 Dynamic light scattering

DLS is used to determine the size distribution profile of small particles in suspension or macromolecules in solution.

DLS is based on a monochromatic light source, usually a laser, which illuminates a sample (see figure 6.6). The scattered light is projected onto a screen. The resulting image is known as a speckle pattern. Molecules or particles (for example, RBCs) in the solution are hit with the light and diffract the light in all directions. The

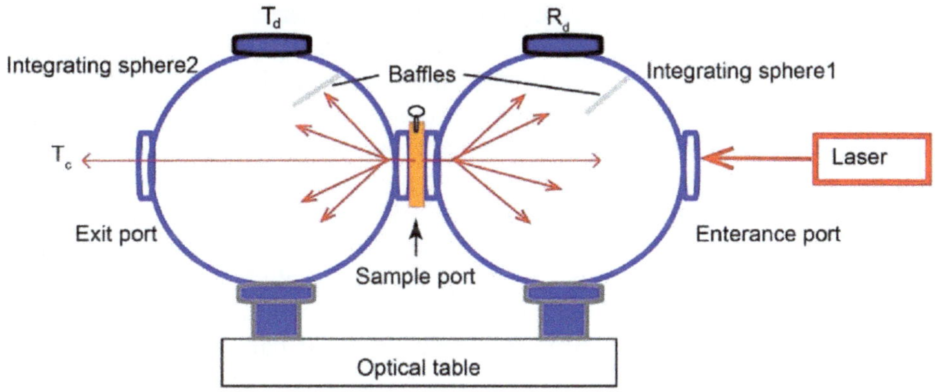

Figure 6.5. Experimental setup to measure the reflectance and transmittance of the biological sample, which are subsequently used in an analytic model to calculate the sample's optical properties. Light passes through the entrance port and hits biological samples. The diffuse reflection or transmission is measured at the port R_d and T_d port, respectively. Modified from [32], Copyright (2020), with permission from Elsevier.

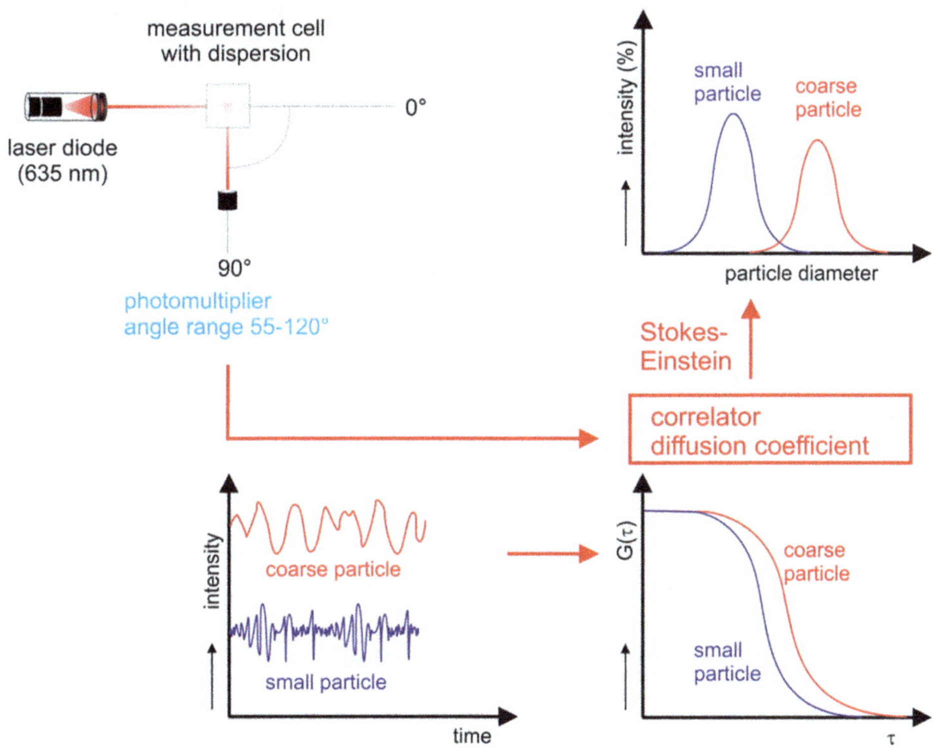

Figure 6.6. DLS measurement principles. Reproduced with permission from [33], copyright 2025 by 3P Instruments.

diffracted light from all the molecules or particles can interfere constructively (bright regions) or destructively (dark regions). An autocorrelator analyzes the resulting set of speckle patterns and compares the light intensity at each spot over time.

In a typical scenario, the photodetector (typically, a photomultiplier) is set at a certain position with respect to the incident light and measures changes in the scattering light over time. The position of the photodetector can be optimized for a particular task. Backscattering detection (e.g., 173° or 175°) is used for turbid and highly concentrated samples containing large particles. Side scattering detection (90°) is recommended for weakly scattering samples, including small particles and transparent samples. Finally, forward scattering detection (e.g., 13° or 15°) is suitable for detecting samples containing mostly small particles with a few large particles.

A typical setup includes two polarizers (one for incoming light and one for scattered light), which can be adjusted independently. In a vertical/vertical (VV) geometry, the second polarizer allows light to pass through in the same direction as the primary polarizer. In vertical/horizontal (VH) geometry, the second polarizer is rotated to be perpendicular to the polarization of the incident light.

The time-dependent scattering intensity (intensity trace) is recorded during a DLS experiment. The dynamic information of the particles is derived from the autocorrelation of the intensity trace recorded during the experiment. An intensity correlation function (or second-order correlation function) is generated from the intensity trace using time averaging (denoted by angular brackets) as follows:

$$G_2(\tau) = <I(t)I(t+\tau)> \tag{6.8}$$

Here, τ is the delay time, I is the intensity, and $G_2(\tau)$ is often normalized as

$$g_2(\tau) = \frac{<I(t)I(t+\tau)>}{<I(t)>^2} \tag{6.9}$$

The correlation decays exponentially. This exponential decay is related to the motion of the particles, and the diffusion coefficient may be obtained. For example, if the sample is monodisperse, then the decay is simply a single exponential:

$$g_2(\tau) = 1 + \beta \exp\left(-2D_T q^2 \tau\right) \tag{6.10}$$

Here, q is the scattering wave vector $q = 4\pi/\lambda \sin(\theta/2)$ and θ is the scattering angle, D_T is the size-dependent translational diffusion coefficient and β is the coherence factor that depends on detector area, optical alignment, and particle or macromolecule scattering properties.

The translational diffusion coefficient D_T for spheres can be found from the Stokes–Einstein equation:

$$D_T = \frac{k_B T}{6\pi\eta R_h} \tag{6.11}$$

Here, T is the temperature, η is the viscosity, and R_h is the hydrodynamic radius of the particle.

6.2.3 Scattering-based techniques in medicine and biomedical research

Multiple scattering-based techniques are used in biomedical research and clinical practice. Their primary utility is measuring particle size, size distribution, shape complexity (flow cytometry and optical coherence tomography (OCT)), and velocity (Doppler- and DLS-based techniques).

6.2.3.1 Wavelength-based methods

LSS is based on detecting a light scattering spectrum of single scattered photons that depends on particle size and refractive index [25]. LSS typically utilizes the convenient approximation of assuming that the particles can be adequately modeled as spheres of unknown size and refractive index. Analysis of spectral oscillations yields parameters like the size distributions of nuclei, their population density, and relative refractive index [34]. In traditional implementations of LSS, light from a broadband source is linearly polarized and illuminates the tissue or cell monolayer surface to be analyzed. The scattered light is passed through an analyzer to the detector plane (polarization-gated LSS [35]).

Elastic scattering spectroscopy (ESS) or diffuse reflectance spectroscopy is based on multiple scattering in biological tissues. In typical implementations of ESS, light from a broadband source is coupled into a multimode fiber, and the distal end is placed in direct contact with the tissue to be analyzed. A secondary fiber or fibers near the illumination spot collects diffusely scattered photons, which are coupled into a spectrometer for data analysis.

6.2.3.2 Flow cytometry

Flow cytometry uses hydrodynamic focusing in combination with light scattering or fluorescence emission (from autofluorescence or if the particle is labeled with a fluorophore) to study the particle's properties.

Light scattering flow cytometry determines a particle's size and provides information about the complexity of the particle's shape.

The standard approach in light scattering flow cytometry is to measure forward scatter (FSC) and side scatter (SSC) amplitudes.

Light scattered in the forward direction after interacting with a particle and collected by a photodetector (photomultiplier or photodiode) is known as the FSC channel. The FSC measurement can estimate a particle's size, with larger particles refracting more light than smaller particles. However, it can depend on several factors, such as the sample, the wavelength of the laser, the collection angle, and the refractive index of the sample and sheath fluid.

Light measured at a 90° angle to the excitation light is called SSC. The SSC can provide information about a cell or particle's relative complexity (for example, granularity and internal structures); however, like FSC, interpretation depends on various factors. Both FSC and SSC are unique for every particle, and a combination of the two may be used to roughly differentiate cell types in a heterogeneous population such as blood.

Scanning flow cytometry (SFC) can determine standard FSC and SSC amplitudes but is also capable of measuring angle-resolved light-scattering patterns of individual particles [36].

Ektacytometry is a laser diffraction viscometry technique to measure the deformability of RBCs. It is a small-angle light scattering technique based on the inability of rigid cells to align in response to shear stress properly. This inability results in a distorted diffraction pattern [37]. Measuring the degree of distortion provides a reliable indicator of the deformability and heterogeneity of the erythrocytes in blood. However, despite being considered the reference technique, this technique is rarely used as a routine diagnosis tool for RBC membrane disorders due to its limited availability [38].

6.2.3.3 Doppler-based techniques

In the presence of moving blood cells, the incident monochromatic light becomes Doppler-broadened to a degree determined by the concentration and velocity of the moving scatterers. Since the backscattered light is spectrally broadened about its carrier frequency, the light intensity pattern formed on the detector surface constitutes a fluctuating speckle with the local intensity variations mainly determined by tissue perfusion [39].

Laser Doppler flowmetry (single point measurement) and laser Doppler perfusion Imaging (wide field of view technique) are based on recording the Doppler shifts that photons undergo when scattered in moving blood cells. The method allows continuous and noninvasive recording of microvascular tissue perfusion, defined as the product of average velocity and concentration of blood cells in the illuminated tissue volume. These techniques require oblique illumination so that flow is not perpendicular to the beam, complicating correct velocity assessment.

Laser Doppler perfusion imaging (LDPI) is a scanning technique that combines laser Doppler flowmetry principles with imaging technology to visualize and quantify blood flow in tissues in a spatially resolved manner. Unlike traditional laser Doppler flowmetry, which measures blood flow at a single point, LDPI provides two-dimensional or three-dimensional images of the distribution and dynamics of blood flow across a tissue or organ.

6.2.3.4 DLS-based techniques

There are several DLS-based techniques that are used to determine the velocity of particles, which can be used for perfusion and blood velocity measurements in biomedical applications.

Laser speckle imaging (LSI) or laser speckle contrast Imaging (LSCI) is a wide field of view, a non-scanning optical technique used to observe blood flow [40]. LSI uses the core concept of DLS: monochromatic and polarized light interference on small particles (speckle formation). Since ordered (flow) and disordered (Brownian motion) motions have different velocity distribution profiles (Gaussian and Lorentzian profiles, respectively), information about flow velocity can be extracted. Because RBCs are the primary moving scatterers in tissue, the blood velocity in microcirculation can be determined.

The spatial resolution (~10 μm) and temporal resolution (10 ms to 10 s) of LSCI can be tailored to the application [40].

6.2.3.5 Optical coherence tomography

OCT is an interferometry-based imaging technique that measures the backscattering properties of tissues [41]. OCT can obtain a micrometer-level resolution of the subsurface morphology of biological tissues. It uses a low coherence length light source and transverse scanning of the light beam to form two- and three-dimensional images from light reflected from within biological tissue or other scattering media.

OCT-based techniques are widely used in various medical fields, with several adaptations focusing on characterizing blood flow, particularly in ophthalmology. One such adaptation is Doppler OCT (D-OCT), which combines OCT with Doppler-based methods to visualize and quantify blood flow. Traditional Doppler OCT can measure blood velocity along the direction of the OCT beam, but accurate blood flow measurements also require knowledge of the angle between the blood vessel and the light beam, known as the Doppler angle.

Several improvements have been proposed to address this issue. For example, blood vessels can be visualized using Doppler OCT in conjunction with time-domain OCT by extracting and comparing the A-scan phase changes related to the Doppler frequency shift, a method known as optical Doppler tomography [42]. Haindl *et al* [43] proposed a three-beam D-OCT technique to further enhance this approach.

The ability to provide information about flow is a key feature of OCT angiography (OCTA). Braaf *et al* [44] discussed the utility of OCT-based velocimetry for retinal blood flow quantification.

More details on OCT applications for blood can be found in chapter 10 (Optical coherence tomography and polarimetry of blood).

6.2.3.6 Microscopic techniques

There are multiple scattering-based microscopic techniques to analyze biological tissues and small particles, including blood components.

For example, dark-field microscopy is widely used in alternative and complementary medicine for blood analysis (so-called Enderlein's dark-field analysis of live blood). Teut *et al* [45] tested the interobserver reliability and test–retest reliability of Enderlein's dark-field analysis and found low interobserver reliability (0.35, 95% CI: 0.27–0.43) and the test–retest reliability (0.44, 95% CI: 0.36–0.53).

Verebes *et al* [46] proposed a hyperspectral-enhanced dark-field microscopy. They analyzed RBCs and WBCs and found that this technique can detect changes in the light scattering property of blood cells due to their morphological properties.

Bernhardt *et al* [47] used digital holographic microscopy to investigate the sedimentation of intact RBCs.

6.2.3.7 Fourier-domain-based techniques

Fourier transform light scattering (FTLS) was reported by Ding *et al* in 2008 [48]. FTLS is based on diffraction phase microscopy (DPM) [49] to acquire a wavefront image near the microscope's image plane. Park *et al* [50] used FTLS to study the static and dynamic light scattering on RBCs during the metabolic remodeling of the membrane.

Spatial frequency-domain imaging (SFDI) is another example of a Fourier domain-based technique. The technique was proposed by Cuccia *et al* in 2005 [51]. It encodes frequency-domain interrogation into the illumination to extract the tissue's absorption and reduced scattering coefficients. Applegate *et al* [52] used multispectral SFDI to monitor hyperspectral changes in the optical absorption and reduced scattering spectra of blood exposed to air over 24 h.

6.3 Scattering by blood and blood components

Blood primarily consists of plasma (55% of blood by volume) and RBCs (45% of blood by volume), which are the primary cell components of blood. However, there are multiple other cell types, which can be broadly grouped into leucocytes (WBCs) and thrombocytes (platelets).

6.3.1 Plasma

The scattering properties of pure plasma are expected to be described by Rayleigh scattering of protein molecules, resulting in a scattering cross-section that decreases with increasing wavelength ($\sim\lambda^{-4}$) (see equation (6.1)) and isotropic scattering. However, Meinke *et al* [23] found that the scattering anisotropy factor for the plasma is about 0.2, indicating a slightly forward scattering and a scattering coefficient that was much higher than expected by Rayleigh scattering, based on calculations for a 10% albumin solution. Based on Mie's theory, they estimated that particles with a size of approximately 100 nm and a total concentration of 10% must be present to explain the deviation from Rayleigh scattering. They attributed these particles to protein aggregates and lipids or cell components, which the centrifugation procedure could not remove.

6.3.2 Red blood cells

Human RBCs are anucleate cells containing a dense Hb solution, which is believed to be the primary component for the scattering and absorption of the UV, blue, and green spectral ranges of light [53].

A typical RBC shape is biconcave. However, depending on ambient factors (for example, moving in blood vessels), the RBC shape can deviate from the biconcave. In addition, RBCs are able to undergo shape change from the 'normal' discocyte to either echinocytes or stomatocytes, depending on a large variety of membrane and cytoplasmic parameters.

6.3.2.1 Shear rate

In flow, some rheological transformations of blood components may occur. In particular, changes may depend on the shear rate, defined as the slope of the velocity profile. This rate is high when the flow velocity is high, and the vessel diameter is

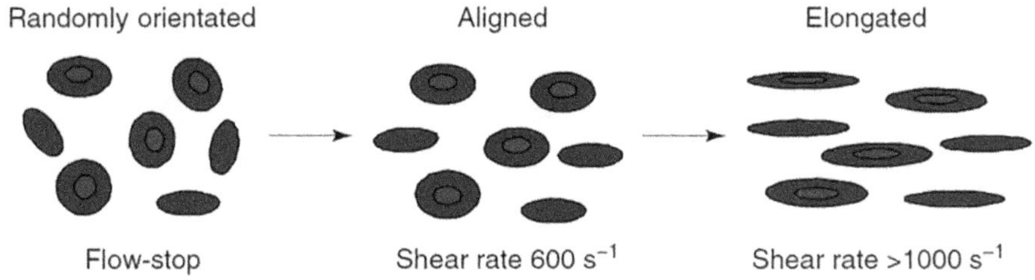

Figure 6.7. Illustration of shear rate influences on RBCs in physiological saline solution. Reproduced from [54] John Wiley & Sons. Copyright 2011 Wiley-VCH Verlag GmbH & Co. KGaA.

small; conversely, the shear rate is low when the flow velocity is low and the vessel diameter is large. For example, reversible aggregation may occur at lower shear rates, while erythrocytes are deformed into ellipsoids under higher shear rates (see figure 6.7.).

The shear rate also impacts alignment (see figure 6.7).

The shear rate in blood vessels can vary depending on the location, vessel size, and blood flow rate. For example, the wall shear rates in large veins can be as low as 10 s^{-1}, while in arteries, it can be as high as 1000 s^{-1}, and in pathology, it can be above 5000 s^{-1} [55].

6.3.2.2 Deformability

RBCs deform (e.g., elongate) as they traverse capillaries that are sometimes smaller in diameter than the RBC itself. RBC deformation is thought to be an important stimulus for ATP export from RBCs and allows them to dilate arterioles and readily traverse capillaries [56]. The RBC deformability can be measured by several methods, including micropipette, filterability, ektacytometry, and using optical tweezers [57]. For example, in the optical tweezer technique, optical force is applied to opposite ends of a visualized cell, and one of the laser beams is moved inward, deforming the cell. To quantify deformability, the elongation index (EI), which is the ratio of length to width of the RBC, is reported as a function of stress.

Changes in deformability can be associated with certain diseases. For example, Agrawal *et al* [58] used optical tweezers to study the deformability of RBCs from type 2 diabetes mellitus (T2DM) patients with or without diabetic retinopathy compared to matched healthy controls. They found that deformability was modestly but significantly lower in both groups of T2DM patients than in the healthy controls.

6.3.2.3 Osmolarity

The composition of the surrounding medium of the cells can disturb the iso-osmotic balance of 300 $mOsm\,l^{-1}$, as illustrated in figure 6.8. In a medium of low osmolarity ($<$ 300 $mOsm\,l^{-1}$), the cells start to swell by diffusion of water into the cell, leading to spherically formed cells, which become full to the point of bursting. In a hyperosmolar medium ($>$ 300 $mOsm\,l^{-1}$), cells shrink due to water outflow, resulting in characteristically shaped cells called spinocytes. These variations in osmolarity change not

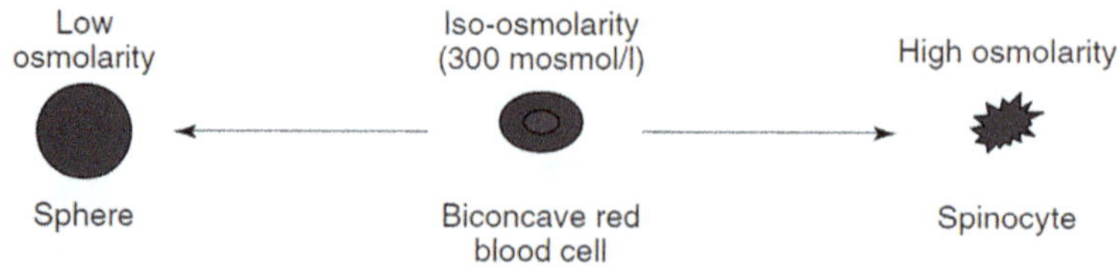

Figure 6.8. Illustration of osmolarity influences on RBCs in physiological saline solution. Reproduced from [54] John Wiley & Sons. Copyright 2011 Wiley-VCH Verlag GmbH & Co. KGaA.

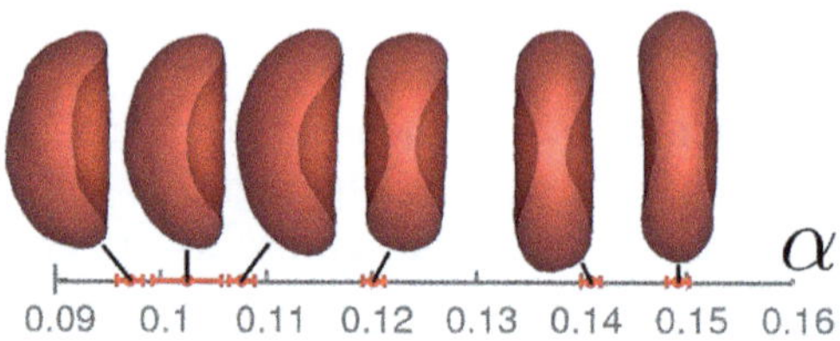

Figure 6.9. RBC shapes and associated asphericity α that characterizes the deviation from a spherical shape. Reproduced from [60] CC BY 4.0.

only the shape and volume of the cells but also the inner cell Hb concentration. As a result, the complex refractive index inside the cell increases due to increased Hb concentration.

Roggan *et al* [59] found that increasing osmolarity increases absorption while scattering and anisotropy decrease.

RBC shapes can be characterized by their asphericity α, which describes the deviation from a spherical shape. Asphericity ranges from 0.1 for a stomatocyte (or a cup-like shape) to 0.15 for a biconcave (or discocyte) shape (see figure 6.9).

Mauer *et al* [60] used the Rayleigh–Gans–Debye approximation to perform numerical calculations of SLS and DLS for a single RBC. Their results showed that the static scattering function averaged over many possible orientations of a diffusing RBC is not highly sensitive to changes in RBC membrane properties, such as shear elasticity and bending rigidity, or to moderate variations in RBC shapes (e.g., biconcave versus stomatocyte). Based on this, they concluded that orientationally-averaged SLS measurements are unlikely to be practical for detecting changes in RBC shape. However, they found that DLS, which analyzes the temporal correlations of instantaneous scattering amplitudes, can effectively reveal the diffusive behavior of an RBC and its membrane properties.

6.3.2.4 Static light scattering

Mauer *et al* [60], using a triangulated discocyte model of the RBC, calculated the SLS on RBC using two mesoscopic hydrodynamics approaches, multi-particle collision dynamics (MPCD) [61] and dissipative particle dynamics (DPD) [62].

The calculated scattering intensities of the RBC for different orientations are depicted in figure 6.10. One can see that the scattering intensities of RBC for small wave vectors $q = R_0/h_0$ are like those of short cylinders. They start to diverge only

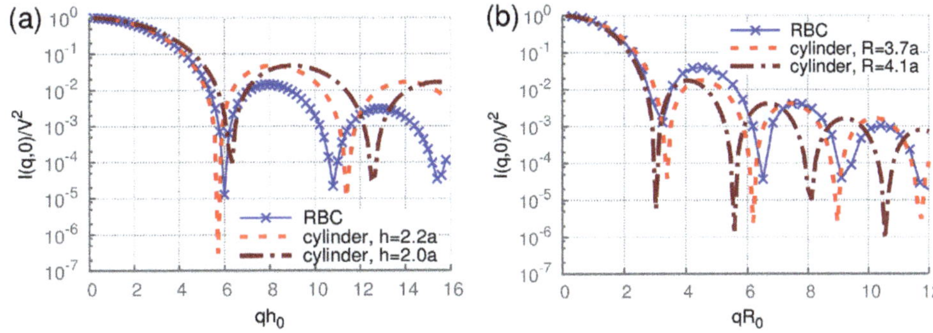

Figure 6.10. Static scattering by an RBC with a fixed orientation. The scattering intensity of a rigid discocyte for wave vectors q (a) parallel and (b) perpendicular to the RBC axis of rotational symmetry. $h_0 = 2a$. Analytical solutions for cylinders with different radii R_0 and heights h_0 are also plotted for comparison. Reproduced from [60] CC BY 4.0.

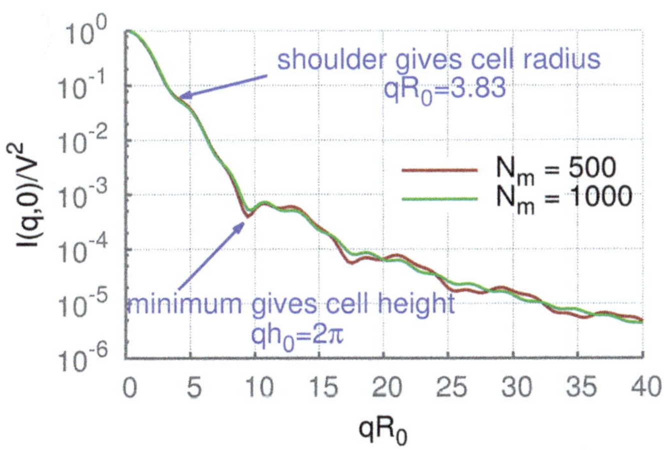

Figure 6.11. Orientationally-averaged static scattering functions of RBCs using the DPD method can be used to find cell height and radius. Simulation results converge, as shown by simulations with different numbers of triangles that approximate the shape ($N_m = 500$ and 1000). V is the cell volume. Reproduced from [60] CC BY 4.0.

for larger wave vectors q. Thus, the first and second minima for RBC shape intensity can be matched with the theory to produce estimates of the height h and radius R of the discocyte.

In figure 6.11, one can see the static scatting intensity averaged over multiple directions.

The orientationally-averaged scattering intensity is obviously different from the case of a fixed orientation; however, characteristic features are still visible. Firstly, a shoulder in the scattering intensity at $qR_0 = 3.83$ is clearly visible in all cases, corresponding to the RBC radius. Secondly, the scattering curves have a local minimum at $qh_0 = 2\pi$ related to the thickness of RBCs. Thus, RBCs' two main geometrical characteristics remain visible in the orientationally-averaged scattering intensities.

However, Mauer *et al* [60] found that differences in the static scattering function for biconcave and stomatocytic RBC shapes are not very pronounced. Therefore, the orientationally-averaged SLS function is not expected to be sensitive to changes in membrane properties and moderate alterations in cell shapes.

6.3.2.5 Dynamic light scattering

DLS provides information about the cell dynamics and membrane properties.

Mauer *et al* [60] used computer simulations of DLS to calculate translational diffusion of normal and deformed RBCs.

Park *et al* [50] used FTLS to study the static and dynamic light scattering on RBCs during the metabolic remodeling of the membrane. Using dynamic scattering, they found that the alterations in mechanical properties of the RBC membranes are ATP-dependent.

6.3.2.6 Multiple-scattering effects

In whole blood, the concentration of RBCs may be as high as 50%, and multiple-scattering effects must be considered.

For large ensembles of erythrocytes (like whole blood), approaches to account for the contribution of multiple scattering effects will be discussed in section 6.3.6.

Some simple conclusions can be derived for the smaller groups of RBCs (e.g., hundreds or thousands of RBCs). For example, due to the strong forward-scattering nature of scattering on cellular blood components, one could expect that the contribution of multiple-scattering effects will be relatively small. This notion was confirmed indirectly by He *et al* [63], who investigated the interaction of light with multiple RBCs using the finite-difference time-domain (FDTD) method [64], the superposition approximation, the Rytov approximation [65], and the discrete dipole approximation (DDA) [66]. Their simulations showed that the lateral multiple scattering between RBCs is very weak and that the polarization has an almost insignificant influence on the distribution of the scattered light.

6.3.3 Leukocytes

Leukocytes contain nuclei (often multi-lobe); thus, light experiences additional scattering at the cytoplasm/nucleus interface.

Meinke *et al* [23] found that the existence of physiological concentrations of leukocytes has no measurable influence on the optical properties of plasma and, therefore, on the optical parameters of whole blood.

The primary interest in scattering properties of leukocytes lies in discrimination between different types of leukocytes and their counting in flow cytometry.

Regular flow cytometry allows measuring the forward and side scattering from single cells, which can be used to discriminate lymphocytes, monocytes, and granulocytes [67]. Terstappen *et al* [68] reported the correlation between the fraction of cells with significant side scattering and the fraction of cytotoxic lymphocytes,

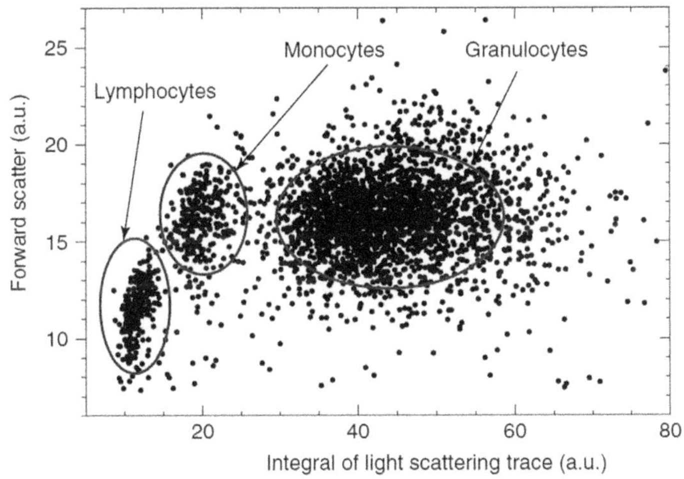

Figure 6.12. Light scattering cytogram of leukocytes. Reproduced from [72] John Wiley & Sons. Copyright 2011 Wiley-VCH Verlag GmbH & Co. KGaA.

which can be potentially used to determine the latter fraction from light scattering only.

Angle-resolved light-scattering measurements of single mononuclear cells using optical traps were performed for human lymphocytes by Doornbos *et al* [69] and for human monocytes by Watson *et al* [70]. Zharinov *et al* [71] studied the light scattering profile (LSP) of individual WBCs using proprietary-developed SFC. The same group [72] proposed to use absolute values of the integrated whole light-scattering trace instead of side scattering for cell discrimination (see figure 6.12). Even though monocytes and lymphocytes can be discriminated this way, it was impossible to determine whether a lymphocyte is T- or B-, using only its morphological characteristics determined from LSP.

In flow cytometers, granulocytes can be discriminated from other leukocytes by their higher forward and side scattering, except the basophils found in the light-scattering region of lymphocytes [73]. However, using only LSP, granulocytes cannot be discriminated into sub-types [72].

Dannhauser *et al* [74] used an LSP to discriminate T-, B-lymphocytes, and monocytes using LSP analysis of individual mononuclear bloodstream cells in-flow. A distinctive optical signature for each viscoelastically aligned cell was obtained.

6.3.4 Platelets

Blood platelets play a central role in hemostasis and are involved in many pathophysiological processes, including thrombosis, hemorrhage, inflammation, and cancer [75].

Platelets are anucleate cells. Unactivated (resting) platelets circulate in the blood as small disc-shaped cells whose cell size varies significantly. The aspect ratio (diameter/thickness) also varies from cell to cell within a wide range from 2 to 8 [76].

Upon activation, the platelet becomes a spiny sphere with pseudopodia. Excluding pseudopodia, an activated platelet can be described as spheroid with an aspect ratio slightly larger than 1.

Meinke *et al* [53] found that platelets do not change the absorption but increase the scattering of the blood. This increase in scattering is proportional to the platelet concentration.

Mean platelet volume (MPV) and platelet distribution width (PDW) are considered clinically important parameters [77]. However, despite a platelet undergoing dramatic shape change during activation, the standard flow cytometric techniques (forward- versus side-light-scattering maps, FSC-SSC) for resting and activated platelets differ slightly [78].

Moskalensky *et al* [79] demonstrated that unactivated (resting) and activated platelets can be distinguished by measuring the angle-resolved light-scattering pattern of blood platelets using a SFC. The platelet characteristics were determined from the solution of the inverse light-scattering problem using the precomputed database of theoretical LSPs, which were calculated using the discrete dipole approximation (DDA).

Maurer-Spurej *et al* [80] proposed the DDLS platelet monitor (DLS-PM) for the quality of platelet concentrates for transfusion to extend the current 5-day shelf life of platelet concentrates. The DLS-PM measures platelet size, the number of platelet-derived microparticles, and the response of platelets to temperature changes, which are combined to calculate a platelet quality score.

6.3.5 Scattering by whole blood

6.3.5.1 Scaling on hematocrit

Let's assume that the space with the total volume V_T contains N identical particles with a scattering cross-section σ_s. Then, ignoring the interaction between particles, the scattering coefficient of this ensemble can be found as

$$\mu_{s,ind} = \frac{N}{V_T}\sigma_s = \frac{hct}{V_P}\sigma_s \tag{6.12}$$

where hct is the hematocrit [%] or the volume percentage of RBCs in the blood and V_P is the particle's volume. In the case of RBCs, V_P is typically assumed to be 90 μm^3 [6].

Since the hematocrit (volume fraction) of blood is on average 40% for adult women and 45% for adult men, the interaction between scattering fields of individual particles cannot be ignored. This situation is often referred to as *dependent scattering*, which occurs when particles (RBCs in this case) are closely spaced, or a correlation exists between their positions. The phase relation between the fields scattered from different particles cannot be ignored for dependent scattering. Therefore, the scattering fields should be added instead of the scattering intensities.

The scattering coefficient for the dependent scattering can be expressed (see, for example [81]) through the scattering coefficient for the independent scattering

$$\mu_{s,d} = \gamma(hct)\mu_{s,ind} \tag{6.13}$$

Where $\gamma(hct)$ is a hematocrit-dependent scaling factor between the scattering cross-section for dependent and independent scattering. The scaling factor γ can be found as [81]

$$\gamma(hct) = 2\pi \int_0^{\pi} S(\theta, hct) p_s(\theta) \sin\theta d\theta \tag{6.14}$$

where $p_s(\theta)$ is the scattering phase function of the individual scatterer and $S(\theta, hct)$ is the structural factor, which can be found as [82]

$$S(\theta, hct) = 1 + 2\pi \frac{hct}{V_p} \int_0^{\infty} (G(r) - 1) r^2 \frac{\sin qr}{qr} dr \tag{6.15}$$

where $q = 4\pi/\lambda \sin(\theta/2)$ and $G(r)$ is the radial distribution function that characterizes the probability of finding two particles over a distance r.

Thus, the scaling factor γ can be found if we know both the scattering phase function of the individual scatterer and the radial distribution function.

In particular, solutions were derived by Twersky [83] in the case of isotropic scattering ($p_s(\theta) = 1/4\pi$) for a gas

$$\gamma_{T-g}(hct) = 1 - hct \tag{6.16}$$

And non-deformable spheres

$$\gamma_{T-s}(hct) = \frac{(1 - hct)^4}{(1 + 2hct)^2} \tag{6.17}$$

Steinke found [6] that equations (6.16) and (6.17) have limited accuracy in describing scattering for whole blood and proposed the empirical expression

$$\gamma_S(hct) = (1 - hct)(1.4 - hct) \tag{6.18}$$

More recently, Bosschaart *et al* [81], using the Mie scattering phase function and the Percus–Yevick radial distribution function for non-deformable spheres [84], obtained the following approximation

$$\gamma_B(hct) = (1 - hct)^2 \tag{6.19}$$

Douplik and Loschenov measured the optical properties of the whole blood as a function of hematocrit [85]. They found a decrease in scattering with the *hct* increase of over 50% as the blood cells started to contact each other. The erythrocytes begin to adhere and to be deformed by each other. Blood-like media with 'islands of erythrocytes and its aggregates within plasma' transform into the media 'particles of plasma between erythrocytes.' In the limit $hct \rightarrow 100\%$, the 'plasma particles' disappear, and μ_s of blood should approach zero [86]. The absorption and reduced scattering coefficients are shown in figure 6.13. The decrease in scattering is consistent with the scaling model equation (6.12) combined with the scaling factor provided by equations (6.18) or (6.19).

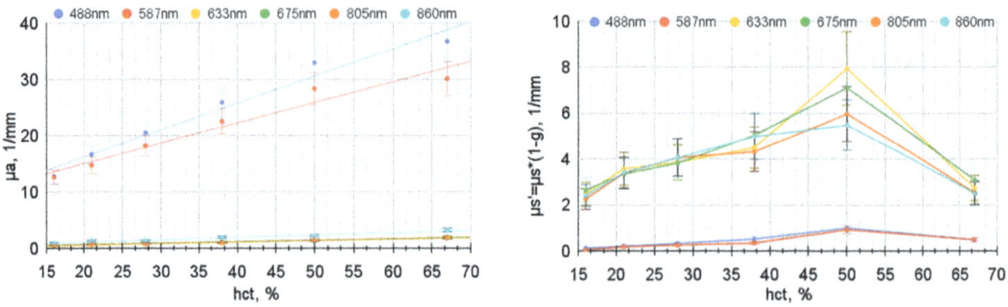

Figure 6.13. Whole blood absorption and reduced scattering coefficients as a function of hematocrit. The oxygen saturation (sO_2) was 99% with an optical path of 140 μm (modified with permission from [85], copyright (1996) Society of Photo-Optical Instrumentation Engineers (SPIE)).

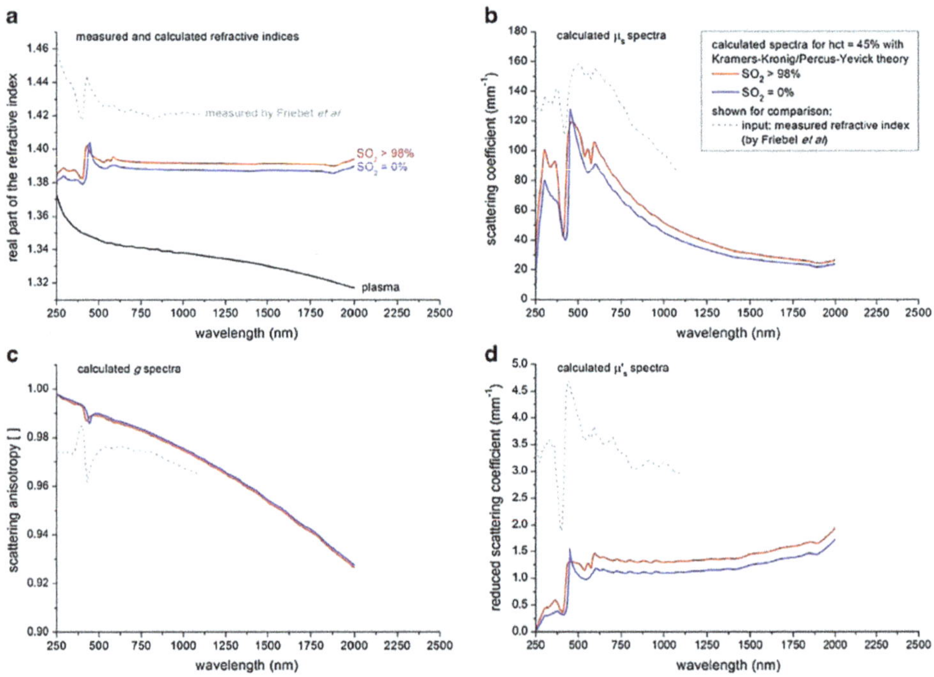

Figure 6.14. Theoretical estimates of the optical properties of whole blood:(a) The real part of the refractive index, (b) scattering coefficient, (c) scattering anisotropy factor, and (d) reduced scattering coefficient. Reproduced from [81] CC BY 4.0.

The optical properties of the whole blood, including scattering, were reviewed by Bosschaart *et al* [81]. This review contains tabulated data for the optical properties of whole blood, $hct = 45\%$, in the 250–2000 nm range, using the scaling factor provided by equation (6.19). In addition to optical properties compiled from the literature, they also estimated optical properties based on the Kramers–Kronig relation (see figure 6.14) in the 250–2000 nm range. This tabulated data is provided in table 6.1.

Table 6.1. Tabulated data for the optical property spectra of whole blood, hct = 45%. Reproduced with modifications from [81] CC BY 4.0.

	Compiled averages from literature spectra				Kramers–Kronig/Percus–Yevick theory			
Wavelength, [nm]	μ_a, $sO_2 > 98\%$, [mm^{-1}]	μ_a, $sO_2 = 0\%$, [mm^{-1}]	μ_s, $sO_2 > 98\%$, [mm^{-1}]	g, $sO_2 >$ 98%, [–]	μ_s, $sO_2 > 98\%$, [mm^{-1}]	μ_s, $sO_2 = 0\%$, [mm^{-1}]	g, $sO_2 >$ 98%, [–]	g, $sO_2 = 0\%$, [–]
251	44.02	48.32	58.64	0.8088	22.47	7.00	0.9980	0.9981
252	42.29	48.89	58.61	0.8126	36.69	16.92	0.9978	0.9980
254	43.58	49.47	58.35	0.8147	41.34	21.01	0.9977	0.9979
256	44.89	50.26	58.00	0.8164	44.97	24.41	0.9976	0.9978
258	46.38	50.95	57.36	0.8187	48.07	27.57	0.9975	0.9978
260	47.89	51.57	56.99	0.8200	50.90	30.60	0.9974	0.9977
262	49.48	52.19	56.60	0.8202	53.52	33.55	0.9973	0.9976
264	51.00	52.81	56.04	0.8202	56.00	36.45	0.9972	0.9976
266	52.22	53.32	55.26	0.8204	58.41	39.31	0.9971	0.9975
268	53.29	53.83	54.94	0.8205	60.81	42.15	0.9970	0.9974
270	54.13	54.34	54.63	0.8210	63.40	45.01	0.9969	0.9973
272	54.59	54.63	54.35	0.8222	66.14	48.01	0.9967	0.9972
274	54.99	54.32	54.42	0.8235	68.80	51.06	0.9966	0.9971
276	54.97	53.92	54.63	0.8251	71.26	53.47	0.9965	0.9970
278	54.63	53.56	54.82	0.8281	73.30	55.28	0.9964	0.9970
280	54.14	53.19	54.99	0.8324	75.64	57.11	0.9963	0.9969
282	53.34	52.77	55.18	0.8374	77.96	59.03	0.9962	0.9968
284	52.30	52.03	55.38	0.8428	80.44	61.16	0.9961	0.9967
286	50.45	50.67	55.56	0.8497	82.95	63.32	0.9960	0.9967
288	48.22	48.72	56.00	0.8578	85.69	65.87	0.9960	0.9966
290	46.13	45.94	56.72	0.8648	87.56	68.80	0.9959	0.9965
292	43.58	43.08	57.56	0.8713	90.11	71.14	0.9958	0.9965
294	40.50	40.29	58.46	0.8798	93.61	73.39	0.9957	0.9964

(Continued)

Table 6.1. (*Continued*)

	Compiled averages from literature spectra				Kramers–Kronig/Percus–Yevick theory			
Wavelength, [nm]	μ_a, $sO_2 > 98\%$, [mm^{-1}]	μ_a, $sO_2 = 0\%$, [mm^{-1}]	μ_s, $sO_2 > 98\%$, [mm^{-1}]	g, $sO_2 > 98\%$, [–]	μ_s, $sO_2 > 98\%$, [mm^{-1}]	μ_s, $sO_2 = 0\%$, [mm^{-1}]	g, $sO_2 > 98\%$, [–]	g, $sO_2 = 0\%$, [–]
296	37.82	37.45	59.36	0.8889	96.38	76.05	0.9957	0.9964
298	35.12	34.81	60.11	0.8976	98.85	78.16	0.9956	0.9963
300	32.52	33.15	60.64	0.9035	100.27	79.57	0.9956	0.9963
302	30.99	32.12	61.01	0.9084	100.50	79.87	0.9955	0.9962
304	30.01	31.25	61.36	0.9142	100.33	80.00	0.9955	0.9962
306	29.69	30.47	61.59	0.9159	99.79	79.89	0.9955	0.9962
308	29.75	30.28	61.28	0.9165	99.31	79.22	0.9954	0.9961
310	30.03	30.95	60.80	0.9159	98.78	78.45	0.9954	0.9961
312	30.73	32.10	60.24	0.9146	97.73	77.5	0.9953	0.9961
314	31.49	33.25	59.59	0.9129	96.70	76.71	0.9953	0.9960
316	32.45	34.43	58.90	0.9088	95.68	76.03	0.9952	0.9960
318	33.76	35.61	58.15	0.9029	94.81	75.40	0.9952	0.9959
320	35.15	36.86	57.50	0.8975	93.96	74.72	0.9951	0.9959
322	36.61	38.22	56.85	0.8938	93.08	74.02	0.9950	0.9958
324	38.03	39.50	56.31	0.8901	92.22	73.43	0.9950	0.9957
326	39.49	40.67	55.96	0.8861	91.40	72.96	0.9949	0.9957
328	40.94	41.70	55.59	0.8830	90.62	72.64	0.9948	0.9956
330	42.29	42.61	55.22	0.8797	89.98	72.41	0.9947	0.9955
332	43.46	43.51	54.73	0.8773	89.49	72.12	0.9947	0.9955
334	44.48	44.45	54.40	0.8758	89.26	71.74	0.9946	0.9954
336	45.42	45.94	54.19	0.8743	89.25	71.05	0.9945	0.9954
338	46.02	47.50	53.98	0.8735	89.20	70.45	0.9944	0.9953
340	46.46	48.90	53.80	0.8727	89.17	70.12	0.9943	0.9952
342	46.86	49.89	53.71	0.8720	89.22	70.02	0.9942	0.9951
344	47.23	50.81	53.63	0.8719	89.37	69.86	0.9942	0.9951

346	47.14	51.73	53.59	0.8724	89.94	69.68	0.9941	0.9950
348	46.73	52.68	53.54	0.8734	90.44	69.44	0.9940	0.9949
350	46.29	53.76	53.59	0.8750	90.96	69.11	0.9939	0.9949
352	45.80	54.73	53.84	0.8770	91.25	68.58	0.9939	0.9948
354	45.24	55.68	54.09	0.8793	91.48	68.10	0.9938	0.9947
356	44.37	56.62	54.37	0.8816	91.90	67.72	0.9938	0.9947
358	43.36	57.20	54.70	0.8841	92.56	67.64	0.9937	0.9946
360	42.38	57.74	54.59	0.8863	92.92	67.52	0.9937	0.9945
362	41.67	58.10	54.34	0.8881	93.05	67.39	0.9937	0.9945
364	41.22	58.43	54.08	0.8897	93.03	67.25	0.9937	0.9944
366	40.86	58.76	53.68	0.8913	92.66	67.07	0.9936	0.9944
368	40.72	59.10	53.23	0.8920	92.06	66.84	0.9936	0.9943
370	41.14	59.44	52.88	0.8922	90.92	66.57	0.9936	0.9943
372	42.09	59.74	52.49	0.8915	89.19	66.26	0.9936	0.9942
374	43.14	60.04	52.00	0.8902	87.52	65.93	0.9936	0.9941
376	44.26	60.34	51.33	0.8879	85.78	65.56	0.9936	0.9941
378	45.87	60.67	50.59	0.8851	83.85	65.15	0.9936	0.9941
380	47.86	61.28	49.79	0.8798	81.57	64.71	0.9935	0.9940
382	50.38	61.73	48.64	0.8741	79.10	64.17	0.9935	0.9940
384	54.31	62.83	47.42	0.8675	76.48	62.97	0.9935	0.9940
386	57.72	64.26	46.07	0.8603	73.63	61.59	0.9935	0.9939
388	62.58	65.75	44.93	0.8474	70.24	60.16	0.9934	0.9939
390	68.33	67.75	43.94	0.8379	66.26	58.39	0.9934	0.9938
392	73.62	71.01	43.03	0.8257	62.72	56.43	0.9932	0.9937
394	79.07	74.09	42.33	0.8127	59.85	54.90	0.9931	0.9937
396	84.00	76.95	41.77	0.7967	57.77	53.61	0.9929	0.9936
398	88.56	79.78	41.17	0.7863	56.09	52.39	0.9928	0.9935
400	93.07	82.54	40.12	0.7734	54.32	51.16	0.9926	0.9934
402	97.40	85.59	41.27	0.7866	52.31	49.55	0.9925	0.9933

(Continued)

Table 6.1. *(Continued)*

	Compiled averages from literature spectra				Kramers–Kronig/Percus–Yevick theory			
Wavelength, [nm]	μ_a, $sO_2 > 98\%$, [mm^{-1}]	μ_a, $sO_2 = 0\%$, [mm^{-1}]	μ_s, $sO_2 > 98\%$, [mm^{-1}]	g, $sO_2 >$ 98%, [–]	μ_s, $sO_2 > 98\%$, [mm^{-1}]	μ_s, $sO_2 = 0\%$, [mm^{-1}]	g, $sO_2 >$ 98%, [–]	g, $sO_2 = 0\%$, [–]
404	101.82	89.21	40.25	0.7769	49.52	47.83	0.9924	0.9932
406	106.16	92.73	39.49	0.7726	45.77	46.47	0.9922	0.9930
408	110.73	96.09	38.90	0.7657	42.83	45.36	0.9916	0.9929
410	113.81	99.87	38.60	0.7604	42.44	44.39	0.9910	0.9927
412	116.09	104.21	38.95	0.7575	42.74	43.43	0.9904	0.9926
414	117.97	108.92	39.87	0.7585	43.62	42.46	0.9896	0.9924
416	118.04	114.03	41.09	0.7606	45.59	41.74	0.9890	0.9922
418	117.22	119.62	42.38	0.7657	47.68	41.18	0.9883	0.9919
420	115.39	125.10	43.91	0.7742	51.35	40.78	0.9876	0.9916
422	111.45	131.52	46.42	0.7896	56.08	40.43	0.9872	0.9914
424	106.30	139.37	49.90	0.802	61.93	40.06	0.9870	0.9910
426	100.61	145.30	52.74	0.8141	68.03	40.40	0.9869	0.9906
428	94.94	151.01	55.61	0.8290	74.00	40.72	0.9870	0.9901
430	89.18	155.62	57.55	0.8390	79.94	40.89	0.9870	0.9896
432	82.69	159.31	60.51	0.8568	85.95	41.69	0.9871	0.9889
434	74.61	158.30	62.65	0.8710	95.79	43.48	0.9873	0.9882
436	66.95	156.93	64.74	0.8820	102.94	45.58	0.9877	0.9873
438	58.47	133.73	66.40	0.8928	105.63	50.05	0.9880	0.9865
440	51.07	118.33	68.83	0.9026	109.27	57.64	0.9882	0.9862
442	46.60	107.88	70.39	0.9220	111.29	63.54	0.9883	0.9860
444	42.24	88.84	72.82	0.9302	113.65	73.81	0.9885	0.9861
446	38.21	74.30	73.79	0.9343	114.47	81.66	0.9886	0.9862
448	34.26	54.74	75.05	0.9392	116.38	94.61	0.9887	0.9863
450	31.48	33.81	77.20	0.9447	116.55	118.29	0.9888	0.9869
452	29.42	25.94	78.01	0.9488	117.24	125.06	0.9888	0.9878

454	27.66	19.82	78.82	0.9520	118.02	128.16	0.9889	0.9884
456	26.00	17.04	79.42	0.9544	118.52	127.52	0.9889	0.9888
458	24.47	13.61	80.17	0.9567	118.65	126.75	0.9890	0.9890
460	22.82	11.45	80.31	0.9587	118.94	125.60	0.9890	0.9892
462	21.33	10.37	80.37	0.9611	119.16	124.50	0.9890	0.9894
464	20.10	9.64	80.85	0.9634	119.13	123.31	0.9890	0.9895
466	18.97	9.12	81.74	0.9651	119.26	122.08	0.9890	0.9896
468	17.93	8.65	82.77	0.9665	119.26	120.90	0.9890	0.9897
470	17.05	8.29	82.61	0.9677	119.15	119.73	0.9891	0.9897
472	16.30	7.99	83.21	0.9684	119.01	118.60	0.9891	0.9898
474	15.71	7.79	83.50	0.9690	118.85	117.42	0.9891	0.9898
476	15.16	7.60	83.81	0.9695	118.63	116.30	0.9891	0.9898
478	14.63	7.44	84.99	0.9700	118.38	115.20	0.9890	0.9898
480	14.15	7.31	86.13	0.9705	118.12	114.14	0.9890	0.9898
482	13.67	7.43	86.48	0.9714	117.80	113.05	0.9890	0.9899
484	13.30	7.56	86.75	0.9723	117.42	112.00	0.9890	0.9899
486	12.92	7.69	86.80	0.9731	117.03	110.99	0.9890	0.9899
488	12.54	7.86	86.81	0.9738	116.65	110.00	0.9890	0.9899
490	12.23	8.10	87.02	0.9743	116.26	108.96	0.9890	0.9898
492	11.94	8.35	87.52	0.9748	115.89	107.96	0.9889	0.9898
494	11.65	8.60	88.31	0.9752	115.52	106.99	0.9889	0.9898
496	11.37	8.87	88.75	0.9756	115.13	106.04	0.9889	0.9898
498	11.19	9.17	88.87	0.9759	114.73	105.10	0.9888	0.9898
500	11.05	9.50	88.63	0.9761	114.28	104.16	0.9888	0.9898
502	10.90	9.88	88.23	0.9762	113.83	103.25	0.9888	0.9897
504	10.74	10.25	87.75	0.9762	113.35	102.36	0.9888	0.9897
506	10.59	10.64	86.35	0.9762	112.88	101.49	0.9888	0.9897
508	10.52	10.99	85.75	0.9762	112.32	100.65	0.9887	0.9896
510	10.55	11.41	85.43	0.9763	111.71	99.82	0.9887	0.9896

(Continued)

Table 6.1. (*Continued*)

	Compiled averages from literature spectra				Kramers–Kronig/Percus–Yevick theory			
Wavelength, [nm]	μ_a, $sO_2 > 98\%$, [mm^{-1}]	μ_a, $sO_2 = 0\%$, [mm^{-1}]	μ_s, $sO_2 > 98\%$, [mm^{-1}]	g, $sO_2 > 98\%$, [–]	μ_s, $sO_2 > 98\%$, [mm^{-1}]	μ_s, $sO_2 = 0\%$, [mm^{-1}]	g, $sO_2 > 98\%$, [–]	g, $sO_2 = 0\%$, [–]
512	10.74	11.91	85.03	0.9764	111.05	99.01	0.9887	0.9896
514	11.09	12.42	84.54	0.9765	110.29	98.21	0.9886	0.9895
516	11.59	12.92	83.74	0.9765	109.41	97.44	0.9886	0.9895
518	12.34	13.43	82.61	0.9763	108.32	96.68	0.9886	0.9894
520	13.26	13.98	81.42	0.9760	107.15	95.93	0.9886	0.9894
522	14.36	14.50	79.88	0.9756	105.81	95.16	0.9886	0.9894
524	15.62	15.22	78.06	0.9751	104.37	94.37	0.9885	0.9893
526	17.17	16.04	76.69	0.9744	102.87	93.59	0.9885	0.9893
528	19.20	16.96	75.28	0.9728	101.37	92.83	0.9884	0.9892
530	20.91	17.82	73.83	0.9707	99.91	92.08	0.9883	0.9892
532	22.48	18.66	72.78	0.9687	98.65	91.34	0.9883	0.9891
534	23.91	19.51	71.83	0.9668	97.67	90.60	0.9882	0.9891
536	25.17	20.37	71.10	0.9650	96.93	89.88	0.9881	0.9890
538	26.22	21.25	70.59	0.9637	96.44	89.18	0.9880	0.9890
540	27.13	22.13	70.14	0.9627	96.27	88.50	0.9879	0.9889
542	27.31	23.19	69.93	0.9625	96.43	87.87	0.9878	0.9888
544	26.79	24.01	69.89	0.9625	96.98	87.30	0.9877	0.9887
546	26.06	24.77	70.34	0.9627	97.79	86.81	0.9876	0.9887
548	25.15	25.45	70.86	0.9633	98.80	86.45	0.9875	0.9886
550	23.86	25.99	71.49	0.9642	99.80	86.20	0.9874	0.9885
552	22.54	26.38	72.27	0.9652	100.46	85.89	0.9874	0.9884
554	21.34	26.70	73.12	0.9664	100.86	85.66	0.9874	0.9884
556	20.29	26.80	73.70	0.9677	100.98	85.56	0.9874	0.9883
558	19.55	26.71	74.10	0.9690	100.71	85.54	0.9874	0.9883
560	19.12	26.56	74.13	0.9694	100.25	85.59	0.9873	0.9882

562	19.47	26.00	73.63	0.9696	99.50	85.77	0.9873	0.9881
564	20.14	25.38	72.90	0.9693	98.42	85.97	0.9873	0.9880
566	21.04	24.74	72.04	0.9687	97.07	86.17	0.9873	0.9880
568	22.56	24.06	70.98	0.9681	95.53	86.39	0.9872	0.9879
570	24.38	23.29	70.02	0.9677	93.95	86.59	0.9872	0.9879
572	25.62	22.38	69.20	0.9674	92.53	86.76	0.9871	0.9878
574	26.70	21.43	68.82	0.967	91.56	86.91	0.9870	0.9878
576	27.20	20.49	68.84	0.9666	91.44	87.14	0.9869	0.9878
578	26.87	19.64	69.09	0.9663	92.37	87.45	0.9867	0.9877
580	25.75	18.87	70.07	0.9662	94.28	87.72	0.9865	0.9876
582	23.29	18.08	72.11	0.9669	96.77	87.97	0.9864	0.9876
584	20.06	17.27	74.68	0.9680	99.53	88.24	0.9863	0.9875
586	16.51	16.33	77.42	0.9692	101.95	88.55	0.9862	0.9874
588	12.68	15.30	79.88	0.9708	103.81	88.96	0.9862	0.9874
590	9.72	14.21	81.67	0.9724	105.02	89.50	0.9862	0.9873
592	7.32	13.12	83.13	0.9743	105.69	90.03	0.9862	0.9872
594	5.66	11.92	84.67	0.9759	105.95	90.54	0.9862	0.9872
596	4.48	10.60	85.58	0.9774	105.94	90.98	0.9862	0.9871
598	3.60	9.29	86.21	0.9784	105.74	91.35	0.9862	0.9871
600	2.62	7.53	86.88	0.9794	105.49	91.56	0.9861	0.9871
605	1.51	5.55	87.89	0.9809	104.02	90.96	0.9861	0.9870
610	0.88	4.07	88.09	0.9815	102.49	90.12	0.9860	0.9869
615	0.63	3.27	88.09	0.982	101.04	89.04	0.9860	0.9869
620	0.46	2.82	88.28	0.9823	99.64	87.85	0.9859	0.9868
625	0.35	2.48	88.50	0.9824	98.30	86.66	0.9859	0.9867
630	0.28	2.27	88.55	0.9826	97.50	86.01	0.9857	0.9866
635	0.24	2.10	88.63	0.9827	96.75	85.38	0.9856	0.9864
640	0.20	1.98	88.84	0.9827	96.01	84.75	0.9854	0.9863
645	0.17	1.89	88.55	0.9826	95.30	84.15	0.9853	0.9862

(Continued)

Table 6.1. (*Continued*)

	Compiled averages from literature spectra				Kramers–Kronig/Percus–Yevick theory			
Wavelength, [nm]	μ_a, $sO_2 > 98\%$, [mm^{-1}]	μ_a, $sO_2 = 0\%$, [mm^{-1}]	μ_s, $sO_2 > 98\%$, [mm^{-1}]	g, $sO_2 > 98\%$, [–]	μ_s, $sO_2 > 98\%$, [mm^{-1}]	μ_s, $sO_2 = 0\%$, [mm^{-1}]	g, $sO_2 > 98\%$, [–]	g, $sO_2 = 0\%$, [–]
650	0.16	1.80	88.01	0.9825	94.61	83.56	0.9852	0.9861
655	0.16	1.71	87.72	0.9825	93.44	82.50	0.9851	0.9859
660	0.15	1.64	87.61	0.9826	92.29	81.45	0.9850	0.9858
665	0.14	1.58	87.51	0.9828	91.16	80.44	0.9849	0.9857
670	0.14	1.51	87.25	0.9832	90.06	79.45	0.9848	0.9856
675	0.14	1.43	86.82	0.9830	88.98	78.47	0.9847	0.9855
680	0.14	1.35	86.61	0.9831	87.91	77.51	0.9846	0.9854
685	0.14	1.26	86.57	0.9834	86.87	76.57	0.9845	0.9853
690	0.13	1.17	86.35	0.9835	85.84	75.63	0.9843	0.9852
695	0.13	1.10	86.18	0.9835	84.83	74.71	0.9842	0.9850
700	0.14	1.00	85.70	0.9836	83.86	73.82	0.9841	0.9849
705	0.14	0.93	83.70	0.9837	83.35	73.40	0.9840	0.9848
710	0.17	0.87	83.33	0.9841	82.87	73.00	0.9838	0.9847
715	0.17	0.80	82.99	0.9840	82.40	72.61	0.9837	0.9845
720	0.18	0.75	82.57	0.9839	81.94	72.22	0.9835	0.9843
725	0.19	0.72	82.18	0.9839	81.46	71.82	0.9833	0.9841
730	0.20	0.70	81.64	0.9839	80.57	70.99	0.9831	0.9840
735	0.21	0.70	81.09	0.9839	79.67	70.13	0.9831	0.9839
740	0.22	0.72	80.66	0.9839	78.78	69.29	0.9830	0.9838
745	0.23	0.76	80.40	0.9838	77.90	68.45	0.9829	0.9837
750	0.24	0.81	80.22	0.9837	77.04	67.62	0.9827	0.9836
755	0.26	0.85	79.85	0.9836	76.19	66.84	0.9826	0.9834
760	0.27	0.84	79.41	0.9835	75.36	66.10	0.9824	0.9832
765	0.29	0.80	78.93	0.9835	74.54	65.39	0.9823	0.9831
770	0.30	0.73	78.42	0.9833	73.73	64.69	0.9822	0.9830

775	0.31	0.66	78.00	0.9832	72.95	64.01	0.9821	0.9829
780	0.33	0.59	77.61	0.9832	72.59	63.73	0.9819	0.9827
785	0.34	0.54	77.19	0.9832	72.25	63.47	0.9818	0.9826
790	0.36	0.51	76.82	0.9832	71.92	63.20	0.9816	0.9824
795	0.37	0.48	76.77	0.9831	71.59	62.94	0.9814	0.9822
800	0.38	0.47	76.73	0.9833	71.27	62.68	0.9812	0.9820
805	0.39	0.46	76.47	0.9832	70.53	62.00	0.9810	0.9818
810	0.40	0.45	76.10	0.9833	69.80	61.33	0.9809	0.9817
815	0.42	0.44	75.70	0.9833	69.08	60.66	0.9808	0.9816
820	0.43	0.44	75.48	0.9834	68.36	60.00	0.9807	0.9815
825	0.45	0.43	75.27	0.9835	67.66	59.35	0.9806	0.9814
830	0.46	0.43	75.06	0.9835	66.96	58.72	0.9804	0.9812
835	0.47	0.43	74.83	0.9834	66.28	58.09	0.9803	0.9811
840	0.48	0.43	74.65	0.9834	65.61	57.48	0.9801	0.9809
845	0.48	0.43	74.51	0.9833	64.95	56.87	0.9799	0.9807
850	0.49	0.42	74.20	0.9832	64.33	56.30	0.9798	0.9806
855	0.51	0.43	73.58	0.9831	64.06	56.08	0.9796	0.9804
860	0.51	0.43	72.87	0.9831	63.82	55.88	0.9794	0.9803
865	0.52	0.43	72.43	0.9831	63.58	55.69	0.9793	0.9801
870	0.53	0.43	72.29	0.9830	63.35	55.50	0.9791	0.9799
875	0.55	0.43	72.12	0.9829	63.09	55.29	0.9789	0.9797
880	0.56	0.44	71.63	0.9828	62.50	54.76	0.9788	0.9796
885	0.56	0.45	70.79	0.9828	61.90	54.20	0.9786	0.9794
890	0.56	0.45	70.07	0.9826	61.30	53.66	0.9784	0.9792
895	0.56	0.46	69.41	0.9824	60.72	53.12	0.9782	0.9791
900	0.56	0.46	68.86	0.9824	60.14	52.59	0.9781	0.9789
905	0.57	0.47	68.35	0.9823	59.57	52.07	0.9780	0.9788
910	0.57	0.47	68.07	0.9820	59.00	51.56	0.9778	0.9787
915	0.57	0.47	67.82	0.9820	58.44	51.05	0.9777	0.9786

(Continued)

Table 6.1. (*Continued*)

	Compiled averages from literature spectra				Kramers–Kronig/Percus–Yevick theory			
Wavelength, [nm]	μ_a, $sO_2 > 98\%$, [mm^{-1}]	μ_a, $sO_2 = 0\%$, [mm^{-1}]	μ_s, $sO_2 > 98\%$, [mm^{-1}]	g, $sO_2 >$ 98%, [–]	μ_s, $sO_2 > 98\%$, [mm^{-1}]	μ_s, $sO_2 = 0\%$, [mm^{-1}]	g, $sO_2 >$ 98%, [–]	g, $sO_2 = 0\%$, [–]
920	0.57	0.47	67.54	0.9819	57.89	50.55	0.9776	0.9784
925	0.65	0.46	67.24	0.9818	57.38	50.09	0.9774	0.9783
930	0.65	0.45	66.86	0.9815	57.18	49.93	0.9772	0.9780
935	0.65	0.44	66.42	0.9812	57.01	49.81	0.9770	0.9778
940	0.65	0.43	66.08	0.9811	56.84	49.66	0.9768	0.9776
945	0.65	0.41	65.67	0.9810	56.67	49.55	0.9766	0.9774
950	0.65	0.39	65.21	0.9808	56.47	49.40	0.9763	0.9772
955	0.65	0.38	64.78	0.9805	55.99	48.97	0.9762	0.9770
960	0.66	0.36	64.38	0.9801	55.48	48.51	0.9760	0.9769
965	0.68	0.34	63.95	0.9800	54.97	48.06	0.9759	0.9767
970	0.69	0.32	63.58	0.9799	54.48	47.62	0.9758	0.9766
975	0.69	0.31	63.20	0.9798	53.99	47.18	0.9756	0.9765
980	0.68	0.29	62.68	0.9798	53.51	46.74	0.9755	0.9763
985	0.67	0.26	62.27	0.9798	53.04	46.31	0.9754	0.9762
990	0.66	0.25	62.09	0.9798	52.58	45.89	0.9752	0.9760
995	0.65	0.23	62.00	0.9800	52.11	45.47	0.9750	0.9758
1000	0.64	0.22	61.83	0.9801	51.66	45.04	0.9748	0.9756
1005	0.66	0.31	61.69	0.9801	51.32	44.74	0.9746	0.9754
1010	0.65	0.28	61.62	0.9801	51.01	44.46	0.9744	0.9752
1015	0.63	0.28	61.57	0.9800	50.69	44.18	0.9742	0.9750
1020	0.61	0.28	61.46	0.9800	50.38	43.90	0.9740	0.9748
1025	0.60	0.27	61.18	0.9800	50.07	43.62	0.9738	0.9747
1030	0.58	0.24	60.85	0.9800	49.76	43.35	0.9737	0.9745
1035	0.56	0.24	60.49	0.9800	49.46	43.08	0.9736	0.9744
1040	0.53	0.23	60.35	0.9800	49.16	42.81	0.9734	0.9743

1045	0.50	0.22	60.31	0.9800	48.86	42.55	0.9733	0.9741
1050	0.49	0.22	60.15	0.9800	48.56	42.28	0.9731	0.9739
1055	0.48	0.22	59.87	0.9800	48.27	42.02	0.9729	0.9737
1060	0.46	0.21	59.53	0.9799	47.97	41.77	0.9727	0.9735
1065	0.45	0.20	59.26	0.9799	47.69	41.52	0.9724	0.9732
1070	0.42	0.19	59.04	0.9799	47.41	41.27	0.9722	0.9730
1075	0.40	0.19	58.73	0.9800	47.13	41.02	0.9720	0.9728
1080	0.37	0.18	58.34	0.9802	46.85	40.78	0.9718	0.9726
1085	0.35	0.17	58.08	0.9801	46.58	40.54	0.9716	0.9724
1090	0.34	0.17	57.98	0.9802	46.30	40.30	0.9714	0.9722
1095	0.34	0.16	57.89	0.9804	46.02	40.06	0.9712	0.9721
1100	0.35	0.15	57.81	0.9797	45.74	39.82	0.9711	0.9719
1105	0.33	0.15	57.58	0.9834	45.48	39.59	0.9709	0.9718
1110	0.33	0.16	57.66	0.9832	45.21	39.36	0.9708	0.9716
1115	0.33	0.15	57.67	0.9832	44.95	39.13	0.9706	0.9715
1120	0.31	0.14	57.72	0.9832	44.69	38.90	0.9704	0.9713
1125	0.32	0.14	57.53	0.9829	44.43	38.68	0.9703	0.9711
1130	0.31	0.13	57.26	0.9828	44.18	38.45	0.9700	0.9709
1135	0.30	0.15	57.78	0.9832	43.92	38.23	0.9698	0.9706
1140	0.30	0.16	57.93	0.9835	43.67	38.01	0.9696	0.9704
1145	0.29	0.18	57.72	0.9834	43.43	37.79	0.9694	0.9702
1150	0.30	0.19	57.51	0.9832	43.18	37.58	0.9691	0.9699
1155	0.31	0.21	57.33	0.9830	42.94	37.37	0.9689	0.9697
1160	0.32	0.21	57.05	0.9829	42.69	37.16	0.9687	0.9695
1165	0.32	0.21	56.82	0.9828	42.46	36.96	0.9685	0.9693
1170	0.32	0.21	56.55	0.9827	42.22	36.76	0.9683	0.9691
1175	0.32	0.21	56.21	0.9827	41.99	36.56	0.9681	0.9689
1180	0.33	0.21	55.55	0.9827	41.76	36.36	0.9679	0.9688
1185	0.33	0.21	55.41	0.9827	41.54	36.17	0.9677	0.9686

(Continued)

Table 6.1. (*Continued*)

	Compiled averages from literature spectra				Kramers–Kronig/Percus–Yevick theory			
Wavelength, [nm]	μ_a, $sO_2 > 98\%$, [mm^{-1}]	μ_a, $sO_2 = 0\%$, [mm^{-1}]	μ_s, $sO_2 > 98\%$, [mm^{-1}]	g, $sO_2 > 98\%$, [–]	μ_s, $sO_2 > 98\%$, [mm^{-1}]	μ_s, $sO_2 = 0\%$, [mm^{-1}]	g, $sO_2 > 98\%$, [–]	g, $sO_2 = 0\%$, [–]
1190	0.34	0.21	55.48	0.9827	41.31	35.97	0.9676	0.9684
1195	0.35	0.20	55.37	0.9827	41.09	35.78	0.9674	0.9683
1200	0.36	0.20	55.20	0.9826	40.88	35.59	0.9672	0.9681
1205	0.37	0.20	55.16	0.9826	40.70	35.40	0.9671	0.9679
1210	0.20	0.20	50.16	0.9784	40.48	35.22	0.9669	0.9677
1215	0.20	0.20	49.98	0.9784	40.25	35.03	0.9667	0.9675
1220	0.20	0.19	49.81	0.9784	40.04	34.85	0.9665	0.9673
1225	0.19	0.19	49.43	0.9784	39.82	34.67	0.9663	0.9671
1230	0.18	0.17	49.21	0.9784	39.61	34.49	0.9660	0.9668
1235	0.18	0.17	49.25	0.9784	39.40	34.31	0.9658	0.9666
1240	0.18	0.17	49.19	0.9783	39.19	34.13	0.9655	0.9664
1245	0.18	0.17	47.97	0.9782	38.99	33.96	0.9653	0.9661
1250	0.17	0.17	47.51	0.9781	38.79	33.78	0.9651	0.9659
1255	0.17	0.17	48.18	0.9781	38.58	33.61	0.9648	0.9656
1260	0.17	0.17	48.64	0.9783	38.38	33.44	0.9646	0.9654
1265	0.17	0.15	47.36	0.9781	38.19	33.27	0.9643	0.9652
1270	0.15	0.14	46.50	0.9775	37.99	33.10	0.9641	0.9650
1275	0.16	0.15	47.09	0.9774	37.79	32.93	0.9639	0.9648
1280	0.18	0.16	47.91	0.9778	37.59	32.76	0.9638	0.9646
1285	0.17	0.16	47.13	0.9778	37.40	32.59	0.9636	0.9645
1290	0.16	0.16	46.21	0.9778	37.21	32.43	0.9634	0.9643
1295	0.18	0.18	45.77	0.9778	37.01	32.26	0.9633	0.9641
1300	0.19	0.20	45.36	0.9779	36.82	32.09	0.9631	0.9640
1305	0.20	0.21	44.79	0.978	36.63	31.93	0.9629	0.9638
1310	0.21	0.22	44.21	0.9776	36.44	31.76	0.9628	0.9636

1315	0.22	0.23	43.95	0.9772	36.25	31.60	0.9626	0.9634
1320	0.24	0.26	43.91	0.9769	36.06	31.43	0.9624	0.9632
1325	0.26	0.29	43.64	0.9766	35.87	31.27	0.9622	0.9630
1330	0.29	0.31	43.38	0.9768	35.68	31.11	0.9619	0.9627
1335	0.32	0.34	43.85	0.9771	35.49	30.95	0.9617	0.9625
1340	0.35	0.37	44.37	0.9775	35.31	30.80	0.9614	0.9622
1345	0.37	0.37	44.02	0.9775	35.13	30.65	0.9611	0.9619
1350	0.39	0.38	43.68	0.9771	34.95	30.49	0.9609	0.9617
1355	0.42	0.41	43.00	0.9764	34.76	30.33	0.9606	0.9614
1360	0.45	0.43	42.32	0.9754	34.58	30.17	0.9603	0.9611
1365	0.50	0.51	41.09	0.9744	34.38	29.99	0.9601	0.9609
1370	0.59	0.65	40.31	0.9736	34.18	29.81	0.9598	0.9607
1375	0.72	0.78	40.80	0.9738	33.97	29.64	0.9596	0.9604
1380	0.88	0.92	41.69	0.9741	33.77	29.48	0.9594	0.9602
1385	1.07	1.05	41.21	0.9743	33.57	29.32	0.9592	0.9600
1390	1.30	1.20	40.43	0.9741	33.37	29.16	0.9590	0.9599
1395	1.46	1.35	39.59	0.9733	33.20	29.01	0.9588	0.9597
1400	1.62	1.49	39.21	0.9725	33.04	28.86	0.9586	0.9595
1405	1.78	1.71	39.09	0.9715	32.90	28.74	0.9585	0.9594
1410	1.94	1.83	38.98	0.9707	32.78	28.63	0.9583	0.9592
1415	2.04	1.94	39.09	0.9699	32.67	28.53	0.9581	0.9590
1420	2.13	2.08	39.08	0.9695	32.56	28.43	0.9579	0.9588
1425	2.24	2.27	38.20	0.9694	32.45	28.33	0.9577	0.9586
1430	2.33	2.36	38.15	0.9697	32.35	28.26	0.9575	0.9584
1435	2.38	2.43	38.11	0.9692	32.26	28.19	0.9573	0.9582
1440	2.38	2.50	38.01	0.9686	32.18	28.12	0.9571	0.9579
1445	2.40	2.51	37.53	0.9683	32.10	28.07	0.9568	0.9576
1450	2.41	2.48	37.05	0.9685	32.02	28.01	0.9565	0.9574
1455	2.40	2.44	37.24	0.9686	31.94	27.96	0.9563	0.9571

(Continued)

Table 6.1. (*Continued*)

	Compiled averages from literature spectra				Kramers–Kronig/Percus–Yevick theory			
Wavelength, [nm]	μ_a, $sO_2 > 98\%$, [mm^{-1}]	μ_a, $sO_2 = 0\%$, [mm^{-1}]	μ_s, $sO_2 > 98\%$, [mm^{-1}]	g, $sO_2 >$ 98%, [–]	μ_s, $sO_2 > 98\%$, [mm^{-1}]	μ_s, $sO_2 = 0\%$, [mm^{-1}]	g, $sO_2 >$ 98%, [–]	g, $sO_2 = 0\%$, [–]
1460	2.38	2.37	37.36	0.9685	31.86	27.91	0.9560	0.9568
1465	2.40	2.35	37.11	0.9682	31.78	27.84	0.9557	0.9565
1470	2.34	2.33	36.85	0.9684	31.72	27.78	0.9554	0.9562
1475	2.27	2.29	36.77	0.9689	31.65	27.72	0.9551	0.9559
1480	2.20	2.24	36.72	0.9693	31.59	27.67	0.9548	0.9556
1485	2.06	2.17	36.32	0.9684	31.54	27.61	0.9545	0.9553
1490	1.89	2.07	35.91	0.9681	31.48	27.57	0.9542	0.9550
1495	1.78	1.95	35.70	0.9682	31.39	27.52	0.9539	0.9548
1500	1.71	1.82	35.56	0.9683	31.31	27.46	0.9537	0.9545
1505	1.63	1.73	35.19	0.9685	31.23	27.39	0.9534	0.9543
1510	1.50	1.63	35.07	0.9687	31.15	27.32	0.9531	0.9540
1515	1.39	1.54	34.99	0.9690	31.06	27.25	0.9529	0.9538
1520	1.34	1.49	34.98	0.9693	30.97	27.18	0.9527	0.9536
1525	1.27	1.42	34.88	0.9688	30.87	27.11	0.9525	0.9534
1530	1.21	1.33	34.72	0.9683	30.78	27.04	0.9523	0.9532
1535	1.15	1.23	34.54	0.9686	30.68	26.97	0.9521	0.9530
1540	1.11	1.14	34.33	0.9688	30.59	26.90	0.9519	0.9528
1545	1.07	1.09	34.11	0.9685	30.49	26.81	0.9517	0.9526
1550	1.03	1.05	33.98	0.9683	30.40	26.73	0.9514	0.9524
1555	0.97	1.01	33.90	0.9686	30.31	26.65	0.9513	0.9522
1560	0.91	0.97	33.82	0.9683	30.22	26.57	0.9510	0.9520
1565	0.85	0.92	33.73	0.9685	30.12	26.49	0.9508	0.9518
1570	0.82	0.87	33.63	0.9694	30.02	26.42	0.9506	0.9515
1575	0.79	0.82	33.53	0.9691	29.92	26.34	0.9504	0.9513
1580	0.75	0.78	33.37	0.9688	29.82	26.25	0.9502	0.9511

1585	0.73	0.75	32.93	0.9684	29.73	26.17	0.9499	0.9508
1590	0.72	0.71	32.60	0.9683	29.63	26.09	0.9497	0.9506
1595	0.70	0.69	32.55	0.9682	29.53	26.01	0.9495	0.9503
1600	0.69	0.67	32.48	0.9681	29.43	25.93	0.9492	0.9501
1605	0.67	0.65	32.44	0.9681	29.36	25.87	0.9489	0.9498
1610	0.66	0.64	32.40	0.9682	29.28	25.81	0.9486	0.9495
1615	0.64	0.62	32.32	0.9683	29.21	25.74	0.9483	0.9492
1620	0.64	0.62	32.21	0.9684	29.14	25.68	0.9480	0.9489
1625	0.63	0.61	31.76	0.9684	29.06	25.62	0.9477	0.9486
1630	0.63	0.61	31.50	0.9685	28.99	25.56	0.9474	0.9483
1635	0.62	0.61	31.38	0.9685	28.92	25.50	0.9471	0.9480
1640	0.62	0.61	31.21	0.9685	28.85	25.45	0.9468	0.9477
1645	0.62	0.60	31.08	0.9684	28.78	25.39	0.9465	0.9473
1650	0.60	0.59	31.02	0.9682	28.71	25.33	0.9462	0.9470
1655	0.58	0.57	31.10	0.9681	28.64	25.28	0.9459	0.9467
1660	0.57	0.56	31.17	0.9679	28.57	25.22	0.9456	0.9465
1665	0.57	0.56	30.97	0.9671	28.50	25.16	0.9453	0.9462
1670	0.57	0.56	30.75	0.9663	28.42	25.10	0.9450	0.9459
1675	0.57	0.56	30.48	0.9663	28.35	25.04	0.9447	0.9456
1680	0.57	0.56	30.23	0.9663	28.28	24.98	0.9444	0.9454
1685	0.57	0.57	30.02	0.9662	28.21	24.93	0.9442	0.9451
1690	0.58	0.58	29.81	0.9660	28.14	24.87	0.9439	0.9449
1695	0.59	0.58	29.66	0.9660	28.07	24.81	0.9437	0.9446
1700	0.60	0.59	29.65	0.9660	28.00	24.75	0.9434	0.9444
1705	0.60	0.59	29.75	0.9660	27.93	24.69	0.9432	0.9442
1710	0.61	0.60	29.75	0.9660	27.86	24.64	0.9430	0.9440
1715	0.61	0.61	29.40	0.9660	27.79	24.58	0.9428	0.9437
1720	0.62	0.61	29.08	0.9659	27.72	24.52	0.9425	0.9435
1725	0.62	0.62	28.89	0.9658	27.65	24.46	0.9423	0.9433

(Continued)

Table 6.1. *(Continued)*

	Compiled averages from literature spectra				Kramers–Kronig/Percus–Yevick theory			
Wavelength, [nm]	μ_a, $sO_2 > 98\%$, [mm^{-1}]	μ_a, $sO_2 = 0\%$, [mm^{-1}]	μ_s, $sO_2 > 98\%$, [mm^{-1}]	g, $sO_2 >$ 98%, [–]	μ_s, $sO_2 > 98\%$, [mm^{-1}]	μ_s, $sO_2 = 0\%$, [mm^{-1}]	g, $sO_2 >$ 98%, [–]	g, $sO_2 = 0\%$, [–]
1730	0.64	0.63	28.71	0.9657	27.58	24.41	0.9421	0.9431
1735	0.65	0.64	28.55	0.9655	27.50	24.35	0.9419	0.9429
1740	0.67	0.65	28.49	0.9653	27.43	24.29	0.9417	0.9427
1745	0.69	0.66	28.56	0.9651	27.36	24.23	0.9415	0.9425
1750	0.71	0.68	28.62	0.9650	27.29	24.17	0.9413	0.9423
1755	0.74	0.72	28.43	0.9652	27.22	24.10	0.9411	0.9420
1760	0.76	0.75	28.23	0.9649	27.15	24.04	0.9408	0.9418
1765	0.78	0.79	28.00	0.9640	27.08	23.99	0.9406	0.9416
1770	0.81	0.81	27.76	0.9633	27.01	23.93	0.9404	0.9413
1775	0.83	0.82	27.59	0.9634	26.94	23.88	0.9401	0.9410
1780	0.84	0.83	27.49	0.9635	26.87	23.82	0.9398	0.9407
1785	0.86	0.84	27.55	0.9646	26.80	23.77	0.9395	0.9404
1790	0.88	0.84	27.60	0.9663	26.74	23.71	0.9392	0.9401
1795	0.88	0.84	27.37	0.9651	26.67	23.66	0.9389	0.9398
1800	0.87	0.84	27.14	0.9639	26.61	23.60	0.9386	0.9395
1805	0.86	0.83	26.89	0.9628	26.56	23.56	0.9383	0.9392
1810	0.84	0.84	26.65	0.9629	26.51	23.51	0.9379	0.9388
1815	0.83	0.84	26.55	0.9630	26.46	23.46	0.9376	0.9385
1820	0.81	0.84	26.57	0.9639	26.40	23.41	0.9372	0.9381
1825	0.79	0.85	26.65	0.9647	26.34	23.36	0.9369	0.9378
1830	0.78	0.88	26.56	0.9643	26.27	23.29	0.9365	0.9374
1835	0.78	0.90	26.33	0.9640	26.19	23.23	0.9362	0.9370
1840	0.80	0.94	26.11	0.9630	26.11	23.15	0.9358	0.9367
1845	0.80	0.97	25.97	0.9610	26.01	23.07	0.9355	0.9364
1850	0.87	1.02	25.75	0.9622	25.89	22.97	0.9351	0.9360

1855	1.10	1.21	25.52	0.9619	25.75	22.84	0.9348	0.9357
1860	1.40	1.81	25.23	0.9610	25.59	22.68	0.9345	0.9355
1865	1.78	2.19	24.79	0.9591	25.43	22.53	0.9342	0.9352
1870	2.16	2.65	24.35	0.9597	25.26	22.41	0.9339	0.9349
1875	3.03	3.24	23.96	0.9615	25.05	22.27	0.9337	0.9346
1880	3.90	3.99	23.57	0.9597	24.89	22.13	0.9334	0.9344
1885	4.60	5.05	23.77	0.9540	24.77	22.01	0.9332	0.9341
1890	5.30	5.89	24.16	0.9479	24.68	21.96	0.9329	0.9339
1895	6.16	6.56	24.03	0.9421	24.61	21.98	0.9326	0.9336
1900	7.10	7.00	23.90	0.9361	24.58	22.02	0.9324	0.9333
1905	7.40	7.33	23.96	0.9326	24.63	22.08	0.9321	0.9330
1910	7.69	7.41	24.27	0.9244	24.69	22.18	0.9318	0.9327
1915	8.01	7.41	24.48	0.9156	24.77	22.26	0.9315	0.9325
1920	8.08	7.41	24.25	0.9096	24.86	22.33	0.9312	0.9322
1925	8.13	7.57	24.15	0.9113	24.95	22.38	0.9309	0.9320
1930	8.17	7.70	24.26	0.9122	25.04	22.44	0.9307	0.9317
1935	8.22	7.84	24.03	0.9081	25.14	22.51	0.9304	0.9314
1940	7.97	7.73	23.75	0.9052	25.27	22.62	0.9301	0.9312
1945	7.79	7.57	23.54	0.9141	25.38	22.72	0.9298	0.9309
1950	7.58	7.41	23.32	0.9197	25.49	22.82	0.9296	0.9306
1955	7.34	7.25	23.06	0.9159	25.58	22.91	0.9293	0.9304
1960	7.11	7.07	22.69	0.9110	25.68	23.00	0.9290	0.9301
1965	6.87	6.85	22.63	0.9147	25.77	23.10	0.9287	0.9298
1970	6.63	6.63	22.63	0.9206	25.86	23.19	0.9284	0.9295
1975	6.40	6.41	22.32	0.9267	25.95	23.29	0.9282	0.9292
1980	6.17	6.19	22.15	0.9282	26.05	23.38	0.9279	0.9289
1985	6.00	6.04	22.24	0.9269	26.16	23.50	0.9275	0.9286
1990	5.86	5.88	22.27	0.9291	26.30	23.64	0.9272	0.9282
1995	5.72	5.73	22.26	0.9349	26.53	23.88	0.9268	0.9278

As shown in figure 6.14, blood is characterized by a very high scattering anisotropy coefficient. Very high anisotropy implies strongly forward scattering with interesting implications. Despite the presence of the scattering, the scattering has a minor impact on the light propagation trajectory. So, from this perspective, the scattering can be ignored entirely in certain situations. Thus, for example, the light intensity in a slab can be approximated well by the Beer–Lambert law with absorption only

$$I(z) = I_0 e^{-\mu_a z} \tag{6.20}$$

Here, μ_a is the absorption coefficient; z is the distance from the slab's surface. Thus, despite relatively strong scattering, absorption will determine the attenuation. These considerations align with estimations provided by Bosschaart *et al* [81].

Additionally, one can conclude that polarization degradation, which is sensitive to the number of scattering events, is high. Thus, polarization should not play an important role in the whole blood optical measurements, which is in line with simulations by He *et al* [63].

6.3.6 Scattering by blood in vessels

Roggan *et al* [59] investigated the optical properties of circulating human blood at 633 nm using a DIS technique and Monte Carlo simulations. Pertinent to scattering, they found that (a) scattering and absorption increased linearly with hematocrit when $hct < 50\%$, (b) absorption and scattering decreased slightly with increasing shear rate, (c) the deformation of erythrocytes had no significant impact on the optical properties if volume and hemoglobin content were kept constant, (d) increasing osmolarity leads to an increase of absorption while both scattering and anisotropy decreased, (e) Mie calculations on spherical equivalents provided a precise estimation of the RBC scattering behavior, (f) increasing hemolysis led to a reduction in absorption and scattering and (g) oxygenation had no impact on scattering properties. Douplik *et al* observed a modulation in the absorption and scattering coefficients influenced by the shear rate, which could not be solely attributed to the orientation of erythrocytes within the flow [87]. This phenomenon is likely also associated with the deformation of RBCs.

6.3.7 Pathology

While there are multiple blood pathologies, we will consider just several examples: sickled cells and bacteria presence, which can be relevant for early detection of blood infections and sepsis.

6.3.7.1 Sickled cells

Sickle cell disease (SCD) is a condition in which RBCs deform abnormally into an elongated shape under low oxygen conditions, impairing blood circulation. This disease is caused by a mutant form of HB, known as hemoglobin S (HbS), resulting from substituting a single amino acid in the hemoglobin protein.

Kim *et al* [88] measured light scattering spectra along two independent axes of elongated-shaped sickle RBCs with arbitrary orientation by introducing the anisotropic Fourier transform light scattering (aFTLS) technique. They measured both static and dynamic anisotropic light scattering. In particular, they classified the sickle RBCs in accordance with the morphology: echinocyte (type II), discocyte (type III), and crescent-shaped irreversibly sickled cell (type IV; ISC). In SLS, the sickle RBCs in type IV showed significantly different angular scattering signals along long and short axes. In contrast, sickle RBCs in types II–III did not show statistically different light scattering signals along those two axes. The crescent and elongated shapes can explain these anisotropic scattering signals in type IV sickle RBCs.

Light scattering techniques were used to study the process of HbS polymerization, which occurs under low oxygen pressure and causes distortion and increased rigidity of the sickle RBC, leading to blockage of the capillaries and a host of resulting complications. Goktas *et al* [89] showed that the angle-resolved light scattering approach using image-based flow cytometry provides reliable quantitative data to define the change in morphology of large populations of sickled RBCs when the cells are exposed for different times to low oxygen.

6.3.7.2 Bacteria

Qui *et al* [90] used LSS to detect and identify bacteria in the whole blood. They used visible range LSS and were able to distinguish between four common bacteria responsible for 80% of sepsis worldwide [91]: *Pseudomonas aeruginosa, Escherichia coli, Klebsiella pneumonia*, and *Staphylococcus aureus*. They found that species-level identification can be based on bacteria concentration of approximately 10^3 CFU ml^{-1} without observing entire colonies or performing susceptibility testing.

6.4 Additional topics

6.4.1 Scattering by blood substitutes

Several oxygen-carrying alternatives to blood have been proposed since the first administration of a Hb-saline solution in 1947 [92]. The various blood substitutes have different components of different sizes (see figure 6.15). Thus, their light scattering differs significantly. While larger components like microparticle-based Hb-based oxygen carrier (HBOC) or cell-based HBOCs have sizes comparable to RBCs and

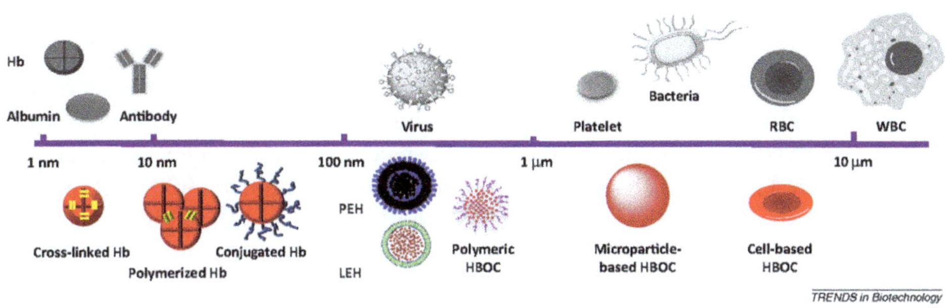

Figure 6.15. The relative size of artificial blood substitutes compared to typical biological components found in blood. Abbreviations: Hb—hemoglobin, HBOC—hemoglobin-based oxygen carrier, KEH—liposome-encapsulated hemoglobin, PEH—polymersome-encapsulated hemoglobin. Reprinted from [93], Copyright (2014), with permission from Elsevier. All rights reserved.

the associated Mie scattering, other blood substitutes (like cross-linked, polymerized, and conjugated Hbs) have much smaller sizes. Thus, they are predominantly Rayleigh scatterers.

6.4.2 Optical clearing

Scattering occurs due to mismatches in refractive indices. In biological tissues, these mismatches are mainly caused by the low refractive index of water, the primary component of extracellular fluids (ECFs) and cytoplasm, contrasted with the higher refractive indices of lipids and proteins.

The use of optical clearing agents (OCAs) has been proposed to change the light scattering properties of tissues reversibly (tissue optical clearing, TOC) [94]. While optical clearing is typically applied to superficial turbid tissues, like skin, it can also be applied to blood.

Upon introducing OCAs into the blood, the refractive index of the blood plasma increases and becomes comparable with that of RBCs. For example, when 6.5% glycerol solution was added to whole blood diluted by saline to twice its volume, the optical penetration depth at 820 nm was correspondingly increased by 17% [95]. For the other tested agents (glucose, dextrans, propylene glycol, and Trazograf), the penetration enhancement was around 20%–50% [96]. It was shown that minimal light scattering also occurs at a glucose concentration in blood of 0.65 $\mathrm{g\,ml^{-1}}$. In this case, blood is wholly immersed. However, residual scattering remains due to differences in spectral dependences of refractive indices of glucose solution and RBCs [96]. Evidently, such large concentrations of glucose could only be applied locally and briefly to avoid damage to blood cells and vessel wall tissue. However, endoscopic optical imaging techniques (OCT or confocal microscopy) and controllable injection of small amounts of glucose in the vessel lumen can help to image an atherosclerotic plaque through a bloodless layer with high contrast. There is also the possibility of applying a small amount of Hb within the vessel area near the endoscopic optical probe as an immersion agent [97]. A 30%–40% reduction of the scattering coefficient of blood in the spectral range 400–1000 nm due to the local hemolysis (up to 20% of RBC in the close vicinity of the optical probe) was demonstrated theoretically [98] as well as experimentally [98].

An optical clearing effect has been proposed for glucose sensing using OCT. For example, Larin *et al* [99] measured the OCT signal in healthy volunteers while administering glucose (glucose drink). They found that decreases and increases in the OCT followed the changes in blood glucose concentration. The slopes changed significantly (by 17%) with changes in glucose concentration from 90 to 140 $\mathrm{mg\,dl^{-1}}$.

Apart from the above, the optical clearing and increase of the light transmission in the blood can be found at hematocrits greater than 50%, as shown by Douplik *et al* [85].

6.4.3 Open questions

Despite significant efforts in blood optics, there are still numerous open questions.

The nature of light scattering on blood cells has yet to be clarified. Even though the calculations of scattering amplitudes can be done numerically, the complexity of calculations masks the dominant mechanisms of scattering. Notably, there are still conflicting accounts of the primary source of scattering. For example, in [100], the light scattering in blood is attributed primarily to the refractive index mismatch between blood plasma and erythrocyte cytoplasm, which depends on Hb concentration [59]. Similarly, in addition to scattering on the cell membrane interface with surrounding media, the elastic light scattering may originate from the cell nucleus and other intracellular structures (e.g., mitochondria). This determination can be done by measuring scattering from cells in media with different indices of refraction. The underlying principle of these experiments is that when the index of refraction difference between the scatterer and the surrounding media is reduced, the scattering intensity will be reduced. Therefore, when the index of refraction of the medium outside a cell is increased so that it is closer to that of the cell, scattering from the interface between the cell and the external medium will be reduced. Scattering from internal cellular structures, however, will not be affected. Thus, the decrease in scattering in the optical clearing experiments supports the notion of scattering on the cellular membranes.

An indirect confirmation of membrane-based origins of the scattering came from Roggan *et al* [59], who investigated the dependence of the scattering on the hemolysis rate. They found that the scattering coefficient μ_s showed a distinct (close to linear) decrease with increasing hemolysis. At complete hemolysis, μ_s amounted to 18% of the value measured for intact blood.

Another open question is the behavior of scattering of the whole blood for large hematocrit. It is well established that at high hematocrit, the scattering decreases as hematocrit increases. However, where this infliction point occurs is the question of debate. While some authors (e.g., Douplik *et al* [85]) claim that it occurs above 50%, other authors (e.g., Roggan *et al* [59]) report the values as low as 33%. This question can be boiled down to the scaling factor (equation (6.14)). In particular, if the simple scaling factor for gas (see equation (6.16)) holds true, then infliction occurs at 50%. If, however, the scaling factor provided by Bosschaart *et al* [81] (see equation (6.19)) is more accurate, then the infliction point will be 33%.

Another open question is the aggregation of RBCs and its impact on scattering. It is well-known that aggregation of RBCs occurs under certain conditions. In particular, the erythrocyte sedimentation rate (ESR) is a standard hematology test, which is a non-specific measure of inflammation. ESR measures the rate at which red blood cells in anticoagulated whole blood descend in a standardized tube over a period of one hour.

RBC aggregation has a significant impact on the optical properties of blood. In particular, the relationship between the RBC aggregation and optical signal has been well known and studied for many years *in vitro* [101–104].

It is known that blood sedimentation occurs primarily due to rouleau formation. Fine *et al* [105] proposed that the RBC aggregation process by rouleau formation can explain the optical signal (e.g., photoplethysmographic or PPG signal, including pulse oximetry) behavior *in vivo*. Later, Fine and Kaminsky [106] elaborated the model and proposed a model of RBC aggregation, which can be qualitatively described as follows: The dynamic balance between the destruction and formation of RBC aggregates is determined by the blood velocity and shear rate. The size of RBC aggregates is inversely proportional to the magnitude of the shear rate [107]. The increase in shear rate results in the breakup of large aggregates into smaller ones or individual RBCs. All RBC aggregates for shear rates exceeding 50 s^{-1} are dissociated into single erythrocytes [108]. Under normal conditions, a periodic pulse wave causes oscillations in velocity and shear forces, modulating the aggregate size. Hence, the oscillation in the shear forces of blood flow is the main rheological factor leading to observed variations in the measured optical signals (for example, PPG signal).

However, this hypothesis requires further verification. Firstly, the aggregation of RBCs is prevented by Coulomb forces, as RBCs are negatively charged due to the presence of the carboxyl group of sialic acids in the cell membrane [109]. As such, these charges create a repulsive electric zeta potential between cells. Secondly, in the ESR test, the blood sedimentation caused by rouleau formation occurs on a long time scale (1 h in the clinical test). Thus, the ability to rapidly aggregate and disaggregate during pulse wave propagation also requires further verification.

The impact of oxygenation on scattering is also being debated. Some authors (see, for example, [59]) claim that whole blood scattering does not depend on oxygenation, but there are some reasons to expect that oxygenation affects scattering. Specifically, oxygenation changes the membrane potential, which may impact the aggregation of RBCs. Thus, aggregation (e.g., via the rouleau formation mentioned above) and sedimentation can be oxygenation-dependent. This reasoning aligns with Bosschaart *et al* [81], who found a significant difference in scattering between oxygenated and deoxygenated blood using the Kramers–Kronig relations.

6.5 Conclusions

The light scattering in blood arises primarily from a mismatch between the refractive indexes of the plasma and the cell membranes.

Blood consists of several types of cells, which have a broad distribution in shapes and sizes. As light scattering is sensitive to the shape and size of the particles, light scattering plays an important role in studying blood and blood components. Light scattering techniques are used to characterize the shapes, sizes, and distribution of cells in the blood. Light can also be used to characterize their hydrodynamic properties and speed.

The optical properties of blood (including scattering) are dominated by RBCs, whose absorption and scattering are two to three orders of magnitude larger than those of the other blood components [23].

The selection of a medium for measuring the optical properties of blood components is critically important, especially when the absolute values are reported. The slightly higher refractive index of plasma than that of saline solutions can change the effective scattering of RBCs by up to 100% when substituting plasma with saline solution [23].

Since Lord Rayleigh's pioneering experiments in the 19th century, various light scattering techniques have been developed, many of which have become standard tools in biomedical research and hematology laboratories.

With the rapid developments in artificial intelligence (AI) and machine learning (ML) techniques, it is expected that the next big step in developing light scattering techniques for blood analysis will be their integration with ML/AI tools. This integration will create methodologies with high throughput, sensitivity, and specificity.

References

[1] https://my.clevelandclinic.org/health/diagnostics/17683-hematocrit

[2] https://sciencenotes.org/leukocytes-or-white-blood-cells/

[3] Liu S, Deng Z, Li J *et al* 2019 Measurement of the refractive index of whole blood and its components for a continuous spectral region *J. Biomed. Opt.* **24** 1–5

[4] Sumathi J, Jaleeli Z A, Jaleeli K A and Ahmad A 2022 To Investigate the refractive index of blood plasma suspended in various tonicity solutions *J. Res. Appl. Sci. Biotech.* **1** 216–21

[5] Meyer R A 1979 Light scattering from biological cells: dependence of backscatter radiation on membrane thickness and refractive index *Appl. Opt.* **18** 585–8

[6] Steinke J M and Shepherd A P 1988 Comparison of Mie theory and the light scattering of red blood cells *Appl. Opt.* **27** 4027–33

[7] Bohren C F and Huffman D R 1983 *Absorption and Scattering of Light by Small Particles* (New York: Wiley)

[8] Mie G 1908 Beiträge zur Optik trüber Medien, speziell kolloidaler Metallösungen *Ann. Phys.* **330** 377–445

[9] https://en.wikipedia.org/wiki/Mie_scattering

[10] Brock B C 2016 *Bistatic and monostatic radar cross section of radially inhomogeneous spheres* Sandia Report SAND2016–2087 https://osti.gov/servlets/purl/1618259

[11] Graaff R, Aarnoudse J G, Zijp J R *et al* 1992 Reduced light-scattering properties for mixtures of spherical-particles—a simple approximation derived from Mie calculations *Appl. Opt.* **31** 1370–6

[12] Bohren C F and Huffman D R 2010 *Absorption and Scattering of Light by Small Particles* (New York: Wiley-Interscience)

[13] Argentin C, Berg M J, Mazur M *et al* 2021 Assessing the limits of Rayleigh–Debye–Gans theory: phasor analysis of a biosphere *J. Quant. Spectrosc. Radiat. Transf.* **264** 107550

[14] Garcia-Lopez A C, Snider A D and Garcia-Rubio L H 2006 Rayleigh–Debye–Gans as a model for continuous monitoring of biological particles: part I, assessment of theoretical limits and approximations *Opt. Express* **14** 8849–65

[15] Garcia-Lopez A C and Garcia-Rubio L H 2008 Rayleigh–Debye–Gans as a model for continuous monitoring of biological particles: part II, development of a hybrid model *Opt. Express* **16** 4671–87

[16] van de Hulst H 1957 *Light Scattering by Small Particles* (New York: Wiley)

[17] Farone W A and Robinson M J 3rd 1968 The range of validity of the anomalous diffraction approximation to electromagnetic scattering by a sphere *Appl. Opt.* **7** 643–5

[18] Sharma S K and Banerjee S 2012 On the validity of the anomalous diffraction approximation in light-scattering studies of soft biomedical tissues *J. Mod. Opt.* **59** 701–9

[19] Streekstra G, Hoekstra A, Nijhof E-J and Heethaar R 1993 Light scattering by red blood cells in ektacytometry: Fraunhofer versus anomalous diffraction *Appl. Opt.* **32** 2266–72

[20] Jacques S L, Alter C A and Prahl S A 1987 Angular dependence of HeNe laser light scattering by human dermis *Lasers Life Sci.* **1** 309–33
[21] Yaroslavsky L A N, Yaroslavsky I V, Goldbach T and Schwarzmaier H J 1996 The optical properties of blood in the near infrared spectral range *Proc. SPIE* **2678** 314–24
[22] Friebel L M, Roggan A, Müller G and Meinke M 2006 Determination of optical properties of human blood in the spectral range 250–1100 nm using Monte Carlo simulations with hematocrit-dependent effective scattering phase functions *J. Biomed. Opt.* **11** 031021
[23] Meinke M, Müller G, Helfmann J and Friebel M 2007 Optical properties of platelets and blood plasma and their influence on the optical behavior of whole blood in the visible to near infrared wavelength range *J. Biomed. Opt.* **12** 014024
[24] Steelman Z A, Ho D S, Chu K K and Wax A 2019 Light-scattering methods for tissue diagnosis *Optica* **6** 479–89
[25] Perelman L T, Backman V, Wallace M *et al* 1998 Observation of periodic fine structure in reflectance from biological tissue: a new technique for measuring nuclear size distribution *Phys. Rev. Lett.* **80** 627
[26] Gurjar R, Backman V, Perelman L *et al* 2001 Imaging human epithelial properties with polarized light-scattering spectroscopy *Nat. Med.* **7** 1245–8
[27] Cheong W-F, Prahl S A and Welch A J 1990 A review of the optical properties of biological tissues *IEEE J. Quantum Electr.* **26** 2166–85
[28] Roggan A, Albrecht H J, Doerschel K *et al* 1995 Experimental set-up and Monte-Carlo model for the determination of optical tissue properties in the wavelength range 330 to 1100 nm *Laser Interaction with Hard and Soft Tissue II* **vol 2323** (SPIE) pp 21–36
[29] Prahl S A, van Gemert M J C and Welch A J 1993 Determining the optical properties of turbid media by using the adding-doubling method *Appl. Opt.* **32** 559–68
[30] Pickering J W, Prahl S A, van Wieringen N *et al* 1993 Double-integrating-sphere system for measuring the optical properties of tissue *Appl. Opt.* **32** 399–410
[31] Lemaillet P, Bouchard J-P, Hwang J and Allen D W 2015 Double-integrating-sphere system at the National Institute of Standards and Technology in support of measurement standards for the determination of optical properties of tissue-mimicking phantoms *J. Biomed. Opt.* **20** 121310
[32] Rehman A U, Ahmad I and Qureshi S A 2020 Biomedical applications of integrating sphere: a review *Photodiagn. Photodyn. Ther.* **31** 101712
[33] https://3p-instruments.com/measurement-methods/dynamic-light-scattering/
[34] Gurjar R S, Backman V, Perelman L T *et al* 2001 Imaging human epithelial properties with polarized light-scattering spectroscopy *Nat. Med.* **7** 1245–8
[35] Siegel M P, Kim Y L, Roy H K *et al* 2006 Assessment of blood supply in superficial tissue by polarization-gated elastic light-scattering spectroscopy *Appl. Opt.* **45** 335–42
[36] Maltsev V P 2000 Scanning flow cytometry for individual particle analysis *Rev. Sci. Instrum.* **71** 243–55
[37] Parrow N L, Violet P C, Tu H *et al* 2018 Measuring deformability and red cell heterogeneity in blood by ektacytometry *J. Vis. Exp.* **12** 56910
[38] Da Costa L, Suner L, Galimand J *et al* 2016 Diagnostic tool for red blood cell membrane disorders: assessment of a new generation ektacytometer *Blood Cells Mol. Dis.* **56** 9–22
[39] Wardell K, Jakobsson A and Nilsson G E 1993 Laser Doppler perfusion imaging by dynamic light scattering *IEEE Trans. Biomed. Eng.* **40** 309–16

[40] Senarathna J, RegeA L N and Thakor N V 2013 Laser Speckle contrast imaging: theory, instrumentation and applications *IEEE Rev. Biomed. Eng.* **6** 99–110
[41] Huang D, Swanson E A, Lin C P *et al* 1991 Optical coherence tomography *Science* **254** 1178–81
[42] Zhao Y, Chen Z, Saxer C *et al* 2000 Phase-resolved optical coherence tomography and optical Doppler tomography for imaging blood flow in human skin with fast scanning speed and high velocity sensitivity *Opt. Lett.* **25** 114–6
[43] Haindl R, Trasischker W, Wartak A *et al* 2016 Total retinal blood flow measurement by three beam Doppler optical coherence tomography *Biomed. Opt. Express* **7** 287–301
[44] Braaf B, Gräfe M G O, Uribe-Patarroyo N *et al* 2019 OCT-based velocimetry for blood flow quantification *High Resolution Imaging in Microscopy and Ophthalmology: New Frontiers in Biomedical Optics* ed J F Bille (Cham: Springer) ch 7 Available from: https://ncbi.nlm.nih.gov/books/NBK554059/
[45] Teut M, Lüdtke R and Warning A 2006 Reliability of Enderlein's darkfield analysis of live blood *Altern. Ther. Health Med.* **12** 36–41
[46] Verebes G S, Melchiorre M, Garcia-Leis A *et al* 2013 Hyperspectral enhanced dark field microscopy for imaging blood cells *J. Biophotonics* **6** 960–7
[47] Bernhardt I, Ivanova L, Langehanenberg P *et al* 2008 Application of digital holographic microscopy to investigate the sedimentation of intact red blood cells and their interaction with artificial surfaces *Bioelectrochemistry* **73** 92–6
[48] Ding H, Wang Z, Nguyen F *et al* 2008 Fourier transform light scattering of inhomogeneous and dynamic structures *Phys. Rev. Lett.* **101** 238102
[49] Popescu G, Ikeda T, Dasari R R and Feld M S 2006 Diffraction phase microscopy for quantifying cell structure and dynamics *Opt. Lett.* **31** 775–7
[50] Park Y, Best-Popescu C A, Dasari R R and Popescu G 2011 Light scattering of human red blood cells during metabolic remodeling of the membrane *J. Biomed. Opt.* **16** 011013
[51] Cuccia D J, Bevilacqua F, Durkin A J and Tromberg B J 2005 Modulated imaging: quantitative analysis and tomography of turbid media in the spatial-frequency domain *Opt. Lett.* **30** 1354–6
[52] Applegate M B, Spink S S and Roblyer D 2020 Dual-DMD hyperspectral spatial frequency domain imaging (SFDI) using dispersed broadband illumination with a demonstration of blood stain spectral monitoring *Biomed. Opt. Express* **12** 676–88
[53] Meinke M C, Friebel M and Helfmann J 2011 Optical properties of flowing blood cells *Advanced Optical Flow Cytometry: Methods and Disease Diagnoses* ed V V Tuchin (Weinheim: Wiley-VCH) pp 95–132
[54] Tuchin V V (ed) 2011 *Advanced Optical Flow Cytometry: Methods and Disease Diagnoses* 1st edn (Weinheim: Wiley-VCH) p 99
[55] Casa L D C, Deaton D H and Ku D N 2015 Role of high shear rate in thrombosis *J Vasc. Surg.* **61** 1068–80
[56] McMahon T J 2019 Red blood cell deformability, vasoactive mediators, and adhesion *Front. Physiol.* **10** 1417
[57] Musielak M 2009 Red blood cell-deformability measurement: review of techniques *Clin. Hemorheol. Microcirc.* **42** 47–64
[58] Agrawal R, Smart T, Nobre-Cardoso J *et al* 2016 Assessment of red blood cell deformability in type 2 diabetes mellitus and diabetic retinopathy by dual optical tweezers stretching technique *Sci. Rep.* **6** 15873

[59] Roggan A, Friebel M, Dorschel K *et al* 1999 Optical properties of circulating human blood in the wavelength range 400–2500 nm *J. Biomed. Opt.* **4** 36–46
[60] Mauer J, Peltomäki M, Poblete S *et al* 2017 Static and dynamic light scattering by red blood cells: a numerical study *PLoS One* **12** e0176799
[61] Gompper G, Ihle T, Kroll D M and Winkler R G 2009 Multi-particle collision dynamics: a particle-based mesoscale simulation approach to the hydrodynamics of complex fluids *Adv. Polym. Sci.* **221** 1–87
[62] Español P and Warren P 1995 Statistical mechanics of dissipative particle dynamics *Europhys. Lett.* **30** 191–6
[63] He J, Karlsson A, Swartling J and Andersson-Engels S 2004 Light scattering by multiple red blood cells *J. Opt. Soc. Am.* A **21** 1953–61
[64] Drezek R, Dunn A and Richards-Kortum R 1999 Light scattering from cells: finite-difference time-domain simulations and goniometric measurements *Appl. Opt.* **38** 3651–61
[65] Kak A C and Slaney M 1988 *Principles of Computerized Tomographic Imaging* (Piscataway, NJ: IEEE Press)
[66] Draine B T and Flatau P J 1994 Discrete-dipole approximation for scattering calculations *J. Opt. Soc. Am.* A **11** 1491–9
[67] Terstappen L W M M, de Grooth B G, Visscher K *et al* 1988 Four-parameter white blood cell differential counting based on light scattering measurements *Cytometry* **9** 39–43
[68] Terstappen L W, de Grooth B G, Ten Napel C H *et al* 1986 Discrimination of human cytotoxic lymphocytes from regulatory and B-lymphocytes by orthogonal light scattering *J. Immunol. Methods* **95** 211–6
[69] Doornbos R M P, Schaeffer M, Hoekstra A G *et al* 1996 Elastic light-scattering measurements of single biological cells in an optical trap *Appl. Opt.* **35** 729–34
[70] Watson D, Hagen N, Diver J *et al* 2004 Elastic light scattering from single cells: orientational dynamics in optical trap *Biophys. J.* **87** 1298–306
[71] Zharinov A E, Tarasov P A, Shvalov A N *et al* 2006 A study of light scattering of mononuclear blood cells with scanning flow cytometry *J. Quant. Spectrosc. Radiat. Transfer* **102** 121–8
[72] Maltsev V P, Hoekstra A G and Yurkin M A 2011 Optics of white blood cells: Optical models, simulations, and experiments *Advanced Optical Flow Cytometry* ed V V Tuchin (Weinheim: Wiley-VCH)
[73] Terstappen L W M M, Johnson D, Mickaels R A *et al* 1991 Multidimensional flow cytometric blood cell differentiation without erythrocyte lysis *Blood Cells* **17** 585–602
[74] Dannhauser D, Rossi D, Ripaldi M *et al* 2017 Single-cell screening of multiple biophysical properties in leukemia diagnosis from peripheral blood by pure light scattering *Sci. Rep.* **7** 12666
[75] Michelson A D 2006 *Platelets* 2nd edn (San Diego: Academic)
[76] Frojmovic M M and Panjwani R 1976 Geometry of normal mammalian platelets by quantitative microscopic studies *Biophys. J.* **16** 1071–89
[77] Kim K Y, Kim K E and Kim K H 1986 Mean platelet volume in the normal state and in various clinical disorders *Yonsei Med. J.* **27** 219–26
[78] Maurer-Spurej E and Chipperfield K 2007 Past and future approaches to assess the quality of platelets for transfusion *Transfus. Med. Rev.* **21** 295–306
[79] Moskalensky A E, Yurkin M A, Konokhova A I *et al* 2013 Accurate measurement of volume and shape of resting and activated blood platelets from light scattering *J. Biomed. Opt.* **18** 017001

[80] Maurer-Spurej E, Labrie A and Brown K 2008 Routine quality testing of blood platelet transfusions with dynamic light scattering *Part. Part. Syst. Charact.* **25** 99–104
[81] Bosschaart N, Edelman G J, Aalders M C *et al* 2014 A literature review and novel theoretical approach on the optical properties of whole blood *Lasers Med. Sci.* **29** 453–79 Erratum in:Bosschaart N, Edelman G J, Aalders M C G, van Leeuwen T G and Faber D J 2022 Correction to: A literature review and novel theoretical approach on the optical properties of whole blood *Lasers Med. Sci.* **37** 691
[82] Hespel L, Mainguy S and Greffet J J 2001 Theoretical and experimental investigation of the extinction in a dense distribution of particles: nonlocal effects *J. Opt. Soc. Am.* A **18** 3072–6
[83] Twersky V 1970 Absorption and multiple scattering by biological suspensions *JOSA* **60** 1084–93
[84] Percus J K and Yevick G J 1958 Analysis of classical statistical mechanics by means of collective coordinates *Phys. Rev.* **110** 1
[85] Douplik A and Loschenov V 1996 Identification of spectroscopic and optical parameters of whole blood depending on its concentration and layer thickness *SPIE* **2624** 165–76
[86] Ishimaru A 2017 Bio-optics, optical absorption and scatteringin blood *Electromagnetic Wave Propagation, Radiation, and Scattering, From Fundamentals to Applications* The IEEE Press Series on Electromagnetic Wave Theory 2nd edn (IEEE)
[87] Douplik A, Loschenov V, Malinin V *et al* 1996 Changes of optical parameters of moving whole blood depending on shear rate *Proc. SPIE* **2923** 35–43
[88] Kim Y, Higgins J M, Dasari R R *et al* 2012 Anisotropic light scattering of individual sickle red blood cells *J. Biomed. Opt.* **17** 040501
[89] Goktas P, Sukharevsky I O, Larkin S *et al* 2019 Image-based flow cytometry and angle-resolved light scattering to define the sickling process *Cytometry* A **95** 488–98
[90] Qiu L, Zhang L, Horowitz G L *et al* 2021 Rapid detection and identification of bacteria directly from whole blood with light-scattering spectroscopy-based biosensor *Sens. Actuators* B **346** 130489
[91] Ani C, Farshidpanah S, Stewart A B and Nguyen H B 2015 Variations in organism-specific severe sepsis mortality in the United States: 1999–2008 *Crit. Care Med.* **43** 65–77
[92] Amberson W R 1947 Clinical experience with hemoglobin-saline solutions [Letter] *Science* 117
[93] Tao Z and Ghoroghchian P P 2014 Microparticle, nanoparticle, and stem cell-based oxygen carriers as advanced blood substitutes *Trends Biotechnol.* **32** 466–73
[94] Tuchin V V, Maksimova I L, Zimnyakov D A *et al* 1996 Light propagation in tissues with controlled optical properties *SPIE* **2925** 118–42
[95] Tuchin V V 2006 *Optical Clearing of Tissues and Blood* **154** (Bellingham, WA: SPIE Press)
[96] Tuchin V V, Xu X and Wang R K 2002 Dynamic optical coherence tomography in studies of optical clearing, sedimentation, and aggregation of immersed blood *Appl. Opt.* **41** 258–71
[97] Tuchin V V, Zhestkov D, Bashkatov A and Genina E 2004 Theoretical study of immersion optical clearing of blood in vessels at local hemolysis *Opt. Exp.* **12** 2966–71
[98] Popescu G, Ikeda T, Best C A *et al* 2005 Erythrocyte structure and dynamics quantified by Hilbert phase microscopy *J. Biomed. Opt.* **10** 060503
[99] Larin K V, Eledrisi M S, MotamediM and Esenaliev R O 2002 Noninvasive blood glucose monitoring with optical coherence tomography—a pilot study in human subjects *Diabetes Care* **25** 2263–7

[100] Tuchin V V 2007 *Tissue Optics: Light Scattering Methods and Instruments for Medical Diagnosis* 2nd edn (Bellingham, WA: SPIE)
[101] Klose H, Volger E, Brechtelsbauer H *et al* 1972 Microrheology and light transmission of blood *Pfluegers Arch.* **333** 126–39
[102] Donner M, Siadat M and Stoltz J F 1988 Erythrocyte aggregation: approach by light scattering determination *Biorheology* **25** 367–76
[103] Priezzhev A V, Ryaboshapka O M, Firsov N N and Sirko I V 1999 Aggregation and disaggregation of erythrocytes in whole blood: study by backscattering technique *J. Biomed. Opt.* **4** 76–84
[104] Tsinopoulos S V, Sellountos E J and Polyzos D 2002 Light scattering by aggregated red blood cells *Appl.Opt.* **41** 1408–17
[105] Fine I, Fikhte B and Shvartsman L D 2000 Occlusion spectroscopy as a new paradigm for non-invasive blood measurements *Proc. SPIE* **4263** 122–30
[106] Fine I and Kaminsky A 2019 Possible error in reflection pulse oximeter readings as a result of applied pressure *J. Healthc. Eng.* **2019** 1–7
[107] Bishop J J, Nance P R, Popel A S *et al* 2004 Relationship between erythrocyte aggregate size and flow rate in skeletal muscle venules *Am. J. Physiol.—Heart Circ. Physiol.* **286** H113–20
[108] Hoeks A P, Samijo S K, Brands P J and Reneman R S 1995 Noninvasive determination of shear-rate distribution across the arterial lumen *Hypertension* **26** 26–33
[109] Eylar E H, Madoff M A, Brody O V and Oncley J L 1962 The contribution of sialic acid to the surface charge of the erythrocyte *J. Biol. Chem.* **237** 1992–2000

Chapter 7

Fluorescence spectroscopy and imaging of blood

Meiyun Cao and Alexandre Douplik

This chapter delves into the diverse applications of the fluorescence across various biological systems, with a particular focus on a foundational overview of the biological sources of autofluorescence in the blood, including whole blood, blood plasma, blood serum, red blood cells (RBCs), white blood cells (WBCs), blood pigment, blood platelets, as well as the pathological modification of the fluorescence properties of blood and a brief review of the external fluorescent dyes for intravenous (IV) administration for the clinical applications.

7.1 Introduction

Autofluorescence is the intrinsic emission of light by biological tissues and emitted by certain biomolecules [1] when excited by specific wavelengths usually matching the biomolecules' optical absorption maxima [2]. The autofluorescence spectra are broad for biomolecules reflecting their multi-component content. Researchers study via the fluorescence the structure and function of cells and tissues in their native state, providing insights that are minimally invasive [3, 4].

7.2 Autofluorescence properties of whole blood

7.2.1 Main fluorophores of whole blood

In the context of whole blood, autofluorescence provides critical insights into the physiological and pathological states of blood components [5], including RBCs, WBCs, platelets, and plasma. The ability to monitor these characteristics in real time without the need for external dyes or stains makes autofluorescence a valuable approach for studying cellular functions, diagnosing diseases, and guiding therapeutic interventions.

The autofluorescence of whole blood is predominantly driven by the presence of endogenous fluorophores, such as nicotinamide adenine dinucleotide (NADH) [6], flavins [7], porphyrins [8], and certain aromatic amino acids like tryptophan [9].

doi:10.1088/978-0-7503-4806-5ch7

Table 7.1. Endogenous fluorophores of blood [4]. John Wiley & Sons. Copyright 2021 Wiley Periodicals LLC.

Fluorophores	Excitation (nm)	Emission (nm)	Source	Implicated pathologies/unexplored potential impactful pathologies
Porphyrins	400–450	630–700	Plasma, RBC	Thalassemia, cancers/sickle cell anemia, acute intermittent porphyria, porphyria cutanea tarda [8, 17]
Amino acid	240–280, 280–350, 488	520–620	RBC, WBC, plasma	Acute coronary syndrome [18], lung cancer [19]
Phenylalanine	258 (max)	280 (max)	Plasma	Metabolic characterization [20]
Tryptophan, Tyrosine	280 (max), 275 (max)	250–310, 300 (max)	Plasma	Aging, inflammation [21]
FAD	410–450	510–560	WBC	Select cancers [15]
FMN	440–450	540		Eosinophil-associated inflammation and cytotoxicity [22]
Riboflavin	444 (max), 410–500	558 (max), 510–590, 520–750	Plasma	Oxidative stress, metabolic dysfunction [15, 21, 23]
NADH	330–380	440/462 (bound/free)	WBC	Diabetes [6], select cancers [15], liver disease [24]
NAD(P)H	290, 351, 340, 336	440, 460–480	Plasma	
Lipopigments	340–395, 400–500	430–460, 540, 480–700	Plasma, RBC	Neurodegenerative diseases [25]
Elastin	290, 325	340, 400	Tissue	Lung cancer/Marfan syndrome [26]
Keratin	280–325	495–525	Tissue	Squamous cell carcinoma [27]
Collagen	330–340, 350–420	400–410, 420–510	Tissue/plasma	Osteogenesis imperfecta, Ehlers–Danlos syndrome [28]
Fatty acid	330–350	470–480	Tissue	MCAD deficiency [29]
Retinol	327 (max)	510 (max)	Tissue, plasma	Xerophthalmia [30]
Vitamin K	335 (max)	480 (max)	Tissue, plasma	Disorder of coagulation factor [31]
Vitamin D	390 (max)	480 (max)	Tissue, plasma	Bone metabolic disorders [32–34]
Vitamin B12	275 (max)	305 (max)	Tissue, plasma	Pernicious anemia, lupus [35]
Melanin	300–800	440, 520, 575	Tissue, plasma	Skin disorders [36]
Bilirubin	350–520	480–650	Plasma	Jaundice, Gilbert's disease [37]

A summary of fluorophores, including their types, associated diseases, and an example of their absorption, emission, and excitation spectra are presented as table 7.1. List of some endogenous fluorophores along with their autofluorescence spectral range and their origin in either blood components or tissue (copied from Shrirao *et al* with permission) [4, 10–12], and figure 7.1.

7.2.2 Clinical diagnostics using autofluorescence spectroscopy in whole blood

Wolfbeis and Leiner [13] laid the groundwork by characterizing human blood serum components through total fluorescence mapping. Their study identified key fluorophores, including tryptophan, NAD(P)H, and bilirubin, demonstrating that

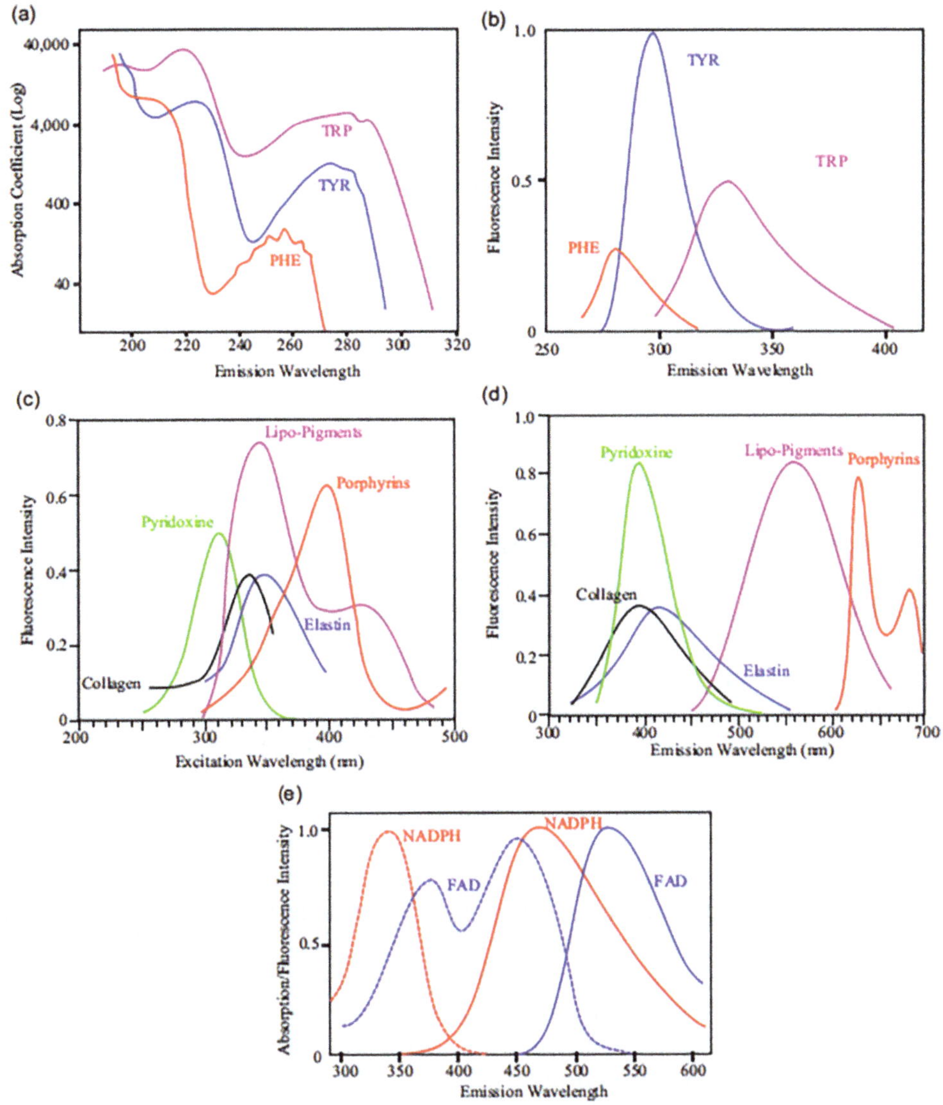

Figure 7.1. Absorption, emission, and excitation spectra endogenous fluorophores. (a) Absorption [38], (b) Emission spectra of aromatic amino acids tryptophan, tyrosine, and phenylaniline [39]. (c) Excitation spectra and (d) emission spectra of collagen (black), elastin (blue), porphyrins (red), lipo-pigments (cyan) and pyridoxine (green) [40]. (e) Absorption (dotted line) and emission (solid line) spectra of NADH (red) and FAD (blue) [41] (copied from Shrirao *et al* with permission) [4] John Wiley & Sons. Copyright 2021 Wiley Periodicals LLC.

variations in fluorescence could indicate pathological states. Porphyrins, which are heme precursors found in RBCs, contribute to the autofluorescence signal and are also important markers in various pathological conditions. Clinically, changes in the autofluorescence profile of blood can serve as early indicators of diseases such as cancer [14, 15], diabetes [6], and lung disease [16], often before these conditions manifest clinically.

For example, the altered metabolic activity [42] in cancer cells leads to distinct changes in NADH and flavin fluorescence, which can be detected in blood samples.

Additionally, in conditions like diabetes, the accumulation of advanced glycation end-products (AGEs) can alter the autofluorescence properties of blood, providing a potential diagnostic marker. In the realm of disease detection, Atkins *et al* [43] examined the use of autofluorescence imaging for detecting blood abnormalities, positioning it as a potential diagnostic tool for various blood disorders. Their research demonstrated that autofluorescence imaging could identify subtle changes in blood cells indicative of disease, often earlier than conventional tests. Further exploring diagnostic applications, Masilamani *et al* [17] investigated blood autofluorescence as a diagnostic tool for diseases like diabetes and cancer stage, suggesting that these changes of porphyrin derivatives, such as Photofrin II, could serve as early biomarkers for gastric cancer, breast cancer and Hodgkin's lymphoma. Based on their spectral analysis, they found that the strength for 590 and 630 nm bands are stronger in gastric cancer patients than healthy subjects. Similarly, blood autofluorescence as a tool for identifying metabolic and hematological disorders at subclinical stages was studied by Kamińska *et al* [44], who employed photoluminescence spectroscopy to identify distinct autofluorescence patterns correlated with early stages of diseases like diabetes and anemia, suggesting their potential as early biomarkers.

Lowndes [12], Lan *et al* [23], and Peng and Liu [45] explored blood autofluorescence focusing on its spectral properties, interference effects, and mechanistic shifts. Lan *et al* investigated how different excitation sources (LED, Ar laser, He–Ne laser) influenced fluorescence spectra of whole blood. The excitation wavelengths for LED, Ar Laser and He–Ne laser are 457, 457.9 and 632.8 nm, respectively, revealing wavelength-dependent variations in emission intensity. Lowndes' group examined blood autofluorescence as an interfering factor in intraoperative fluorescence-guided tumor resection, showing that oxyhemoglobin absorption (541 and 577 nm) disrupts diagnostic signals, necessitating saline rinsing to improve accuracy. Peng and Liu analyzed the red-shift phenomenon in blood fluorescence, attributing it to self-absorption and fluorophore interactions, with shorter excitation wavelengths enhancing this effect. Weber *et al* investigated menstrual bloodstains using steady-state fluorescence spectroscopy to monitor biochemical changes, which shows that oxidative phosphorylation, metabolic changes, and drying effects influence fluorescence intensity. Weber *et al* [21], Schmitz *et al* [46] and Gao *et al* [47] also presented the main fluorophores identified as tryptophan, NADH, and flavins. The fluorescence signatures for these biomolecules are shown in figure 7.2, highlighting their spectral properties and diagnostic relevance.

With the method similar to that of Gao's group, Weber *et al* examined the biochemical aging of peripheral and menstrual bloodstains, which focuses on the degradation of tryptophan to determine post-deposition changes. They also reviewed advances in autofluorescence spectroscopy, particularly its integration with machine learning for clinical diagnostics. This combination significantly

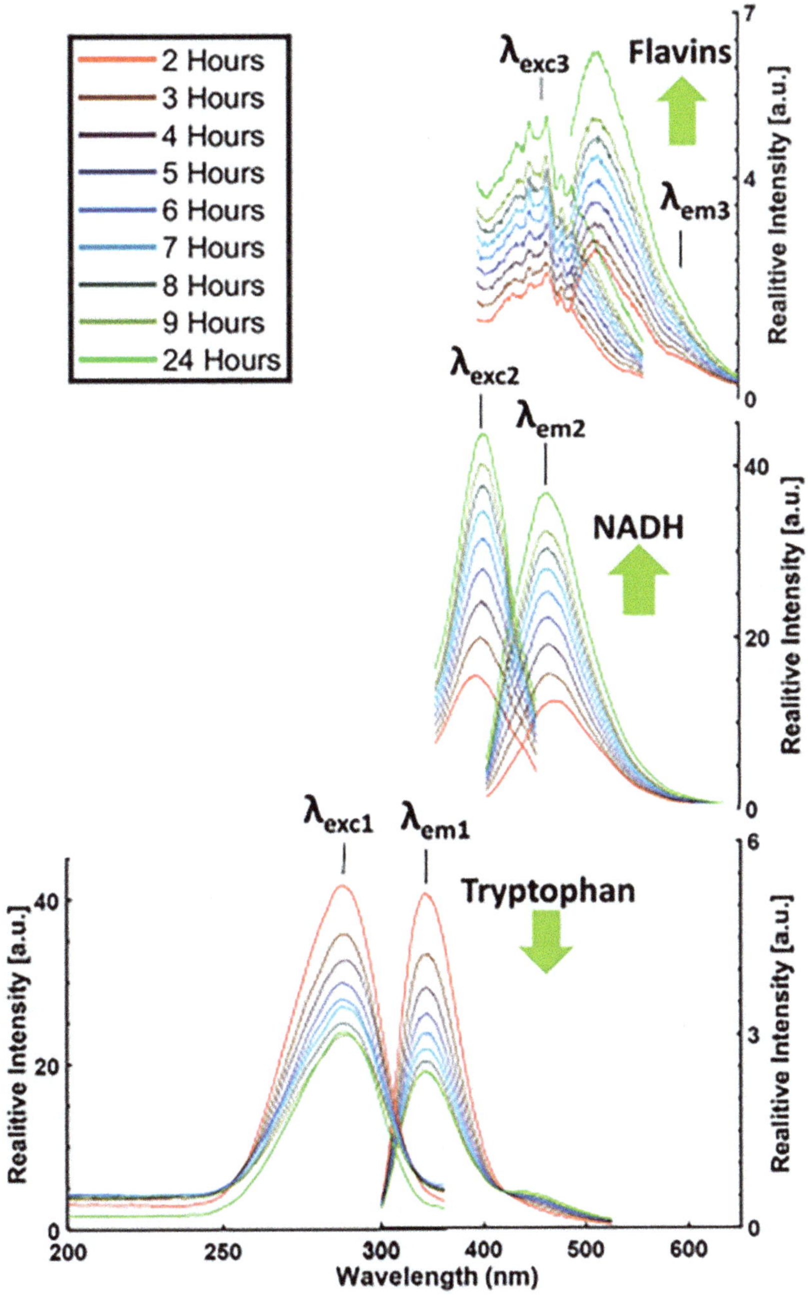

Figure 7.2. Changes in the peripheral bloodstain fluorescence with time since deposition. Excitation and emission spectra collected over the first 24 hours after deposition of one peripheral blood sample obtained from Donor 1. Black lines indicate the values of excitation wavelengths applied to measure emission spectra, respectively, $\lambda_{exc1} = 285$ nm, $\lambda_{exc2} = 350$ nm, $\lambda_{exc3} = 465$ nm, and emission wavelengths fixed for the collection of excitation spectra, respectively, $\lambda_{em1} = 340$ nm, $\lambda_{em2} = 460$ nm, $\lambda_{em3} = 600$ nm. Green arrows indicate the direction of intensity changes. For interpretation of the references to color in this figure legend, the reader is referred to the web version of the article [21], copyright (2021) reprinted with permission froom Elsevier B.V. All rights reserved.

improved the accuracy of diagnosing early-stage diseases, such as cancer and cardiovascular diseases.

While the integration of artificial intelligence with spectroscopy offers enhanced diagnostic precision, the study also noted that the requirement for large datasets and substantial computational resources remains a barrier to broader implementation in clinical settings.

Gao *et al* analyzed the changes in porphyrin fluorescence, associated with heme metabolism, serve as critical indicators of hematological disorders, and the fluorescence properties. McLaughlin *et al* [48] made significant strides in applying fluorescence and Raman spectroscopy to blood component analysis.

7.2.3 Forensic applications: species identification and blood typing

In a forensic context, Seyedi *et al* [49] focused on the spectroscopic analysis of blood antigens and antibodies, emphasizing their autofluorescence properties. The study characterized the optical properties of various blood groups and antibodies, discovering unique autofluorescence characteristics that could improve blood typing accuracy and disease diagnosis.

7.2.4 Integration of fluorescence spectroscopy of whole blood with machine learning

Lemler *et al* [50] focused on the spectral analysis of blood autofluorescence for clinical diagnostics, aiming to establish spectral fingerprints of various blood components for disease diagnosis. The study identified distinct spectral patterns correlated with different pathological conditions, demonstrating the potential of autofluorescence as a tool for early disease detection. Weber and Lednev [51] reviewed recent advancements in autofluorescence spectroscopy techniques, particularly their application in disease diagnosis in their later studies. By integrating advanced spectroscopic methods with machine learning, the study significantly improved the accuracy of diagnosing conditions such as cancer and cardiovascular diseases. The research highlighted the potential of combining computational tools with traditional spectroscopic methods to overcome the limitations of manual analysis, though it also noted the challenges associated with large, well-curated datasets needed to effectively train machine learning models. Fluorescence spectroscopy is also integrated into a deep belief neural network model to classify blood species by Gan *et al* [52], which shows remarkable accuracy (97.5%) in species classification. Their study demonstrated the effectiveness of combining deep learning with spectroscopy, particularly in forensic science, wildlife management, and food safety.

7.3 Autofluorescence properties of blood plasma and blood serum

7.3.1 Clinical diagnostics using autofluorescence spectroscopy in blood plasma and blood serum

Blood plasma and blood serum are essential components of human blood, each playing a crucial role in various physiological processes [53]. Blood plasma is the liquid portion of the blood, comprising about 55% of its overall content [54]. It is primarily composed of water, proteins, electrolytes, hormones, and waste products. Plasma serves as the medium for transporting nutrients, hormones, and proteins to different parts of the body. Blood serum, on the other hand, is the fluid that remains after blood has coagulated and the clotting factors, such as fibrinogen, have been removed [55]. Serum contains many of the same components as plasma, excluding the clotting proteins.

Blood plasma and serum exhibit distinct autofluorescence properties due to their unique biochemical compositions. Early foundational studies, such as Xu *et al* [56], identified characteristic fluorescence profiles in the serum of cancer patients. The study found distinct fluorescence peaks at 630 and 690 nm in cancer patients' serum, which were absent in healthy controls, suggesting that serum fluorescence could be indicative of cancerous conditions. Plasma, the liquid portion of blood, contains fluorophores [57] such as NADH [58], flavins [59], and porphyrins [59] emit fluorescence (figure 7.1). Wolfbeis and Leiner [13] provided foundational insights into the fluorescence properties of human blood serum by mapping its total fluorescence. The study identified key fluorophores such as tryptophan, NADH, and bilirubin, and examined how factors like pH affect their fluorescence profiles. While the research highlighted the potential of using serum fluorescence for diagnosing pathological states, it also pointed out the challenges posed by the dependency on pH and interference from non-fluorescent components.

Changes in the concentration or state of certain fluorophores can reflect alterations in metabolic activity or the presence of disease, such as cancer [60]. Autofluorescence analysis has the potential to serve as a powerful tool for early disease detection, monitoring disease progression, and evaluating the effectiveness of treatments [61]. By understanding the autofluorescence properties of blood plasma and serum, researchers and clinicians can develop diagnostic techniques that are less invasive, more cost-effective, and potentially more sensitive than traditional methods [62]. Li *et al* [19] contributed to this body of work by focusing on the use of laser-induced autofluorescence spectra of serum to differentiate lung cancer patients from healthy controls. As shown in figure 7.3, the spectral profiles of normal individuals and lung cancer patients exhibit distinct differences, highlighting the potential of autofluorescence as a diagnostic tool [19]. In addition, they identified specific fluorescence intensity ratios that achieved a diagnostic accuracy of 83.3%, indicating the technique's promise for non-invasive cancer screening, although limitations related to fluorescence sensitivity and the need for further refinement to enhance accuracy were acknowledged.

Bakun *et al* [63] and Lin *et al* [64] employed distinct fluorescence-based techniques for blood plasma analysis in disease detection, focusing on endometriosis and cancer, respectively. Bakun *et al* utilized Jones-matrix laser autofluorescence imaging to detect early signs of endometriosis by assessing the optical anisotropy of polycrystalline protein networks in blood plasma films. Their study demonstrated significant differences in fluorescence intensity distributions between control groups and patients with endometriosis, underscoring the potential of this method as a non-invasive diagnostic tool. In addition, Lin *et al* also mentioned that protein–

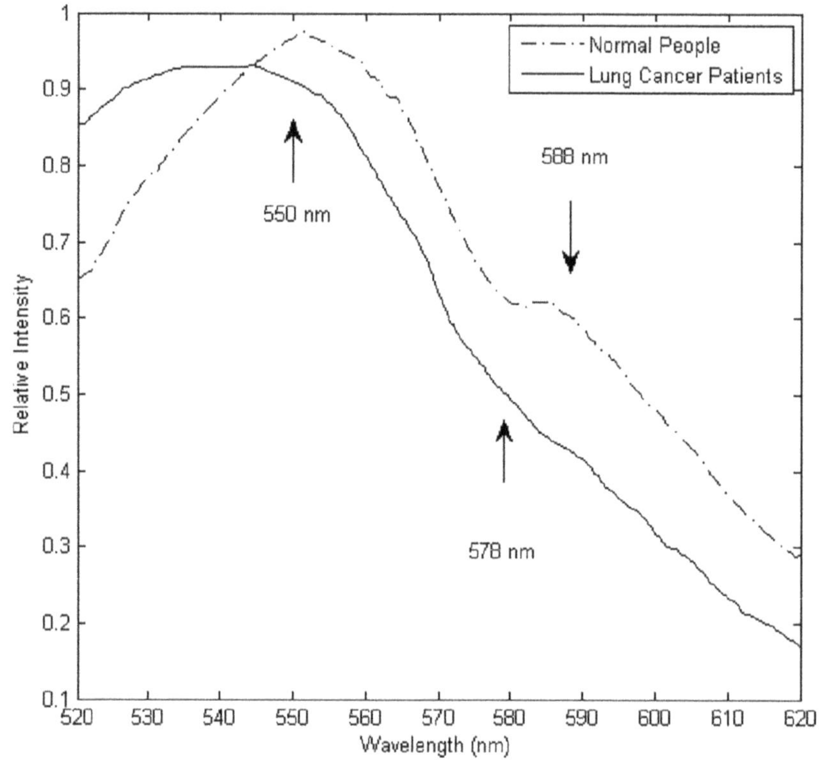

Figure 7.3. Typical autofluorescence spectra of normal and lung cancer patients. Copyright (2011) IEEE. Reprinted, with permission, from [19].

nanoparticle interactions enhance spectral sensitivity for cancer biomarker detection based on the absorption spectrum of albumin–Ag NP mixtures.

Croce and Bottiroli [3] provided an overview of fluorescence spectroscopy and imaging techniques with rate models, emphasizing the utility of autofluorescence in liver and systemic disease diagnosis. The study explored the spectral properties of NAD(P)H, flavins, lipopigments, and bilirubin, correlating their autofluorescence signals with mitochondrial metabolism and oxidative stress. In the same study, they investigated how individual endogenous fluorophores contribute to distinct spectral profiles, forming the basis for such diagnostic applications. They also identified distinct autofluorescence signatures, particularly in NADH and flavins, which could serve as biomarkers for early cancer detection illustrating an example of spectral fitting analysis applied to an autofluorescence spectrum collected *in vivo*, and demonstrating how such techniques can be employed for real-time metabolic assessments.

Building on these approaches, they explored blood plasma autofluorescence to monitor metabolic disorders like diabetes in 2018 [65]. In their more recent study Croce *et al* [66] extended the use of autofluorescence to drug action monitoring in a rat model of liver ischemia and reperfusion (I/R) injury. They explored the role of fluorescing fatty acids (arachidonic, linoleic, and oleic acids), retinoids, and bilirubin as intrinsic serum biomarkers of liver functionality. The study highlighted the excitation-emission spectral characteristics of these fluorophores, emphasizing the impact of obeticholic acid (OCA), a Farnesoid-X Receptor (FXR) agonist, in modulating their fluorescence property.

7.3.2 Integration of fluorescence spectroscopy of blood plasma and blood serum with machine learning

The integration of machine learning algorithms with autofluorescence spectroscopy enhances diagnostic accuracy by analyzing complex fluorescence data patterns. Similarly, Wang *et al* [16] and Yue *et al* [67] integrated machine learning with autofluorescence spectroscopy for blood plasma analysis revealing distinct spectral patterns and intensity of fluorophores between tuberculosis (TB) patients and healthy controls (table 7.2, figure 7.4) to differentiate disease states.

Table 7.2. Main fluorescence emission peaks in normal blood plasma. Reprinted from [16], copyright 2020, with permission from Elsevier GmbH. All rights reserved.

Fluorescence peak positions (nm)	Fluorophores
440	NAD(P)H
470	NADPH
500–520	Vitamin A, Riboflavin, Bilirubin
520	FAD
540	Flavins, Phospholipids
560	Phospholipids
590	Zpp
625	HpD, PpIX

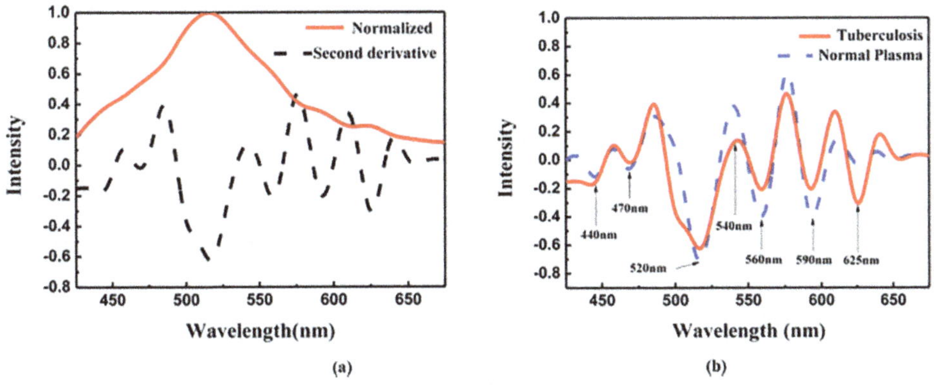

Figure 7.4. (a) The normalized fluorescence and second derivative emission spectra of typical TB blood plasma samples. (b) The second derivative fluorescence of typical TB and normal blood plasma samples. Reprinted from [16], copyright 2020, with permission from Elsevier GmbH. All rights reserved.

7.3.3 Surface-enhanced fluorescence (SERS) in autofluorescence spectroscopy of blood plasma and blood serum

The application of surface-enhanced Raman Spectroscopy (SERS), which leverages nanostructured metallic surfaces from the nanoparticles [68] to significantly amplify weak Raman signals offers a powerful strategy for enhancing biomolecular detection sensitivity. It has demonstrated an increased detection sensitivity. Feng *et al* [69] pioneered the use of SERS to improve the sensitivity of detecting fluorescence signals from plasma proteins for nasopharyngeal cancer diagnostics.

7.3.4 Autofluorescence of blood plasma and blood serum for gastrointestinal disease diagnosis

Tomečková *et al* [61] applied autofluorescence and atomic force microscopy to analyze blood serum in the diagnosis of bowel diseases. By correlating structural and fluorescence characteristics of serum with various bowel diseases, the study revealed significant differences in fluorescence intensity and serum surface structure between patients and health controls. Tomečková *et al* extend the correlation between serum fluorescence intensity and bowel disease markers, suggesting potential non-invasive diagnostic applications. These methods hold potential for improving patient outcomes through earlier intervention and more sensitive disease monitoring.

7.4 Autofluorescence properties of blood pigments

7.4.1 Autofluorescence and excitation-emission properties of hemoglobin

The study of autofluorescence properties of blood pigments, including hemoglobin [70, 71] porphyrins [72], and other related biomolecules, has garnered significant interest in both clinical and research settings.

The primary blood pigments (chromoproteins responsible for color and function) in human blood *in vivo* are the following [73]:

1. *Hemoglobin (Hb) (structure: tetramer (2*α *+ 2*β *subunits) with heme (*Fe^{2+}*-protoporphyrin IX) types:*
   a) Oxyhemoglobin (HbO_2): Bright red (bound to O_2, R-state).
   b) Deoxyhemoglobin (Hb): Dark red/purple (no O_2, T-state).
   c) Methemoglobin (MetHb): Brown (Fe^{3+}, non-functional, <1% in healthy blood).
   d) Carboxyhemoglobin (COHb): Cherry red (bound to CO, toxic).
   e) Glycated hemoglobin (HbA1c): Pinkish (glucose-bound, diabetes marker).
2. *Heme derivatives (breakdown products of hemoglobin)*
   a) Bilirubin: Yellow (heme catabolism, bound to albumin; elevated in jaundice).
   b) Biliverdin: Green (intermediate in heme → bilirubin conversion, minimal in blood).
   c) Hemosiderin: Golden-brown (iron-storage complex in macrophages after hemorrhage).

3. *Other hemoglobin pigments (rare/pathological)*
   a) Sulfhemoglobin (SulfHb): Greenish (sulfur-bound, irreversible, drug-induced).
   b) Cyanmethemoglobin: Bright red (Fe^{3+}–CN, lab artifact for hemoglobin measurement).
   c) Myoglobin (Mb): Red (muscle-derived, leaks into blood after trauma/rhabdomyolysis).
4. *Hemoglobin precursors and derivates*
   a) Porphyrins (protoporphyrin IX, PPIX, <1.0 $\mu g\,dL^{-1}$ in healthy blood, primarily located in erythrocytes, they are intermediates in heme biosynthesis, iron free)
   b) Zinc-PPIX (ZPP, <2.5 $\mu g\,dL^{-1}$ in healthy blood, primarily located in erythrocytes when iron (Fe^{2+}) is unavailable (e.g., iron deficiency or lead poisoning), the enzyme ferrochelatase substitutes zinc (Zn^{2+}) into protoporphyrin IX (PPIX), forming ZnPP, not functional for oxygen transport (only Fe^{2+}-PPIX binds O_2), marker of impaired heme synthesis
   c) Coproporphyrin (<2.0 $\mu g\,dL^{-1}$ in healthy blood, primarily located in plasma, Intermediate metabolites in heme biosynthesis, iron free)
   d) Uroporphyrin (<1.0 $\mu g\,dL^{-1}$ in healthy blood, primarily located in plasma, Intermediate metabolites in heme biosynthesis, iron free).

Hemoglobin fluorescence is largely attributed to the porphyrin ring of the heme prosthetic group. Porphyrins are aromatic macrocycles capable of absorbing and emitting photons due to their conjugated double-bond structure, resulting in intrinsic fluorescence properties [74]. Hemoglobin generally displays significant excitation in the Soret band region (~400–420 nm), with weaker excitation peaks (Q-bands) appearing around 500–600 nm. Fluorescence emission typically occurs in the red to near-infrared range (~600–700 nm), influenced by oxidation state and environmental conditions [4]. Intrinsic fluorescence from hemoglobin is weak compared to other endogenous fluorophores (e.g., NAD(P)H, flavins, collagen), posing challenges in its direct measurement and application. Native hemoglobin fluorescence is rarely detectable *in vivo* due to the low signal-to-noise ratio [75].

This intrinsic autofluorescence is notably weak, with a low quantum yield, meaning that only a small fraction of hemoglobin-absorbed photons is re-emitted as fluorescence (0.001–0.01). This low quantum yield is attributed to efficient non-radiative decay processes within the heme structure, where the energy absorbed is predominantly dissipated through non-fluorescent pathways [76], with the iron in hemoglobin that strongly quenches fluorescence, making hemoglobin a poor emitter, and the reabsorption effects due to hemoglobin's high molar absorptivity (~$10^5\ M^{-1}\ cm^{-1}$ at Soret band). However, a secondary excitation in the UV region (~280 nm) may produce emission due to tryptophan/tyrosine in globin (protein contribution) [77]. The quantum yield of hemoglobin can vary between its conformational states. Studies have shown that in the T-state (tense state, lower oxygen affinity, stabilized structure), the apparent quantum yield can be higher compared to the R-state (relaxed state, higher oxygen affinity, conformationally altered due to oxygen binding). This difference is thought to be due to structural variations affecting the heme environment and its electronic properties [78].

Chemical modifications, such as glycation, can also impact hemoglobin's fluorescence properties. Advanced glycation end-products (AGEs) formed on hemoglobin have been reported to exhibit increased autofluorescence. Despite the presence of the heme group, which typically quenches fluorescence, glycated hemoglobin has shown a quantum yield of approximately 0.19. This enhancement is likely due to the fluorescent nature of the AGE adducts formed on the protein [79, 80]. Factors such as pH, temperature, and solvent polarity can affect the quantum yield by altering the structural conformation of hemoglobin and the electronic environment of the heme group [81, 82].

Hemoglobin's autofluorescence was extensively studies by Saytashev *et al* [83], Sun *et al* [84], Petrich *et al* [85], Clay *et al* [86] and Dong *et al* [87]. Typical hemoglobin autofluorescence spectra are shown in figure 7.5. Saytashev *et al* demonstrated the superior resolution of third-harmonic generation microscopy (THG) in non-invasive imaging of RBCs and Sun *et al* identified the heme group as the key contributor to hemoglobin's fluorescence under two-photon excitation. Petrich *et al* provided a detailed characterization of hemoglobin's intrinsic fluorescence under controlled physiological conditions, emphasizing the importance of experimental factors such as pH and temperature. This research established a foundation for using hemoglobin fluorescence as a marker for oxygenation status and other physiological parameters in clinical diagnostics. Clay *et al* discovered significant two-photon absorptivity in the near-infrared range, positioning hemoglobin as a promising autofluorescence contrast agent for nonlinear optical imaging. Dong *et al* identified unique autofluorescence properties within intact RBCs, emphasizing the importance of controlling physiological variables such as oxygenation and pH to ensure accurate fluorescence measurements presenting the fluorescence spectra of hemoglobin and glycated hemoglobin (HbA1c) under 447 nm excitation, showing spectral shifts due to glycation. Expending from the previous studies, Li *et al* [88] and Gryczynski *et al* [89] both emphasize the potential of

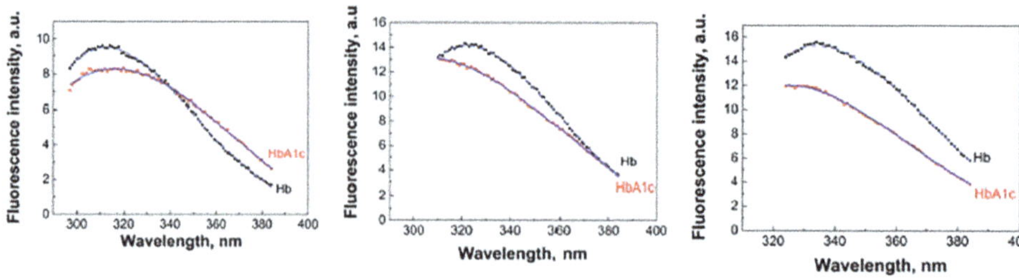

(a) (b) (c)

Figure 7.5. Fluorescence spectra of hemoglobin and HbA1c solutions with optical density of 0.1 at excitation wavelengths: (a) 260 nm; (b) 270 nm; (c) 280 nm (Hb—■ (Black squares), HbA1c—• (Red circles), Gaussian analysis—Blue lines). Reproduced from [93] CC BY 4.0.

hemoglobin fluorescence in medical diagnostics, particularly for imaging and monitoring purposes. Li *et al* demonstrated that hemoglobin's two-photon excited fluorescence (TPEF) could be used to visualize microvascular structures *in vivo*, suggesting its applicability in non-invasive imaging techniques for assessing microcirculatory health. Gryczynski *et al* extended this concept by showing that hemoglobin's fluorescence lifetime varies with its oxygenation state, indicating that time-resolved fluorescence could be employed to monitor blood oxygenation non-invasively, which is critical for clinical diagnostics. Another important aspect of hemoglobin's fluorescence properties is its sensitivity to environmental factors such as pH, oxygenation, and oxidative stress. Asghari-Khiavi *et al* [90] and Hennig *et al* [91] further explored the sensitivity of hemoglobin fluorescence to environmental factors, such as pH and oxygenation state. Hennig *et al* developed a dual-wavelength excitation method to separate fluorescence contributions from zinc protoporphyrin IX (ZnPP) and free protoporphyrin IX (PPIX), minimizing background fluorescence interference. Their difference spectrum approach demonstrated improved detection of ZnPP and PPIX relevant for monitoring heme metabolism disorders.

7.4.2 Excitation/emission spectroscopy of hemoglobin variants

Different hemoglobin variants exhibit distinct excitation and emission spectra, making fluorescence spectroscopy useful for hemoglobinopathy diagnosis. Hirsch *et al* [92] provided groundbreaking insights into the intrinsic fluorescence of oxyhemoglobin, challenging the long-held belief that heme proteins do not exhibit detectable fluorescence. They identified significant fluorescence in oxyhemoglobin, largely due to tryptophan residues, suggesting that this fluorescence could be used to study hemoglobin's conformational dynamics under normal physiological conditions. Hirsch *et al* also presented the comprehensive excitation and emission spectra, including HbA and HbRC, HbH, HbF, HbA, and HbRC, respectively.

Similarly, Lazareva *et al* [93] explored the excitation spectra of hemoglobin and HbA1c with a fluorescence peak at 275 nm, and their corresponding fluorescence emission spectra with optical density of 0.1 at various excitation wavelengths, such as 260, 270, and 280 nm, as shown in figure 7.5 highlighted the distinct emission spectra associated with these pigments and underscored the challenges for accurate interpretation.

Gryczynski *et al* provided a comprehensive analysis of the intrinsic fluorescence properties of heme and non-heme blood components, offering critical data that could enhance the accuracy of fluorescence-based diagnostic tools. The emission spectra of carbonmonoxyhemoglobin under different pressure conditions was presented by Gryczynski *et al* [94] showing how hemoglobin's fluorescence properties change with environmental factors. The distinct fluorescence spectra identified by Gryczynski *et al*, as shown in figure 7.6, are particularly relevant for improving the specificity and sensitivity of these diagnostic methods. Foundational insights into the fluorescence spectra of hemoglobin under different oxygenation states were provided by Rousseau and Ondrias [95] and Rusciano *et al* [96] showing that

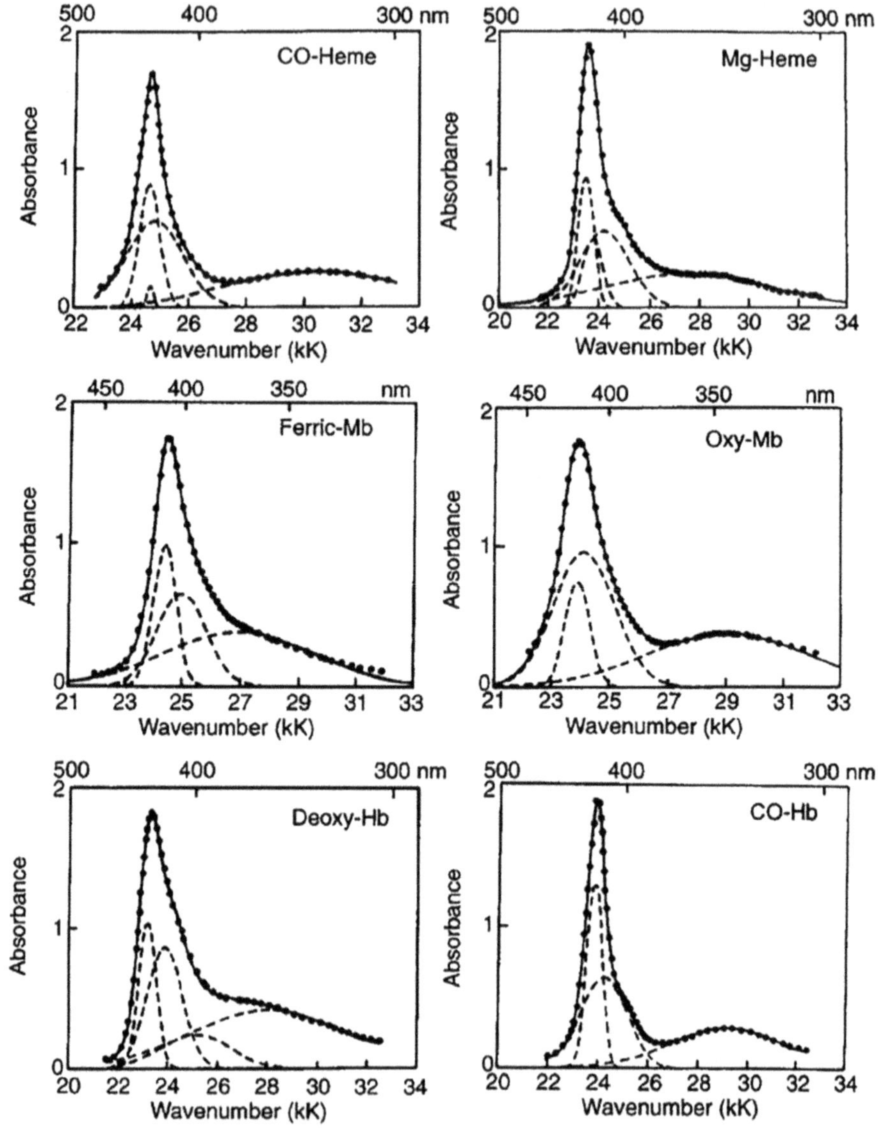

Figure 7.6. Absorption spectra in the near-UV and Soret range of CO-heme and Mg-heme in isotropic polyvinyl alcohol (PVA) film, myoglobin and hemoglobin derivatives in 0.05 phosphate buffer, pH 7.0, at room temperature. The measured values are given by filled circles and the Gaussian components by dashed lines. Reprinted from [94], copyright 1997, with permission from Elsevier Inc.

structural modifications affect heme coordination and fluorescence characteristics. Both studies identified distinct fluorescence patterns for oxyhemoglobin and deoxyhemoglobin, laying the groundwork for using fluorescence spectroscopy to monitor blood oxygenation levels non-invasively. These findings have significant implications for clinical diagnostics and research, as they establish a method for assessing blood oxygenation without invasive procedures.

Studies done by Chakraborty *et al* [97], Hirsch and Nagel [98], Nagababu and Rifkind [99], and Sebba *et al* [100] explored how the fluorescence of hemoglobin is affected by its structure and formation process. Specifically, Chakraborty *et al* and Hirsch and Nagel both emphasized the relationship between hemoglobin's structural state and its fluorescence characteristics. Chakraborty *et al* used time-resolved fluorescence spectroscopy and molecular dynamics simulations to show that conformational changes in hemoglobin significantly affect its fluorescence properties.

Similarly, Hirsch and Nagel explored the sensitivity of hemoglobin's intrinsic fluorescence, particularly tryptophan fluorescence, to detect conformational changes associated with different liganded states exploring potential applications in studying hemoglobinopathies. Nagababu and Rifkind explored the formation and properties of fluorescent heme degradation products and porphyrin-globin, respectively, as a marker for oxidative stress in RBCs, while Sebba *et al* confirmed strong fluorescence from porphyrin-globin, contributing to the understanding of intrinsic fluorescence in hemoglobin and its potential use in biomedical imaging.

7.4.3 Fluorescence quenching and oxidative modifications in hemoglobin

The fluorescence properties of hemoglobin are also influenced by molecular interactions, such as quenching effects and oxidation processes.

Chakraborty *et al* [97] investigated the quenching effect of hesperetin on hemoglobin fluorescence, revealing that ligand binding affects the fluorescence intensity of tryptophan residues. This underscores the potential of fluorescence-based drug interaction studies for therapeutic monitoring. Chen and Hirsch [101] expanded on this by developing a spectroscopic method to simultaneously detect multiple fluorescent species related to heme metabolism in RBCs. Their fluorescence excitation and emission spectra showed that oxidative stress alters hemoglobin's fluorescence, highlighting its potential for assessing oxidative damage in blood disorders. To confirm the assumption, they demonstrated distinct fluorescence emissions of FHDP (466 nm), ZnPP (594 nm), and PPIX (626 nm), which agreed with the fluorescence spectrum of hemoglobin under different oxidative stress done by Sebban *et al* [100] showing that the oxidative stress condition increases the relative fluorescence peak from 280 to 506 nm. These results reinforce the diagnostic utility of fluorescence markers for hemoglobinopathies.

In addition, Chakraborty *et al* also explored fluorescence quenching effects by studying the interaction of hesperitin with HbA fluorescence. The reduction in fluorescence intensity indicated ligand-binding-induced conformational changes, reinforcing the potential for fluorescence-based drug binding studies. Fluorescence titration studies were carried out by Chen and Hirsch, who demonstrated how incremental additions of PPIX and ZnPP significantly altered the fluorescence spectra of hemoglobin, providing insights into the dynamic interactions between these molecules in the blood. Their dose-dependent fluorescence variations indicate that fluorescence spectroscopy can be applied to quantify abnormal heme metabolism in diseases such as sickle cell disease, beta-thalassemia, and erythropoietic protoporphyria.

Alpert *et al* [102] and Nagababu *et al* [103] also investigated the intrinsic fluorescence properties of hemoglobin and its derivatives, focusing on their structural dynamics and response to oxidative stress. They explored the fluorescence emission of tryptophan residues in hemoglobin, revealing its potential as an intrinsic probe for studying hemoglobin dynamics under various conditions. Similarly, Nagababu *et al* highlighted how oxidative modifications significantly alter hemoglobin's fluorescence properties, suggesting that these changes could serve as indicators of oxidative stress, which is crucial for developing diagnostic tools to monitor blood-related oxidative conditions. Pundir and Chawla [104] identified distinct fluorescence signatures associated with oxidative stress, reinforcing the diagnostic potential of blood pigment fluorescence in the early diagnosis and monitoring blood disorders. This body of work underscores the broad applicability of fluorescence spectroscopy in studying hemoglobin's role in health and disease, providing a foundation for future research and the development of non-invasive diagnostic tools.

7.4.4 Glycated hemoglobin detection via the fluorescence and Raman spectroscopy

In addition to fluorescence studies, the differentiation between normal hemoglobin and HbA1c, a key marker for diabetes, was further explored by Lazareva *et al* [93] and Barman *et al* [105]. Both studies demonstrated that optical properties, such as fluorescence and Raman spectra, could distinguish between normal and glycated hemoglobin, supporting the potential of these techniques in non-invasive diabetes diagnostics. They introduced Raman spectroscopy as a sensitive and specific tool for detecting HbA1c, an important biomarker for long-term glycemic control in diabetes. Utilizing the drop coating deposition Raman (DCDR) technique, their study leveraged the coffee-ring effect to enhance Raman signals, enabling precise quantification of HbA1c in hemolysate models [105].

The distinct Raman spectral changes between glycated and non-glycated hemoglobin, as shown in figure 7.7, demonstrated high specificity and reproducibility of this method. This spectral differentiation underscores the method's capability in distinguishing between glycated and non-glycated hemoglobin, demonstrating its high specificity and reproducibility. Lastly, Loannou and Varotsis [106] explored how external factors, such as dietary glyco-products, affect hemoglobin fluorescence, highlighting the impact of the Maillard reaction on hemoglobin function and its potential as a diagnostic tool.

7.5 Autofluorescence properties of red blood cells (or erythrocytes)

7.5.1 Hemoglobin autofluorescence and oxygenation states

RBCs, or erythrocytes, are integral to human physiology, primarily responsible for the transportation of oxygen from the lungs to tissues and the return of carbon dioxide for exhalation [107]. These cells, devoid of nuclei and packed with hemoglobin, have garnered significant research interest not only for their essential biological roles but also for their unique optical properties, particularly autofluorescence [108]. This intrinsic fluorescence can provide critical insights into the

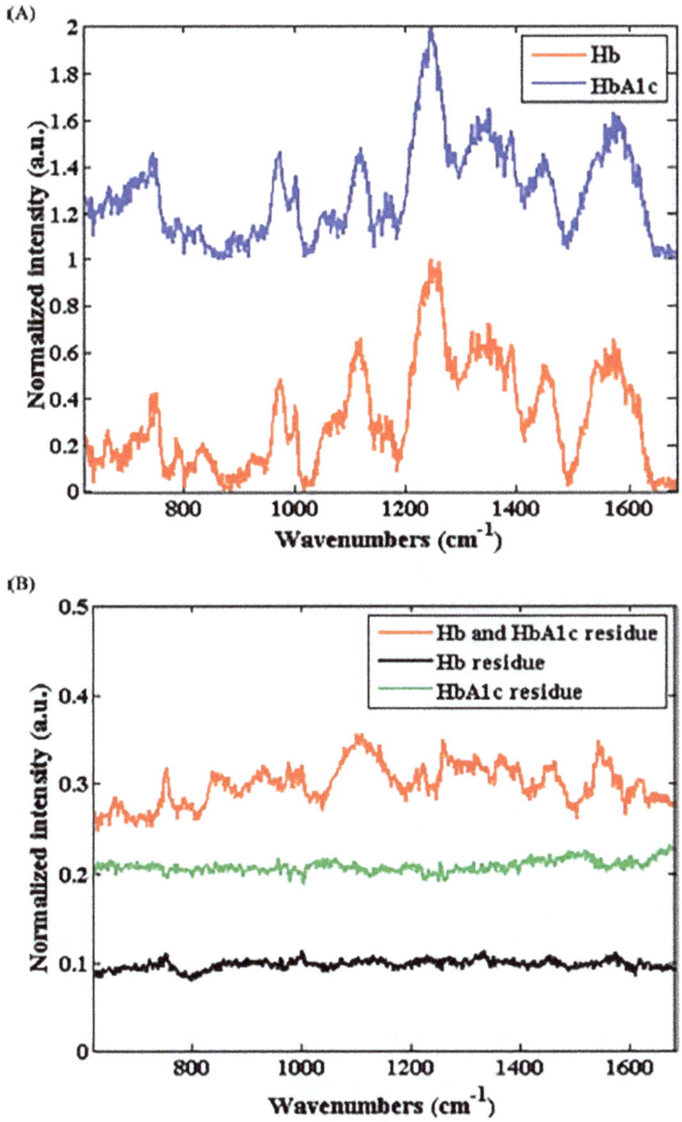

Figure 7.7. (A) Raman spectra acquired from the drop-coated single-protein hemoglobin and HbA1c samples derived from ca. 39 and 34 μM solutions, respectively (the spectra are normalized and offset for the sake of clarity). (B) Spectra computed from the difference between normalized hemoglobin (39 μM) and HbA1c (34 μM) spectra shown in panel A (red); normalized hemoglobin spectra from drop-coated rings derived from 39 and 19.5 μM (green); normalized HbA1c spectra from drop-coated rings derived from 34 and 17 μM (black). Reprinted with permission from [105], copyright 2012 American Chemical Society.

biochemical and structural state of RBCs, offering a non-invasive window into cellular health and function [109].

Early investigations by Hamly *et al* [110] laid the foundational understanding of hemoglobin fluorescence within RBCs, identifying the weak yet measurable

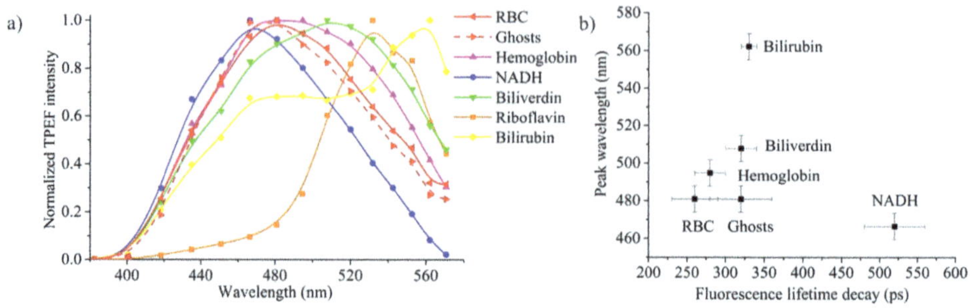

Figure 7.8. TPEF (800 nm, 15 fs) emission spectra for RBCs, erythrocyte ghosts and reagentgrade fluorophores. Reproduced with permission from [83].

fluorescence emission influenced by the oxygenation state of hemoglobin reviewed in section 7.4. Wood *et al* [111] used Raman spectroscopy to identify spectroscopic changes in hemoglobin during oxygenation. Subsequent studies by Saytashev *et al* [83], Shirshin *et al* [112], and Hertz *et al* [113] further demonstrated that hemoglobin's autofluorescence properties shift with oxygenation state, pH, and membrane integrity. Collectively, these findings support the potential of hemoglobin autofluorescence as a non-invasive biomarker for assessing RBC function. Figure 7.8 presents two-photon excited fluorescence (TPEF) spectra (800 nm, 15 fs) for RBCs and their components, revealing how hemoglobin's fluorescence characteristics vary with oxygenation state and membrane integrity [83].

In a related domain, Dasgupta *et al* [114] explored the fluorescence characteristics of RBC membranes, particularly under oxidative stress. This study identified specific fluorescence changes associated with oxidative damage, which could serve as biomarkers for RBC health. While this research primarily focused on fluorescence rather than mechanical properties, it complements the findings of the other studies by providing a different perspective on RBC health, linking fluorescence changes to membrane damage and oxidative stress.

7.5.2 Diagnostic applications of autofluorescence in disease and oxidative stress

In recent years, the autofluorescence of RBCs has been explored as a potential diagnostic tool [115]. Researchers have investigated how changes in RBC autofluorescence can be correlated with different health conditions, leading to the development of techniques that could allow for real-time monitoring of blood oxygenation levels [116], the detection of malaria [117], and the assessment of RBC health in various diseases. Studies employing techniques such as fluorescence spectroscopy, Raman spectroscopy, and time-resolved fluorescence imaging have shown promise in distinguishing between healthy and diseased cells based on their autofluorescence signatures.

The fluorescence properties of RBCs have been leveraged for diagnosing blood disorders and oxidative stress-related conditions. Adak *et al* [118] and Bankapur *et al* [119] studied RBC autofluorescence in sickle cell disease, correlating fluorescence signatures with oxidative states and membrane deformability. Their findings emphasize the diagnostic potential of fluorescence spectroscopy, albeit with challenges in differentiating oxidation states. Adak *et al* explored the fluorescence characteristics of normal and sickle RBCs, revealing distinct fluorescence signatures that correlate with the oxidative states and membrane properties of the cells. Similarly, Bankapur *et al* employed optical tweezers combined with fluorescence spectroscopy to study RBC elasticity, particularly in sickle cell anemia.

Bukara *et al* [120] demonstrated that oxidative stress leads to significant changes in hemoglobin fluorescence lifetime, suggesting that autofluorescence can serve as an early marker for RBC damage. Amor *et al* [121] and Bloom *et al* [122] extended the investigation of RBC autofluorescence to diabetic patients, identifying specific autofluorescence patterns that correlated with glucose levels and disease progression. Lin *et al* [123] concentrated on lipid variations in erythrocyte membranes as a marker for diabetic conditions, utilizing Raman spectroscopy to detect significant spectral differences. These findings, coupled with resonance Raman spectroscopy studies by Sydor *et al* [124], Zhurova *et al* [125] and Hennig *et al* [126], further support the utility of fluorescence techniques in detecting pathological changes in RBCs, where Sydor *et al* investigated the effects of aging and oxidative stress on RBC autofluorescence, identifying similar diagnostic potential for detecting oxidative damage; Zhurova *et al* employed resonance Raman spectroscopy to explore the structural changes in hemoglobin that correspond to shifts in autofluorescence during oxygenation and deoxygenation, with additional insights into the effects of pH on hemoglobin's structure and fluorescence; Hennig *et al* explored the fluorescence properties of hemoglobin, particularly in relation to its oxygenation state, considering the potential for non-invasive monitoring of blood oxygenation.

7.5.3 Spectroscopy of red blood cell autofluorescence and blood product quality

Tougan *et al* [127] investigated autofluorescence-emitting RBCs focusing on the diagnostic potential of hemoglobin's autofluorescence for detecting abnormal forms like methemoglobin. Figure 7.9 presents fluorescence intensity spectra of RBC lysates treated with aminolaevulinic acid (ALA) after 72 h, distinguishing between treated and non-treated RBCs [127]. Khodabux *et al* [128] investigated the fluorescence properties of umbilical cord blood (UCB) RBCs, particularly during storage for transfusion purposes. The study found that UCB RBCs maintain stable fluorescence properties for up to 21 days, supporting their use in neonatal care.

7.5.4 Red blood cell elasticity and deformability via optical techniques

A significant body of research has focused on RBC deformability, an essential factor in microcirculation and disease progression. For instance, Brandao *et al* [129] and Henon *et al* [130] utilized optical tweezers to measure RBC elasticity in sickle cell disease, revealing significantly lower deformability in sickle cell patients compared to healthy individuals. This study provided insights into how hemoglobin's autofluorescence correlates with cell deformability, offering potential diagnostic applications in assessing RBC health. Bambardekar *et al* [131] and Bankapur *et al* [119]

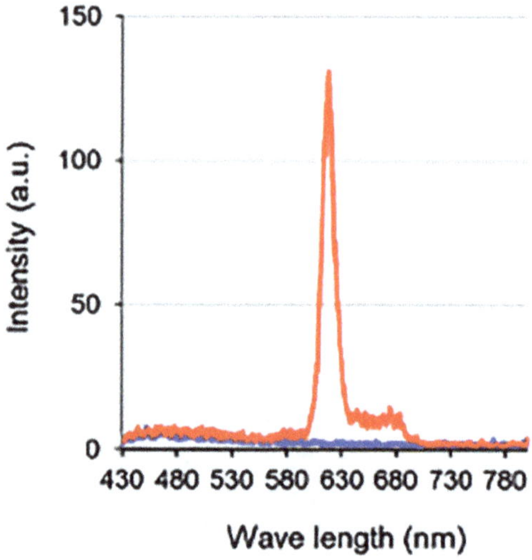

Figure 7.9. Spectrometry data of the RBC lysates treated with ALA after 72 h. Red and blue lines indicate fluorescence intensities from ALA-treated and non-treated RBC lysates, respectively. Reproduced from [127] CC BY 4.0.

employed fluorescence microscopy and optical trapping techniques to assess RBC deformability, particularly in malaria-infected cells. Their research demonstrated that infected RBCs exhibit altered fluorescence and reduced flexibility. Similarly, Bransky *et al* [132] developed an automated rheoscope to assess RBC deformability, linking it to conditions such as hemolytic anemia and malaria exploiting a high-speed camera for precise measurements of RBC deformation under shear stress.

7.5.5 Autofluorescence in hemoglobin derivatives

The autofluorescence of RBCs is primarily driven by the hemoglobin molecule and its various derivatives, which exhibit distinct fluorescence characteristics depending on their state of oxygenation [133] and chemical modifications [134]. Hemoglobin, a metalloprotein, undergoes conformational changes during oxygen binding and release, which in turn alters its autofluorescence properties. These fluorescence variations are of considerable interest because they can reflect the physiological and pathological conditions of RBCs, such as oxidative stress, anemia, and the presence of abnormal hemoglobin derivatives like methemoglobin and carboxyhemoglobin [135].

Wood and McNaughton [136] examined excitation wavelength effects on Raman scattering and autofluorescence in hemoglobin, proposing that specific vibrational modes are enhanced due to excitonic coupling between hemoglobin molecules. Parshina *et al* [137] focused on the autofluorescence of bilirubin in blood plasma, demonstrating its utility in diagnosing liver-related disorders like jaundice. This study highlights the characteristic fluorescence of bilirubin. Wang *et al* [138] investigated hemoglobin fluorescence variations with oxygenation levels, further emphasizing autofluorescence as a non-invasive blood oxygenation monitoring tool.

Tougan *et al* [127] and Wood *et al* [139] studied hemoglobin autofluorescence under different excitation conditions, for detecting abnormal hemoglobin forms, such as methemoglobin.

7.6 Autofluorescence properties of white blood cells (or leucocytes)

7.6.1 Metabolic and functional states of WBCs

WBCs, or leukocytes, play a vital role in the immune system by protecting the body against infections, foreign substances, and various diseases [140, 141]. Understanding the autofluorescence properties of WBCs is crucial as it provides a non-invasive means of studying their behavior, function, and interactions under different physiological and pathological conditions [142]. Autofluorescence is observed in various cellular components of WBCs, including endogenous fluorophores [143], like NADH [143], flavin adenine dinucleotide (FAD) [143], and tryptophan [143].

Fluorescence microscopy and spectroscopy have been exploited for detailed analysis of WBC autofluorescence, providing insights into cellular metabolism, oxidative stress, and immune cell trafficking [144]. By leveraging the unique fluorescence signatures of WBCs, researchers can distinguish between different leukocyte subtypes, assess their activation states, and monitor their responses to various stimulus, such as infections or inflammation [145].

The studies summarized here highlight the diverse applications of WBC autofluorescence, ranging from monitoring immune responses and oxidative stress to detecting infectious diseases like malaria [146]. These cells include diverse subtypes such as lymphocytes, monocytes, neutrophils, eosinophils, and basophils, each performing specialized functions in immune surveillance and response [147]. Li *et al* [142] focused on the two-photon-excited tryptophan fluorescence for imaging leukocyte trafficking *in vivo*, particularly under normal and inflammatory conditions. Li *et al* presented the two-photon excitation spectrum of tryptophan in phosphate buffer solution, demonstrating its potential for non-invasive imaging and its role in visualizing leukocyte movement and interaction with vascular endothelium. Buchwalow *et al* [148] explored NADH and FAD autofluorescence in lymphocytes and macrophages, revealing that these signals increase with immune cell activation, underscoring the role of metabolic changes in modulating WBC autofluorescence as a marker for cell activation and immune response.

7.6.2 Oxidative stress and granulocyte autofluorescence

The significance of WBC autofluorescence lies in its ability to provide real-time insights into cellular processes without the need for external labeling, which can alter cell behavior or viability. For example, FAD and NADH, which are involved in oxidative phosphorylation and other metabolic pathways, emit fluorescence that can be detected and measured to assess cellular energy status, redox state, and metabolic activity [149].

Apart, changes in the autofluorescence of granulocytes could signal an acute inflammatory response, while alterations in lymphocyte autofluorescence might indicate changes in immune activation or suppression [150].

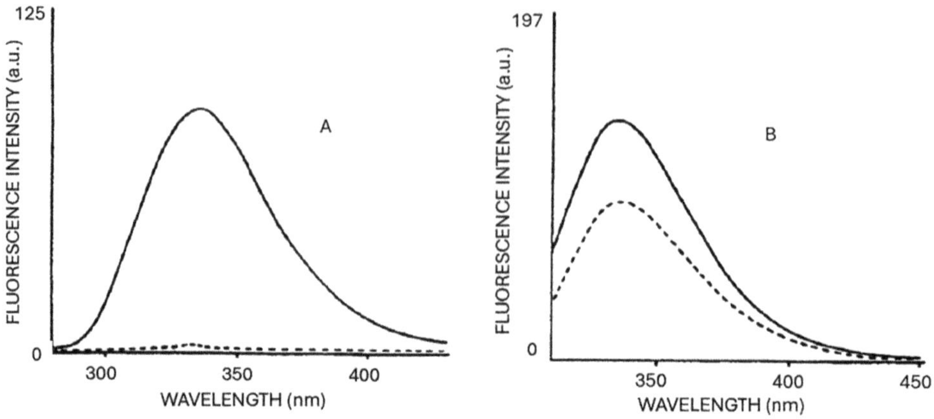

Figure 7.10. Fluorescence emission spectra recorded on human agranulocyte suspensions (–) and human granulocyte suspensions (-) on excitation at 255 nm (A) and 295 nm (B). Reprinted from [20], copyright 1995, with permission from Elsevier B.V.

Lymphocytes show variations in NADH and FAD fluorescence during activation, reflecting shifts in their metabolic demands. Granulocytes, such as neutrophils and eosinophils, display increased autofluorescence in response to oxidative stress, correlating with the production of reactive oxygen species (ROS), which are key to their function in pathogen destruction [151]. Hoeger *et al* [152] further complement these findings by focusing on granulocytes, where oxidative stress and the production of ROS significantly alter autofluorescence. The study demonstrated that granulocytes under oxidative stress exhibit increased autofluorescence, primarily due to the accumulation of oxidized molecules. Figure 7.10 from Monici *et al* illustrates these spectral differences, showing fluorescence emission and excitation spectra recorded on human agranulocyte and granulocyte suspensions [20].

7.6.3 Leukocyte autofluorescence as a non-invasive diagnostic tool

Studying WBC autofluorescence makes it particularly valuable for longitudinal studies, where repeated measurements over time are needed to track disease progression or response to therapy [153]. Lee *et al* [154], Mayeno *et al* [22], and Monici *et al* [20] also converged on the exploration of leukocyte autofluorescence. Lee *et al* focused on how metabolic disorders, particularly diabetes, alter the autofluorescence profiles of leukocytes, revealing significant changes in NADH and FAD signals that reflect shifts in glucose metabolism, thereby positioning autofluorescence as a potential biomarker for metabolic health. Mayeno *et al* identified FAD as the primary fluorophore responsible for eosinophil autofluorescence, linking it to the cells' role in immune responses, particularly in producing ROS. Monici *et al* further extended this understanding by investigating how metabolic changes during cell activation affect the autofluorescence of lymphocytes, showing that activated lymphocytes exhibit increased autofluorescence due to enhanced NADH and flavoprotein signals, which correlate with heightened metabolic activity.

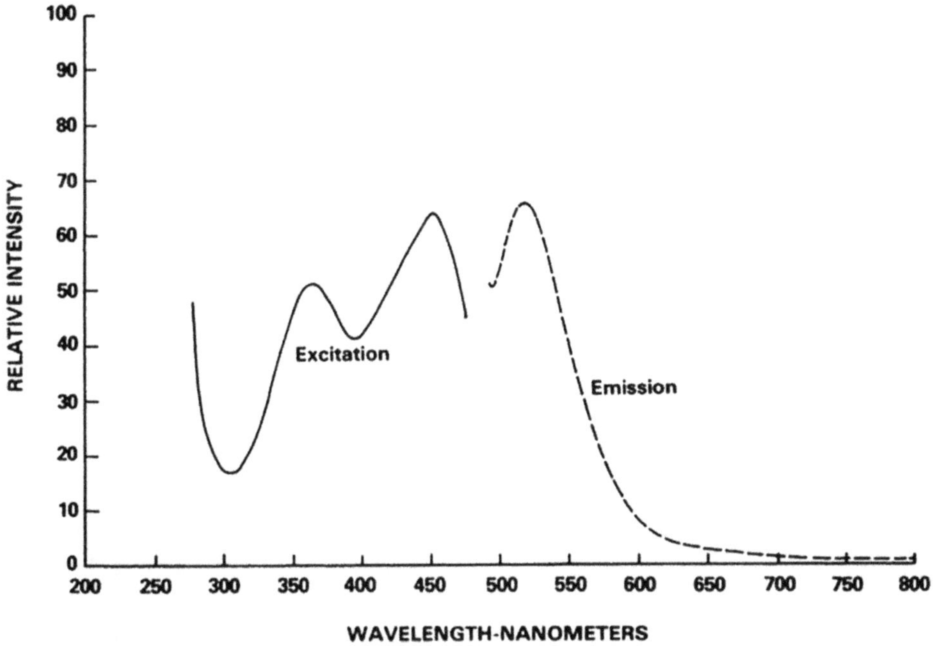

Figure 7.11. Excitation and emission spectra of eosinophil extracts. Excitation spectrum (solid line) recorded at 25 °C for emission of 520 nm. The emission spectrum (dashed line) recorded for excitation of 450 nm. Reprinted from [150], copyright 1981, with permission from American Society of Hematology.

7.6.4 Autofluorescence-based identification of eosinophils and neutrophils

Ozkan *et al* [155], Rehan *et al* [156], and Weil and Chused [150] focused on the diagnostic potential of autofluorescence in different types of WBCs such as eosinophils and neutrophils. Ozkan *et al* investigated the autofluorescence of neutrophils under oxidative stress, highlighting the relationship between neutrophil activation, ROS production, and increased autofluorescence, suggesting these changes could serve as markers for inflammation and oxidative stress in clinical settings. Figure 7.11 from Weil and Chused presents excitation and emission spectra of eosinophil extracts, emphasizing the bright autofluorescence of eosinophils and its potential for distinguishing these cells from other leukocytes.

Weil and Chused also utilized eosinophil autofluorescence for high-purity sorting using flow microfluorometry, suggesting its intensity could be linked to cell function and used diagnostically in conditions like eosinophilia. Rehan *et al* extended these ideas by applying automated hematology analyzers to generate WBC differential fluorescence (WDF) scattergrams, which showed high sensitivity and specificity in detecting malaria.

7.6.5 Advanced optical techniques for leukocyte characterization

Methods such as flow cytometry [157], fluorescence microscopy [158], and more recently, THG microscopy [159] enable researchers to differentiate between various

WBC subtypes, monitor their activation states, and assess their functional responses to different stimuli, providing a wealth of information that is invaluable in both research and clinical settings. The studies by Wu *et al* [159] and Yakimov *et al* [160] both highlight the diagnostic potential of autofluorescence in leukocytes, particularly under normal and stress-induced conditions. Wu *et al* focused on the use of THG microscopy to differentiate major WBC types, such as neutrophils, monocytes, and lymphocytes, based on their autofluorescence characteristics, achieving high accuracy without needing external labels. Yakimov *et al* explored the autofluorescence properties of neutrophils and monocytes in response to metabolic changes associated with oxidative stress and immune activation, revealing that these cells exhibit increased autofluorescence under stress, correlating with heightened metabolic activity.

7.7 Autofluorescence properties of blood platelets (thrombocytes)

7.7.1 Fluorescence spectra of thrombocytes (blood platelets)

Blood platelets, also known as thrombocytes, are small, anucleate cell fragments that play a crucial role in hemostasis—the process that stops bleeding by forming clots at sites of vascular injury [161]. Understanding the behavior and function of platelets is essential for diagnosing and treating a range of cardiovascular and hematological disorders [161]. This intrinsic fluorescence can be harnessed to study various aspects of platelet function, including activation, aggregation, and interaction with other cells [162]. Ryningen and Holmsen [163] explored these biochemical pathways, emphasizing the role of fluorescent phospholipid markers and actin-binding proteins in platelet adhesion and aggregation. As the platelet-derived microparticles (PMPs) have been identified as potent contributors to the coagulation process, Sinauridze *et al* [164] demonstrated that PMPs exhibit 50–100 times higher procoagulant activity than activated platelets due to their increased surface expression of phosphatidylserine and coagulation factor-binding sites. Using flow cytometry and coagulation assays, the study measured elevated densities of CD61, CD62P, and factor X on PMPs, highlighting their ability to accelerate thrombin generation and clot formation.

7.7.2 Flow cytometry and fluorescence-based measurement of platelet activation

The autofluorescence of platelets provides a unique window into the dynamic processes that occur during platelet activation [165]. During this process, platelets undergo significant biochemical and structural changes, including the reorganization of the cytoskeleton, degranulation, and the exposure of surface receptors that facilitate aggregation [166].

Flow cytometry has revolutionized platelet function assessment, allowing real-time monitoring of platelet activation and aggregation. Ault *et al* [167] developed a two-color flow cytometry technique to simultaneously measure platelet release and aggregation in whole blood. Their method utilized monoclonal antibodies against GMP-140 (P-selectin) and glycoprotein Ib (GPIb), which enabled the detection of single platelets, aggregates, and platelet–leukocyte interactions. Similarly, Michelson [168] expanded on flow cytometry's clinical applications, detailing its ability to detect platelet hyperreactivity and circulating activated platelets in conditions such as myocardial infarction, stroke, and diabetes. This study emphasized the use of activation-dependent monoclonal antibodies (MoAbs) that bind only to activated platelets, such as those targeting GPIIb–IIIa, P-selectin, and thrombin-induced binding sites. The study also introduced fluorescence-based detection of platelet surface antigen expression, enabling a highly sensitive, non-radioactive alternative to traditional platelet function tests.

Challenges such as fluorescence quenching and the necessity for precise probe calibration require careful methodological consideration to ensure accurate results [169, 170].

Studies also delve into the biochemical and morphological changes associated with platelet activation, such as pseudopod formation, degranulation, and cytoskeletal reorganization, which are vital for the formation of a hemostatic plug at sites of injury [171]. The methodological emphasis includes the synthesis of fluorescein derivatives like azidofluorescein and their application in real-time studies of platelet cytoskeletal dynamics.

7.7.3 Fluorescence polarization and cytoskeletal dynamics

A foundational study by Rotman and Heldman [172] utilized fluorescence polarization techniques to monitor changes in intracellular viscosity during platelet activation. This work provided early and significant insights into cytoskeletal reorganization, notably the rearrangement of actin filaments, a critical process that underlies platelet aggregation and secretion. Wolberg provided significant insights into cytoskeletal reorganization, notably the rearrangement of actin filaments, a critical process that underlies platelet aggregation and secretion [173]. These findings emphasized the importance of actin dynamics in the functional responses of platelets.

7.7.4 Fluorescence techniques for platelet-activating factor (PAF) studies

Key findings from these studies include the observation of a rapid decrease in intracellular viscosity during platelet activation, the effectiveness of fluorescein-based probes in monitoring the kinetics of activation, and the critical role of PAF in inflammatory signaling [174]. These discoveries not only enhance our understanding of platelet biology but also highlight the potential therapeutic implications, particularly in the treatment of thrombotic and inflammatory diseases.

Further advancing our understanding of platelet biology, Lorant *et al* [174] and Pinckard *et al* [175] examined the role of PAF in mediating interactions between platelets and leukocytes, with a particular focus on inflammation. Their research demonstrated that PAF-induced integrin activation facilitates leukocyte adhesion to endothelial cells, underscoring its pivotal role in inflammatory responses [176]. This work was complemented by the research of Kenneth *et al*, who integrated flow cytometry with fluorescent markers to enable the simultaneous observation of platelet activation and aggregation within whole blood. This methodological advancement provided a more nuanced understanding of platelet behavior in physiological conditions, moving beyond bulk response measurements to capture the complexity of platelet function *in vivo* [177].

Moreover, research on PAF underscores its complex role as a signaling molecule, influencing diverse cellular functions that must be carefully considered in therapeutic development. Targeting PAF in inflammatory conditions holds significant promise for managing excessive inflammation, particularly in autoimmune and vascular diseases, offering potential avenues for novel therapeutic interventions [176].

7.7.5 Application of fluorescence markers in platelet imaging

Xia *et al* [178] employed fluorescein-based probes, including azidofluorescein, to trace intracellular events within platelets. One of the pivotal contributions of their work was the use of FITC-labeled fibrinogen to investigate the binding dynamics of fibrinogen to its receptor GPIIb–IIIa on activated platelets. Through this approach, Xia and colleagues provided deeper insights into the molecular mechanisms driving thrombus formation for understanding the pathophysiology of thrombotic diseases.

Montague *et al* [161] reviewed current and emerging imaging methods, including fluorescence microscopy, intravital microscopy, and microfluidic imaging, exploring platelet adhesion, aggregation, and thrombus formation. They summarized the *in vitro* research in platelet/cell imaging as table 7.3. The study discussed challenges associated with visualizing platelet dynamics due to their small size ($\sim$2 μm) and rapid activation and explored innovative solutions such as label-free imaging technologies (optical coherence tomography and third-harmonic generation microscopy).

7.8 Pathological modification of autofluorescence properties of blood

The exploration of autofluorescence properties of blood pigments, such as porphyrins [197], bilirubin [198], cytochromes [199], myoglobin [200] and hemoglobin [201] presents an avenue for non-invasive diagnostics across various pathological conditions, including cancer [202], liver fibrosis [203], malaria [204], anemia [205], and cardiovascular disorders. Moreover, emerging understanding of COVID-19's multifaceted impact on human health has led to an increased focus on how the disease modifies the biological properties of blood and vascular systems [3]. This chapter section also summarizes the pathological changes in blood fluorescence properties, including how they relate to the broader systemic complications of COVID-19, including coagulopathies, immune dysregulation, and vascular dysfunction.

7.8.1 Cancer diagnostics and blood pigments

Courrol *et al* [206] investigated the spectral profiles of blood porphyrins, particularly Protoporphyrin IX, as a potential biomarker for tumor progression in renal cell carcinoma. The study revealed a significant increase in the fluorescence intensity of Protoporphyrin IX in tumor-induced mice compared to healthy controls, suggesting that blood porphyrin fluorescence could serve as a valuable marker for tracking tumor growth. Research by Courrol *et al* [207] and Devanesan *et al* [208] both explored the potential of fluorescence in cancer diagnostics. Figure 7.12(A) illustrates the emission spectra of porphyrins in normal and tumor blood samples, highlighting distinct spectral differences between cancerous and healthy blood [207]. Additionally, figure 7.12(B) presents the excitation spectrum of blood porphyrin, which was obtained by fixing

Table 7.3. Imaging techniques and applications for platelet research *in vitro*. Reproduced from [161] CC BY 4.0.

Imaging method	Key points	Resolution	Platelet/cell imaging applications (references)	Limitations
Conventional/ Bright-field/ Widefield	Uses visible light or high-intensity light sources to illuminate a sample	$L = 200$–300 nm $Ax = 500$–800 nm	Thrombus formation; microfluidics; large platelet aggregates [179]	Low resolution; not suitable for single-cell evaluation
Confocal/CLSM	Uses light to illuminate a sample through a pinhole to improve optical resolution Uses spatial filtering to block out-of-focus light	$L = \sim 200$ nm (reflection) > 250 nm (fluorescence)	Thrombus formation; platelet spreading; surface receptor information; controls versus patients' samples; wild type mice versus knockout mice differences [179–181]	Limited by wavelength of light; need specific dyes; minimal information on cytoskeleton
GPM/DHM	Generates quantitative measurements from shifts in phase	$L = > 270$ nm	Volumetric measurements of thrombus [182–187]	No receptor profile details; post-image analysis
CLEM/3D cryoEM	Approaching atomic level analysis of ultrastructural changes, adhesion, and granule secretion	$L < 1$ nm	Platelet secretion megakaryocyte positioning in sinusoids and platelet production (applied in *in vitro* setting) [186–189]	Samples need to be mounted on a grid; precise solvent protocol requirements
STED	Confocal excitation beam combined with stimulated emission at target area	$L = 50$–60 nm	Platelet protein distribution when co-incubated with other cells; platelet protein storage [189–192]	Deconvolution required; need specific STED dyes; decreased spatial resolution; increased acquisition time
SMLM/SIM/ PALM/STORM/ Paint	Illuminate the sample to single molecule switching by stochastic excitation Switching on/off of a fluorophore by stochastic excitation	$L = \sim 20$ nm $Ax = \sim 50$ nm	Platelet cytoskeleton proteins; actin nodules/tubulin; megakaryocyte surface and function; synapses platelet receptor co-localization and receptor clustering [193–196]	Computer power/software and storage; post-data analysis and complex image processing; photo-switchable and photostable fluorescent probes

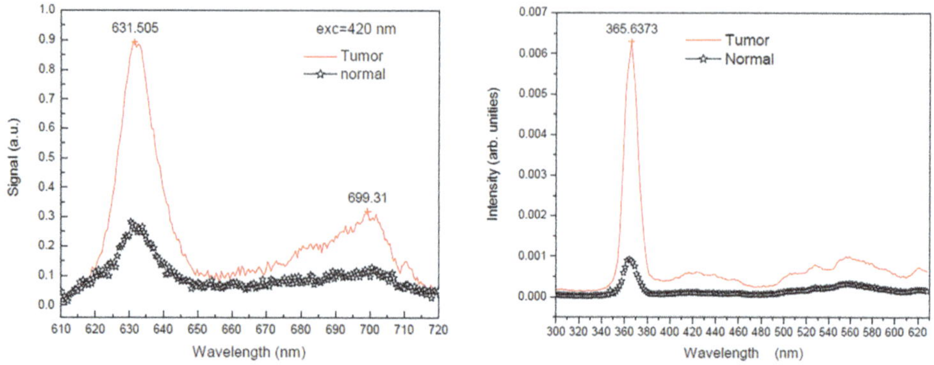

Figure 7.12. (A) Emission spectra of porphyrins of normal and tumor blood samples; (B) Excitation spectrum of blood porphyrin obtained fixing emission at 700 nm. Reprinted with permission from [207], copyright (2007) Society of Photo-Optical Instrumentation Engineers (SPIE).

emission at 700 nm, further emphasizing its potential for diagnostic applications [207]. Devanesan *et al* conducted a fluorescence spectroscopy analysis of RBC acetone extracts, urine samples, and blood plasma to differentiate between normal individuals and cancer patients. The results show an increase in porphyrin fluorescence intensity in RBC extracts, elevated FAD-related fluorescence in urine, and a decrease in NADH-associated fluorescence in blood plasma among cancer patients. These spectral variations indicate metabolic alterations linked to malignancy, suggesting that fluorescence spectroscopy can effectively detect biochemical changes associated with cancer progression. Their study demonstrates that this technique has a sensitivity of 75%, highlighting its potential as a non-invasive preliminary screening tool for early cancer detection.

Further enhancing the application of fluorescence in cancer diagnostics, Ushenko *et al* [209], Wang *et al* [210], and Ding *et al* [211] explored the enhancement and advanced application of the fluorescence for cancer diagnostics. Ushenko *et al* developed a laser polarization autofluorescence technique, demonstrating its ability to differentiate malignant from benign tissues, particularly in the cervix uteri and myocardium. Wang *et al* proposed an RBC-based multimodal probe that enabled precise NIR II fluorescence image-guided tumor resection and enhanced photodynamic therapy (PDT) through laser-triggered oxygen release. Ding *et al* identified specific autofluorescence patterns in blood plasma that correlated with cancerous conditions, suggesting that these patterns could serve as reliable biomarkers for non-invasive cancer detection. These ideas were further validated by Ricci *et al* [212], who confirmed the effectiveness of autofluorescence and polarization microscopy in distinguishing cancerous tissues, making it a promising non-invasive diagnostic tool with strong clinical potential.

7.8.2 Blood disorders and blood protein autofluorescence

The studies by Mauritz *et al* [213], Kirilova *et al* [214], and Saytashev *et al* [83] collectively contribute to the understanding of blood protein autofluorescence at blood disorders. Mauritz *et al* examined hemoglobin autofluorescence in conditions like anemia and thalassemia, finding significant variations that could serve as diagnostic markers. Kirilova *et al* investigated influence of ionizing radiation on fluorescence spectral characteristics of human blood plasma employing hydrophobic fluorescent probe ABM (benzanthrone derivative) and albumin autofluorescence. Figure 7.13 and table 7.4 compared the spectral characteristics in blood plasma from healthy donor and epilepsy patients exploring incidence of albumin pathologic alterations [214].

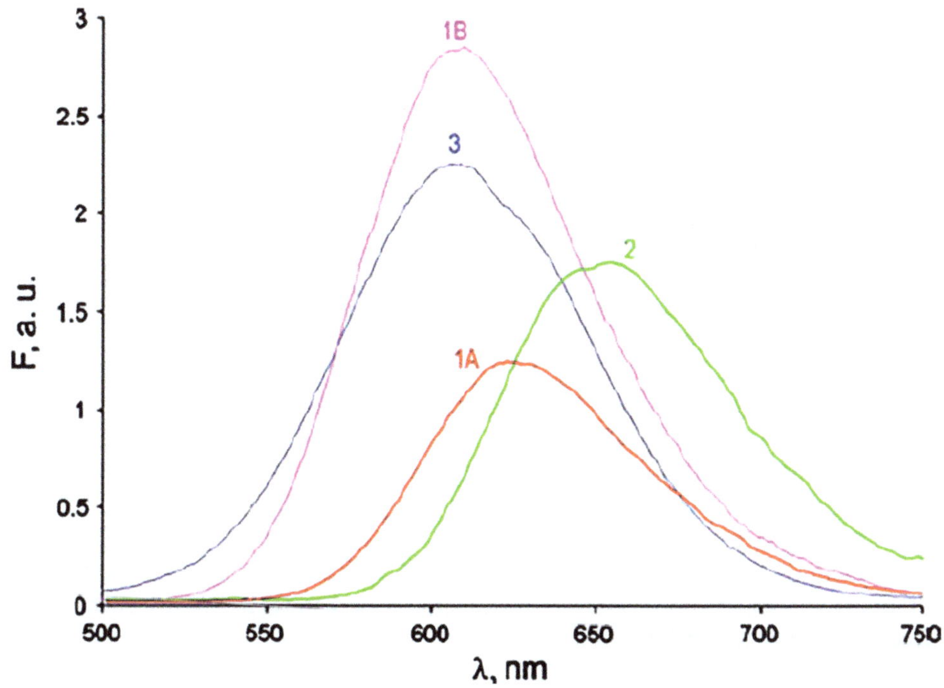

Figure 7.13. Spectral characteristics of ABM in human blood plasma: 1A-acidic expansion; 1B-N-F transition; 2-healthy donors, 3-patients with epilepsy. Reprinted with permission from [214], with permission from Springer Nature.

Table 7.4. Spectral characterization of albumin from Chernobyl clean-up workers' blood plasma. Reproduced from [214], with permission from Springer Nature.

	Probe ABM		Albumin autofluorescence	
Groups of patients	Emission max, nm	F, a.u.	Emission max, nm	F, a.u
1 A. (acidic expansion)	620–630	1.24 ± 0.07	311–318	2.15 ± 0.04
1B. (N-F transition)	600–620	2.85 ± 0.07	309–311	1.85 ± 0.06
2.Healthy	650	1.74 ± 0.06	330	2.48 ± 0.04
3.Epilepsy	604–614	2.25 ± 0.07	309–311	1.38 ± 0.07
Control	630	2.11 ± 0.06	330	2.96 ± 0.05

7.8.3 Porphyria

Veenashree *et al* [215] used autofluorescence in the case of congenital erythropoietic porphyria (CEP) to detect porphyrin accumulation in a patient with acute scleritis. By employing immunofluorescent microscopy and spectroscopic analysis, the study highlighted the potential of autofluorescence as a non-invasive diagnostic method, revealing significant ocular inflammation and porphyrin buildup [216]. Similarly, Enerbäck and Lundvall [217] demonstrated the effectiveness of fluorescence microscopy in diagnosing porphyria cutanea tarda (PCT) by observing porphyrin accumulation in liver biopsies.

7.8.4 Liver and cardiovascular diseases

Pan *et al* [218] and Yuwen *et al* [219] investigated the use of blood and serum autofluorescence as non-invasive markers for liver and cardiovascular diseases. Pan *et al* found that serum autofluorescence intensity increased with the severity of liver fibrosis, suggesting its potential as an alternative to invasive liver biopsies. Pan *et al* illustrated fluorescence emission variations under different oxygenation conditions, demonstrating the relevance of blood autofluorescence in assessing liver and metabolic function. Yuwen *et al* expanded this approach to cardiovascular diseases, identifying distinct fluorescence patterns in whole blood that could serve as diagnostic markers for cardiovascular health. Their study developed a quencher-based autofluorescence suppression strategy using inner filter effect (IFE) mechanisms, allowing for high-sensitivity quantification of trace analytes. They also highlighted the efficiency of this approach, particularly in detecting hydrogen sulfide (H_2S) levels in blood, which are crucial for cardiovascular disease assessment. Hennig *et al* [91] extended the application of autofluorescence to other chronic conditions, such as liver fibrosis and cardiovascular diseases. Hennig *et al* also validated a spectral fitting procedure that used to separate the ZnPP and PPIX fluorescence from the tissue and found shifts in fluorescence intensity between samples with and without these elements in the blood.

7.8.5 Malaria

Research by Rehan *et al* [156] and Wybranowski *et al* [5] focused on the application of fluorescence-based techniques in malaria diagnostics. In the realm of infectious diseases, Rehan *et al* explored the use of abnormal WBC differential fluorescence scattergrams for the early detection of malaria. By utilizing an automated hematology analyzer to detect changes in WBC fluorescence indicative of malarial parasites, the study achieved a sensitivity of 80% and specificity of 93.26%. This scattergram approach demonstrates considerable potential as a reliable diagnostic tool, particularly in resource-limited settings where rapid and accurate malaria diagnosis is crucial. Wybranowski *et al* focused on enhancing the diagnostic accuracy of malaria through improved autofluorescence imaging to amplify the weak autofluorescence signals from malaria-infected blood cells.

7.8.6 Diabetes

Al Salhi *et al* [24] explored the use of blood serum autofluorescence for monitoring diabetes revealing significant differences in fluorescence intensity between diabetic and non-diabetic samples.

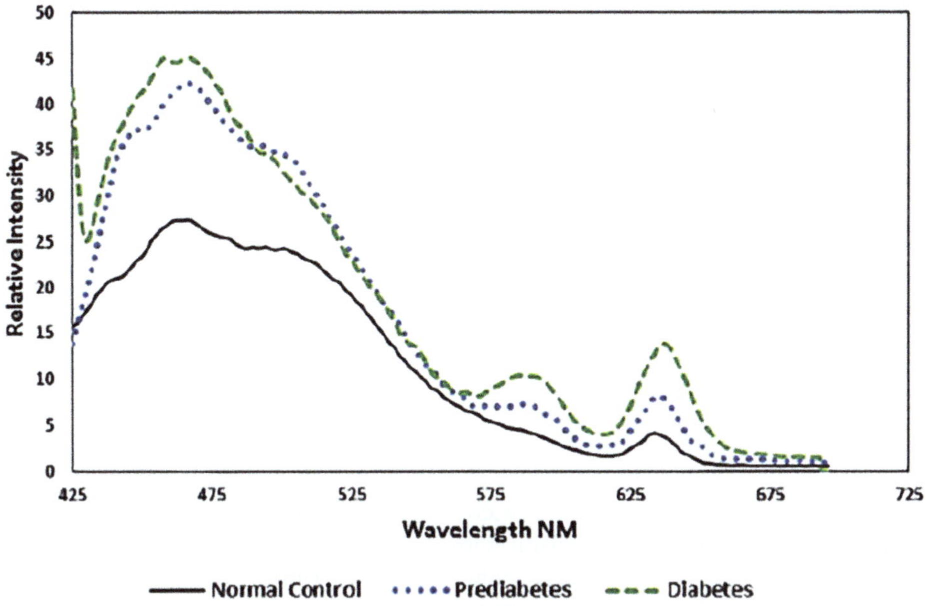

Figure 7.14. The fluorescence emission spectra of acetone extract of the RBCs of (a) normal control, (b) pre-diabetic subjects, and (c) diabetic patients. Reproduced from [24] CC BY 4.0.

Their study highlights the potential of fluorescence biomarkers as non-invasive alternatives to traditional glucose monitoring methods. Figure 7.14 shows a comparison of fluorescence emission spectra between normal, pre-diabetic, and diabetic samples, which demonstrates clear spectral shifts between these conditions.

These results were validated with synchronous emission spectra (SES) of the same example groups. These spectral variations suggest that changes in fluorescent biomolecule concentrations, such as NADH, FAD, and porphyrins, could be used as markers for diabetes progression. They also found that the R2 ratio (I525/I360), representing oxidative stress levels, was markedly increased in diabetic patients, indicating a correlation between diabetes progression and metabolic imbalances. Studies also explored the use of RBCs and lysed hemoglobin autofluorescence as potential biomarkers for diabetic complications. Additionally, significant variations in hemoglobin autofluorescence were observed despite relatively constant HbA1c levels, indicating that hemoglobin autofluorescence could serve as a more sensitive long-term glycemic marker for diabetic complications [220, 221].

7.8.7 Effects of COVID-19

Song *et al* [222] explored the potential disruption of the blood-brain barrier (BBB) in COVID-19 patients and its role in neurological symptoms, using hybridization chain reaction (HCR) RNA fluorescence *in situ* hybridization (RNA-FISH) to detect viral RNA and immunohistochemistry to assess fibrinogen leakage as a marker of BBB integrity. Their post-mortem neuropathological studies revealed that while no SARS-CoV-2 RNA was detected in brain tissues, significant BBB disruption was evident in all COVID-19 patients, with fibrinogen extravasation being more pronounced than in aging or neurodegenerative disease (NDD) cases. This suggests that neurological symptoms in COVID-19 are likely caused by systemic inflammation and vascular injury rather than direct viral invasion of the brain. Fortier *et al* [223] introduced neutrophil side fluorescence (NEU-SFL) as a predictive biomarker for COVID-19 mortality, demonstrating that increased neutrophil autofluorescence correlates with severe disease outcomes. The study utilized automated fluorescence signal measurement in hematology analyzers, enabling rapid and reliable patient stratification for cardiovascular complications related to severe infections.

In two related studies, published by Pretorius *et al* [224] and Kelly *et al* [225] investigated the presence of amyloid blood clots in COVID-19 patients and their role in coagulopathies. Using thioflavin T staining and fluorescence microscopy, the researchers detected significantly elevated levels of amyloid clots in plasma samples from COVID-19 patients, correlating with disease severity. The first study demonstrated that amyloid clots were prominent in COVID-19 patients and contributed to the coagulopathies often seen in severe cases. The findings suggest a therapeutic potential for anti-clotting agents to alleviate these symptoms, laying the groundwork for rapid phenotypic tests to assess disease severity. Their second study further examined amyloid clots in patients with both COVID-19 and Type 2 Diabetes Mellitus (T2DM), revealing a higher prevalence of amyloid structures in these patients compared to healthy controls. Their research highlighted the heightened risk T2DM patients face in developing amyloid clots, exacerbating COVID-19 complications. The findings underscore the need for tailored anti-clotting treatments for patients with dual risks, such as COVID-19 and diabetes, to better manage coagulopathies.

7.8.8 Blood lesion and x-ray dose

Saytashev *et al* [83] and Tungjai *et al* [226] focused on the application of advanced fluorescence imaging techniques for blood analysis. Saytashev *et al* used multi-photon excited hemoglobin fluorescence and THG microscopy to assess the health of stored blood (blood lesions) non-invasively. Tungjai *et al* investigated the effects of medical diagnostic x-rays on the fluorescence anisotropy of RBCs, concluding that standard x-ray doses do not significantly alter RBC membrane integrity.

7.9 External fluorescent dyes for IV clinical administration

The external fluorescent dyes have gained significant attention as versatile tools in clinical diagnostics, therapeutic monitoring, and surgical guidance. The use of intravenous (IV) administered fluorescent dyes, particularly in the field of near-infrared (NIR) fluorescence imaging [227], has revolutionized various aspects of modern medicine. Intravenously (IV) administered fluorescent dyes, particularly those operating in the NIR spectrum, have significantly advanced the field of medical imaging [228]. Their ability to provide high sensitivity, specificity, and real-time visualization has transformed how diseases are diagnosed, monitored, and treated.

NIR fluorescent dyes, such as indocyanine green (ICG) [229] and fluorescein sodium [230], are widely used due to their favorable optical properties, including deep tissue penetration and low background signal interference [231]. These properties make them highly valuable in a range of applications, from enhancing the precision of cancer surgeries through sentinel lymph node mapping and tumor margin detection to enabling non-invasive monitoring of disease progression in conditions like cardiovascular and liver disorders. For instance, ICG is extensively utilized in vascular imaging, hepatic function assessment, and fluorescence-guided oncological surgeries.

Recent advancements in external fluorescent dye technology include targeted fluorescent probes for molecular imaging and theranostic agents that combine diagnostic and therapeutic functions [232]. The use of fluorescent dyes has significantly enhanced molecular biology and genetic research, particularly in DNA detection and sequencing applications. Panchuk-Voloshina *et al* [233] revolutionized molecular biology by introducing SYBR Green I for enhanced DNA detection. Comparing to ethidium bromide, SYBR Green I exhibited 25 to 100 times greater sensitivity, making it invaluable for clinical diagnostics and genetic research.

The study also examined fluorescent Alexa dyes, demonstrating how their absorption and emission spectra shift slightly in conjugated forms while retaining strong fluorescence properties. The absorption and emission properties for Alexa dyes are presented in figure 7.15.

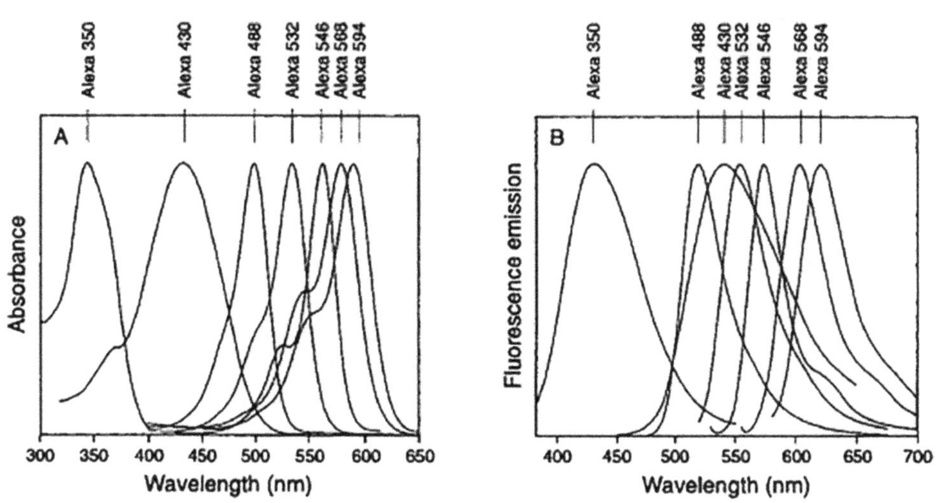

Figure 7.15. Normalized absorption, (A) and emission (B) spectra of the Alexa dyes conjugated to GAM. Except for few-nm shift of the excitation/emission maxima towards the red region of the spectrum, the profile of the conjugates' spectra closely resembles that of the free Alexa dyes. Reprinted with permission from [233], copyright 1999, Sage Publications.

7.10 Summary

This chapter has provided a comprehensive exploration of the fluorescence characteristics of blood, emphasizing both the intrinsic and extrinsic contributors to its optical signatures. From the fundamental photophysical behavior of hemoglobin and its derivatives to the impact of glycation, the discussion has highlighted the fluorescent signals embedded within blood's complex composition.

Advanced imaging strategies, including wavelength-resolved techniques, were outlined as crucial tools for extracting meaningful diagnostic information from weak endogenous fluorescence. In particular, the emerging applications of fluorescence in vascular diagnostics and metabolic monitoring assessment underscore the growing translational potential of this approach.

As fluorescence spectroscopy continues to evolve—with improved instrumentation sensitivity, spectral resolution, and data analysis methods—it is increasingly capable of revealing pathophysiological states through minimally invasive means.

References

[1] Richards-Kortum R and Sevick-Muraca E 1996 Quantitative optical spectroscopy for tissue diagnosis *Annu. Rev. Phys. Chem.* **47** 555–606

[2] Delori F C, Dorey C K, Staurenghi G, Arend O, Goger D G and Weiter J J 1995 *In vivo* fluorescence of the ocular fundus exhibits retinal pigment epithelium lipofuscin characteristics *Invest. Ophthalmol. Vis. Sci.* **36** 718–29

[3] Croce A C and Bottiroli G 2014 Autofluorescence spectroscopy and imaging: a tool for biomedical research and diagnosis *Eur. J. Histochem.* **58** 2461

[4] Shrirao A B, Schloss R S, Fritz Z, Shrirao M V, Rosen R and Yarmush M L 2021 Autofluorescence of blood and its application in biomedical and clinical research *Biotechnol. Bioeng.* **118** 4550–76

[5] Wybranowski T, Ziomkowska B, Cyrankiewicz M, Pyskir J, Bosek M, Napiórkowska M, Pilaczyńska-Cemel M, Przybylski G and Kruszewski S 2023 Time-resolved fluorescence spectroscopy of blood, plasma and albumin as a potential diagnostic tool for acute inflammation in COVID-19 pneumonia patients *Int. J. Mol. Sci.* **24** 14703

[6] Shirshin E A, Cherkasova O P, Tikhonova T, Berlovskaya E, Priezzhev A V and Fadeev V 2015 Native fluorescence spectroscopy of blood plasma of rats with experimental diabetes: Identifying fingerprints of glucose-related metabolic pathways *J. Biomed. Opt.* **20** 1–6

[7] Reichert D *et al* 2023 Flavin fluorescence lifetime and autofluorescence optical redox ratio for improved visualization and classification of brain tumors *Front. Oncol.* **13** 1105648

[8] Devanesan S, AlShebly M, Kalaivani R, Sivaji K, Farhat K, AlSalhi M S, AlAtawi M, Rabah D and Masilamani V 2017 Fluorescence spectral features of blood components of pregnant women *Curr. Sci.* **113** 457–61

[9] Li B, Zhang Z, Xie S and Chen R 2006 Three-dimensional fluorescence spectra of human blood *Proc. SPIE 6026, ICO20: Biomedical Optics* p 60261F

[10] de Oliveira Silva F R, Bellini M H, Tristao V R, Schor N, Vieira N D Jr. and Courrol L C 2010 Intrinsic fluorescence of protoporphyrin IX from blood samples can yield information on the growth of prostate tumours *J. Fluoresc.* **20** 1159–65

[11] Datta R, Heaster T M, Sharick J T, Gillette A A and Skala M C 2020 Fluorescence lifetime imaging microscopy: fundamentals and advances in instrumentation, analysis, and applications *J. Biomed. Opt.* **25** 1–43

[12] Lowndes S 2010 Blood interference in fluorescence spectrum: Experiment, analysis and comparison with intraoperative measurements on brain tumor *BSc Thesis* Linköping University p42

[13] Wolfbeis O S and Leiner M 1985 Mapping of the total fluorescence of human blood serum as a new method for its characterization *Anal. Chim. Acta* **167** 203–15

[14] AlSalhi M, Mehmadi A M A, Abdo A A, Prasad S and Masilamani V 2012 Diagnosis of liver cancer and cirrhosis by the fluorescence spectra of blood and urine *Technol. Cancer Res. Treat.* **11** 345–51

[15] Lawaetz A J, Bro R, Kamstrup-Nielsen M, Christensen I J, Jørgensen L N and Nielsen H J 2012 Fluorescence spectroscopy as a potential metabonomic tool for early detection of colorectal cancer *Metabolomics* **8** 111–21

[16] Wang Y, Zhu J and Chen X 2020 Autofluorescence spectroscopy of blood plasma with multivariate analysis methods for the diagnosis of pulmonary tuberculosis *Optik* **224** 165446

[17] Masilamani V, Al-Zhrani K, Al-Salhi M, Al-Diab A and Al-Ageily M 2004 Cancer diagnosis by autofluorescence of blood components *J. Lumin.* **109** 143–54

[18] Zalesskaya G A and Maslova T O 2010 Fluorescence spectra of blood plasma treated with ultraviolet irradiation *in vivo J. Appl. Spectrosc.* **77** 574–81

[19] Li X, Wang R and Lei M 2011 Analysis on data for detection of lung cancer using serum auto-fluorescence *2011 IEEE Int. Symp. on IT in Medicine and Education* vol 1 (Piscataway, NJ: IEEE) pp 554–6

[20] Monici M, Pratesi R, Bernabei P A, Caporale R, Ferrini P R, Croce A C, Balzarini P and Bottiroli G 1995 Natural fluorescence of white blood cells: spectroscopic and imaging study *J. Photochem. Photobiol.,* B **30** 29–37

[21] Weber A, Wójtowicz A and Lednev I K 2021 Post deposition aging of bloodstains probed by steady-state fluorescence spectroscopy *J. Photochem. Photobiol.,* B **221** 112251

[22] Mayeno A N, Hamann K J and Gleich G J 1992 Granule-associated flavin adenine dinucleotide (FAD) is responsible for eosinophil autofluorescence *J. Leukoc. Biol.* **51** 172–5

[23] Lan X, Gao S, Peng C, Liu Y and Ni X W 2003 Fluorometric determination of whole blood with various excitation wavelengths *Third Int. Conf. on Photonics and Imaging in Biology and Medicine* vol 5254 (SPIE) pp 336–41

[24] Al Salhi M S, Devanesan S, Al Zahrani K E, AlShebly M, Al-Qahtani F, Farhat K and Masilamani V 2018 Impact of diabetes mellitus on human erythrocytes: atomic force microscopy and spectral investigations *Int. J. Environ. Res. Public Health* **15** 2368

[25] Hawkins E P, Hawkins H K and Armstrong D 1986 Lymphocyte autofluorescence: a screening procedure for neurodegenerative diseases *Pediatr. Neurol.* **2** 160–6

[26] Masilamani V, Trinka V, Salhi M A, Elangovan M, Raghavan V, Diab A R A, Hajjar W, Ainia M, Al-Mustafa A and Al-Nachawati H 2011 A new lung cancer biomarker—a preliminary report *Photomed. Laser Surg.* **29** 161–70

[27] Scheer M, Fuss J, Derman M A, Kreppel M, Neugebauer J, Rothamel D, Drebber U and Zoeller J E 2016 Autofluorescence imaging in recurrent oral squamous cell carcinoma *Oral Maxillofac. Surg.* **20** 27–33

[28] Kiss N *et al* 2018 *Ex vivo* nonlinear microscopy imaging of Ehlers–Danlos syndrome-affected skin *Arch. Dermatol. Res.* **310** 463–73

[29] Amaral A U, Cecatto C, da Silva J C, Wajner A, dos Santos Godoy K, Ribeiro R T and Wajner M 2016 cis-4-decenoic and decanoic acids impair mitochondrial energy, redox and Ca2 + homeostasis and induce mitochondrial permeability transition pore opening in rat brain and liver: possible implications for the pathogenesis of MCAD deficiency *Biochim. Biophys. Acta (BBA)—Bioenerg.* **1857** 1363–72
[30] Yung M, Klufas M A and Sarraf D 2016 Clinical applications of fundus autofluorescence in retinal disease *Int. J. Retina Vit.* **2** 1–25
[31] Coppinger J A, Cagney G, Toomey S, Kislinger T, Belton O, McRedmond J P, Cahill D J, Emili A, Fitzgerald D J and Maguire P B 2004 Characterization of the proteins released from activated platelets leads to localization of novel platelet proteins in human atherosclerotic lesions *Blood* **103** 2096–104
[32] Krul-Poel Y H M, Agca R, Lips P, van Wijland H, Stam F and Simsek S 2015 Vitamin D status is associated with skin autofluorescence in patients with type 2 diabetes mellitus: a preliminary report *Cardiovasc. Diabetol.* **14** 1–7
[33] Yavuz D G and Apaydin T 2022 Skin autofluorescence is associated with low bone mineral density in type 2 diabetic patients *J. Clin. Densitom.* **25** 373–9
[34] Liu H, Wang G, Wu T, Hu J, Mu Y and Gu W 2022 Association of skin autofluorescence with low bone density/osteoporosis and osteoporotic fractures in type 2 diabetes mellitus *J. Diabetes* **14** 571–85
[35] Benjilali L, Tazi-Mezalek Z, Harmouche H, Lebbar K, Aouni M, Adnaoui M and Maaouni A 2007 Pernicious anemia in a young man with systemic lupus erythematosus *Lupus* **16** 827–9
[36] Han X, Lui H, McLean D I and Zeng H 2009 Near-infrared autofluorescence imaging of cutaneous melanins and human skin *in vivo J. Biomed. Opt.* **14** 024017
[37] Cebecauerova D, Jirasek T, Budisova L, Mandys V, Volf V, Novotna Z, Subhanova I, Hrebicek M, Elleder M and Jirsa M 2005 Dual hereditary jaundice: simultaneous occurrence of mutations causing Gilbert's and Dubin-Johnson syndrome *Gastroenterology* **129** 315–20
[38] Wetlaufer D B 1963 Ultraviolet spectra of proteins and amino acids *Adv. Protein Chem.* **17** 303–90
[39] Albani J R 2004 Fluorophores: descriptions and properties *Structure and Dynamics of Macromolecules: Absorption and Fluorescence Studies* ed J R Albani (Elsevier Science) ch 3 pp 99–140
[40] Wagnieres G A, Star W M and Wilson B C 1998 *In vivo* fluorescence spectroscopy and imaging for oncological applications *Photochem. Photobiol.* **68** 603–32
[41] Islam M S, Honma M, Nakabayashi T, Kinjo M and Ohta N 2013 pH dependence of the fluorescence lifetime of FAD in solution and in cells *Int. J. Mol. Sci.* **14** 1952–63
[42] Bess S N, Igoe M J, Denison A C *et al* 2023 Autofluorescence imaging of endogenous metabolic cofactors in response to cytokine stimulation of classically activated macrophages *Cancer Metab* **11** 22
[43] Atkins C G, Buckley K, Blades M W and Turner R F 2017 Raman spectroscopy of blood and blood components *Appl. Spectrosc.* **71** 767–93
[44] Kamińska A, Kowalska A, Albrycht P, Witkowska E and Waluk J 2016 ABO blood groups' antigen–antibody interactions studied using SERS spectroscopy: towards blood typing *Anal. Methods* **8** 1463–72
[45] Peng C and Liu J 2013 Studies on red-shift rules in fluorescence spectra of human blood induced by LED *Appl. Phy. Res* **5** 1–6

[46] Schmitz R L *et al* 2023 Autofluorescence lifetime imaging classifies human lymphocyte activation and subtype *bioRxiv*
[47] Gao S, Peng C and Liu Y 2005 Study on ultraviolet-light-excited blood fluorescence spectra characteristics *Optics in Health Care and Biomedical Optics: Diagnostics and Treatment II* **vol 5630** (SPIE) pp 553–7
[48] McLaughlin G, Doty K C and Lednev I K 2014 Raman spectroscopy of blood for species identification *Anal. Chem.* **86** 11628–33
[49] Seyedi S S, Parvin P, Jafargholi A, Hashemi N, Tabatabaee S M, Abbasian A and Khorrami A 2020 Spectroscopic properties of various blood antigens/antibodies *Biomed. Opt. Express* **11** 2298–312
[50] Lemler P, Premasiri W R, DelMonaco A and Ziegler L D 2014 NIR Raman spectra of whole human blood: effects of laser-induced and *in vitro* hemoglobin denaturation *Anal. Bioanal. Chem.* **406** 193–200
[51] Weber A and Lednev I K 2022 Brightness of blood: review of fluorescence spectroscopy analysis of bloodstains *Front. Anal. Sci.* **2** 906532
[52] Gan J, Zhou L, Cui J, Man B, Jia X, Shi S and Liu L 2019 Classification of blood species using fluorescence spectroscopy combined with deep learning method *J. Appl. Math. Phys.* **7** 2324
[53] Lakowicz J R (ed) 2006 *Principles of Fluorescence Spectroscopy* (Boston, MA: Springer US)
[54] Schaller J, Gerber S, Kaempfer U, Lejon S and Trachsel C 2008 *Human Blood Plasma Proteins: Structure and Function* (New York: Wiley)
[55] Issaq H J, Xiao Z and Veenstra T D 2007 Serum and plasma proteomics *Chem. Rev.* **107** 3601–20
[56] Xu X, Meng J, Hou S, Ma H and Wang D 1988 The characteristic fluorescence of the serum of cancer patients *J. Lumin.* **40** 219–20
[57] Scully P, O'Kennedy R and Groarke A 2001 Autofluorescence of human blood plasma: effect of assay format *J. Immunol. Methods* **248** 31–43
[58] Chance B and Thorell L 1970 *Fluorescence Measurements of NADH as an Indicator of Tissue Oxygenation* (Berlin: Springer)
[59] Plavskii V Y, Sobchuk A N, Mikulich A V, Dudinova O N, Plavskaya L G, Tretyakova A I and Leusenka I A 2024 Identification by methods of steady-state and kinetic spectrofluorimetry of endogenous porphyrins and flavins sensitizing the formation of reactive oxygen species in cancer cells *Photochem. Photobiol.* **100** 1310–27
[60] Madhuri S, Vengadesan N, Aruna P, Koteeswaran D, Venkatesan P and Ganesan S 2003 Native fluorescence spectroscopy of blood plasma in the characterization of oral malignancy *Photochem. Photobiol.* **78** 197–204
[61] Tomečková V *et al* 2018 Analysis of bowel diseases from blood serum by autofluorescence and atomic force microscopy techniques: autofluorescence & atomic force microscopy in bowel disease diagnosis *Open Chem.* **16** 238–45
[62] Zhan Y-T, Li L, Weng J, Song X, Yang S-Q and An W 2012 Serum autofluorescence, a potential serum marker for the diagnosis of liver fibrosis in rats *Int. J. Mol. Sci.* **13** 12130–9
[63] Bakun O V, Voloshynovych N S, Dudka Y A, Lisnianska N V, Kolesnik O V, Slobodian K V and Pradatu A 2022 The informativeness of the Johns-matrix image of laser autofluorescence in blood plasma films for early diagnosis of endometriosis associated with infertility *J. Med. Life* **15** 1511

[64] Lin J, Chen R, Feng S, Pan J, Li Y, Chen G, Cheng M, Huang Z, Yu Y and Zeng H 2011 A novel blood plasma analysis technique combining membrane electrophoresis with silver nanoparticle-based SERS spectroscopy for potential applications in noninvasive cancer detection *Nanomed. Nanotechnol. Biol. Med.* **7** 655–63
[65] Croce A C, Bottiroli G, Di Pasqua L G, Berardo C, Siciliano V, Rizzo V, Vairetti M and Ferrigno A 2018 Serum and hepatic autofluorescence as a real-time diagnostic tool for early cholestasis assessment *Int. J. Mol. Sci.* **19** 2634
[66] Croce A C, Ferrigno A, Palladini G, Mannucci B, Vairetti M and Di Pasqua L G 2023 Fatty acids and bilirubin as intrinsic autofluorescence serum biomarkers of drug action in a rat model of liver ischemia and reperfusion *Molecules* **28** 3818
[67] Yue F, Li S, Wu L, Chen X and Zhu J 2024 Rapid diagnosis of latent and active pulmonary tuberculosis by autofluorescence spectroscopy of blood plasma combined with artificial neural network algorithm *Photodiagn. Photodyn. Ther.* **50** 104426
[68] Bonifacio A, Dalla Marta S, Spizzo R, Cervo S, Steffan A, Colombatti A and Sergo V 2014 Surface-enhanced Raman spectroscopy of blood plasma and serum using Ag and Au nanoparticles: a systematic study *Anal. Bioanal. Chem.* **406** 2355–65
[69] Feng S, Chen R, Lin J, Pan J, Chen G, Li Y, Cheng M, Huang Z, Chen J and Zeng H 2010 Nasopharyngeal cancer detection based on blood plasma surface-enhanced Raman spectroscopy and multivariate analysis *Biosens. Bioelectron.* **25** 2414–9
[70] Roussel C, Bellamy V, Bertil G and Thiennot P 2010 Hemoglobin autofluorescence as a diagnostic tool for anemia *Clin. Hematol. Int.* **4** 127–33
Mauritz J M, Simmons J and Kovacs M 2018 Hemoglobin autofluorescence in blood disorders *Hematology* **15** 37–42
[71] Kirilova G, Chaldakov G and Simeonova S 2011 Autofluorescence characteristics of hemoglobin derivatives in disease diagnosis *J. Clin. Pathol.* **64** 587–93
[72] AlSalhi M S, Masilamani V, Al Obaid S A and Atif M 2018 Autofluorescence as a diagnostic tool for metabolic disorders *Spectrochim. Acta, Part* A **189** 119–25
[73] Means R T, Arber D A, Glader B E, Appelbaum F R *et al* 2023 *Wintrobe's Clinical Hematology* 15th edn (Lippincott Williams & Wilkins (LWW))
[74] Boscencu R, Radulea N, Manda G, Machado I F, Socoteanu R P, Lupuliasa D, Burloiu A M, Mihai D P and Ferreira L F V 2023 Porphyrin macrocycles: general properties and theranostic potential *Molecules* **28** 1149
[75] Hegyi J, Hegyi V, Ruzicka T, Arenberger P and Berking C 2011 New developments in fluorescence diagnostics *JDDG: J. Dtsch. Dermatol. Ges.* **9** 368–72
[76] Min W, Lu S, Chong S, Roy R, Holtom G R and Xie X S 2009 Imaging chromophores with undetectable fluorescence by stimulated emission microscopy *Nature* **461** 1105–9
[77] Anand B S and Sujatha N 2012 Fluorescence quenching effects of hemoglobin on simulated tissue phantoms in the UV–Vis range *Meas. Sci. Technol.* **23** 025502
[78] Morris R J and Gibson Q H 1984 The apparent quantum yield of T-state human hemoglobin. Contribution of protein and heme to rates of oxygen reactions *J. Biol. Chem.* **259** 365–71
[79] Vigneshwaran N, Bijukumar G, Karmakar N, Anand S and Misra A 2005 Autofluorescence characterization of advanced glycation end products of hemoglobin *Spectrochim. Acta, Part* A **61** 163–70
[80] Guo H W, Tseng T Y, Lin C J and Dong C Y 2021 Hemoglobin autofluorescence as potential long-term glycemic marker in the rat animal model *J. Biophotonics* **14** e202000389

[81] Stirban A and Heinemann L 2014 Skin autofluorescence–a non-invasive measurement for assessing cardiovascular risk and risk of diabetes *Eur. Endocrinol.* **10** 106

[82] Vigneshwaran N, Bijukumar G, Karmakar N, Anand S and Misra A 2003 Fluorescence and biochemical characterization of glycated hemoglobin *Macromolecular Symposia* **vol 193** (Weinheim: Wiley-VCH) pp 119–28

[83] Saytashev I, Glenn R, Murashova G A, Osseiran S, Spence D, Evans C L and Dantus M 2016 Multiphoton excited hemoglobin fluorescence and third harmonic generation for non-invasive microscopy of stored blood *Biomed. Opt. Express* **7** 3449–60

[84] Sun Q, Zheng W, Wang J, Luo Y and Qu J Y 2015 Mechanism of two-photon excited hemoglobin fluorescence emission *J. Biomed. Opt.* **20** 105014–4

[85] Petrich J W, Poyart C and Martin J L 1988 Photophysics and reactivity of heme proteins: a femtosecond absorption study of hemoglobin, myoglobin, and protoheme *Biochemistry* **27** 4049–60

[86] Clay G O, Schaffer C B and Kleinfeld D 2007 Large two-photon absorptivity of hemoglobin in the infrared range of 780–880nm *J. Chem. Phys.* **126**

[87] Dong P T, Lin H, Huang K C and Cheng J X 2019 Label-free quantitation of glycated hemoglobin in single red blood cells by transient absorption microscopy and phasor analysis *Sci. Adv.* **5** eaav0561

[88] Li D, Zheng W, Zeng Y, Luo Y and Qu J Y 2011 Two-photon excited hemoglobin fluorescence provides contrast mechanism for label-free imaging of microvasculature *in vivo Opt. Lett.* **36** 834–6

[89] Gryczynski Z, Beretta S, Lubkowski J, Razynska A, Gryczynski I and Bucci E 1997 Time-resolved fluorescence of hemoglobin species *Biophys. Chem.* **64** 81–91

[90] Asghari-Khiavi M, Mechler A, Bambery K R, McNaughton D and Wood B R 2009 A resonance Raman spectroscopic investigation into the effects of fixation and dehydration on heme environment of hemoglobin *Raman Spectrosc.* **40** 1668–74

[91] Hennig G, Gruber C, Vogeser M, Stepp H, Dittmar S, Sroka R and Brittenham G M 2014 Dual-wavelength excitation for fluorescence-based quantification of zinc protoporphyrin IX and protoporphyrin IX in whole blood *J. Biophotonics* **7** 514–24

[92] Hirsch R E, Zukin R S and Nagel R L 1980 Intrinsic fluorescence emission of intact oxy hemoglobins *Biochem. Biophys. Res. Commun.* **93** 432–9

[93] Lazareva E, Zyubin A, Dikht N, Bucharskaya A, Samusev I, Slezhkin V, Kochubey V I and Tuchin V 2022 Optical properties of glycated and non-glycated hemoglobin–Raman/fluorescence spectroscopy and refractometry *J. Biomed. Photon. Eng.* **8** 020303–9

[94] Gryczynski Z, Lubkowski J and Bucci E 1997 Intrinsic fluorescence of hemoglobins and myoglobins *Methods Enzymol.* **278** 538–69

[95] Rousseau D L and Ondrias M R 1983 Resonance Raman scattering studies of the quaternary structure transition in hemoglobin *Annu. Rev. Biophys. Bioeng.* **12** 357–80

[96] Rusciano G, De Luca A C, Pesce G and Sasso A 2008 Raman tweezers as a diagnostic tool of hemoglobin-related blood disorders *Sensors* **8** 7818–32

[97] Chakraborty S, Chaudhuri S, Pahari B, Taylor J, Sengupta P K and Sengupta B 2012 A critical study on the interactions of hesperitin with human hemoglobin: Fluorescence spectroscopic and molecular modeling approach *J. Lumin.* **132** 1522–8

[98] Hirsch R E and Nagel R L 1981 Conformational studies of hemoglobins using intrinsic fluorescence measurements *J. Biol. Chem.* **256** 1080–3

[99] Nagababu E and Rifkind J M 1998 Formation of fluorescent heme degradation products during the oxidation of hemoglobin by hydrogen peroxide *Biochem. Biophys. Res. Commun.* **247** 592–6
[100] Sebban P, Coppey M, Alpert B, Lindqvist L and Jameson D M 1980 Fluorescence properties of porphyrin-globin from human hemoglobin *Photochem. Photobiol.* **32** 727–31
[101] Chen Q and Hirsch R E 2006 A direct and simultaneous detection of zinc protoporphyrin IX, free protoporphyrin IX, and fluorescent heme degradation product in red blood cell hemolysates *Free Radic. Res.* **40** 285–94
[102] Alpert B, Jameson D M and Weber G 1980 Tryptophan emission from human hemoglobin and its isolated subunits *Photochem. Photobiol.* **31** 1–4
[103] Nagababu E, Chrest F J and Rifkind J M 2000 The origin of red cell fluorescence caused by hydrogen peroxide treatment *Free Radical Biol. Med.* **29** 659–63
[104] Pundir C S and Chawla S 2014 Determination of glycated hemoglobin with special emphasis on biosensing methods *Anal. Biochem.* **444** 47–56
[105] Barman I, Dingari N C, Kang J W, Horowitz G L, Dasari R R and Feld M S 2012 Raman spectroscopy-based sensitive and specific detection of glycated hemoglobin *Anal. Chem.* **84** 2474–82
[106] Ioannou A and Varotsis C 2019 Probing hemoglobin glyco-products by fluorescence spectroscopy *RSC Adv.* **9** 37614–9
[107] Sydor A M *et al* 2021 Autofluorescence properties of red blood cells under varying physiological conditions *J. Fluoresce.* **31** 243–50
[108] Bouffard N A, Lee K, DeLance N M, Clason T, Chatterjee N and Taatjes D J 2023 Novel post-acquisition image processing to attenuate red blood cell autofluorescence for quantitative image analysis *Histochem. Cell Biol.* **159** 119–25
[109] Wesełucha-Birczyńska A *et al* 2014 Human erythrocytes analyzed by generalized 2D Raman correlation spectroscopy *J. Mol. Struct.* **1069** 305–12
[110] Hamly D H, Hummer G J and Sheard C 1947 Fluorescence of red blood cells *Science* **106** 169–70
[111] Wood B R, Stoddart P R and McNaughton D 2011 Molecular imaging of red blood cells by raman spectroscopy *Aust. J. Chem.* **64** 593–9
[112] Shirshin E A, Yakimov B P, Rodionov S A, Omelyanenko N P, Priezzhev A V, Fadeev V V and Darvin M E 2018 Formation of hemoglobin photoproduct is responsible for two-photon and single photon-excited fluorescence of red blood cells *Laser Phys. Lett.* **15** 075604
[113] Hertz L *et al* 2019 The evolution of erythrocytes becoming red in respect to fluorescence *Front. Physiol.* **10** 753
[114] Dasgupta R, Ahlawat S, Verma R S, Uppal A and Gupta P K 2010 Hemoglobin degradation in human erythrocytes with long-duration near-infrared laser exposure in Raman optical tweezers *J. Biomed. Opt.* **15** 055009
[115] Tougan T *et al* 2020 Diagnostic potential of hemoglobin autofluorescence: Applications in detecting abnormal hemoglobin derivatives *J. Biomed. Opt.* **25** 095003
[116] Taylor-Williams M, Spicer G, Bale G and Bohndiek S E 2022 Noninvasive hemoglobin sensing and imaging: optical tools for disease diagnosis *J. Biomed. Opt.* **27** 080901
[117] Wood B R *et al* 2011 Raman spectroscopy for molecular imaging of red blood cells: Implications for malaria diagnostics *J. Raman Spectrosc.* **42** 524–30

[118] Adak S, Chowdhury S and Bhattacharyya M 2008 Dynamic and electrokinetic behavior of erythrocyte membrane in diabetes mellitus and diabetic cardiovascular disease *Biochim. Biophys. Acta (BBA)—Gen. Subj.* **1780** 108–15
[119] Bankapur A, Zachariah E, Chidangil S, Valiathan M and Mathur D 2010 Raman tweezers spectroscopy of live, single red and white blood cells *PLoS One* **5** e10427
[120] Bukara K, Jovanić S, Drvenica I T, Stančić A, Ilić V, Rabasović M D, Pantelić D, Jelenković B, Bugarski B and Krmpot A J 2017 Mapping of hemoglobin in erythrocytes and erythrocyte ghosts using two photon excitation fluorescence microscopy *J. Biomed. Opt.* **22** 026003
[121] Amor R, Mahajan S, Amos W B and McConnell G 2014 Standing-wave-excited multi-planar fluorescence in a laser scanning microscope reveals 3D information on red blood cells *Sci. Rep.* **4** 7359
[122] Bloom S M and Spaide R F 2022 Autofluorescence and yellowing subhyaloid blood with proliferative diabetic retinopathy *Retinal Cases Brief Rep.* **16** 401–2
[123] Lin J, Zeng Y, Lin J, Wang J, Li L, Huang Z, Li B, Zeng H and Chen R 2014 Erythrocyte membrane analysis for type II diabetes detection using Raman spectroscopy in high-wavenumber region *Appl. Phys. Lett.* **104**
[124] Sydor M J, Anderson D S, Steele H B, Ross J A and Holian A 2021 Fluorescence lifetime imaging microscopy and time-resolved anisotropy of nanomaterial-induced changes to red blood cell membranes *Methods. Appl. Fluoresc.* **9** 035002
[125] Zhurova M, Olivieri A, Holt A and Acker J P 2014 A method to measure permeability of red blood cell membrane to water and solutes using intrinsic fluorescence *Clin. Chim. Acta* **431** 103–10
[126] Hennig G *et al* 2016 Non-invasive detection of iron deficiency by fluorescence measurement of erythrocyte zinc protoporphyrin in the lip *Nat. Commun.* **7** 1–8
[127] Tougan T, Itagaki S, Toya Y, Uchihashi K and Horii T 2020 Implementation of a red blood cell-optical (RBO) channel for detection of latent iron deficiency anaemia by automated measurement of autofluorescence-emitting red blood cells *Sci. Rep.* **10** 15605
[128] Khodabux C M, van Beckhoven J M, Scharenberg J G, El Barjiji F, Slot M C and Brand A 2011 Processing cord blood from premature infants into autologous red-blood-cell products for transfusion *Vox Sang.* **100** 367–73
[129] Brandao M M, Fontes A, Barjas-Castro M L, Barbosa L C, Costa F F, Cesar C L and Saad S T O 2003 Optical tweezers for measuring red blood cell elasticity: application to the study of drug response in sickle cell disease *Eur. J. Haematol.* **70** 207–11
[130] Henon S, Lenormand G, Richert A and Gallet F 1999 A new determination of the shear modulus of the human erythrocyte membrane using optical tweezers *Biophys. J.* **76** 1145–51
[131] Bambardekar K, Dharmadhikari A K, Dharmadhikari J A, Mathur D and Sharma S 2008 Measuring erythrocyte deformability with fluorescence, fluid forces, and optical trapping *J. Biomed. Opt.* **13** 064021
[132] Bransky A, Korin N, Nemirovski Y and Dinnar U 2006 An automated cell analysis sensing system based on a microfabricated rheoscope for the study of red blood cells physiology *Biosens. Bioelectron.* **22** 165–9
[133] Gifford S C, Derganc J, Shevkoplyas S S, Yoshida T and Bitensky M W 2006 A detailed study of time-dependent changes in human red blood cells: from reticulocyte maturation to erythrocyte senescence *Br. J. Haematol.* **135** 395–404

[134] Wood B R and McNaughton D 2007 Resonance Raman spectroscopy of red blood cells: Autofluorescence and hemoglobin oxidation states *J. Raman Spectrosc.* **38** 1345–53

[135] Semenov A N *et al* 2020 The oxidation-induced autofluorescence hypothesis: red edge excitation and implications for metabolic imaging *Molecules* **25** 1863

[136] Wood B R and McNaughton D 2002 Raman excitation wavelength investigation of single red blood cells *in vivo J. Raman Spectrosc.* **33** 517–23

[137] Parshina E Y, Sarycheva A S, Yusipovich A I, Brazhe N A, Goodilin E A and Maksimov G V 2013 Combined Raman and atomic force microscopy study of hemoglobin distribution inside erythrocytes and nanoparticle localization on the erythrocyte surface *Laser Phys. Lett.* **10** 075607

[138] Wang J *et al* 2013 Morphologically homogeneous red blood cells present a heterogeneous response to hormonal stimulation *PLoS One* **8** e67697

[139] Wood B R, Caspers P, Puppels G J, Pandiancherri S and McNaughton D 2007 Resonance Raman spectroscopy of red blood cells using near-infrared laser excitation *Anal. Bioanal. Chem.* **387** 1691–703

[140] Minors D S 2004 Physiology of red and white blood cells *Anaesth. Intensive Care Med.* **5** 174–8

[141] Fu H, Li J, Zhang C, Du P, Gao G, Ge Q, Guan X and Cui D 2024 Aβ-Aggregation-generated blue autofluorescence illuminates senile plaques as well as complex blood and vascular pathologies in Alzheimer's disease *Neurosci. Bull.* **40** 1115–26

[142] Li C, Pastila R K, Pitsillides C, Runnels J M, Puoris' haag M, Côté D and Lin C P 2010 Imaging leukocyte trafficking *in vivo* with two-photon-excited endogenous tryptophan fluorescence *Opt. Express* **18** 988–99

[143] Buchwalow I B *et al* 2017 NADH and FAD autofluorescence in immune cells *Immunol. Lett.* **190** 79–86

[144] Yakimov A *et al* 2019 Autofluorescence properties of neutrophils and monocytes under oxidative stress and immune activation *Cell Biochem. Biophys.* **77** 213–21

[145] Zeming K K, Lu R, Woo K L, Sun G, Quek K Y, Cheow L F, Chen C H, Han J and Lim S L 2021 Multiplexed single-cell leukocyte enzymatic secretion profiling from whole blood reveals patient-specific immune signature *Anal. Chem.* **93** 4374–82

[146] Hoeger P H *et al* 2004 Granulocyte autofluorescence under oxidative stress *Clin. Immunol.* **110** 362–9

[147] Zhang X, Zink F, Hezel F *et al* 2020 Metabolic substrate utilization in stress-induced immune cells *ICMx* **8** 28

[148] Buchwalow I, Atiakshin D, Samoilova V, Boecker W and Tiemann M 2018 Identification of autofluorescent cells in human angioimmunoblastic T-cell lymphoma *Histochem. Cell Biol.* **149** 169–77

[149] Kolenc O I and Quinn K P 2019 Evaluating cell metabolism through autofluorescence imaging of NAD(P)H and FAD *Antioxid. Redox Signal.* **30** 875–89

[150] Weil G J and Chused T M 1981 Eosinophil autofluorescence and its use in isolation and analysis of human eosinophils *Blood* **57** 1099–104

[151] Araźna M, Pruchniak M P and Demkow U 2014 Reactive oxygen species, granulocytes, and NETosis *Respiratory Virology and Immunogenicity. Advances in Experimental Medicine and Biology* **vol 836** ed M Pokorski (Cham: Springer)

[152] Hoeger B, Koellner B, Kotterba G, Van Den Heuvel M R, Hitzfeld B and Dietrich D R 2004 Influence of chronic exposure to treated sewage effluent on the distribution of white

blood cell populations in rainbow trout (Oncorhynchus mykiss) spleen *Toxicol. Sci.* **82** 97–105

[153] Niwa Y, Kasama T, Miyachi Y and Kanoh T 1989 Neutrophil chemotaxis, phagocytosis and parameters of reactive oxygen species in human aging: cross-sectional and longitudinal studies *Life Sci.* **44** 1655–64

[154] Lee D H, Li X, Ma N, Digman M A and Lee A P 2018 Rapid and label-free identification of single leukemia cells from blood in a high-density microfluidic trapping array by fluorescence lifetime imaging microscopy *Lab Chip* **18** 1349–58

[155] Özkan H, Akkoç N, Aydın A, Kavukçu S, Olgun N, Irken G, Akyol F and Çevik N T 1995 Relationship between serum unconjugated bilirubin levels and the autofluorescence of white blood cells in neonatal jaundice *Neonatology* **68** 100–3

[156] Rehan M, Khalid A and Nasreen F 2022 White blood cell differential fluorescence abnormal scattergram: a useful indicator for early detection of malarial parasite *Pak. J. Med. Sci.* **38** 687

[157] Seliger C, Schaerer B, Kohn M, Pendl H, Weigend S, Kaspers B and Härtle S 2012 A rapid high-precision flow cytometry-based technique for total white blood cell counting in chickens *Vet. Immunol. Immunopathol.* **145** 86–99

[158] García M J, Kamaid A and Malacrida L 2023 Label-free fluorescence microscopy: revisiting the opportunities with autofluorescent molecules and harmonic generations as biosensors and biomarkers for quantitative biology *Biophys. Rev.* **15** 709–19

[159] Wu C H, Wang T D, Hsieh C H, Huang S H, Lin J W, Hsu S C, Wu H T, Wu Y M and Liu T M 2016 Imaging cytometry of human leukocytes with third harmonic generation microscopy *Sci. Rep.* **6** 37210

[160] Yakimov B P, Gogoleva M A, Semenov A N, Rodionov S A, Novoselova M V, Gayer A V and Shirshin E A 2019 Label-free characterization of white blood cells using fluorescence lifetime imaging and flow-cytometry: molecular heterogeneity and erythrophagocytosis *Biomed. Opt. Express* **10** 4220–36

[161] Montague S J, Lim Y J, Lee W M and Gardiner E E 2020 Imaging platelet processes and function—current and emerging approaches for imaging *in vitro* and *in vivo Front. Immunol.* **11** 78

[162] Lohmann W and Lohmann C 1988 Native fluorescence of platelets from patients with occlusive arterial disease *Biochem. Biophys. Res. Commun.* **152** 1410–5

[163] Ryningen A, Jensen B O and Holmsen H 1999 Role of autocrine stimulation on the effects of cyclic AMP on protein and lipid phosphorylation in collagen-activated and thrombin-activated platelets *Eur. J. Biochem.* **260** 87–96

[164] Sinauridze E I, Kireev D A, Popenko N Y, Pichugin A V, Panteleev M A, Krymskaya O V and Ataullakhanov F I 2007 Platelet microparticle membranes have 50-to 100-fold higher specific procoagulant activity than activated platelets *Thromb. Haemost.* **97** 425–34

[165] Panzera A 2011 Novel blood platelet diagnostic platform *PhD Dissertation* Dublin City University

[166] Duran-Padilla M, Serrano-Loyola R, Perez-Garcia A, Carrillo-Betancourt R, Campos-García Rojas C, Reyes-Alberto M, Franco W, Hernandez-Ruiz J and Gutierrez-Herrera E 2024 Tryptophan intrinsic fluorescence from wound healing correlates with re-epithelialization in a rabbit model *Skin Res. Technol.* **30** e13834

[167] Ault K A, Rinder H M, Mitchell J G, Rinder C S, Lambrew C T and Hillman R S 1989 Correlated measurement of platelet release and aggregation in whole blood *Cytometry* **10** 448–55

[168] Michelson A D 1996 Flow cytometry: a clinical test of platelet function *Blood* **87** 4925–36

[169] Lakowicz J R and Lakowicz J R 1999 Introduction to fluorescence *Principles of Fluorescence Spectroscopy* (Springer) pp 1–23

[170] Lakowicz J R 2006 Plasmonics in biology and plasmon-controlled fluorescence *Plasmonics* **1** 5–33

[171] Lyberg I A H T 2000 Blood platelet activation evaluated by flow cytometry: optimised methods for clinical studies *Platelets* **11** 137–50

[172] Rotman A and Heldman J 1981 Intracellular viscosity changes during activation of blood platelets: studies by fluorescence polarization *Biochemistry* **20** 5995–9

[173] Wolberg A S 2007 Thrombin generation and fibrin clot structure *Blood Rev.* **21** 131–42

[174] Lorant D E, Mclntyre T M, Prescott S M and Zimmerman G A 1999 Platelet-activating factor: a signaling molecule for leukocyte adhesion *Vascular Adhesion Molecules and Inflammation* (Basel: Birkhäuser Basel) pp 81–107

[175] Pinckard R N, Woodard D S, Weintraub S T and McManus L M 1997 Qualitative and quantitative assessment of platelet activating factors *Platelets and Their Factors* (Berlin: Springer) pp 507–27

[176] Prescott S M, Zimmerman G A, Stafforini D M and McIntyre T M 2000 Platelet-activating factor and related lipid mediators *Annu. Rev. Biochem.* **69** 419–45

[177] Michelson A D 2004 Platelet function testing in cardiovascular diseases *Circulation* **110** e489–93

[178] Xia Z, Wong T, Liu Q, Kasirer-Friede A, Brown E and Frojmovic M M 1996 Optimally functional fluorescein isothiocyanate-labelled fibrinogen for quantitative studies of binding to activated platelets and platelet aggregation *Br. J. Haematol.* **93** 204–14

[179] van Geffen J P *et al* 2018 High-throughput elucidation of thrombus formation reveals sources of platelet function variability *Haematologica* **104** 1256

[180] Cardo L, Thomas S G, Mazharian A, Pikramenou Z, Rappoport J Z, Hannon M J and Watson S P 2015 Accessible synthetic probes for staining actin inside platelets and megakaryocytes by employing Lifeact peptide *Chem. Bio. Chem.* **16** 1680–8

[181] Celi A, Merrill-Skoloff G, Gross P, Falati S, Sim D S, Flaumenhaft R, Furie B C and Furie B 2003 Thrombus formation: direct real-time observation and digital analysis of thrombus assembly in a living mouse by confocal and widefield intravital microscopy *J. Thromb. Haemost.* **1** 60–8

[182] Park Y, Depeursinge C and Popescu G 2018 Quantitative phase imaging in biomedicine *Nat. Photonics* **12** 578–89

[183] Lee K, Kim K, Jung J, Heo J, Cho S, Lee S, Chang G, Jo Y, Park H and Park Y 2013 Quantitative phase imaging techniques for the study of cell pathophysiology: from principles to applications *Sensors* **13** 4170–91

[184] He X, Montague S J, Tao X, Gardiner E E and Lee W M 2018 Quantifying embolism: label-free volumetric mapping of thrombus structure and kinesis in a microfluidic system with optical holography *Adv. Biosyst.* **2** 1800089

[185] Ma Y, Guo S, Pan Y, Fan R, Smith Z J, Lane S and Chu K 2019 Quantitative phase microscopy with enhanced contrast and improved resolution through ultra-oblique illumination (UO-QPM) *J. Biophoton.* **12** e201900011

[186] Scandola C, Erhardt M, Rinckel J Y, Proamer F, Gachet C and Eckly A 2020 Use of electron microscopy to study megakaryocytes *Platelets* **31** 589–98

[187] Brown E, Carlin L M, Nerlov C, Celso C L and Poole A W 2018 Multiple membrane extrusion sites drive megakaryocyte migration into bone marrow blood vessels *Life Sci. Alliance* **1** e201800061

[188] Eckly A, Rinckel J Y, Proamer F and Gachet C 2018 High-resolution 3D imaging of megakaryocytes using focused ion beam-scanning electron microscopy *Methods Mol. Biol.* **1812** 217–31

[189] Engberts K B, Seinen C, Geerts W J and Heijnen H F 2018 Electron tomography and correlative approaches in platelet studies *Methods Mol. Biol.* **1812** 55–79

[190] Ronnlund D, Xu L, Perols A, Gad A K, Eriksson Karlström A, Auer G and Widengren J 2014 Multicolor fluorescence nanoscopy by photobleaching: concept, verification, and its application to resolve selective storage of proteins in platelets *ACS Nano* **8** 4358–65

[191] Vicidomini G, Bianchini P and Diaspro A 2018 STED super-resolved microscopy *Nat. Methods* **15** 173–82

[192] Bergstrand J, Xu L, Miao X, Li N, Öktem O, Franzén B, Auer G, Lomnytska M and Widengren J 2019 Super-resolution microscopy can identify specific protein distribution patterns in platelets incubated with cancer cells *Nanoscale* **11** 10023–33

[193] Poulter N S *et al* 2017 Clustering of glycoprotein VI (GPVI) dimers upon adhesion to collagen as a mechanism to regulate GPVI signaling in platelets *J. Thromb. Haemost.* **15** 549–64

[194] Poulter N S *et al* 2015 Platelet actin nodules are podosome-like structures dependent on Wiskott–Aldrich syndrome protein and ARP2/3 complex *Nat. Commun.* **6** 7254

[195] Kahr W H *et al* 2017 Loss of the Arp2/3 complex component ARPC1B causes platelet abnormalities and predisposes to inflammatory disease *Nat. Commun.* **8** 14816

[196] Miklosi A G, Del Favero G, Marko D, Harkany T and Lubec G 2018 Resolution matters: correlating quantitative proteomics and nanoscale-precision microscopy for reconstructing synapse identity *Proteomics* **18** 1800139

[197] Rimington C 1939 Porphyrins and their relation to the metabolism of blood pigments *Proc. R. Soc. Med.* **32** 1268–75

[198] Haga Y, Kay H D, Tempero M A and Zetterman R K 1992 Flow cytometric measurement of intracellular bilirubin in human peripheral blood mononuclear cells exposed to unconjugated bilirubin *Clin. Biochem.* **25** 277–83

[199] Campbell J M, Gosnell M, Agha A, Handley S, Knab A, Anwer A G, Bhargava A and Goldys E M 2024 Label-free assessment of key biological autofluorophores: material characteristics and opportunities for clinical applications *Adv. Mater.* **36** 2403761

[200] Oellingrath I M and Slinde E 1985 Color, pigment and iron content of meat loaves with blood, blood emulsion, or mechanically deboned meat added *J. Food Sci.* **50** 1551–5

[201] Redmond J R 1964 The role of blood pigments in the delivery of oxygen to tissues *Helgol. Mar. Res.* **9** 303–11

[202] Sharma V, Olweny E O, Kapur P, Cadeddu J A, Roehrborn C G and Liu H 2014 Prostate cancer detection using combined auto-fluorescence and light reflectance spectroscopy: *ex vivo* study of human prostates *Biomed. Opt. Express* **5** 1512–29

[203] Larsen A K, Simón-Santamaría J, Elvevold K, Ericzon B G, Mortensen K E, McCourt P, Smedsrød B and Sørensen K K 2021 Autofluorescence in freshly isolated adult human liver sinusoidal cells *Eur. J. Histochem.: EJH* **65**

[204] Bellemare M J, Bohle D S, Brosseau C N, Georges E, Godbout M, Kelly J, Leimanis M L, Leonelli R, Olivier M and Smilkstein M 2009 Autofluorescence of condensed heme

aggregates in malaria pigment and its synthetic equivalent hematin anhydride (β-hematin) *J. Phys. Chem.* B **113** 8391–401

[205] Lekha T, Safiya P and Narasimham D 2017 Fundus autofluorescence imaging of subinternal limiting membrane hemorrhage in anemic retinopathy *Indian J. Ophthalmol.* **65** 1021–2

[206] Courrol L C, de Oliveira Silva F R, Coutinho E L, Piccoli M F, Mansano R D, Vieira Júnior N D and Bellini M H 2007 Study of blood porphyrin spectral profile for diagnosis of tumor progression *J. Fluoresc.* **17** 289–92

[207] Courrol L C, de Oliveira Silva F R, Bellini M H, Mansano R D, Schor N and Vieira N D Jr 2007 Blood porphyrin luminescence and tumor growth correlation *Optical Methods for Tumor Treatment and Detection: Mechanisms and Techniques in Photodynamic Therapy XVI* **vol 6427** (SPIE) pp 209–16

[208] Devanesan S, Masilamani V, AlSalhi M S, Prasad S, Alshebly M M, Alqahtany F S and Aljaafreh M J 2021 Cancer screening by fluorescence spectra of blood and urine–a double blind study *J. King Saud Univ.-Sci.* **33** 101456

[209] Ushenko Y A, Arkhelyuk A D, Sidor M I, Bachynskyi V T and Wanchuliak O Y 2014 Laser polarization autofluorescence of endogenous porphyrins of optically anisotropic biological tissues and fluids in diagnostics of necrotic and pathological changes of human organs *Appl. Opt.* **53** B181–91

[210] Wang P, Wang X, Luo Q, Li Y, Lin X, Fan L, Zhang Y, Liu J and Liu X 2019 Fabrication of red blood cell-based multimodal theranostic probes for second near-infrared window fluorescence imaging-guided tumor surgery and photodynamic therapy *Theranostics* **9** 369

[211] Ding L, Wu Y, Wu M, Zhao Q, Li H, Liu J, Zhang X and Zeng Y 2021 Engineered red blood cell biomimetic nanovesicle with oxygen self-supply for near-infrared-II fluorescence-guided synergetic chemo-photodynamic therapy against hypoxic tumors *ACS Appl. Mater. Interfaces* **13** 52435–49

[212] Ricci A, Guida C C, Manzini P, Cuoghi C and Ventura P 2021 Kidney involvement in acute hepatic porphyrias: pathophysiology and diagnostic implications *Diagnostics* **11** 2324

[213] Mauritz J M, Esposito A, Tiffert T, Skepper J N, Warley A, Yoon Y Z, Cicuta P, Lew V L, Guck J R and Kaminski C F 2010 Biophotonic techniques for the study of malaria-infected red blood cells *Med. Biol. Eng. Comput.* **48** 1055–63

[214] Kirilova E M, Kalnina I, Zvagule T, Gabruseva N, Kurjane N and Solomenikova I I 2011 Fluorescent study of human blood plasma albumin alterations induced by ionizing radiation *J. Fluoresc.* **21** 923–7

[215] Veenashree M P, Sangwan V S, Vemuganti G K and Parthasaradhi A 2002 Acute scleritis as a manifestation of congenital erythropoietic porphyria *Cornea* **21** 530–1

[216] Venkatesh R *et al* 2024 Role of fundus autofluorescence imaging in the management of submacular hemorrhage *BMC Ophthalmol.* **24** 440

[217] Enerbäck L and Lundvall O 1970 Properties and distribution of liver fluorescence in porphyria cutanea tarda (PCT) *Virchows Arch.* A **350** 293–302

[218] Pan L, Wang X, Yang S, Wu X, Lee I, Zhang X, Rupp R A and Xu J 2012 Ultraviolet irradiation-dependent fluorescence enhancement of hemoglobin catalyzed by reactive oxygen species *PLoS ONE* **7** e44142

[219] Yuwen Z, Zeng Q, Ye Q, Zhao Y, Zhu J, Chen K, Liu H and Yang R 2023 A quencher-based blood-autofluorescence-suppression strategy enables the quantification of trace analytes in whole blood *Angew. Chem.* **135** e202302957

[220] Evans N D, Gnudi L, Rolinski O J, Birch D J S and Pickup J C 2005 Glucose-dependent changes in NAD (P) H-related fluorescence lifetime of adipocytes and fibroblasts *in vitro*: potential for non-invasive glucose sensing in diabetes mellitus *J. Photochem. Photobiol.,* B **80** 122–9

[221] Choudhuri S, Mandal L K, Paine S K, Sen A, Dutta D, Chowdhury I H, Mukherjee A, Saha A, Bhadhuri G and Bhattacharya B 2013 Role of hyperglycemia-mediated erythrocyte redox state alteration in the development of diabetic retinopathy *Retina* **33** 207–16

[222] Song H *et al* 2023 Detection of blood–brain barrier disruption in brains of patients with COVID-19, but no evidence of brain penetration by SARS-CoV-2 *Acta Neuropathol.* **146** 771–5

[223] Fortier M, Chea M, Aïn C, Loyens M, Boudemaghe T, Gris J C and Bouvier S 2022 Direct blood fluorescence signal intensity of neutrophils (NEU-SFL): a predictive marker of death in hospitalized COVID-19 patients? *Front. Med.* **9** 1062112

[224] Pretorius E, Venter C, Laubscher G J, Lourens P J, Steenkamp J and Kell D B 2020 Prevalence of readily detected amyloid blood clots in 'unclotted' Type 2 diabetes mellitus and COVID-19 plasma: a preliminary report *Cardiovasc. Diabetol.* **19** 1–8

[225] Kell D B, Laubscher G J and Pretorius E 2022 A central role for amyloid fibrin microclots in long COVID/PASC: origins and therapeutic implications *Biochem. J.* **479** 537–59

[226] Tungjai M, Phathakanon N, Ketnuam P, Tinlapat J and Kothan S 2018 Determination of hemolysis, osmotic fragility and fluorescence anisotropy on irradiated red blood cells as a function of kV of medical diagnostic X-rays *Int. J. Radiat. Res.* **16** 123–7

[227] van der Vorst J R *et al* 2013 Near-infrared fluorescence imaging of colorectal liver metastases in humans *Clin. Cancer Res.* **19** 5746–54

[228] Sevick-Muraca E M 2012 Translation of near-infrared fluorescence imaging technologies: emerging clinical applications *Annu. Rev. Med.* **63** 217–31

[229] Agrawal R, Balne P K, Tun S B B, Sia Wey Y, Khandelwal N and Barathi V A 2017 Fluorescent dye labeling of erythrocytes and leukocytes for studying the flow dynamics in mouse retinal circulation *J. Vis. Exp.* **125** e55495

[230] Li C Q and Li Y Q 2010 Endomicroscopy of intestinal metaplasia and gastric cancer *Gastroenterol. Clin.* **39** 785–96

[231] Kravchenko Y, Sikora K, Wireko A A and Lyndin M 2024 Fluorescence visualization for cancer detection: experience and perspectives *Heliyon* **10** e24390

[232] Liu Y, Bhattarai P, Dai Z and Chen X 2019 Photothermal therapy and photoacoustic imaging via nanotheranostics in fighting cancer *Chem. Soc. Rev.* **48** 2053–108

[233] Panchuk-Voloshina N, Haugland R P, Bishop-Stewart J, Bhalgat M K, Millard P J, Mao F, Leung W Y and Haugland R P 1999 Alexa dyes, a series of new fluorescent dyes that yield exceptionally bright, photostable conjugates *J. Histochem. Cytochem.* **47** 1179–88

Chapter 8

Raman scattering of blood

Anuradha Ramoji, Hulya Yilmaz, Susanne Pahlow and Juergen Popp

Blood evaluation is highly significant in clinical diagnostics, with the hemogram forming a crucial part of routine clinical analysis. The morphological, chemical and physical aspects of the blood and its components provide insights into human vitality and are therefore attracting keen interest from the research community. With advancements in optical techniques, utilizing light to extract relevant diagnostic biochemical information from human samples has thrived in recent years. One promising emerging technique is Raman spectroscopy, an analytical method that allows probing the sample in its native state. It is based on inelastic scattering of light and thereby provides highly specific chemical information on the sample. By combining the technique with a microscope, morphological, structural, and physical information can be obtained. Hence, Raman spectroscopy has a high potential in clinical diagnostics. This chapter discusses Raman scattering of blood and its components. It covers various aspects of blood sampling and examination methods, as well as the fundamental properties of blood as revealed by Raman spectroscopy. Additionally, the chapter explores the application of Raman spectroscopy in biomedical diagnostics and reviews novel studies on using the Raman spectral signature of blood for disease diagnosis, drug monitoring and therapy. The chapter also highlights various specialized Raman spectroscopy techniques used in blood investigation and offers a future perspective on blood diagnostics.

Abbreviations

AD	Alzheimer's disease
ALT	alanine aminotransferase
AST	aspartate aminotransferase
ATP	adenosine triphosphate
BACS	Buoyancy-activated cell sorting
CA125	Cancer antigen 125
CARS	coherent anti-Stokes Raman spectroscopy

doi:10.1088/978-0-7503-4806-5ch8

CBC	Complete blood count
CCD	charge-coupled device
CD40	Cluster of differentiation 40
CGM	Continuous glucose monitoring
CMP	comprehensive metabolic panel
CRP	C-reactive protein
CTC	Circulating tumour cell
DCLS	direct classical least squares
deoxyHb	deoxygenated haemoglobin
DHM	digital holographic images
DLB	Dementia with Lewy bodies
DRRS	diffuse resonance Raman spectroscopy
ECDL	External cavity diode laser
FACS	fluorescence-activated cell sorting
FT	Fourier transform
IL-4	Interleukin 4
IL-6	Interleukin 6
kNN	k-nearest neighbour
LDH	Lactate dehydrogenase
LPS	lipopolysaccharide
MACS	magnetic-activated cell sorting
Mfsd2a	Major facilitator superfamily domain-containing protein 2
NAD+	oxidized nicotinamide adenine dinucleotide
NADH	reduced nicotinamide adenine dinucleotide
NET	neutrophil extracellular trap
NIPALS	Non-linear iterative partial least squares
NIR	near-infrared
NNLS	non-negative least squares
oxyHb	oxygenated haemoglobin
PBMC	Peripheral blood mononuclear cells
PCA	principal component analysis
PCT	procalcitonin
PHA	phytohaemagglutinin
PLS	partial least squares
PMA	phorbol 12-myristate 13-acetate
PRP	Platelet-rich plasma
PVC	polyvinyl chloride
PVP	polyvinylpyrrolidone
RBC	Red blood cell
RNA	ribonucleic acid
SARS-CoV-2	Severe acute respiratory syndrome coronavirus type 2
SERS	surface-enhanced Raman spectroscopy
SORS	Spatially offset Raman spectroscopy
SRS	stimulated Raman scattering
SVM	Support vector machine
TCR	T cell receptor
THP1 cells	Tohoku Hospital Pediatrics-1 Cells
TLR	Toll-like receptor
TNF-alpha	Tumour necrosis factor alpha
TTP	Thrombotic thrombocytopenic purpura

UV-VIS	ultraviolet-visible
vWF	von Willebrand factor
WBC	White blood cell

8.1 Introduction

Blood, often referred to as life's essential fluid, plays a critical role in clinical diagnostics and healthcare. It is a complex and specialized connective tissue composed of various cellular components suspended in a fluid called plasma. These cellular elements primarily include red blood cells (RBCs), also known as erythrocytes, white blood cells (WBCs) or leucocytes, and platelets (thrombocytes), each serving distinct functions. RBCs represent the most abundant cellular component in whole blood. Their primary responsibility is the transport of oxygen, a function made possible by the presence of haemoglobin, a protein that binds to and carries oxygen from the lungs to every cell in the body. The iron content of haemoglobin gives blood its characteristic red colour. The efficient oxygen-carrying capacity of RBCs is vital for fuelling cellular respiration, the process through which cells generate energy [1]. WBCs, or leucocytes, are crucial components of the immune system. They play a central role in defending the body against infections, viruses, bacteria, and other intruders. These remarkable cells come in various types, each specializing in different aspects of immune response. Neutrophils, for instance, are the first responders to infections, while lymphocytes play a pivotal role in immune memory and antibody production. The heterogeneous WBC population ensures that the body can effectively combat a wide range of health threats [2]. Platelets, or thrombocytes, are essential for blood clotting, or coagulation. When blood vessels are damaged, platelets are the first to arrive at the site and initiate the clotting process. They adhere to the injured vessel walls and release clotting factors to form a plug that prevents excessive bleeding. This rapid and precise clot formation is vital for preventing haemorrhages and maintaining blood vessel integrity. In addition to its cellular components, blood plasma is a pale-yellow liquid that constitutes approximately 55% of the total blood volume. Plasma is composed of water, electrolytes, hormones, waste products, and various proteins, including albumin and globulins. These proteins play a pivotal role in maintaining osmotic pressure, transporting substances such as hormones and lipids, and contributing to the immune response [3–5]. The analysis of blood samples provides invaluable information about a patient's health status. A multitude of blood tests yield data on diverse health parameters, including blood cell counts, biomarkers, and physical properties.

Blood counts are used to identify conditions such as anaemia, infections, and blood disorders. For example, a low RBC count may indicate anaemia, while an elevated WBC count might signal an ongoing infection [6, 7]. Biomarkers, such as glucose levels, offer diagnostic clues for conditions like diabetes and provide a window into organ function. Elevated glucose levels in the blood may be indicative of diabetes mellitus, a condition characterized by impaired blood sugar regulation. Furthermore, biomarkers associated with liver function, kidney function, and cardiac health are evaluated in blood tests, which assist in the identification and monitoring of a wide range of medical conditions [8]. Blood tests also assess physical characteristics such as viscosity, coagulation properties, and oxygen-carrying capacity, which illuminate various physiological processes and medical conditions. Abnormalities in blood coagulation can indicate conditions such as thrombosis, a potentially dangerous formation of blood clots within blood vessels. Anaemia, a condition characterized by a decreased ability of the blood to carry oxygen, is often detected through assessments of blood composition and its oxygen-carrying capacity [9, 10]. The morphological, chemical, and physical aspects of blood and its components offer a multifaceted perspective on human vitality that has captivated the research community. By investigating the intricate details of blood, researchers aim to gain a comprehensive understanding of human health and disease, leading to advancements in both clinical diagnostics and therapeutic interventions [11, 12]. These insights, in turn, have a profound impact on healthcare, leading to earlier disease detection, more effective treatments, and the development of personalized medicine strategies [13]. In addition to the current clinical diagnostic methods, the necessity for more rapid, precise, cost-effective, and extensive panels of disease biomarkers has prompted the advancement of technological platforms for blood investigations. Biophotonic tools, such as Raman spectroscopy, represent one of the emerging analytical techniques that are being employed extensively for blood investigations. The chapter offers an in-depth examination of the fascinating world of Raman scattering as it is applied to the analysis of blood and its components. The text provides an in-depth exploration of a number of diverse aspects, commencing with an examination of the methods and techniques employed for blood sampling and examination. Furthermore, the chapter reveals the intrinsic qualities of blood that are uncovered through the lens of Raman spectroscopy. Furthermore, the chapter examines the extensive use of Raman spectroscopy in biomedical diagnostics. The chapter presents innovative research that utilizes the Raman spectral signature of blood to diagnose diseases and monitor the effects of drugs and therapies. Furthermore, the chapter offers insight into the bespoke Raman spectroscopy techniques that have been developed for the investigation of blood, providing a comprehensive overview of their applications and advantages. In conclusion, the chapter presents a forward-looking perspective on the future of blood diagnostics through Raman spectroscopy. It highlights the promising developments and potential breakthroughs in this field.

8.2 Blood composition and its therapeutic importance

The cellular composition of the blood exhibits slight inter-individual variability, which may be influenced by factors such as age, sex, and health status. In general, the highest population of cells is that of RBCs, which account for 4.5–6 million cells per microliter. The second most abundant population of cells is that of platelets, which can be found in concentrations of approximately 150000 to 400000 per microliter. In contrast, the WBCs are found in a range of 4.5000–11000 cells per microliter. The WBCs are further subclassified into different types. The liquid component of blood, known as plasma, is composed of 92% water and a variety of

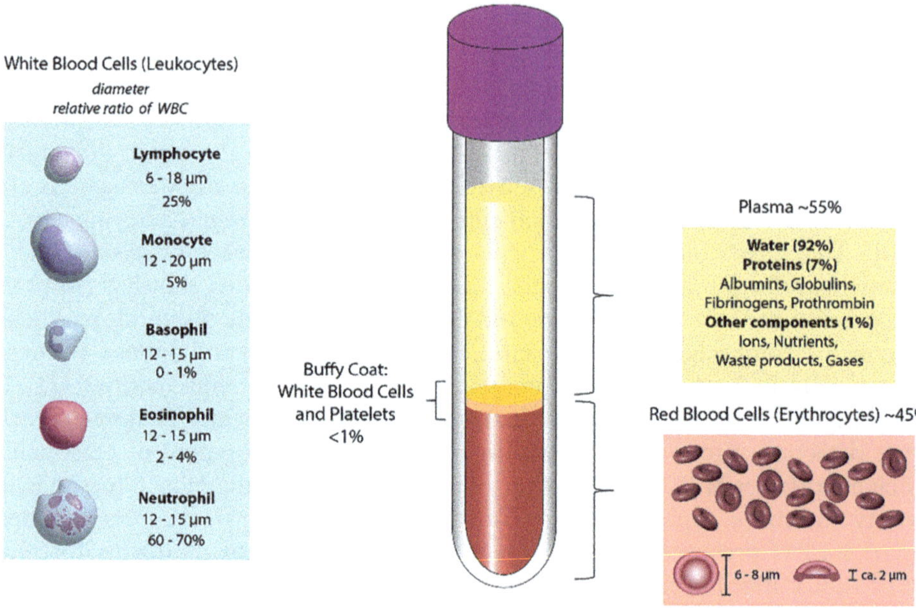

Figure 8.1. Schematic presentation of blood composition.

essential molecules. The remaining 93% of the plasma is composed of a variety of proteins, including albumin, globulin, and fibrinogen, as well as regulatory proteins (enzymes, hormones, and vitamins) and other solutes such as electrolytes (sodium, potassium, bicarbonate, chloride, and calcium), nutrients, gases, and waste products. Plasma devoid of fibrinogen is designated as serum. Figure 8.1 provides a comprehensive overview of the cellular and fluid composition of blood.

Blood cells, plasma, and serum are employed in clinical diagnostics and serve as valuable biomarkers for various diseases. For example, RBCs are of pivotal importance in diagnostic medicine, offering insights into various physiological and pathological conditions. Their abundance in the bloodstream serves to emphasise their diagnostic significance. Erythrocyte parameters, including count, haemoglobin concentration, and haematocrit levels, are of significant importance in routine diagnostic tests such as the complete blood count (CBC). Abnormal values assist in the diagnosis and classification of conditions such as anaemia, polycythaemia and dehydration. Moreover, erythrocyte characteristics are significant in the identification of haematological disorders such as sickle cell disease, thalassaemia and autoimmune haemolytic anaemia. The evaluation of erythrocyte morphology, size and distribution provides valuable diagnostic clues, which guide further investigations and treatment decisions. Furthermore, erythrocytes' role in oxygen transport emphasises their importance in assessing tissue oxygenation and respiratory function. Monitoring changes in erythrocyte parameters over time is an essential aspect of evaluating treatment response and disease progression, thereby ensuring optimal patient care. Consequently, erythrocytes serve as indispensable diagnostic markers, contributing significantly to the comprehensive evaluation of haematological health and overall patient well-being. The diagnostic value of leucocytes is derived from their dynamic functions and unique characteristics in comparison to erythrocytes. In contrast to erythrocytes, leucocytes possess nuclei and organelles, enabling them to exit the bloodstream and migrate to sites of infection in response to chemical signals. This capacity for directed movement allows leucocytes, such as macrophages and lymphocytes, to play crucial roles in immune defence mechanisms within the body's tissues. In clinical practice, differential counts of leucocyte types and their percentages serve as pivotal indicators for diagnosing various conditions. A CBC with differential is a common blood test that can assist in the diagnosis of various medical conditions, including infections, autoimmune diseases, and blood disorders. For example, an increase in the number of neutrophils, designated as neutrophilia, may indicate a bacterial infection, whereas an increase in the number of eosinophils, designated as eosinophilia, may indicate an allergic reaction or parasitic infection. Conversely, a reduction in the number of leucocytes, designated leucopenia, may indicate damage to the bone marrow, whereas an increase in the number of leucocytes, designated leukocytosis, may indicate inflammation or infection. Consequently, differential counts of leucocytes furnish healthcare professionals with crucial data, enabling them to ascertain the root cause of a patient's ailment and to devise an efficacious treatment plan. Platelets, also known as thrombocytes, are not actual cells but fragments of the cytoplasm of a megakaryocyte. Megakaryocytes are large cells that produce platelets and are stimulated by thrombopoietin. Platelets play a pivotal role in haemostasis, limiting blood loss and secreting growth factors essential for tissue growth and repair. Nevertheless, an imbalance in platelet numbers can give rise to serious disorders, such as thrombocytosis or thrombocytopenia. Platelet function tests may include platelet aggregation studies, bleeding time tests, and platelet factor assays. Platelet aggregation studies evaluate the efficacy of platelet clumping in response to a specific stimulus, while bleeding time tests assess the time required for bleeding to cease following a minor incision. Platelet factor assays quantify the concentration of specific clotting factors in the blood, which are essential for platelet functionality. These tests can assist in the diagnosis of platelet-related disorders and in determining the underlying cause of thrombocytosis or thrombocytopenia. Furthermore, platelet counts can fluctuate throughout the day, and may be influenced by various factors, including stress and exercise. Consequently, multiple tests may be required to accurately diagnose platelet-related disorders. In summary, platelets play a vital role in haemostasis and tissue repair. An understanding of platelet function and of platelet counts can assist in the diagnosis and management of platelet-related disorders, ensuring proper treatment and preventing serious complications. Plasma diagnostics play a pivotal role in the diagnosis and management of various diseases and conditions. Thrombotic thrombocytopenic purpura (TTP) is a condition characterized by fever, thrombocytopenia, haemolytic anaemia, renal dysfunction, and neurological dysfunction. The identification of this condition relies on plasma diagnostics, which can be used to identify it through laboratory findings such as anaemia, thrombocytopenia, schistocytes on a peripheral smear, increased lactate dehydrogenase (LDH), and increased creatinine. Plasma exchange with fresh frozen plasma represents a fundamental aspect of treatment for TTP. Similarly, clotting disorders such as haemophilia and von Willebrand disease, which are caused by deficiencies in specific clotting factors, benefit from plasma-derived clotting factors and diagnostic assays such as the von Willebrand factor (vWF)-ristocetin cofactor activity assay. Immunodeficiency disorders, defined by the inability to produce antibodies, are treated with immunoglobulin infusions derived from plasma, which enhance the body's defence against infections. Furthermore, plasma plays a pivotal role in laboratory diagnostics for various diseases and in therapeutic interventions such as plasmapheresis, particularly in autoimmune disorders such as myasthenia gravis and Guillain–Barré syndrome. Platelet-rich plasma (PRP) injections, derived from autologous blood with elevated platelet concentrations, offer promising avenues for the management of musculoskeletal pathologies such as knee osteoarthritis, with superior outcomes compared to traditional treatments in recent studies. Several additional diagnostic tests are conducted utilizing plasma, including a comprehensive metabolic panel (CMP), which is employed to assess the chemical composition of blood. A CMP is a diagnostic test that assesses various metabolic parameters and organ functions. The principal components of a CMP test include the evaluation of blood sugar for diabetes management, the measurement of levels of essential ions to assess electrolyte balance, blood urea nitrogen tests and the assessment of creatinine for kidney functions, the measurement of liver enzymes such as alanine aminotransferase (ALT), aspartate aminotransferase (AST), alkaline phosphatase and total bilirubin for liver function, the measurement of total protein and albumin levels in blood to assess nutritional status and liver function. Consequently, plasma diagnostics not only facilitate the identification of disease but also play a pivotal role in therapeutic interventions across a spectrum of medical conditions. The routine blood diagnostics utilizing different components of the blood are of paramount importance in the diagnosis of various medical conditions and are employed to monitor the effects of treatments and to track changes in a patient's health over time. Physicians utilize the results of blood diagnostics, in conjunction with other clinical data, to inform medical decisions and develop personalized treatment plans for individual patients. Each of the aforementioned investigations of different blood components is conducted using a combination of optical and non-optical devices. These include spectrophotometers, which are used to quantify blood analytes, microscopes, which are employed to investigate the shape, size and morphology of blood cells, mass spectrometers, which are employed to determine the concentration of lipid and protein biomarkers, and so forth. Novel diagnostic platforms are being developed to obtain comprehensive information with minimal blood loss in a rapid and accurate manner. Raman spectroscopy is an emerging analytical technique that is being extensively employed in the field of blood investigations. Its application in this context allows for the acquisition of clinically relevant information, which is then used to assess patients' disease conditions and to provide diagnostic and therapeutic information.

8.3 Raman spectroscopy analysis of blood components

Raman spectroscopy provides information at the molecular level by utilizing the highly specific interactions between molecules present in the sample and the incident photons. When a sample is probed with monochromatic light, a small fraction (approximately 1 in 10^8) of the photons is scattered in an inelastic manner. This results in a frequency shift, which corresponds to specific molecular vibrations. The change in frequency is known as the Raman shift and is an intrinsic property of the molecules involved. In order to link the chemical information on the sample with spatial information, the Raman spectrometer is commonly coupled with a microscope. Raman spectroscopic techniques can be categorized into two main groups: linear and non-linear. The specific choice depends on the absorption properties of the blood and the targeted blood component. Spontaneous or conventional Raman spectroscopy is a linear process in which a small fraction of the incident photons exchanges quanta of vibrational/rotational energy with sample molecules and is incoherently scattered to Stokes or anti-Stokes frequencies. However, the low efficiency of the inelastic scattering process leads to poor sensitivity, and the simultaneous excitation of fluorescence can further mask the Raman signal. One strategy to prevent inference from fluorescence and increase the scattering efficiency is to exploit non-linear processes in techniques such as stimulated Raman scattering (SRS), hyper-Raman or coherent anti-Stokes Raman spectroscopy (CARS). non-linear Raman spectroscopy is based on non-linear optical effects involving Raman-active molecular transitions and is typically achieved by mixing two or more wavelengths emitted by spatially and temporally synchronized pulsed lasers. In addition to these non-linear approaches, there are other possibilities for increasing the signal intensity, such as resonance or plasmonic enhancement. In resonance Raman spectroscopy, the excitation wavelength is chosen in a way that coincides with an absorption band of the analyte. Consequently, the Raman modes associated with the electronic transition are enhanced by several orders of magnitude. This is of particular importance in the case of biological samples. For example, different excitation wavelengths yield different information in the case of proteins. Using a laser in the ultraviolet (UV) region results in the most prominent modes of aromatic amino acid side chains. Even lower wavelengths in the deep UV region can be used to probe information on the secondary structure. The visible region of the spectrum can be employed to enhance the modes of cofactors such as haem, which is responsible for the oxygen-binding capacity of the protein haemoglobin.

Another important variant of Raman spectroscopy is surface-enhanced Raman scattering (SERS), in which the Raman signal of analyte molecules is increased via plasmonic enhancement, mostly using silver or gold metal nanoparticles or nanostructures. The main contribution of the signal enhancement, which is often several orders of magnitude, comes from the excitation of localized surface plasmons in the metal. Of course, the excitation wavelength of the laser has to be tuned to the specific metal of the SERS substrate. Analyte molecules in close vicinity to the metal surface experience a very high electric field due to the coherent oscillation of the electrons in the metal. Below are the most important variants of Raman spectroscopy for blood analysis:

i. **Resonance Raman spectroscopy:** Resonance Raman spectroscopy involves the use of a laser wavelength that matches the absorption peak of specific chromophores, such as haemoglobin. This technique enhances the Raman signal, making it especially useful for studying haemoglobin and haem-related compounds in blood. It can provide insights into haemoglobin conformation and oxygenation states.

ii. **Surface-Enhanced Raman spectroscopy (SERS):** SERS involves the use of metallic nanoparticles (e.g., silver or gold) to enhance the Raman signals of molecules adsorbed onto their surfaces. In the investigation of blood, SERS can increase the sensitivity of Raman measurements, allowing for the detection of low concentrations of biomolecules. It has been applied to study various blood components and analyse blood plasma for disease biomarkers.

iii. **Coherent anti-Stokes Raman scattering (CARS):** CARS is a non-linear Raman spectroscopy technique that offers faster acquisition of Raman spectra. It has been applied to study lipid-rich components in blood, such as lipoproteins. CARS can provide insights into lipid metabolism and cardiovascular disease risk.

iv. **Spontaneous Raman spectral imaging:** This technique combines Raman spectroscopy with imaging capabilities to create chemical maps of blood samples. It enables the analysis of blood components at the spatial level and can be used to visualize cell types, their distribution, and the chemical composition of blood clots.

v. **Time-resolved Raman spectroscopy:** Time-resolved Raman spectroscopy captures the dynamics of molecular vibrations over time. This technique can be used to study fast processes in blood, such as blood coagulation, by tracking the changes in molecular vibrations as they occur.

vi. **Stimulated Raman spectroscopy (SRS):** SRS is a label-free imaging technique that can be used to study vibrational frequencies in blood components with high spatial resolution. It has been employed to visualize and analyze specific molecules within blood samples, including lipids and proteins.

vii. **Raman tweezers:** Raman tweezers combine optical trapping with Raman spectroscopy, allowing for the manipulation and analysis of individual blood cells or particles. This technique can provide information about the biochemical composition of single cells within blood samples. This approach is valuable for the study of blood flow, cell sorting, and the real-time analysis of blood components under various conditions.

viii. **Microfluidic-based Raman spectroscopy:** Integration of microfluidic devices with Raman spectroscopy enables the analysis of blood samples within controlled microscale environments. This approach is of value in the study of blood flow, cell sorting, and the real-time analysis of blood components under a variety of conditions.

These advanced Raman spectroscopy techniques have broadened the scope of blood investigation, enabling researchers and clinicians to gain deeper insights into the chemical composition and structure of blood components. These techniques have applications in understanding blood-related diseases, such as anaemia, coagulation disorders, and cardiovascular diseases, as well as in drug development and personalized medicine. Raman spectroscopy has been extensively applied in blood investigations, either in the context of the whole blood or individual isolated components, including RBCs, WBCs, platelets, plasma, and serum. Atkins *et al.* have provided a comprehensive review of Raman spectroscopy investigations of blood components, including a detailed analysis of haemoglobin, intact RBCs, RBC membranes, WBCs, plasma, and serum platelets. Furthermore, the review encompasses the utilization of Raman spectroscopy for the diagnosis of diseases such as cancer, malaria, blood disorders, and others [14]. The next section will discuss the Raman spectroscopic profile of blood and blood components.

8.3.1 Whole blood

The entire blood sample is analysed in either its liquid state or as a dried spot on a suitable Raman substrate. The majority of the whole blood is composed of RBC, which explains why the Raman spectra acquired from whole blood are primarily influenced by the haemoglobin signal present in the RBC. In addition to the RBC, whole blood contains a variety of other components, as illustrated in figure 8.1. Whole blood has been investigated with Raman spectroscopy using different excitation wavelengths (figure 8.2). For example, Atkins *et al.* have reported Raman spectra of whole blood acquired using a 720 nm excitation wavelength,

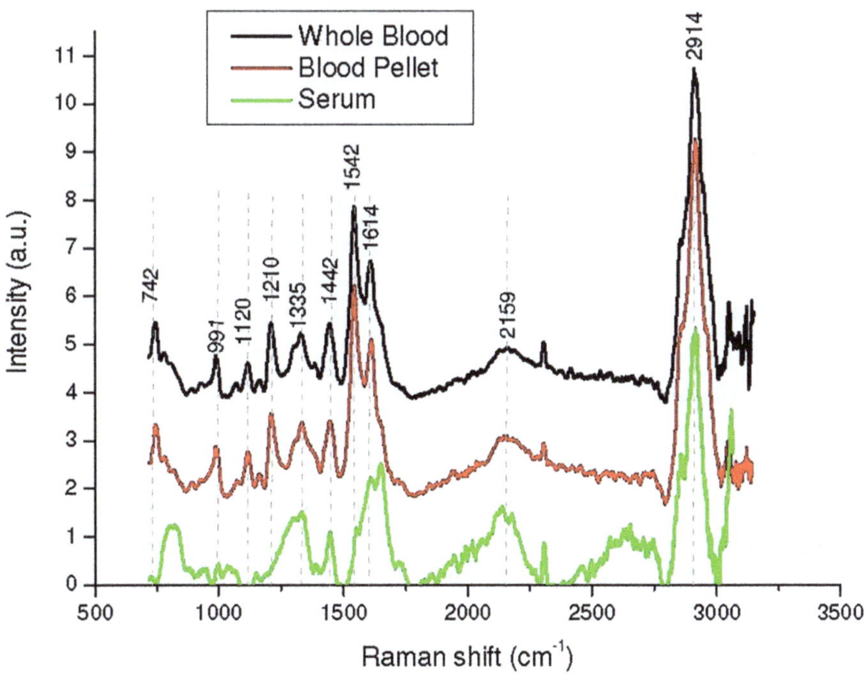

Figure 8.2. Raman spectra of whole blood, blood pellet and serum. The Raman spectra were acquired using 785 nm excitation wavelength. Reprinted with permission from [20], copyright 2011 Optical Society of America.

which yielded strong Raman scattering of carotenoids and protein. Furthermore, the wavelength allows the acquisition of the Raman signal of the haem chromophore without interference from the fluorescence background. The Raman spectra of dried whole blood collected using an excitation wavelength of 785 nm exhibited features of oxygenated haemoglobin (oxyHb) and exhibited higher power than 2 mW, which may result in the aggregation or denaturation of haemoglobin. Further, Raman spectroscopy-based detection and monitoring of blood glucose has been shown possible by many scientists. Enejder *et al.* applied Raman spectroscopy to simultaneously measure multiple analytes, namely, glucose, urea, total protein, albumin, triglycerides, haematocrit and haemoglobin and quantitatively predicted their concentrations [15]. Volkov *et al.* applied Raman spectroscopy in combination with density functional calculations and determined that electronic transitions of the ligand to metal charge transfer are responsible for the colour of the blood [16]. Raman spectroscopy has been extensively applied for forensic purposes such as whole bloodstain identification [17], differentiating human and animal blood [18], race differentiation using bloodstain, etc [19].

Another area of interest for researchers in whole blood investigations is the combination of Raman spectroscopy with different platforms, including microfluidic, sensor-based, and other capture techniques. For instance, Matthiae *et al.* and Chiang *et al.* developed a microfluidic platform combined with Raman spectroscopy for in-line monitoring of blood plasma without the necessity for centrifugation. A special microfluidic design has been proposed for the instantaneous fractionation of plasma, and the suitability of this platform has been demonstrated for the detection of free haemoglobin and beta-carotene in blood plasma [21, 22]. Similarly, Hansson *et al.* developed a flow cell-based Raman spectroscopy technique to overcome the photodegradation in human blood. The researcher demonstrated that the novel flow cell-based setup can detect minute changes in whole blood lysates' spectral features resulting from natural aging. The ageing effect due to natural oxidation does not interfere with Raman spectral measurements when using Raman spectroscopy. Furthermore, hydrogen peroxide-treated blood, which induces oxidative stress, can be discriminated from normal blood with high accuracy (above 90%) [23].

8.3.2 Haemoglobin and RBC

Haemoglobin is one of the most extensively researched components of blood and is a strong Raman scatterer due to its highly conjugated four haem subunits, which enable it to transport up to four oxygen molecules. It is primarily found in RBCs, and isolated haemoglobin is responsible for over 95% of the dry weight of each RBC. Each RBC can contain approximately 300 million haemoglobin molecules, which enables it to bind and transport as many as 1.2 billion oxygen molecules. This makes haemoglobin an essential component of the circulatory system, as it ensures that oxygen is delivered to all parts of the body that require it [24]. The absorption spectra of haemoglobin vary according to the oxygenation status of the molecule, with oxyHb exhibiting a broad absorption band from 300 to 1000 nm and deoxygenated haemoglobin (deoxyHb) displaying a narrower absorption band. Given the broad

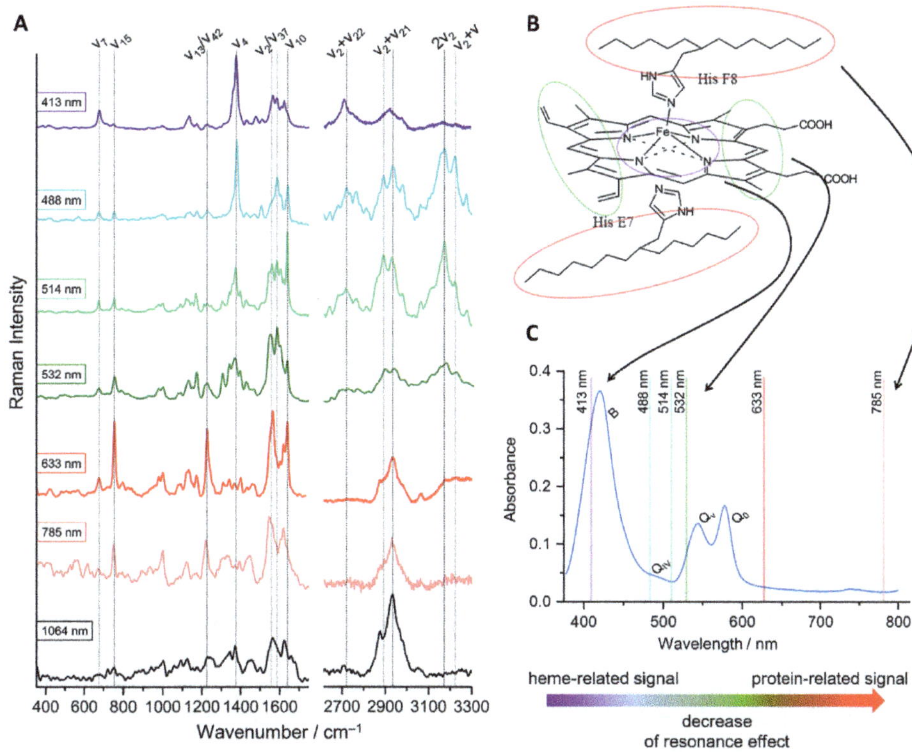

Figure 8.3. (A) Raman spectra of the RBC acquired using different excitation wavelengths. The important haem vibrational modes have been marked with lines. (B) A typical haem structure with marked areas of oscillations involved in resonance mechanism depending on the used excitation wavelength, and (C) UV-VIS absorption spectrum of the isolated RBC with assignments of the bands and marked wavelengths. The colours used to mark excitation wavelengths correspond with each other on all panels. Reproduced from [25] CC BY 4.0.

absorption band, Raman spectra of whole blood are usually dominated by the haemoglobin, especially when investigated using excitation wavelengths in the visible and near-infrared (NIR) region. In figure 8.3, Raman spectra of isolated RBC recorded with various excitation wavelengths are displayed along with UV-VIS absorption spectrum of the isolated RBC.

The strong Raman peaks observed in the haemoglobin spectra arise due to the haem porphyrin ring vibrations and are observed around 756, 1133, and 1600 cm^{-1} [26]. In addition to these peaks, several less intense peaks are observed from ring deformation vibrations, methyl groups, and proteins (1002, 1653 cm^{-1}), among others. A number of studies have demonstrated that the Raman spectra differ between oxyHb and deoxyHb (figure 8.4). Upon excitation with 488 nm, the Raman peak at 1220 cm^{-1} shifts to 1360 cm^{-1} upon transition from oxyHb to deoxyHb [14, 26–30]. Employing resonance Raman spectroscopy (532 nm excitation), investigations of haemoglobin revealed that the Raman peaks in the range 1355 to 1380 cm^{-1} and 1500 to 1650 cm^{-1} are the marker peaks for the haemoglobin oxidation state [26]. The transition of oxyHb to deoxyHb was induced by treating RBCs with a 0.9% saline solution, thereby implicating the role of saline solution during blood transfusion [28].

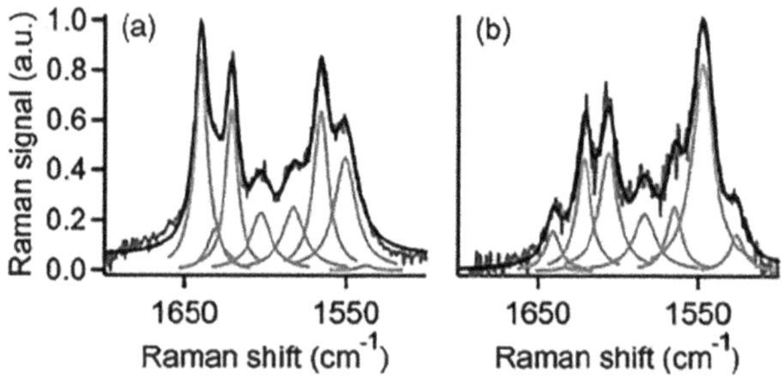

Figure 8.4. Raman spectra of (a) oxygenated and (b) deoxygenated haemoglobin. The solid black line is a least-square fit of a sum of Lorentzian contributions to the data. The individual contributions are shown in grey. Raman spectra were acquired using 633 nm excitation wavelength. Reproduced with permission from [31], copyright (2012) American Chemical Society.

In a separate study by Lukose *et al.*, the Raman marker peaks of deoxyHb were identified to be 1209, 1222, 1544 and 1561 cm^{-1} [28]. Rao *et al.* reported a change in the oxygenation state of haemoglobin due to mechanical stress induced in human RBCs via optical tweezers [27]. The study replicated the stretching and compressing of RBCs that occur when they pass through vessels and smaller capillaries, which induces a change in the oxygenation status of the RBCs. Modelling methods demonstrated that the transition in the oxygenation state of the RBC is due to interactions between haemoglobin and the RBC membrane, as well as between neighbouring haemoglobins. The most prominent Raman peak to a change during the transition was identified as 1625 cm^{-1} (C–C vibration of the polyporphyrin side chain) [32]. The Raman peaks in the region of 1500 cm^{-1} are also affected, which corresponds to the spin-state marker of the centre iron atom in the haem. The 1567 cm^{-1} peak is indicative of low-spin ferrous iron and is characteristic of bound oxygen [33]. For deoxyHb, it is most probable that the iron is in the high-spin state. In this condition, it was demonstrated that the Raman band splits into two, with one band at 1546 cm^{-1} and the other at 1578 cm^{-1} [27]. In a study conducted by Nagatomo *et al.*, using crystallography and density functional theory calculations, the resonance Raman band (excited by 488 and 442 nm wavelengths) arising from ferric haems was assigned to 899 and 876 cm^{-1} [34].

In a study conducted by Dybas *et al.*, resonance Raman and spontaneous Raman imaging were employed to investigate living RBCs. The research team placed a particular emphasis on the cyanohaemoglobin adducts present within RBCs and the active site environment of haem proteins. The results of the resonance Raman studies revealed the occurrence of Fe–CN stretching and bending modes, as well as C–N stretching mode, at 454, 382 and 2123 cm^{-1}, respectively. Furthermore, the studies demonstrate that the conformational arrangement of the Fe–CN fragment is conserved in the isolated cynohaemoglobin. However, in the living RBC, there is a minor difference in the degree of distortion, resulting in a slight change in the ligand geometry. This can be attributed to the high ordering and tight packing of Hb molecules inside the RBC [32]. A comprehensive overview of the biomedical analysis of RBCs is provided in the review article by Dybas *et al.* This covers the details of classical methods applied for RBC characterization and insights into Raman-based techniques applied to obtain information on the molecular level [25]. Lin *et al.* investigated the use of Raman spectroscopy for the detection of diabetes, with the isolation of haemoglobin from RBC and measurement of the latter as a dried spot. The Raman peaks observed at 1228 cm^{-1} (C–H methine deformation and glutathione) exhibited a decrease in intensity with an increase in blood glucose levels. Conversely, the Raman peaks at 1562, 1580 and 1621 cm^{-1} exhibited an increase in intensity [35].

RBCs have also been investigated as a biomarker for a number of different diseases, including diabetes, malaria, dengue, and haematological alterations [36–40]. Another study reports how Raman difference imaging provides insight into cellular biochemistry *in vivo,* as a function of sub-cellular dimensions and the cellular environment. The study examines Raman microscopic images of the distribution of the different haemoglobins in both healthy (discocyte) and unhealthy (echinocyte) blood cells and interprets these images using pre-calculated, accurate pre-resonant Raman tensors for scattering intensities specific to haemoglobins [16]. Furthermore, stimulated Raman scattering microscopy was applied to image blood vessels and RBC with high spatial and temporal resolution [41]. A review article providing an overview of SERS for bioanalysis and diagnosis. The article discusses the potential of SERS for the detection of biomolecules in blood samples, including glucose, cholesterol, and haemoglobin [42]. A broader overview of abnormal RBC morphologies and their associated pathologies that are accessible to Raman imaging is summarized in (table 8.1).

8.3.3 White blood cells

WBCs, also known as leucocytes, constitute a minor fraction of the blood components. Nevertheless, they play a pivotal role in maintaining homeostasis of the human immune system. There are several subpopulations of WBCs. The major subpopulations are illustrated in figure 8.1, namely neutrophils, monocytes, eosinophils, and lymphocytes. Characteristic Raman spectra from the nucleus region and cytoplasm region of neutrophils, monocytes, lymphocytes and eosinophils are displayed figure 8.5. In addition to these, there are other minor subpopulations, including dendritic cells, basophils, and macrophages, among others. Lymphocytes can be further classified into T-cells and B-cells. T-cells can be further classified based on the surface markers they express, such as CD4 and CD8. They can also be divided into different categories based on their role in the immune system, including T-helper cells, cytotoxic cells, and effector cells. Raman spectroscopy has been employed for the characterization and phenotyping of WBC subpopulations. Borek–Dorosz *et al.* applied Raman spectroscopy to differentiate between WBCs and identified specific Raman marker peaks, including those associated with carotenoid and nucleic acid vibrations, which contribute to the discrimination between B and T lymphocytes [43]. Moreover, the majority of carotenoids present in T-cells are beta-carotenoids, which contribute to the differentiation of T lymphocytes from neutrophils [44]. Chen *et al.* employed wavelength-modulated

Table 8.1. List of unusual RBC morphologies and associated pathology that can potentially be studied using different imaging variants of Raman spectroscopy, providing both morphological and chemical insights.

Anisocytosis (variation in size)		Poikilocytosis (variation of shape)	
Microcytosis	Smaller than normal	Sickle cell	Sickle-shaped
Macrocytosis	Larger than normal	Burr Cell (Echinocytes)	RBCs that have evenly distributed sharp protrusions on their surface.
	Haemoglobin distribution	Schistocyte	Triangular or helmet shape, distorted or distorted RBCs, smaller than normal size
Hypochromia	Less colour than normal		
Polychromasia	More immature than normal	Elliptocyte (Ovalocytes)	Long axis twice as long as short axis, oval or elliptical shape.
	Red cell distribution	Spherocyte	Not biconcave but more spherical. There is no central pallor due to cellular dehydration.
Agglutination	Irregularly shaped clumps of RBCs		
Rouleaux	stacked together in long chains.	Stomatocyte	Uniconcave or cup-shaped RBCs with slit like areas of central pallor.
	Inclusions	Target cell (Codocytes)	RBCs are characterized by an area of enhanced increased staining that appears in the area of central pallor.
Howell-Jolly bodies	In the cytoplasm, small, round, inclusions with staining characteristics similar to nuclei. These inclusions are DNA fragments.	Blister cells	Have a vacuole or blister-like area seen in microangiopathic haemolytic anaemia
Heinz bodies	These are denatured haemoglobin (methaemoglobin) within cells and appear as small blue crystals when crystal violet stain, is used.	Tear drop (Dacrocytes)	RBCs are tear drop or pear-shaped. They are typically microcytic and usually hypochromic.
		Bite cells (Degmacytes)	These RBCs have one or more semicircular portions removed, appearing as if 'bitten.' They are seen in conditions involving oxidative damage, such as G6PD deficiency.
Pappenheimer Bodie	These are iron deposits with irregular blue granules that appear in the Wright stain.	Roleaux	Stacks of RBCs resembling coin stacks.
Basophilic stippling	These are large numbers of tiny basophilic inclusions inside RBC, with precipitated ribonucleic acid (RNA).	Acanthocytes	RBCs with irregularly spaced protuberances. They vary in size but usually have rounded ends.
Cabot's ring	Reddish filamentous rings, purple, and are remnants of the nuclear membrane.	Tomatocytes	Red cells with an oblique slit in the centre or stoma. Appear as a mouth-shaped structure in the peripheral smear.

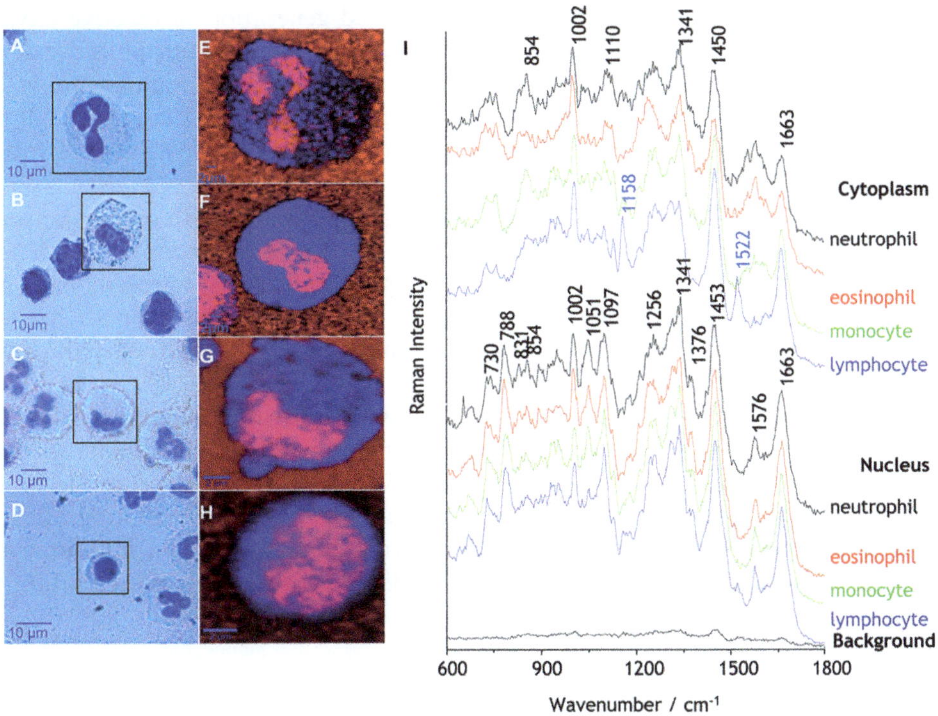

Figure 8.5. Morphological characteristics of the different leucocytes: neutrophil (A and E), eosinophil (B and F), monocyte (C and G), and lymphocyte (D and H). (A–D) white light images after Kimura staining, (E–H) false colour Raman images of the same cell using the intensity at ~788 cm^{-1} to highlight the nucleus (pink) and the intensity of the CH stretching between 2800 and 3050 cm^{-1} to colour code the overall cell area (blue). (I) Averaged Raman spectra of the cytoplasm, nucleus, and background region. Reprinted with permission from [44], copyright (2012) American Chemical Society.

Raman spectroscopy to differentiate T lymphocyte subsets, natural killer cells, and dendritic cells [45]. Neutrophils are of great interest to researchers as they form the first line of defence and employ various strategies to combat pathogens, including phagocytosis, the formation of neutrophil extracellular traps (NETs), and the release of cytokines and enzymes. Atkins *et al.* provide a brief overview of studies involving neutrophils in a review article [14].

Raman spectroscopy imaging was employed at the single-cell level to identify NETs and necrosis as inflammatory responses and to distinguish between the two processes. NETs are networks of extracellular fibres, primarily composed of nucleic acids, which serve the purpose of capturing pathogens. In contrast, necrosis represents a form of cell death that occurs as a consequence of cellular injury. Raman spectra were collected from neutrophils undergoing necrosis and neutrophils that had formed NETs. Principal component analysis was employed to distinguish between the two cellular processes [46]. Golubewa *et al.* demonstrated that exposure to carbon nanotubes leads to the activation of neutrophils, which in turn releases NET. Furthermore, it was demonstrated that the nanotubes are not phagocytosed by the neutrophils, but rather lead to the enhanced generation of reactive oxygen species and chlorine species. The free radicals generated by the neutrophils disrupted the crystal nanostructure of the nanotubes [47]. Similarly, Arzumanyan *et al.* investigated the NETotic transformation of neutrophils and demonstrated the presence of different spectral archetypes of neutrophils during the various activation stages [48].

The study by Dorosz *et al.* highlighted the molecular differences between neutrophils and eosinophils, as observed using Raman spectroscopy, CARS and fluorescence microscopy [49]. Another area of significant interest in recent years has been the differentiation of activated and naïve neutrophils using Raman spectroscopy. This has involved challenging neutrophils with a range of pathogens, including bacteria, fungi and viruses [50–52].

Similarly, monocytes and lymphocytes, the two major subpopulations of WBCs following neutrophils, have been extensively investigated using Raman spectroscopy. Figure 8.6 shows a density plot for a Raman spectral-based model using principal component-based linear discriminant analysis for differentiating infected and non-infected neutrophils, monocytes and lymphocytes, along with accuracy of the different models [50]. Chaudhary *et al.* demonstrated the differentiation of

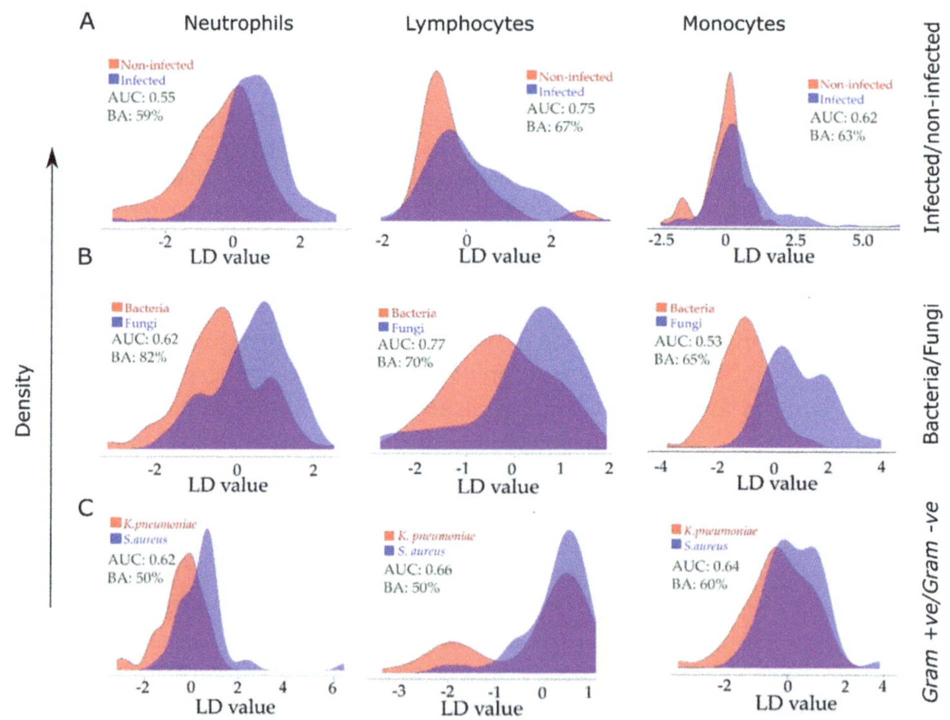

Figure 8.6. Raman spectroscopic analysis of *in vitro* stimulation of leucocyte subpopulations to differentiate (A) infected and non-infected cells, (B) bacteria and fungi (*C. albicans*) infected cells, and (C) Gram-positive (*S. aureus*) and Gram-negative (*K. pneumoniae*) bacteria. In addition, the balanced accuracy (BA) on the sample level and average AUC on cell level as been shown. Adapted from [50] CC BY 4.0.

immune cells using Raman spectroscopy, including both cell lines and primary cells isolated from blood. The performance of the Raman spectral classification model was found to be correlated with the cellular activation level, as measured through the expression of cell-specific cytokines. The targeted WBC subpopulations were monocytes, T-cells, and B-cells, and the corresponding cell lines used were THP1, Jurkat and Raji cells. It was observed that both primary cells and cell lines exhibited a comparable pattern of alterations in their biochemical profiles in response to stimulation. Nevertheless, the spectral profiles and the biochemical changes exhibited by the cells in response to the stimulant vary depending on the cell type. T-cells were activated with phytohaemagglutinin (PHA) and, as a consequence of stimulation, displayed a reduction in nucleic acid signals in line with the increase in protein phosphorylation upon activation. This phenomenon was also observed in activated Jurkat cells. The Raji cells stimulated with ionomycin and phorbol 12-myristate 13-acetate (PMA) also demonstrated a similar trend, with a decrease in nucleic acid signals observed in the Raman spectra. However, the corresponding primary B-cells, which were activated with IL-4 and CD40 ligand, did not exhibit this trend in lower nucleic acids, but rather demonstrated an increase in spectral contribution from TNF-alpha. A probable cause for this discrepancy was attributed to the difference in signalling pathway [53]. This illustrates that the different modes of action of stimulants can be observed using Raman spectroscopy.

A further study on primary monocytes isolated from peripheral blood demonstrated the potential to capture a distinct molecular fingerprint signature of *Chlamydia pneumoniae*-infected monocytes in comparison to lipopolysaccharide (LPS) infection, as observed using Raman spectroscopy. The most notable spectral alterations were observed in the lipid and fatty acid profiles. The study's key findings were that intracellular pathogens induce altered cytokine and chemokine profiles when compared to stimulation with extracellular ligands, such as LPS [54]. The polarization of peripheral blood monocyte-derived macrophages has been investigated by various researchers using Raman spectroscopy. Naumann *et al.* applied Raman spectroscopy for the characterization of macrophage phenotypes, demonstrating the spectral differentiation of M0, M1 and M2. This was correlated with flow cytometry and fluorescence imaging [55]. Similar studies were conducted by Ribeiro *et al.*, where distinct M1 and M2 stages of macrophages were analysed [56].

For investigations of immune cells, Raman spectroscopy can be combined with different platforms, such as digit holographic microscopy. This approach was employed by McReynolds and colleagues, who constructed a multimodal system capable of acquiring single-point Raman spectra and digital holographic images (DHMs) of single cells simultaneously. The multimodal system was employed to identify and differentiate immune cell populations, namely T-cells, B-cells and monocytes. The two techniques are mutually reinforcing, with DHMs relying on the linear elastic scattering of a wave front passing through the sample and Raman spectroscopy relying on the inelastic vibrational scattering from the sample. In order to classify immune cells, the researchers employed a two-pronged approach, utilizing information obtained from both Raman spectroscopy and DHM. The former technique yielded data pertaining to intracellular biochemical information, while the latter provided insights into factors such as differences in the amount of cytoplasm, stippled chromatin, nuclear morphology (size, homogeneity and nuclear folds, thickness of nuclear membrane, and presence and uniformity of nucleoli). This approach was first proposed by McReynolds *et al.* [57]. Similarly, the SERS technique was employed in conjunction with microfluidics for the detection of circulating tumour cells (CTCs) in blood, as described by Niciński *et al.* The CTCs were isolated from whole blood using size-based inertia, as the CTCs are typically larger compared to the healthy immune cells. The isolated CTCs were then passed through an optical chamber coated with a SERS-active platform based on a photovoltaic cell, after which the SERS spectra were collected. The Raman spectral-based model was able to identify and differentiate CTCs from blood cells with an accuracy of 89% [58].

8.3.4 Platelets

Platelets, also known as thrombocytes, play a crucial role in blood coagulation and are involved in the pathogenesis of various diseases, including thrombocytopenia, thrombotic thrombocytopenic purpura, Jacobsen syndrome, and others [59]. Wang *et al.* have reported the Raman spectroscopy characterization of platelets isolated from human, pig, rat and rabbit. The platelets were suspended in solution and trapped with the laser tweezers effect using a 785 nm excitation wavelength, after which Raman spectra were collected. The Raman marker peaks of platelets from humans were observed to be approximately 1157 and 1524 cm^{-1}. In the case of the pig, rat and rabbit, the intensity ratio of the aforementioned vibrations differed from that observed in the human. A multivariate statistical method was employed to demonstrate the potential for differentiating between human and animal platelets [60]. The physiology of platelets varies in disease states compared to healthy conditions. Raman spectroscopy in conjunction with Fourier transform infrared attenuated total reflectance spectroscopy was employed to differentiate between platelets of hypertensive and healthy subjects. The Raman peak of lipids due to C–C vibrations at ~960 cm^{-1} and the amide I peak at ~1658 cm^{-1} exhibited a statistically significant difference. Infrared spectra of proteins (amide I and amide II) revealed the greatest differences between the platelet spectra of healthy and hypertensive individuals (figure 8.7). Modifications in the phosphate-associated bands were observed, which may be related to the phospholipids' behaviour and the phosphorylation of proteins. These changes indicate biochemical changes at the cellular membrane level [61]. SERS has been extensively applied for the investigation of platelets, including the spectral homogeneity of human platelets obtained from individuals and comparisons between healthy and cardiovascular patients, biochemical differences in platelets from healthy and individuals with cardiovascular disease, and the assessment of the chemical composition of platelets between healthy controls, healthy individuals on antiplatelet therapy, and cardiovascular patients on antiplatelet therapy [62–65]. In the context of the SERS study, the 532 nm excitation wavelength was employed in conjunction with either gold nanoparticles or gold-titanium rough surfaces. The characteristic SERS peaks were observed at 960, 1150 and 1520 cm^{-1}. Furthermore, a Raman spectroscopy-based

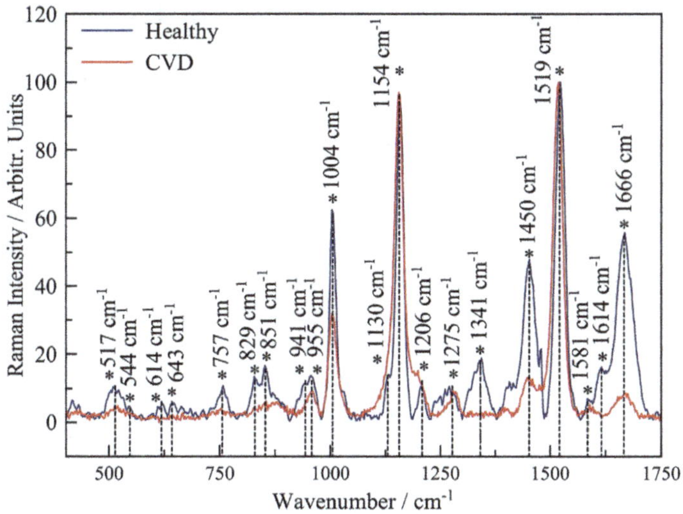

Figure 8.7. Surface enhanced Raman spectra of platelets from healthy (blue line) and individuals with cardiovascular pathology (red line). The Raman spectra were acquired using 532 nm excitation wavelength. Platelets isolated from whole blood were measured in dried condition. Reprinted from [65] CC BY 4.0.

platelet study was conducted on a mouse model of Alzheimer's disease and compared with that of healthy mice. Raman spectra acquired using a 633 nm excitation wavelength indicated the presence of protein vibrations at ~740 and 1654 cm^{-1}, which exhibited differences between healthy and diseased mice [66].

8.3.5 Plasma and serum

Plasma constitutes approximately 50% of the total blood volume, wherein the cells are suspended. As previously stated, 98% of plasma is composed of water, which is a moderately alkaline aqueous fluid. Once the clotting factors have been removed, the remaining fluid is known as serum. Plasma analysis provides insights into the metabolic processes involved, and any changes indicate the presence of disease pathology. Raman spectroscopy has been extensively applied in the investigation of plasma/serum to develop molecular-specific diagnostic platforms for biomarker sensing. The Raman spectra of blood plasma obtained using an excitation wavelength of 514 nm exhibit strong Raman peaks at 1160 and 1520 cm^{-1}, which are attributed to resonant-enhanced conjugated systems of C–C single- and double-bond stretching vibrations. These vibrations were assigned to the beta-carotenoid biochemical present in the blood. Furthermore, it was reported that Raman spectra (using 514 nm excitation) of plasma from patients with infection and other diseases, such as cancer, display a high fluorescence background compared to healthy volunteers [14]. Medipally *et al.* tested different excitation wavelengths (785, 660, 532, and 473 nm) and recorded Raman spectra of plasma [67]. The carotenoid vibrations exhibited strong scattering with excitation wavelengths of 532 and 473 nm, while the 660 nm wavelength exhibited high fluorescence, and a resonance effect was observed for carotenoid [14, 68]. In another study, Fourier transform Raman spectroscopy (1064 nm excitation wavelength) was applied for simultaneous detection of glucose, triglycerides and total cholesterol from 161 human blood samples. The blood was allowed to sediment and the plasma was collected and analyzed in liquid form. The Raman spectral model-based concentration of the detected analytes was compared with the clinically measured values [69].

Both plasma and serum have been investigated in both liquid form and as dried spots. In the case of a dried drop, the biomolecules are not distributed uniformly due to the phenomenon known as the 'coffee-ring' effect [70, 71]. The distribution of biomolecules in a dried sample spot is contingent upon the drying conditions, including temperature and the charge and size of the analyte molecules present in the sample. The low molecular weight and hydrophilic molecules within the sample tend to aggregate at the periphery of the dried spot. In contrast, hydrophobic and high-molecular-weight molecules tend to aggregate at the centre of the dried spot. Huang *et al.* conducted a study in which they analysed plasma samples from three patients with different cardiac conditions using both Raman spectroscopy (with an excitation wavelength of 785 nm) and infrared spectroscopy (figure 8.8). The study demonstrated the significance of acquiring Raman and infrared spectra representative of the inner and outer rings of the dried sample spot for the diagnostic and therapeutic evaluation of cardiac biomarkers in plasma [70]. In a review article, Parachalil *et al.*, summarized recent advances in the investigation of plasma in fluid form, including serum fractionation methods, data collection, and pre-treatment for statistical analysis [68]. Byrne *et al.* advocate for the use of fractionated serum investigations in liquid form, employing Raman spectroscopy for the quantification of high and low molecular weight compounds [72].

The optimization of Raman spectroscopy measurements of liquid plasma and serum samples has been discussed, including the use of different microscope geometries and laser wavelengths. For instance, the use of an excitation wavelength of 785 nm and an inverted geometry with the sample sandwiched between two substrates of calcium fluoride or an excitation wavelength of 532 nm can be employed. The use of a glass coverslip as a substrate has been demonstrated to enhance performance [72]. A summary of the different blood analytes that have been measured using Raman spectroscopy can be found in the work of Atkins *et al.* [14]. In the blood plasma from healthy donors, the concentration of glucose, cholesterol, triglyceride, urea, albumin, and total protein were predicted using Raman spectroscopy (with an excitation wavelength of 830 nm). To facilitate the detection of the selected analytes, the researchers removed the macromolecules that could potentially interfere with the process. Another field that has been extensively researched is the use of Raman spectroscopy for glucose sensing. Spontaneous Raman spectroscopy (532 nm excitation) demonstrated the potential for the detection of low physiopathological glucose levels [73]. The area under the curve of the 1125 cm^{-1} Raman peak is the marker for glucose concentration detection. The study also investigated lactate and urea, where the Raman marker peaks were reported to be 861 and 1005 cm^{-1}, respectively.

SERS has been extensively applied for the quantification of plasma and serum analytes and the ultrasensitive detection of these analytes even in traces [74].

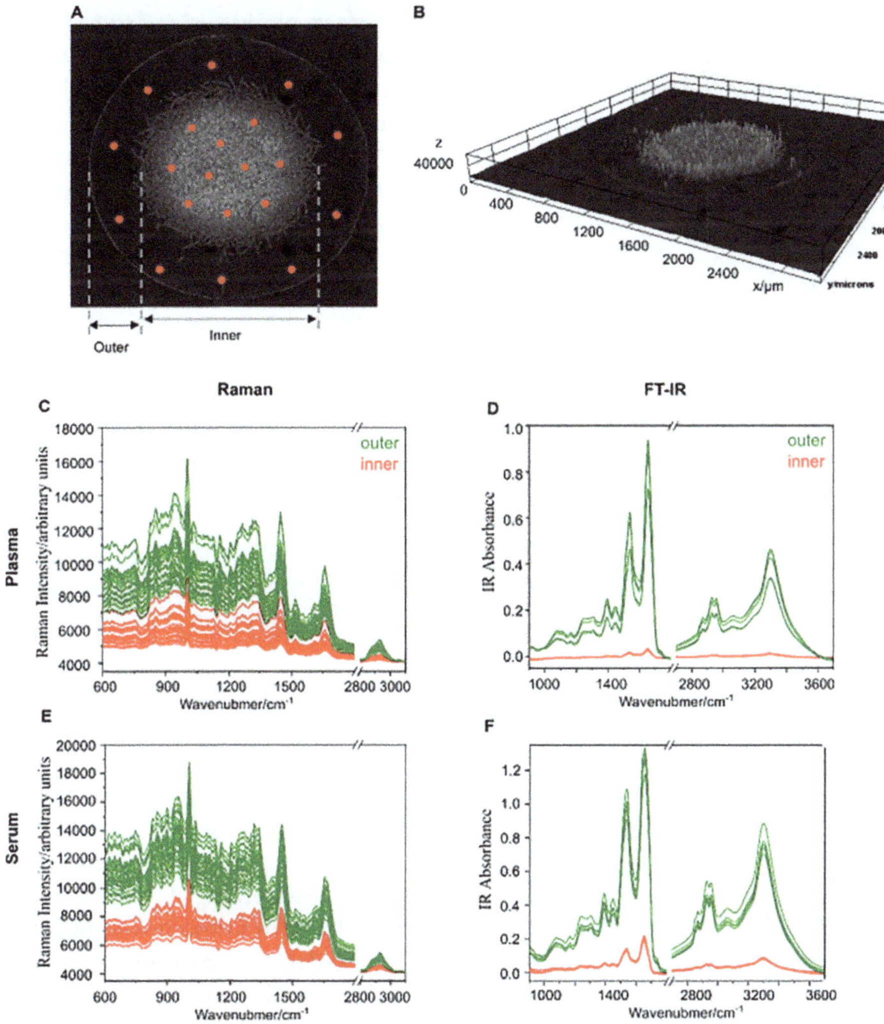

Figure 8.8. Representative image of pattern of a dried sample along and the vibrational spectra collected from different region of the dried droplet. (A) 2D-image showing data collection position from inner and outer region of the dried plasma sample spot of a healthy donor, (B) 3D-image visualizing the crystal pattern formed in the inner region of the dried sample. Scale bar is 200 μm. Unprocessed Raman spectra collected from different regions of the dried (C) plasma and (E) serum droplet. (Healthy donor, $n = 1$). Unprocessed FT-IR spectra collected from different region of the dried (D) plasma and (F) serum droplet. The vibrational spectra collected from the inner region are depicted in red and spectra from the outer-ring region in green. Reprinted from [70] CC BY 4.0.

The detection of drug concentrations in plasma and serum is another widely studied area using Raman spectroscopy. In a study by Parachalil *et al.*, the concentrations of busulfan and methotrexate in human serum were monitored within the therapeutic ranges. Methotrexate was detected at a concentration of approximately 8 μM, while busulfan could be detected in 0.0002 mg ml^{-1} [75]. In a clinical setting,

Startzbichler *et al.* evaluated 38 different biomarkers in blood serum from 328 end-stage liver disease patients using Raman spectroscopy with an excitation wavelength of 780 nm. The low concentration biomarkers, such as creatinine, were challenging to detect, whereas biomarkers such as albumin and glucose could be reliably detected. The detection of calcium and iron was more straightforward than that of sodium and chloride, because calcium and iron are predominantly protein-bound and therefore easier to detect [76]. In a separate experiment, researchers employed SERS gold-nanostar capturing target antibodies in a blood sample to diagnose and treat white matter lesions. The ultrasensitive detection of matrix metalloproteinase, soluble platelet-derived growth factor receptor, and major facilitator superfamily domain-containing Mfsd2a was demonstrated in blood samples, with a detection limit of 1 fg ml^{-1}. It was demonstrated that the aforementioned three biomarkers are specific for white matter lesions [77]. The capacity to analyse these Raman-active molecules in blood can be of significant value in the field of medical diagnostics, disease detection, and the monitoring of various health parameters. Raman spectroscopy represents a valuable tool for researchers and clinicians alike, offering insights into the molecular composition and structural changes of blood components, thereby aiding in healthcare and biomedical research.

8.4 Experimental techniques for Raman scattering of blood

8.4.1 Blood cell isolation

Raman spectroscopy is a highly effective technique for analysing biological and biomedical samples at the molecular level, offering several advantages over conventional methods for blood analysis. However, the complex and heterogeneous composition of blood presents challenges to the investigation of targeted blood components that necessitate effective sample preparation. In numerous applications, including glucose detection, forensic science, and blood drug concentration, blood has been investigated directly, either in dried or liquid form, without the necessity for any sample preparation [69, 78–80]. If the objective of the analytical investigation is to examine individual blood components, the preparation of blood samples for Raman spectroscopy represents a pivotal step in obtaining accurate and reliable results [53, 81]. The conventional techniques for the separation of specific blood components, including WBC, RBC, plasma and serum, include centrifugation, immunocapture and filtration. It is of the utmost importance to gain an understanding of the characteristics of the cell types involved to select the most appropriate isolation method. For example, WBCs comprise several subtypes, including neutrophils, monocytes, eosinophils, basophils, and lymphocytes, each of which exhibits distinct properties. The accurate identification and isolation of these subtypes is of paramount importance for the specific diagnostic and research applications in question. The selection of an appropriate method for blood cell isolation is based on specific needs, taking into account factors such as sensitivity, specificity, throughput, and compatibility with downstream applications. Centrifugation is a widely used technique that separates blood components based on density, particularly useful for isolating plasma or serum from whole blood. The most common techniques for the separation of WBC subpopulations include magnetic-activated cell sorting (MACS), fluorescence-activated cell sorting (FACS), and immunodensity cell isolation. These methods are selected based on the specific requirements of the study. Recent advancements include microfluidic-based Raman-assisted cell sorting for immune cell separation and enrichment, or plasma separation, which offers precise control and efficient handling of small sample volumes [21, 82, 83]. Optimizing blood sample preparation for Raman spectroscopy can significantly enhance its diagnostic capabilities. Pre-treatment methods such as peroxide treatment for haemoglobin elimination or magnetic labelling for leucocyte purification can enhance the accuracy and reliability of Raman spectroscopic analysis. In conclusion, the selection of an appropriate method for blood sample preparation based on specific requirements significantly impacts the quality and usefulness of the results. With the development of innovative techniques and careful consideration of the unique properties of blood components, Raman spectroscopy can be effectively utilized for a wide range of diagnostic and research purposes.

Centrifugation: Centrifugation is a highly efficient and cost-effective method for the sorting of cells based on their physical characteristics. The process entails the application of high-speed spinning, which enables the separation of cells according to their size, density, and shape. This process is based on the principles of gravity and centrifugal force, which are used to sediment different cell fractions. The sedimentation rate is influenced by several factors, including the mass, density, and volume of the cells, the density of the medium, the shape of the cells, and friction. A variety of centrifugation techniques are employed for the separation of blood components, including differential centrifugation and density gradient centrifugation. In contrast to density gradient centrifugation, differential centrifugation does not require any reagents and is based on the mass of the particles. This method is employed for the isolation of buffy coat from whole blood and plasma/serum. In contrast, in density gradient centrifugation, single or multiple reagents with varying densities are employed, depending on the targeted blood component. As cells traverse the gradient, larger cells attain a stable point at an earlier stage than smaller cells. This is because smaller cells must traverse a longer distance through the larger particle zone before reaching a stable position. Consequently, smaller cells require a longer period to traverse the larger particle zone and to settle at a deeper position within the gradient. The time required for this process varies following the size of the cells and may be employed to ascertain the dimensions of the cells. Density gradient centrifugation is a widely employed technique for the separation of blood cellular components. Each cell exhibits distinctive physical characteristics, including size and density (table 8.2), which are fundamental aspects of its biological composition. These characteristics can be employed to separate and isolate individual cells.

Table 8.2. Classification and features of blood cells.

Blood cells		Major subpopulations	Size in diameter (μm)	Density (g ml^{-1})
WBC	Granulocytes	Eosinophils	10–12	1.09–1.1
		Neutrophils	10–12	1.08–1.09
		Basophils	8–10	1.072–1.078
	Mononuclear cells	Monocytes	12–20	1.067–1.077
		Lymphocytes (Natural killer, B, and T-cells)	10–14	1.073–1.077
RBC	Erythrocytes		7–8	1.098
Platelets	Thrombocytes		2–4	

Density gradient reagents: Density gradient reagents are a class of substances that are used in the process of density gradient centrifugation. Density gradient centrifugation is a highly specialized process that employs specific reagents with distinct densities to separate different cell populations from heterogeneous mixtures.

The utilization of such reagents can markedly enhance the efficiency of the process and improve the purity and yield of the isolated cells. The failure to select an appropriate medium can result in the inaccurate separation of cell populations, which may lead to unreliable data and conclusions. It is therefore of the utmost importance to exercise great care when selecting the appropriate medium in order to ensure the effective separation of cells. It is of the utmost importance to prevent the cells from clustering and instead create a well-defined interface to achieve optimal results. The quality of reagents is of paramount importance in this context, as the use of substandard or unsuitable reagents can result in unsatisfactory cell separation and reduced yield. Table 8.3 lists some of the reagents commonly employed for density gradient centrifugation in blood cell isolations.

The choice of density gradient medium is based on the size and density of the targeted cells. For instance, for the isolation of mononuclear cells (PBMCs) from peripheral blood, bone marrow, and cord blood, it is recommended to utilize medium with a density of 1.077 g ml^{-1}, such as Lymphoprep™ or Ficoll-Paque™ [84]. The whole blood (if required, diluted with saline) is then layered on top of the density gradient medium usually with a ratio of 1:2 between medium and blood followed by centrifugation [85]. Similarly, polymorphprep medium is used for the isolation of granulocytes. A combination of media can be used to obtain both mononuclear cells and granulocytes from the whole blood (figure 8.9).

Immunodensity cell isolation: Immunodensity cell separation, erythrocyte rosetting, is a negative selection technique that combines antibody-based labelling with density gradient centrifugation. In this process, antibodies are added to a whole blood sample, which then attaches to unwanted cells and binds them

Table 8.3. Commonly used density gradient reagents for isolating blood cells.

Mediums	Features	Types of cells
LymphoPrep™ and Lympholyte®	The two media are similar in composition, being prepared, sterile, and endotoxin-tested density gradient media, comprising sodium diatrizoate and polysaccharide. The medium is highly effective for purifying human mononuclear cells (monocytes and lymphocytes) from peripheral blood, cord blood, and bone marrow. The density of the medium is 1.077 g ml^{-1}.	PBMC
Percoll®	The solution comprises a colloid of silica particles coated with polyvinylpyrrolidone (PVP). This mixture is employed for the separation of subcellular particles, organelles, viruses, and cells. The density of the substance is 1.131 g ml^{-1}.	All blood cell types
Polymorphprep	This reagent offers a practical and effective method for isolating neutrophils from peripheral blood, which can be employed for investigative purposes. The solution contains 9.1% (w/v) sodium diatrizoate and 5.7% (w/v) polysaccharide.	Neutrophils
Polysucrose 400 or Histopaque	It is a non-ionic synthetic polymer derived from sucrose. The sucrose polymer is combined with sodium diatrizoate to form gradients.	WBCs and RBCs Thrombocyte
Ficoll-Paque®	This is similar to polysucrose, but is osmotically inert, in contrast to polysucrose.	WBCs and RBCs Mononuclear cells and granulocytes
Optiprep®	The composition of the product is iodixanol in water. The Monocytes are of a lower density and larger diameter, allowing them to float more quickly through a density barrier than the lymphocytes.	Monocytes

to RBCs, forming immunorosettes. During centrifugation, the unwanted cells aggregate with the RBC, leaving the target cells in a layer above the density medium. The immunodensity cell separation technique is a straightforward method that can be incorporated into existing density gradient centrifugation protocols, enabling the isolation of specific cell subsets directly from whole blood without the need for additional specialized equipment beyond a centrifuge [86].

Immunomagnetic cell separation (MACS): Immunomagnetic cell separation is a sophisticated and widely utilized technique that employs magnetic particles to selectively isolate particular cell populations of interest from a complex mixture of cells, such as those present in whole blood. The technique effectively and efficiently separates target cells from non-target cells in a

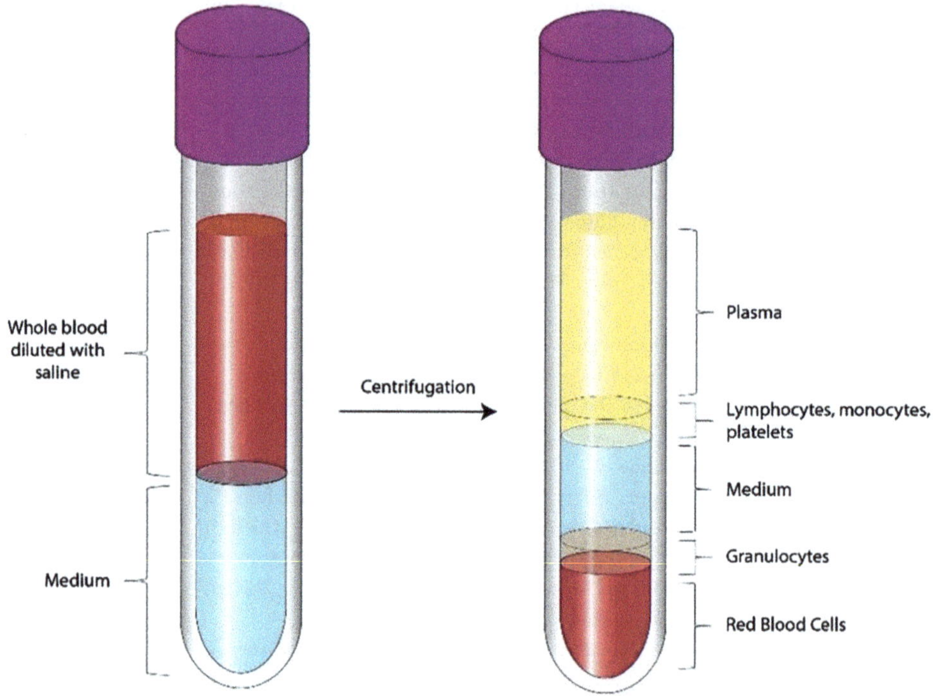

Figure 8.9. Schematic illustration of the cell separation using density gradient centrifugation

heterogeneous cell population by binding magnetic particles to the cell surface proteins of the target cells using antibodies, enzymes, streptavidin, or lectins. The process entails the placement of the sample in an electromagnetic field, which attracts the magnetic particles along with the labelled cells, physically separating them from the remainder of the blood sample and non-target cells. This results in the non-target cells remaining in the supernatant, while the desired cells, labelled cells, can be used either directly or separated from the magnetic beads by cleaving the binding agents. The MACS method allows for the selective separation of positively and negatively labelled cells. The selection method employed is contingent upon several factors, including the desired cell purity, the availability of specific antibodies, and the intended downstream studies. In positive selection, the desired cells are labelled with magnetic particles, which enables them to be captured in an electromagnetic field while the unwanted cells are discarded. Conversely, negative selection involves leaving the desired cells in the supernatant while magnetically removing the undesired cells. In the context of cell separation, positive selection is the preferred method when high purities are required. Conversely, negative selection is the preferred method when untouched cells are desired, or when the binding of an antibody to the desired cell may affect downstream studies. In the context of Raman spectroscopy, the negative selection method is employed to obtain 'untouched cells.' This approach circumvents the potential for interference from magnetic beads and binding agents. This highly precise and efficient technique is widely utilized in medical and research settings for the targeted isolation and purification of cells of interest, thereby enabling the generation of pure populations of cells. This, in turn, facilitates the conduct of precise studies and experiments, which in turn lead to a better understanding of biological processes and advances medical treatments [85, 87].

Flow cytometry: Flow cytometry and its advanced variant, fluorescence-activated cell sorting (FACS), represent highly sophisticated techniques for the identification, sorting, and analysis of individual cells with exceptional precision. Laser technology is employed to measure the unique characteristics of cells, including size, shape, granularity, labelled surface and internal markers. This technique enables the detection and distinction of highly sensitive cells through the use of fluorescent probes, even in heterogeneous cell populations [88]. The choice of blood cell isolation technique is influenced by several factors, including the intended use and the cell types in question. In certain instances, the utilization of multiple techniques in conjunction with one another may prove advantageous in the isolation of a specific cell population, as exemplified in figure 8.10.

Microfluidic cell sorting: Microfluidics, colloquially referred to as 'lab-on-a-chip' devices, represents a category of cell separation methods that manipulate fluids on a microscopic level, to facilitate single-cell isolation. Their compact size offers a multitude of benefits, including the reduced number of samples and reagents needed for operation. Their portability renders them an optimal choice for diagnostic applications in the field. Microfluidic methods can be divided into two categories: active and passive systems. These can be further classified according to the presence or absence of cell labelling. Microfluidics offers a plethora of techniques for the isolation of cells, including acoustophoresis, aqueous two-phase systems, biomimetic microfluidics, cell affinity chromatography, deterministic lateral displacement, electrophoretic sorting, field flow fractionation, gravity and sedimentation, magnetophoresis, microfiltration, and optical sorting (figure 8.11). Acoustophoresis employs sound waves to separate cells based on their size and mechanical properties. Aqueous two-phase systems employ the principle of phase separation to divide cells according to their affinity for different phases of a two-phase liquid. Biomimetic microfluidics emulates physiological conditions for cell growth and differentiation. Cell affinity chromatography employs ligands to facilitate the capture of specific cells. The deterministic lateral displacement method is based on the size-based separation of cells. Electrophoretic sorting is a method of cell separation based on the electrophoretic mobility of the cells in question. In field flow fractionation, a combination of applied field and fluid flow is used to separate cells. The separation of cells based on their density and size is achieved through the application of gravity and sedimentation. It is possible to combine

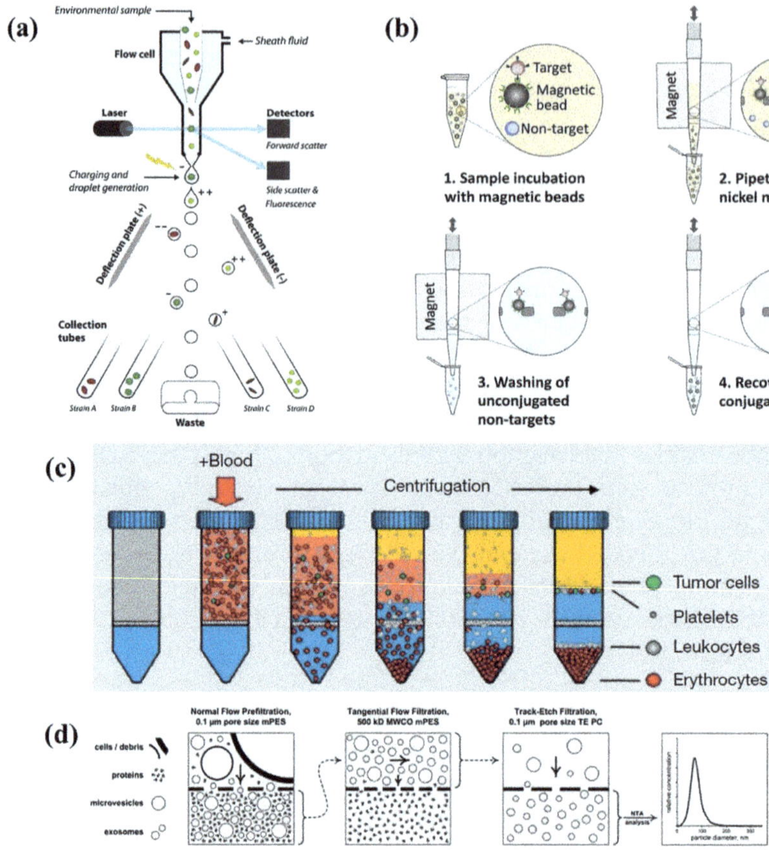

Figure 8.10. Schematic illustration of: (a) Fluorescence-activated cell sorting for sorting different cells. (b) Immunomagnetic separation in a pipette tip by Magnetic-activated cell sorting. (c) Density gradient centrifugation for isolation and detection of cancer cells. (d) Ultrafiltration for isolation and characterization of functional exosomes. Reprinted from [89], copyright (2022), with permission from Elsevier B.V.

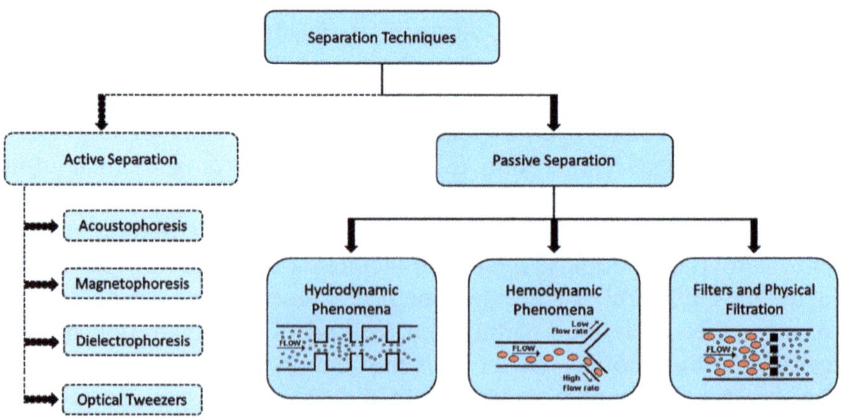

Figure 8.11. Classification of the microfluidic systems. Reproduced from [91] CC BY 4.0.

microfluidic-based cell sorting with Raman spectroscopy-assisted cell sorting. The use of Raman spectral fingerprinting allows for the sorting of cells according to their desired characteristics, thus circumventing the necessity for fluorescence labelling. In the context of Raman-assisted cell sorting, spontaneous Raman spectroscopy and Raman image activation are employed using stimulated Raman scattering technique [90–95].

Buoyancy-activated cell sorting (BACS): BACS represents a highly efficient cell separation technique that has gained considerable popularity in recent years. The technique employs the use of microbubbles, which are formed from glass, and antibodies that are specific to the target cells. Once these microbubbles are introduced into the sample, they bind selectively to the target cells, forming a complex that is denser than the surrounding fluid. The increased buoyancy force causes the microbubbles to rise to the surface of the sample, carrying the target cells with them and thereby separating the target cells from the rest of the sample. This technique is highly efficient and enables the isolation of pure cell populations [96].

Aptamer technology: Single-stranded RNA or DNA oligonucleotides, designated aptamers, exhibit specific structural characteristics that facilitate their capacity to bind to a target with exceptional precision. The systematic evolution of ligands by exponential enrichment (SELEX) technology enables the screening and synthesis of aptamers to target any type of cell with unparalleled accuracy. Aptamers' superior specificity and affinity towards their targets render them an optimal choice for labelling with fluorochromes or magnetic particles for cell separation. Aptamers possess an unparalleled advantage in that they exhibit an unmatched lack of immunogenicity. Fluorophore-labelled aptamers have been demonstrated to be an effective tool for the sorting of mesenchymal stem cells from bone marrow, while RNA aptamers have been employed to isolate mouse embryonic stem cells with unparalleled efficiency [90, 97].

8.4.2 Raman instrumentation for blood investigations

Raman spectroscopy for blood investigations, especially for haematology applications requires sophisticated technology designed to capture and analyse the Raman spectra of blood samples. This process requires precise and sensitive equipment to ensure the accuracy and reliability of the results. Key components include the laser source, optical components, sample holders and detection systems. Laser wavelengths commonly used for blood Raman scattering range from 532 to 1064 nm, with each wavelength offering specific advantages. Optical components such as mirrors, lenses and filters play a critical role in directing and focusing the laser beam onto the blood sample while minimizing signal loss and background noise. Detection systems are typically based on charge-coupled device (CCD) detectors, which capture the scattered Raman signal with high sensitivity and distinguish between weak Raman signals and background noise. Due to the weak nature of Raman scattering, it is essential to deliver sufficient laser power to the sample to generate detectable Raman photons within a reasonable integration time. However, considerations of sample photodamage, instrument stability and the optical properties of the target sample influence the choice of laser wavelength. NIR excitation sources (i.e., 785 nm excitation) are often preferred for blood studies due to their lower attenuation coefficients and reduced fluorescence background. The evolution of Raman instrumentation has seen advances such as the adoption of diode laser technology, which offers smaller, more efficient solutions compared to traditional laser sources. External cavity diode lasers (ECDLs) have proven to be robust and cost-effective light sources for Raman applications, offering stable output and wavelength tunability. Modern Raman systems typically comprise a dispersive Raman detection system with a short focal length imaging spectrograph coupled to a cooled CCD camera, allowing fast spectral acquisition and accurate measurements [98–100].

8.4.3 Raman spectral data acquisition and analysis

8.4.3.1 Collecting Raman images

The process of analysing specific regions of blood components through Raman spectroscopy can be conducted in two distinct ways: mapping and imaging [101].

8.4.3.2 Raman mapping

Mapping necessitates the sequential measurement of each adjacent region's spectrum as the region is positioned within the beam and the spectrum is recorded. The measurement is then repeated until the entire region of interest has been covered. Two mapping methods for analysing the collected data are point-by-point and line-focus mapping.

8.4.3.3 Point focus mapping

The Raman microscope employs a laser beam to focus the laser onto a specific point on the sample. The sample is positioned on a motorized stage that facilitates the movement of the sample beneath the laser beam. The spectrometer collects spectra from a series of points distributed across the sample. The spatial resolution of an image depends on the dimensions of the laser spot and the distance between the acquisition points. A smaller laser spot size is produced by higher magnification and shorter laser wavelengths, which in turn results in a higher resolution. To ensure optimal results, the sample stages must have a sufficiently large travel range and a step size that is smaller than the smallest spot size.

8.4.3.4 Line focus mapping

In contrast to the conventional approach of illuminating a single point on the sample, line illumination is achieved using a laser, which enables the collection of spectra from multiple positions on the sample simultaneously. This approach not only enhances the efficiency of the process but also reduces the overall time required for data acquisition. This approach allows for the utilization of higher total laser powers without the risk of damaging the sample. A more sophisticated technique, designated as line-focus imaging, entails the illumination of a vertical line on the sample. It is of paramount importance to consider the potential consequences of undersampling, which occurs when the laser spot or line is smaller than the spacing between acquisition points, during imaging activities. Throughout the scanning process, the system employs a laser line to traverse the sample along the y-axis. Concurrently, the CCD detector acquires data from a multitude of points on the sample. The width of the laser line is employed as the step size in the x-direction. This scanning method ensures comprehensive coverage of the sample, although it may not be the swiftest alternative available. Nevertheless, the system is adept at acquiring detailed information about the analysed sample.

8.4.3.5 Raman imaging

In contrast, imaging is analogous to taking a digital photograph, necessitating the focused imaging of the sample onto an array detector. The intensity of the radiation passing through each region of the sample is simultaneously measured at each pixel. It is crucial to highlight that mapping experiments, where the sample is moved in both the x and y dimensions, should not be classified as imaging since the spectra have not been acquired by an array detector. Nevertheless, the spectra can be treated in the same manner as if they had been acquired with an array detector. Hybrid mapping/imaging instruments are commercially available, which employ a linear array of detectors to acquire a line map comprising 32 detectors. This is followed by the movement of the sample, after which the process is repeated. In hyperspectral imaging, images are recorded at more than 10 wavelength regions simultaneously with a two-dimensional array detector. The degree of resolution achievable in imaging is significantly influenced by the magnification optics employed in the system and the dimensions of the elements comprising the detector. Nevertheless, it is crucial to acknowledge that these constraints are ultimately determined by the intrinsic wavelike nature of light, which establishes the maximum achievable resolution at a level just below a micrometre.

8.4.3.6 Raman spectra analysis

Raman imaging offers a diverse range of analytical techniques that can be employed based on the software utilized in conjunction with the system. One straightforward approach to displaying Raman data is to visualize the intensity of a single frequency within the spectrum. This method is rapid and straightforward, yet it is susceptible to misinterpretation due to its inability to differentiate between intensities that originate from a Raman band of interest and those associated with broad background fluorescence. An alternative approach is to utilize curve fit parameters to fit a theoretical curve to each Raman band in each spectrum of a Raman image. This method enables the computation of parameters such as the Raman shift, bandwidth, or relative intensity. In Raman images, variations in the Raman shift of a band can indicate the presence of localized stress, while variations in the Raman bandwidth can reveal different degrees of crystallinity.

Multivariate parameters represent a powerful option since they utilize information from the entire spectrum, resulting in higher-quality Raman images with enhanced chemical specificity. In contrast to alternative methodologies that depend on a single Raman band parameter (e.g., intensity at a single frequency or one curve-fitted band), multivariate approaches leverage the entire spectral data set. Multivariate analysis is a valuable tool for the analysis of complex samples containing multiple components. If reference spectra for the chemical components present within a sample are available, Raman images can be generated to illustrate their distribution. In such instances, component analysis techniques such as direct classical least squares (DCLS) or non-negative least squares (NNLS) would be employed, enabling the generation of quantitative concentration estimates. These methods are suitable for the analysis of samples containing known components. In the absence of reference spectra, unsupervised chemometric methods, such as cluster analysis or principal component analysis (PCA), may still be employed. These sophisticated analytical techniques analyse the systematic variance between Raman spectra to predict the spectral components and to detect structures within biological samples, including blood, which often contains no pure biochemicals. In conclusion, Raman imaging offers a range of analysis options, ranging from simple univariate band parameters to complex multivariate methods, depending on the software used with the system and the type of sample being analysed. By using appropriate analysis methods, Raman imaging can provide valuable insights into the chemical composition of a sample and help researchers make informed decisions.

8.4.3.7 Cosmic ray removal

During Raman measurements of extended duration, it is not uncommon to observe abrupt peaks in the spectra that are not directly related to the sample being analysed. These spikes are the consequence of cosmic rays colliding with the detector, which can result in the generation of spurious features that are typically narrower than Raman bands. Cosmic rays are high-energy particles originating from outer space and entering the Earth's atmosphere, resulting in a cascade of secondary cosmic rays. These random and unavoidable events can result in the generation of spurious spikes in the Raman spectra, which can present a challenge for the analysis of the sample being studied. It is therefore of great importance to be aware of the effects of cosmic rays on Raman measurements and to take appropriate measures to mitigate their impact.

The removal of cosmic rays from spectral data offers several benefits. Firstly, the process of data processing and analysis is simplified, which in turn facilitates the interpretation of the data. Furthermore, the removal of these features allows the spectral band shape to be maintained, which is of great importance when analysing the data using unsupervised chemometric methods such as PCA. This approach ensures that the data being analysed is solely sample-related, such as Raman or photoluminescence. Finally, the removal of cosmic rays from images eliminates the presence of artifacts, thereby enhancing the representativeness and visual appeal of the images.

It should be noted that the removal of cosmic rays may be undertaken before and after data collection, depending on the specific Raman system in question. Before data collection, cosmic rays can be removed through the utilization of a filtering option that involves the acquisition of two additional accumulations for each desired spectrum. For each Raman frequency, the median of the three values is calculated, thereby automatically eliminating cosmic rays of all shapes and sizes. This is because cosmic rays will always be an extreme value rather than the median. This method also serves to minimize noise. Although this approach may necessitate a threefold increase in the time required to collect the data, the acquisition time can be reduced, and the number of accumulations can be increased to maintain a relatively short total experiment time. During data collection, it is possible to remove a small number of these cosmic rays through the use of a zap function. This technique involves replacing the affected region with a single line, which effectively addresses the issue of obvious cosmic ray features. However, in instances where multiple spectra are present within a single data file, this method becomes impractical and time-consuming. Consequently, alternative methods may be required to effectively remove cosmic rays from the data.

8.4.3.8 Fluorescent background removal

Background subtraction is an extremely effective data processing technique that is highly recommended to eliminate fluorescence signals that can interfere with Raman spectra. In contrast to alternative methodologies that depend on specific components of the confocal Raman microscope to physically impede the emission of fluorescence, this technique eliminates the fluorescence after the data has been recorded. By selecting a user-defined filter size, the degree to which the background is subtracted can be controlled. The filter size can be adjusted to allow for the degree of background subtraction to be fine-tuned based on the complexity of the sample, thus preventing any unwanted changes or artifacts in the processed spectrum. The filter can be applied to individual spectra or entire data sets comprising Raman maps and kinetic studies. This method is particularly valuable when Raman bands are sufficiently intense to be observed above fluorescence emissions and not completely obscured in the raw spectrum. This method is highly effective and is therefore recommended for the accurate and reliable analysis of Raman spectroscopy data.

8.4.4 Challenges and limitations in Raman spectroscopy blood analysis

Raman spectroscopy has the potential to revolutionize clinical applications, particularly in blood analysis. However, its efficacy is currently constrained by several challenges that demand meticulous attention. It is therefore of the utmost importance to address these challenges to ensure the reliability and clinical relevance of Raman spectroscopy in haematology. One of the principal challenges encountered when acquiring Raman spectra of blood is the low signal-to-noise ratio and signal-to-background ratio. In addition, there is a risk of photodamage due to laser-induced heating. This is particularly pertinent when investigating whole blood, RBCs, isolated haemoglobin, and live WBCs. Furthermore, the Raman signal is accompanied by a substantial non-Raman background, including endogenous sample fluorescence, which affects the reliability of RS measurements. The presence of large fluorescence backgrounds, accompanied by a correspondingly high photon count, is a common phenomenon observed in blood samples. This results in a type of noise known as shot noise, rather than other sources of stochastic noise, such as dark noise or CCD readout noise. Shot noise is typically the most significant source of noise in Raman spectroscopy. The phenomenon of shot noise is attributed to the discrete nature of the detected photon stream. To reduce its impact, it is possible to increase the data acquisition time to maximize the occupied fraction of the dynamic range of the sensor. Furthermore, averaging over multiple spectral accumulations can also be employed to mitigate the effects of shot noise. To obtain a satisfactory Raman signal, it is often necessary to use long exposure times of several seconds. However, this increases the detector's vulnerability to high-energy cosmic rays, which are known to affect CCD sensors. Such anomalies typically manifest as narrow peaks in Raman spectra and, if not removed, can affect regression and discrimination models. Furthermore, the intricacy of Raman spectral data from healthy and diseased blood necessitates the utilization of machine learning and multivariate analysis methodologies. To overcome these challenges, it is essential to employ optimized experimental design and instrumentation [98, 102].

8.5 Clinical applications of Raman spectroscopy in haematology

It is widely acknowledged that Raman spectroscopy represents a valuable tool for clinical diagnostics. This is also reflected in the broad range of diseases that have been covered using this technique. The following section presents a selection of recent studies in which the Raman spectroscopic characterization of whole blood or blood components has enabled the development of alternative diagnostic approaches. For work conducted prior to 2017, we recommend the excellent review by Atkins *et al.* [14]

8.5.1 Cancer

A tumour in the body is associated with characteristic metabolic byproducts, circulating tumour cells or DNA, or, in the case of blood cancer, with alterations in the blood cells themselves. Due to its high specificity towards chemical changes, Raman spectroscopy is able to capture these changes and permit discrimination between healthy and diseased states. Nargis *et al.* were able to differentiate between healthy individuals and patients with different stages of breast cancer by analysing Raman spectra from blood plasma samples [103]. Giamougiannis *et al.* focused their efforts on improving ovarian cancer detection by spectroscopic analysis of urine and blood samples—both plasma and serum were investigated [104]. They were able to confirm findings of similar studies according to which Mucin 16 or Cancer Antigen 125 (CA125) is likely to be a major contributor to the spectral differences between cancerous and benign states. Da Silva *et al.* investigated whole blood as well as plasma samples from leukaemia patients and healthy subjects. Discrimination between the two classes was successful for both sample types using either PCA or partial least squares (PLS) [105]. For increasing the chances of survival, it is vital to catch the cancer as soon as possible. Xu *et al.* developed a biosensor for detecting circular RNA from blood serum, which is characteristic for tumour formation. While the introduced technique utilizes a nucleic acid probe and thus is not label-free, it demonstrates how Raman spectroscopy enables highly sensitive quantification by using plasmonic enhancement [106]. Another work utilizing SERS by Xue *et al.* analyses the Raman signatures of blood sera from patients with oral squamous cell carcinoma. The SERS spectra allowed discriminating between different tumour stages [107]. In a similar fashion, Hong *et al.* acquired SERS spectra from serum samples stemming from patients with colorectal cancer. Using a support-vector machine (SVM) as a classification method, healthy and diseased states were successfully distinguished with 89% accuracy [108]. Koster *et al.* were able to significantly improve the accuracy of their models for identifying head and neck cancer patients from a mixed cohort by combining Raman spectra acquired from plasma and saliva samples [109]. The strategy of combining two sample types that can be gained with minimal additional strain on the patients, but providing a greater depth of information, deserves to be considered for future studies.

8.5.2 Dementia

Dementia is a term that encompasses different diseases associated with cognitive deterioration. With rising age, the probability of developing some form of dementia is increasing. Alzheimer's disease (AD) is the most prevalent form of dementia, but also vascular dementia and dementia with Lewy bodies (DLB) are common. Currently, there is a lack of non-invasive and cost-efficient diagnostic tools to differentiate between them and enable early detection and treatment. To that end, Paraskevaidi *et al.* characterized blood plasma samples of early-stage AD, late-stage AD and DLB patients as well as healthy controls. Using an SVM for classification they were able to differentiate between all groups with a specificity of at least 77%. Importantly, early-stage AD could also be distinguished from healthy controls with 84% sensitivity and 86% specificity [110].

8.5.3 Sepsis and infection

Infectious diseases can be caused by bacterial, viral or fungal pathogens. In the majority of cases, infections are non-lethal and can be effectively treated or successfully fought by a competent immune system. However, if the patient suffers from severe trauma due to surgery or has certain co-morbidities, an infection can develop into a life-threatening condition such as sepsis or septic shock, when the host response becomes dysregulated. An early diagnosis is vital to save the patient's life and prevent permanent organ damage.

We were able to show that the Raman spectroscopic profiles of leucocytes from peripheral blood combined with biomarker levels of C-reactive protein (CRP), procalcitonin (PCT) and Interleukin 6 (IL-6) improve diagnostic accuracy of identifying septic patients [111]. In an *in vitro* study involving leucocytes, we showed how their Raman spectroscopic profiles enable differentiation between fungal and bacterial infection [51]. Leucocytes, more specifically neutrophil granulocytes, also display a typical response upon viral infection. Pistiki *et al.* demonstrated in an *in vitro* study that pre-activated neutrophil granulocytes stimulated with SARS-CoV-2 display a characteristic Raman signature, which is correlated to with the expression of proinflammatory cytokines [52]. In a recent study, Pietruszewska *et al.* characterized lymphocytes via Raman spectroscopy in patients infected with Epstein–Barr virus for a period over 30 days. The spectral data enabled them to observe immunoglobulin activation, which was reached on average at the fourth day of hospitalization [112]. Several approaches, mostly SERS-based, exist for detecting Hepatitis B and C infections using Raman spectroscopy. Nasir *et al.* analyzed RNA extracted from blood samples of Hepatitis C patients and healthy volunteers via SERS and found distinct differences between the spectra of the two groups [113]. Kashif *et al.* analyzed serum samples of Hepatitis C positive and negative individuals, both with Raman spectroscopy and SERS. They found that the SERS approach enables a more reliable quantification of the viral load [114]. Shakeel *et al.* integrated filtration as a sample preparation method in the SERS-based analysis of serum samples for improved differentiation between healthy volunteers and Hepatitis C patients [115]. Ahmad *et al.* determined the viral load of Hepatitis B virus (HBV) in serum using SERS [116], while Khan *et al.* were able to differentiate between healthy and infected individuals using conventional Raman spectroscopy [117]. Another currently highly relevant viral infection is dengue fever. Mahmood *et al.* demonstrated how Raman spectroscopy can be used as a screening tool to detect the dengue virus in blood serum with high accuracy [118]. More detailed information on the potential of vibrational spectroscopy for diagnosis of sepsis and infection can be found in the review by Cornfield *et al.* [119]. Another recent review by Tannert *et al.* focuses on how photonic methods can aid in monitoring treatment for sepsis and infection [120].

8.5.4 Malaria

Malaria is caused by parasites of the genus *Plasmodium*. It is prevalent in tropical and subtropical regions and transmitted to humans through bites of infected mosquitoes. The parasites first settle in the liver, multiply and subsequently infect RBCs. As the parasites induce characteristic chemical changes in the erythrocytes, Raman spectroscopy is well-suited for detection. Chen *et al.* characterized RBCs of malaria patients via SERS and were able to differentiate between different stages of infection [121]. Wang *et al.* established a SERS-based screening method for *Plasmodium falciparum* and *Plasmodium vivax* using whole blood as a sample [122].

8.5.5 Endometriosis

Endometriosis is a painful condition occurring in women due to the growth of endometrial tissue outside the uterus. Mostly, such growth of tissue occurs in the pelvic region, but also other organs can be affected. Depending on the location of the abnormal spread of endometrial tissue, it can be very hard to diagnose, and a biopsy is necessary. Unfortunately, it often takes several years until women receive a correct diagnosis. A non-invasive method would help to significantly shorten this time and alleviate the suffering. As a first step towards this, Parlatan *et al.* have investigated blood serum samples from endometriosis patients and healthy volunteers via Raman spectroscopy. They were able to differentiate between the two groups using k-nearest neighbour (kNN) classification algorithm with high accuracy [123].

8.5.6 Drug monitoring

A critical factor in the successful treatment of infectious diseases is the proper dosage of the antibiotic or anti-infective agent. While an overdose will harm the patient due to increased toxicity and side effects, an underdose will not be able to eradicate the causative pathogen. Accordingly, technologies enabling therapeutic drug monitoring are of great importance. Parachalil *et al.* established a method that allows determining the serum levels of Methotrexate and Busulfan, which are both important anti-cancer drugs [75]. Their approach involves filtration as sample preparation procedure and subsequent Raman spectroscopic characterization of the filtrate. They were able to quantify both drugs in the clinically relevant range. Göksel *et al.* also developed an approach for quantification of Methotrexate in blood serum. For enhancing the Raman signal, they incorporated SERS substrates coated with silver nanoparticles enabling detection of Methotrexate within only 10 min. Increased sensitivity can by obtain by an additional filtration step, which leads to a total analysis time of 40 min [124]. More SERS-based strategies for drug monitoring were developed by Fornasaro *et al.* for Imatinib [125] and by Panikar *et al.* for Paclitaxel and Cyclophosphamide [126]. Adomavičiūtė *et al.* employed SERS as well for determining low concentrations of Aspirin (salicylic acid) in blood serum down to 3 mM [127].

8.5.7 Antibiotic susceptibility testing (AST)

Due to the dramatic rise of antibiotic resistance in the last decades, it has become more and more urgent for physicians not only to identify the bacterial species causing the infection, but also their resistance profiles. While there are well-established protocols based on cultivation, in practice it takes up to 72 h until the final result is available. Especially for critically ill patients this is too large a time span, and alternative approaches need to be developed. Kirchhoff *et al.* were able to determine Ciprofloxacin resistance within less than three hours by combining dielectrophoresis as sample preparation method with Raman spectroscopy for phenotypical characterization of the bacterial strains [128]. Their assay involves an incubation step where the bacterial cells interact with different concentrations of the antibiotic. The metabolic changes induced upon this interaction can be traced via the Raman spectra. Another promising approach for Raman-based AST stems from Han *et al.* They established a protocol that allows analysing bacteria from positive blood cultures. In order to isolate the bacterial cells from the complex sample, selective lysis of the RBCs was performed followed by several washing steps. Subsequently the isolated bacterial cells were treated with the antibiotics oxacillin (*Escherichia coli*) and cefotaxime (*Staphylococcus aureus*). After another purification step the bacterial cells are transferred to a SERS substrate and the spectra are acquired. Resistant and sensitive strains can be identified according to characteristic spectral features [129].

8.5.8 Diabetes and glucose monitoring

Continuous glucose monitoring (CGM) has significantly improved diabetes management [130]. While many commercially available wearable devices rely on enzyme electrodes as sensing technology [131], optical methods are investigated as promising options as well. A fluorescence-based system has already been commercialized [131]. Vibrational spectroscopic techniques, such as Raman and infrared (IR) spectroscopy, provide insights into the chemical composition of the sample and therefore are well suited to identify abnormal deviations of biomarkers in body fluids (interstitial fluid, saliva, tears, sweat, blood, etc) in diabetic individuals. A non-invasive method for monitoring glucose in blood utilizing Raman spectroscopy was introduced by Li *et al.* [132]. They were able to directly measure glucose concentration in the microvessels in the superficial layer of the human nailfold utilizing Raman spectroscopy. Wang *et al.* used Fourier transform Raman spectroscopy to simultaneously quantify glucose, triglycerides, and total cholesterol in whole blood [69]. Non-linear iterative partial least squares (NIPALS) with orthogonal signal correction (OSC) enabled establishing a multivariate model. In a later study, Pian *et al.* investigated the possibilities of neural networks for glucose quantification via FT Raman spectra acquired from whole blood [133]. The amino acids leucine and isoleucine might be useful predictive diabetes type 2 biomarkers. Birech *et al.* were able to demonstrate how Raman spectroscopy can not only detect glucose, but also leucine and isoleucine, and thereby constitutes a promising screening tool for clinical studies that investigate new therapies against diabetes [134]. Further information can be found in the review by Ralbovsky and Lednev, which discusses the potential of vibrational spectroscopy for diabetes diagnostics in detail [135], while the work of Pandey *et al.* focuses specifically on glucose monitoring in blood by means of Raman spectroscopy [136].

8.5.9 Blood transfusion bag quality control

Last but not least, the possibility of non-invasively investigating red blood cells in transfusion bags via Raman spectroscopy has to be mentioned. Despite being stored at 4 °C in a saline solution with stabilizing additives, the red blood cells still undergo biochemical and morphological changes and are therefore not permitted to be used after longer than 42 days [137]. Raman spectroscopy might be an interesting tool for quality control. Buckley *et al.* employed spatially offset Raman spectroscopy (SORS) in order to be able to retrieve spectral information from inside 400 μm thick polyvinyl chloride (PVC) blood-bags. They were able to characterize the oxygenation state of the RBCs in the sealed bags. Later on, Vardaki *et al.* monitored the biochemical changes of RBCs in blood transfusion bags over a period of six weeks using a commercially available SORS system. They found individual behaviour regarding the oxygenation state of haemoglobin for the different donors, though the general trend of increased oxygenation was the same [138]. Another approach was introduced by Gautam *et al*, utilizing diffuse resonance Raman spectroscopy (DRRS). By exploiting the resonance Raman effect, they were also able to assess the degree of degradation of RBCs within a transfusion bag spectroscopically [139].

8.6 Current trend in Raman spectroscopy investigations of blood

Several notable trends have characterized the field of blood Raman spectroscopy research. Researchers have employed the capabilities of Raman spectroscopy to facilitate the advancement of disease diagnosis and monitoring, particularly in conditions such as anaemia, diabetes, and cancer. Haemoglobin and haematocrit measurements, which have historically presented significant challenges, have emerged as a key area of focus. Raman spectroscopy has demonstrated potential as a viable alternative to traditional methods. Moreover, the technique has been applied to monitor blood gases, including oxygen and carbon dioxide levels, and blood pH, which are critical for assessing a patient's respiratory and metabolic health. Furthermore, there has been a growing interest in investigating lipid profiles in relation to cardiovascular diseases. Researchers have endeavoured to comprehend the natural biological variability in Raman spectra and the potential influence of factors such as age, sex, and ethnicity. The application of Raman imaging techniques has enabled the creation of spatially resolved maps of blood components, offering a detailed and localized analysis. The utilization of Raman-active nanoparticles has further augmented the sensitivity for targeted biomarker analysis. Furthermore, the application of artificial intelligence and machine learning has become increasingly crucial in the analysis and interpretation of data. The development of portable, point-of-care Raman devices has the potential to facilitate rapid and convenient blood analysis in non-laboratory settings. Moreover, blood Raman spectroscopy has made a significant contribution to biomedical research and drug development by studying the effects of therapeutic interventions on blood properties. Finally, researchers have investigated multimodal approaches, integrating Raman spectroscopy with other imaging and analytical techniques, with the aim of providing a more comprehensive understanding of blood components and their interactions. These trends collectively demonstrate the versatility and growing importance of blood Raman spectroscopy in healthcare and research.

References

[1] Wang H, Wei H-W, Shen H-C, Li Z-Z, Cheng Y, Duan L-S, Yin L, Yu J and Guo J-R 2020 To study the effect of oxygen carrying capacity on expressed changes of erythrocyte membrane protein in different storage times *Biosci. Rep.* **40** BSR20200799

[2] Alberts B, Johnson A, Lewis J, Raff M, Roberts K and Walter P 2002 *Molecular Biology of the Cell* (Garland Science)

[3] Mathew J, Sankar P and Varacallo M (eds) 2023 *Physiology, Blood Plasma* (StatPearls Publishing)

[4] Belinskaia D A, Voronina P A, Shmurak V I, Jenkins R O and Goncharov N V 2021 Serum albumin in health and disease: esterase, antioxidant, transporting and signaling properties *Int. J. Mol. Sci.* **22** 10318

[5] Hackshaw K V, Miller J S, Aykas D P and Rodriguez-Saona L 2020 Vibrational spectroscopy for identification of metabolites in biologic samples *Molecules* **25**

[6] Turner J, Parsi M and Badireddy M (eds) 2023 *Anemia* (StatPearls Publishing)

[7] Dean L (ed) 2005 *Blood Groups and Red Cell Antigens* (National Center for Biotechnology Information)

[8] Fiala C and Diamandis E P 2018 Utility of circulating tumor DNA in cancer diagnostics with emphasis on early detection *BMC Med.* **16** 166

[9] Haas J D and Brownlie T 2001 Iron deficiency and reduced work capacity: a critical review of the research to determine a causal relationship *J. Nutr.* **131** 676S–88S

[10] Hoffman R (ed) 2018 *Hematology Basic Principles and Practice* 7th edn (Philadelphia, PA: Elsevier)

[11] Goodacre R, Graham D and Faulds K 2018 Recent developments in quantitative SERS: Moving towards absolute quantification *TrAC—Trends Anal. Chem.* **102** 359–68

[12] Bates I and Bain B J 2006 Approach to the diagnosis and classification of blood diseases *Dacie and Lewis Practical Haematology* (Elsevier) ch 23 pp 609–24

[13] Goetz L H and Schork N J 2018 Personalized medicine: motivation, challenges, and progress *Fertil. Steril.* **109** 952–63

[14] Atkins C G, Buckley K, Blades M W and Turner R F 2017 Raman spectroscopy of blood and blood components *Appl. Spectrosc.* **71** 767–93

[15] Enejder A M K, Koo T-W, Oh J, Hunter M, Sasic S, Feld M S and Horowitz G L 2002 Blood analysis by Raman spectroscopy *Opt. Lett.* **27** 2004–6

[16] Volkov V V, McMaster J, Aizenberg J and Perry C C 2021 Mapping blood biochemistry by Raman spectroscopy at the cellular level *Chem. Sci.* **13** 133–40

[17] Kistenev Y V, Borisov A V, Samarinova A A, Colón-Rodríguez S and Lednev I K 2023 A novel Raman spectroscopic method for detecting traces of blood on an interfering substrate *Sci. Rep.* **13** 5384

[18] Doty K C and Lednev I K 2018 Differentiation of human blood from animal blood using Raman spectroscopy: a survey of forensically relevant species *Forens. Sci. Int.* **282** 204–10

[19] Mistek E, Halámková L, Doty K C, Muro C K and Lednev I K 2016 Race differentiation by Raman spectroscopy of a bloodstain for forensic purposes *Anal. Chem.* **88** 7453–6

[20] Huang N, Short M, Zhao J, Wang H, Lui H, Korbelik M and Zeng H 2011 Full range characterization of the Raman spectra of organs in a murine model *Opt. Express* **19** 22892–909

[21] Matthiae M, Zhu X, Marie R and Kristensen A 2019 In-line whole blood fractionation for Raman analysis of blood plasma *Analyst* **144** 602–10

[22] Chiang C-C, Huang S-J, Immanuel P N, Lan J-H, Lo F-Y and Young K-C 2023 Using a 3D silicon micro-channel device and Raman spectroscopy for the analysis of whole blood and abnormal blood *Micromachines* **15**

[23] Hansson B, Allen C H, Qutob S, Behr B, Nyiri B, Chauhan V and Murugkar S 2019 Development of a flow cell based Raman spectroscopy technique to overcome photo-degradation in human blood *Biomed. Opt. Express* **10** 2275–88

[24] Ahmed M H, Ghatge M S and Safo M K 2020 Hemoglobin: structure, function and allostery *Sub-cell. Biochem.* **94** 345–82

[25] Dybas J *et al.* 2022 Trends in biomedical analysis of red blood cells—Raman spectroscopy against other spectroscopic, microscopic and classical techniques *TrAC, Trends Anal. Chem.* **146** 116481

[26] Torres Filho I P, Terner J, Pittman R N, Proffitt E and Ward K R 2008 Measurement of hemoglobin oxygen saturation using Raman microspectroscopy and 532-nm excitation *J. Appl. Physiol.* **104** 1809–17

[27] Rao S, Bálint S, Cossins B, Guallar V and Petrov D 2009 Raman study of mechanically induced oxygenation state transition of red blood cells using optical tweezers *Biophys. J.* **96** 209–16

[28] Lukose J, N M, Mohan G, Shastry S and Chidangil S 2019 Normal saline-induced deoxygenation of red blood cells probed by optical tweezers combined with the micro-Raman technique *RSC Adv.* **9** 7878–84

[29] Brazhe N A, Thomsen K, Lønstrup M, Brazhe A R, Nikelshparg E I, Maksimov G V, Lauritzen M and Sosnovtseva O 2018 Monitoring of blood oxygenation in brain by resonance Raman spectroscopy *J. Biophoton.* **11** e201700311

[30] Marzec K M, Rygula A, Wood B R, Chlopicki S and Baranska M 2015 High-resolution Raman imaging reveals spatial location of heme oxidation sites in single red blood cells of dried smears *J. Raman Spectrosc.* **46** 76–83

[31] Rinia H A, Bonn M, Vartiainen E M, Schaffer C B and Müller M 2006 Spectroscopic analysis of the oxygenation state of hemoglobin using coherent anti-Stokes Raman scattering *J. Biomed. Optics* **11** 50502

[32] Dybas J, Chiura T, Marzec K M and Mak P J 2021 Probing heme active sites of hemoglobin in functional red blood cells using resonance Raman spectroscopy *J. Phys. Chem.* B **125** 3556–65

[33] Kitahama Y, Egashira M, Suzuki T, Tanabe I and Ozaki Y 2014 Sensitive marker bands for the detection of spin states of heme in surface-enhanced resonance Raman scattering spectra of metmyoglobin *Analyst* **139** 6421–5

[34] Nagatomo S *et al.* 2022 Heme-bound tyrosine vibrations in hemoglobin M: resonance Raman, crystallography, and DFT calculation *Biophys. J.* **121** 2767–80

[35] Lin J, Lin J, Huang Z, Lu P, Wang J, Wang X and Chen R 2014 Raman spectroscopy of human hemoglobin for diabetes detection *J. Innov. Opt. Health Sci.* **07** 1350051

[36] Jacob S S *et al.* 2022 Micro-Raman spectroscopy study of optically trapped erythrocytes in malaria, dengue and leptospirosis infections *Front. Med.* **9** 858776

[37] Dasgupta R, Verma R S, Ahlawat S, Uppal A and Gupta P K 2011 Studies on erythrocytes in malaria infected blood sample with Raman optical tweezers *J. Biomed. Opt.* **16** 77009

[38] Chen K, Yuen C, Aniweh Y, Preiser P and Liu Q 2016 Towards ultrasensitive malaria diagnosis using surface enhanced Raman spectroscopy *Sci. Rep.* **6** 20177

[39] Wood B R, Stoddart P R and McNaughton D 2011 Molecular imaging of red blood cells by Raman spectroscopy *Aust. J. Chem.* **64** 593

[40] Bonifacio A, Finaurini S, Krafft C, Parapini S, Taramelli D and Sergo V 2008 Spatial distribution of heme species in erythrocytes infected with Plasmodium falciparum by use of resonance Raman imaging and multivariate analysis *Anal. Bioanal. Chem.* **392** 1277–82

[41] Lee M, Herrington C S, Ravindra M, Sepp K, Davies A, Hulme A N and Brunton V G 2021 Recent advances in the use of stimulated Raman scattering in histopathology *Analyst* **146** 789–802

[42] Tahir M A, Dina N E, Cheng H, Valev V K and Zhang L 2021 Surface-enhanced Raman spectroscopy for bioanalysis and diagnosis *Nanoscale* **13** 11593–634

[43] Borek–Dorosz A *et al.* 2022 Raman-based spectrophenotyping of the most important cells of the immune system *J. Adv. Res.* **41** 191–203

[44] Ramoji A, Neugebauer U, Bocklitz T, Foerster M, Kiehntopf M, Bauer M and Popp J 2012 Toward a spectroscopic hemogram: Raman spectroscopic differentiation of the two most abundant leukocytes from peripheral blood *Anal. Chem.* **84** 5335–42

[45] Chen M, McReynolds N, Campbell E C, Mazilu M, Barbosa J, Dholakia K and Powis S J 2015 The use of wavelength modulated Raman spectroscopy in label-free identification of T lymphocyte subsets, natural killer cells and dendritic cells *PLoS One* **10** e0125158

[46] Lelliott P M *et al.* 2023 Single-cell Raman microscopy with machine learning highlights distinct biochemical features of neutrophil extracellular traps and necrosis *Sci. Rep.* **13** 10093

[47] Golubewa L N, Kulahava T A, Leonik Y S, Shuba M V and Semenkova G N 2021 Application of Raman spectroscopy for studying the mechanisms of neutrophil activation by carbon nanotubes *J. Appl. Spectrosc.* **88** 77–84

[48] Arzumanyan G M, Gur'ev A S, Kravtsunova D E, Mamatkulov K Z, Marchenko A S, Vereshchagin K A and Volkov A 2020 Micro Raman spectroscopy for NETosis detection *J. Raman Spectrosc.* **51** 1960–9

[49] Dorosz A, Grosicki M, Dybas J, Matuszyk E, Rodewald M, Meyer T, Popp J, Malek K and Baranska M 2020 Eosinophils and neutrophils-molecular differences revealed by spontaneous Raman, CARS and fluorescence microscopy *Cells* **9**

[50] Pistiki A *et al.* 2021 Biochemical analysis of leukocytes after *in vitro* and *in vivo* activation with bacterial and fungal pathogens using Raman spectroscopy *Int. J. Mol. Sci.* **22** 10481

[51] Arend N *et al.* 2020 Detection and differentiation of bacterial and fungal infection of neutrophils from peripheral blood using Raman spectroscopy *Anal. Chem.* **92** 10560–8

[52] Pistiki A, Hornung F, Silge A, Ramoji A, Ryabchykov O, Bocklitz T W, Weber K, Löffler B, Popp J and Deinhardt-Emmer S 2022 Raman spectroscopic cellomics for the detection of SARS-CoV-2-associated neutrophil activation after TNF-α stimulation *Clin. Transl. Med.* **12** e1139

[53] Chaudhary N, Nguyen T N Q, Cullen D, Meade A D and Wynne C 2021 Discrimination of immune cell activation using Raman micro-spectroscopy in an in-vitro and ex-vivo model *Spectr. Acta. A, Mol. Biomol. Spectrosc.* **248** 119118

[54] Buchacher T, Wiesinger-Mayr H, Vierlinger K, Rüger B M, Stanek G, Fischer M B and Weber V 2014 Human blood monocytes support persistence, but not replication of the intracellular pathogen *C. pneumoniae BMC Immunol.* **15** 60

[55] Naumann M, Arend N, Guliev R R, Kretzer C, Rubio I, Werz O and Neugebauer U 2023 Label-free characterization of macrophage polarization using Raman spectroscopy *Int. J. Mol. Sci.* **24**

[56] Ribeiro A R B, Silva E C O, Araújo P M C, Souza S T, Da Fonseca E J S and Barreto E 2022 Application of Raman spectroscopy for characterization of the functional polarization of macrophages into M1 and M2 cells *Spectrochim. Acta. A, Mol. Biomol. Spectrosc.* **265** 120328

[57] McReynolds N, Cooke F G M, Chen M, Powis S J and Dholakia K 2017 Multimodal discrimination of immune cells using a combination of Raman spectroscopy and digital holographic microscopy *Sci. Rep.* **7** 43631

[58] Niciński K, Krajczewski J, Kudelski A, Witkowska E, Trzcińska-Danielewicz J, Girstun A and Kamińska A 2019 Detection of circulating tumor cells in blood by shell-isolated nanoparticle—enhanced Raman spectroscopy (SHINERS) in microfluidic device *Sci. Rep.* **9** 9267

[59] Ghoshal K and Bhattacharyya M 2014 Overview of platelet physiology: its hemostatic and nonhemostatic role in disease pathogenesis *Sci. World J.* **2014** 781857

[60] Wang G-W, Yao H-L, He B-J, Peng L-X and Li Y-Q 2007 Raman micro-spectroscopy of single blood platelets *Guangpu* **27** 1347–50

[61] García-Rubio D L, de la Mora M B, Badillo-Ramírez I, Cerecedo D, Saniger J M, Benítez-Benítez J L and Villagrán-Muniz M 2019 Analysis of platelets in hypertensive and normotensive individuals using Raman and Fourier transform infrared-attenuated total reflectance spectroscopies *J. Raman Spectrosc.* **50** 509–21

[62] Zyubin A *et al.* 2022 Spectral homogeneity of human platelets investigated by SERS *PLoS One* **17** e0265247

[63] Samusev I, Zyubin A, Rafalskiy V, Lopatin M, Demishkevich E, Moiseeva E, Kon I, Lyatun I, Khankaev A and Kundalevich A 2023 Study of human platelets spectral homogeneity by SERS technique *Proceedings of the 11th Int. Advances In Applied Physics and Materials Science Congress and Exhibition* (AIP Publishing) p 40012

[64] Zyubin A, Rafalskiy V, Tcibulnikova A, Moiseeva E, Matveeva K, Tsapkova A, Lyatun I, Medvedskaya P, Samusev I and Demin M 2020 Surface-enhanced Raman spectroscopy for antiplatelet therapy effectiveness assessment *Laser Phys. Lett.* **17** 45601

[65] Zyubin A, Rafalskiy V, Tcibulnikova A, Matveeva K, Moiseeva E, Tsapkova A, Samusev I, Bryukhanov V and Demin M 2020 Dataset of human platelets in healthy and individuals with cardiovascular pathology obtained by surface-enhanced Raman spectroscopy *Data Brief* **29** 105145

[66] Wang L J *et al.* 2014 Raman spectroscopy detection of platelet for Alzheimer's disease with predictive probabilities *Laser Phys.* **24** 85702

[67] Medipally D K R, Maguire A, Bryant J, Armstrong J, Dunne M, Finn M, Lyng F M and Meade A D 2017 Development of a high throughput (HT) Raman spectroscopy method for rapid screening of liquid blood plasma from prostate cancer patients *Analyst* **142** 1216–26

[68] Parachalil D R, McIntyre J and Byrne H J 2020 Potential of Raman spectroscopy for the analysis of plasma/serum in the liquid state: recent advances *Anal. Bioanal. Chem.* **412** 1993–2007

[69] Wang Q, Wu G, Pian F, Shan P, Li Z and Ma Z 2021 Simultaneous detection of glucose, triglycerides, and total cholesterol in whole blood by Fourier-transform Raman spectroscopy *Spectrochim. Acta, Part* A **260** 119906

[70] Huang J, Ali N, Quansah E, Guo S, Noutsias M, Meyer-Zedler T, Bocklitz T, Popp J, Neugebauer U and Ramoji A 2021 Vibrational spectroscopic investigation of blood plasma and serum by drop coating deposition for clinical application *Int. J. Mol. Sci.* **22** 2191

[71] Gao S, Lin Y, Zhao X, Gao J, Xie S, Gong W, Yu Y and LIN J 2022 Label-free surface enhanced Raman spectroscopy analysis of blood serum via coffee ring effect for accurate diagnosis of cancers *Spectrochim. Acta A Mol. Biomol. Spectrosc.* **267** 120605

[72] Byrne H J, Bonnier F, McIntyre J and Parachalil D R 2020 Quantitative analysis of human blood serum using vibrational spectroscopy *Clin. Spectrosc.* **2** 100004

[73] Golparvar A, Boukhayma A, Loayza T, Caizzone A, Enz C and Carrara S 2021 Very selective detection of low physiopathological glucose levels by spontaneous Raman spectroscopy with univariate data analysis *Bio. Nano. Sci.* **11** 871–7

[74] Chauhan N, Saxena K, Rawal R, Yadav L and Jain U 2023 Advances in surface-enhanced Raman spectroscopy-based sensors for detection of various biomarkers *Prog. Biophys. Mol. Biol.* **184** 32–41

[75] Parachalil D R, Commerford D, Bonnier F, Chourpa I, McIntyre J and Byrne H J 2019 Raman spectroscopy as a potential tool for label free therapeutic drug monitoring in human serum: the case of busulfan and methotrexate *Analyst* **144** 5207–14

[76] Staritzbichler R, Hunold P, Estrela-Lopis I, Hildebrand P W, Isermann B and Kaiser T 2021 Raman spectroscopy on blood serum samples of patients with end-stage liver disease *PLoS One* **16** e0256045
[77] Song Y, Sun J, Wang M, Gao F, Ni Q, Wang Y, Yang M, Sun B and Zhao P 2023 Quantitative and specific detection of blood biomarkers for accurate prediction of white matter lesions with cognitive dysfunction using dendrite gold nanostar-based surface-enhanced Raman scattering barcode chips *ACS Appl. Nano Mater.* **6** 12686–94
[78] Boyd S, Bertino M F and Seashols S J 2011 Raman spectroscopy of blood samples for forensic applications *Forensic Sci. Int.* **208** 124–8
[79] Boroujerdi R, Paul R and Abdelkader A 2022 Rapid detection of amitriptyline in dried blood and dried saliva samples with surface-enhanced Raman spectroscopy *Sensors* **22** 8257
[80] Zou Y *et al.* 2016 Whole blood and semen identification using mid-infrared and Raman spectrum analysis for forensic applications *Anal. Methods* **8** 3763–7
[81] Jahn I J, Lehniger L, Weber K, Cialla-May D and Popp J 2019 Sample preparation for Raman microspectroscopy *Micro-Raman Spectroscopy: Theory and Application* (De Gruyter) pp 61–80
[82] Rey Gomez L M, Hirani R, Care A, Inglis D W and Wang Y 2023 Emerging microfluidic devices for sample preparation of undiluted whole blood to enable the detection of biomarkers *ACS Sens.* **8** 1404–21
[83] Song Y, Yin H and Huang W E 2016 Raman activated cell sorting *Curr. Opin. Chem. Biol.* **33** 1–8
[84] Kong B S, Lee C and Cho Y M 2022 Protocol for the assessment of human T cell activation by real-time metabolic flux analysis *STAR Protocols* **3** 101084
[85] Graham J M 2002 Separation of monocytes from whole human blood *Sci. World J.* **2** 1540–3
[86] Abhishek K, Louis Sam Titus A S C, Dinh M T P, Mukhamedshin A, Mohan C, Gifford S C and Shevkoplyas S S 2023 Red blood cell rosetting enables size-based separation of specific lymphocyte subsets from blood in a microfluidic device *Lab Chip* **23** 1804–15
[87] Frenea-Robin M and Marchalot J 2022 Basic principles and recent advances in magnetic cell separation *Magnetochemistry* **8** 11
[88] Shields C W, Ohiri K A, Szott L M and López G P 2017 Translating microfluidics: cell separation technologies and their barriers to commercialization *Cytom. Part B, Clin. Cytom.* **92** 115–25
[89] Afsaneh H and Mohammadi R 2022 Microfluidic platforms for the manipulation of cells and particles *Talanta Open* **5** 100092
[90] Dalili A, Samiei E and Hoorfar M 2018 A review of sorting, separation and isolation of cells and microbeads for biomedical applications: microfluidic approaches *Analyst* **144** 87–113
[91] Catarino S O, Rodrigues R O, Pinho D, Miranda J M, Minas G and Lima R 2019 Blood cells separation and sorting techniques of passive microfluidic devices: from fabrication to applications *Micromachines* **10** 593
[92] Gossett D R, Weaver W M, Mach A J, Hur S C, Tse H T K, Lee W, Amini H and Di Carlo D 2010 Label-free cell separation and sorting in microfluidic systems *Anal. Bioanal. Chem.* **397** 3249–67
[93] Yan S, Qiu J, Guo L, Li D, Xu D and Liu Q 2021 Development overview of Raman-activated cell sorting devoted to bacterial detection at single-cell level *Appl. Microbiol. Biotechnol.* **105** 1315–31
[94] Nitta N *et al.* 2020 Raman image-activated cell sorting *Nat. Commun.* **11** 3452

[95] Zhang J, Lin H, Xu J, Zhang M, Ge X, Zhang C, Huang W E and Cheng J-X 2023 High-throughput single-cell sorting by stimulated Raman-activated cell ejection *bioRxiv*

[96] Liou Y-R, Wang Y-H, Lee C-Y and Li P-C 2015 Buoyancy-activated cell sorting using targeted biotinylated albumin microbubbles *PLoS One* **10** e0125036

[97] Guo K-T, SchAfer R, Paul A, Gerber A, Ziemer G and Wendel H P 2006 A new technique for the isolation and surface immobilization of mesenchymal stem cells from whole bone marrow using high-specific DNA aptamers *Stem Cells* **24** 2220–31

[98] Pence I and Mahadevan-Jansen A 2016 Clinical instrumentation and applications of Raman spectroscopy *Chem. Soc. Rev.* **45** 1958–79

[99] Jones R R, Hooper D C, Zhang L, Wolverson D and Valev V K 2019 Raman techniques: fundamentals and frontiers *Nanoscale Res. Lett.* **14** 231

[100] Ciobanu C, Ember K J, Nyiri B J, Rajan S, Chauhan V, Leblond F and Murugkar S 2022 Potential of Raman spectroscopy for blood-based biopsy *IEEE Instrum. Meas. Mag.* **25** 62–8

[101] Zhang Y, Hong H and Cai W 2010 Imaging with Raman spectroscopy *Curr. Pharm. Biotechnol.* **11** 654–61

[102] Kuhar N, Sil S, Verma T and Umapathy S 2018 Challenges in application of Raman spectroscopy to biology and materials *RSC Adv.* **8** 25888–908

[103] Nargis H F *et al.* 2019 Raman spectroscopy of blood plasma samples from breast cancer patients at different stages *Spectrochim. Acta, Part* A **222** 117210

[104] Giamougiannis P, Silva R V O, Freitas D L D, Lima K M G, Anagnostopoulos A, Angelopoulos G, Naik R, Wood N J, Martin-Hirsch P L and Martin F L 2021 Raman spectroscopy of blood and urine liquid biopsies for ovarian cancer diagnosis: identification of chemotherapy effects *J. Biophotonics* **14** e202100195

[105] Da Silva A M, de Siqueira e Oliveira F S A, de Brito P L and Silveira L 2018 Spectral model for diagnosis of acute leukemias in whole blood and plasma through Raman spectroscopy *J. Biomed. Opt.* **23** 107002

[106] Xu L, Chen Y, Ye J, Fan M, Weng G, Shen Y, Lin Z, Lin D, Xu Y and Feng S 2024 Optical nanobiosensor based on surface-enhanced Raman spectroscopy and catalytic hairpin assembly for early-stage lung cancer detection via blood circular RNA *ACS Sens.* **9** 2020–30

[107] Xue L, Yan B, Li Y, Tan Y, Luo X and Wang M 2018 Surface-enhanced Raman spectroscopy of blood serum based on gold nanoparticles for tumor stages detection and histologic grades classification of oral squamous cell carcinoma *Int. J. Nanomed.* **13** 4977–86

[108] Hong Y *et al.* 2020 Label-free diagnosis for colorectal cancer through coffee ring-assisted surface-enhanced Raman spectroscopy on blood serum *J. Biophotonics* **13** e201960176

[109] Koster H J, Guillen-Perez A, Gomez-Diaz J S, Navas-Moreno M, Birkeland A C and Carney R P 2022 Fused Raman spectroscopic analysis of blood and saliva delivers high accuracy for head and neck cancer diagnostics *Sci. Rep.* **12** 18464

[110] Paraskevaidi M, Morais C L M, Halliwell D E, Mann D M A, Allsop D, Martin-Hirsch P L and Martin F L 2018 Raman spectroscopy to diagnose Alzheimer's disease and dementia with lewy bodies in blood *ACS Chem. Neurosci.* **9** 2786–94

[111] Ramoji A *et al.* 2021 Leukocyte activation profile assessed by Raman spectroscopy helps diagnosing infection and sepsis *Crit. Care Explor.* **3** e0394

[112] Pietruszewska M, Biesiada G, Czepiel J, Birczyńska-Zych M, Moskal P, Garlicki A and Wesełucha-Birczyńska A 2024 Raman spectroscopy of lymphocytes from patients with the Epstein–Barr virus infection *Sci. Rep.* **14** 6417

[113] Nasir S *et al.* 2021 Surface enhanced Raman spectroscopy of RNA samples extracted from blood of hepatitis C patients for quantification of viral loads *Photodiagn. Photodyn. Ther.* **33** 102152

[114] Kashif M, Majeed M I, Hanif M A and Rehman A 2020 Surface enhanced Raman spectroscopy of the serum samples for the diagnosis of Hepatitis C and prediction of the viral loads *Spectrochim. Acta, Part* A **242** 118729

[115] Shakeel S *et al.* 2022 Surface-enhanced Raman spectroscopic analysis of centrifugally filtered blood serum samples of hepatitis C patients *Photodiagn. Photodyn. Ther.* **39** 102949

[116] Ahmad S *et al.* 2021 Characterization and prediction of viral loads of Hepatitis B serum samples by using surface-enhanced Raman spectroscopy (SERS) *Photodiagn. Photodyn. Ther.* **35** 102386

[117] Khan S, Ullah R, Khan A, Ashraf R, Ali H, Bilal M and Saleem M 2018 Analysis of hepatitis B virus infection in blood sera using Raman spectroscopy and machine learning *Photodiagn. Photodyn. Ther.* **23** 89–93

[118] Mahmood T *et al.* 2018 Raman spectral analysis for rapid screening of dengue infection *Spectrochim. Acta A Mol. Biomol. Spectrosc.* **200** 136–42

[119] Confield L R, Black G P, Wilson B C, Lowe D J, Theakstone A G and Baker M J 2021 Vibrational spectroscopic analysis of blood for diagnosis of infections and sepsis: a review of requirements for a rapid diagnostic test *Anal. Methods* **13** 157–68

[120] Tannert A, Ramoji A, Neugebauer U and Popp J 2018 Photonic monitoring of treatment during infection and sepsis: development of new detection strategies and potential clinical applications *Anal. Bioanal. Chem.* **410** 773–90

[121] Chen F, Flaherty B R, Cohen C E, Peterson D S and Zhao Y 2016 Direct detection of malaria infected red blood cells by surface enhanced Raman spectroscopy *Nanomed. Nanotechnol. Biol. Med.* **12** 1445–51

[122] Wang W, Dong R, Gu D, He J, Yi P, Kong S-K, Ho H-P, Loo J, Wang W and Wang Q 2020 Antibody-free rapid diagnosis of malaria in whole blood with surface-enhanced Raman spectroscopy using nanostructured gold substrate *Adv. Med. Sci.* **65** 86–92

[123] Parlatan U, Inanc M T, Ozgor B Y, Oral E, Bastu E, Unlu M B and Basar G 2019 Raman spectroscopy as a non-invasive diagnostic technique for endometriosis *Sci. Rep.* **9** 19795

[124] Göksel Y, Zor K, Rindzevicius T, Thorhauge Als-Nielsen B E, Schmiegelow K and Boisen A 2021 Quantification of methotrexate in human serum using surface-enhanced Raman scattering—toward therapeutic drug monitoring *ACS Sens.* **6** 2664–73

[125] Fornasaro S, Bonifacio A, Marangon E, Buzzo M, Toffoli G, Rindzevicius T, Schmidt M S and Sergo V 2018 Label-free quantification of anticancer drug imatinib in human plasma with surface enhanced Raman spectroscopy *Anal. Chem.* **90** 12670–7

[126] Panikar S S, Ramírez-García G, Sidhik S, Lopez-Luke T, Rodriguez-Gonzalez C, Ciapara I H, Castillo P S, Camacho-Villegas T and de La Rosa E 2019 Ultrasensitive SERS substrate for label-free therapeutic-drug monitoring of paclitaxel and cyclophosphamide in blood serum *Anal. Chem.* **91** 2100–11

[127] Adomavičiūtė S, Velička M and Šablinskas V 2020 Detection of aspirin traces in blood by means of surface-enhanced Raman scattering spectroscopy *J. Raman Spectrosc.* **51** 919–31

[128] Kirchhoff J, Glaser U, Bohnert J A, Pletz M W, Popp J and Neugebauer U 2018 Simple ciprofloxacin resistance test and determination of minimal inhibitory concentration within 2 h using Raman spectroscopy *Anal. Chem.* **90** 1811–8

[129] Han Y-Y, Lin Y-C, Cheng W-C, Lin Y-T, Teng L-J, Wang J-K and Wang Y-L 2020 Rapid antibiotic susceptibility testing of bacteria from patients' blood via assaying bacterial metabolic response with surface-enhanced Raman spectroscopy *Sci. Rep.* **10** 12538

[130] Facchinetti A 2016 Continuous glucose monitoring sensors: past, present and future algorithmic challenges *Sensors* **16** 2093

[131] Freckmann G 2020 Basics and use of continuous glucose monitoring (CGM) in diabetes therapy *J. Lab. Med.* **44** 71–9

[132] Li N, Zang H, Sun H, Jiao X, Wang K, Liu T C-Y and Meng Y 2019 A Noninvasive accurate measurement of blood glucose levels with Raman spectroscopy of blood in microvessels *Molecules* **24** 1500

[133] Pian F, Wang Q, Wang M, Shan P, Li Z and Ma Z 2022 A shallow convolutional neural network with elastic nets for blood glucose quantitative analysis using Raman spectroscopy *Spectrochim. Acta, Part* A **264** 120229

[134] Birech Z, Mwangi P W, Bukachi F and Mandela K M 2017 Application of Raman spectroscopy in type 2 diabetes screening in blood using leucine and isoleucine amino-acids as biomarkers and in comparative anti-diabetic drugs efficacy studies *PLoS One* **12** e0185130

[135] Ralbovsky N M and Lednev I K 2021 Vibrational spectroscopy for detection of diabetes: a review *Appl. Spectrosc.* **75** 929–46

[136] Pandey R, Paidi S K, Valdez T A, Zhang C, Spegazzini N, Dasari R R and Barman I 2017 Noninvasive monitoring of blood glucose with Raman spectroscopy *Acc. Chem. Res.* **50** 264–72

[137] Buckley K, Atkins C G, Chen D, Schulze H G, Devine D V, Blades M W and Turner R F B 2016 Non-invasive spectroscopy of transfusable red blood cells stored inside sealed plastic blood-bags *Analyst* **141** 1678–85

[138] Vardaki M Z, Atkins C G, Schulze H G, Devine D V, Serrano K, Blades M W and Turner R F B 2018 Raman spectroscopy of stored red blood cell concentrate within sealed transfusion blood bags *Analyst* **143** 6006–13

[139] Gautam R, Oh J-Y, Patel R P and Dluhy R A 2018 Non-invasive analysis of stored red blood cells using diffuse resonance Raman spectroscopy *Analyst* **143** 5950–8

Chapter 9

Optoacoustic properties of blood

Rajendran Soundararajan and Azhar Zam

Optoacoustic or photoacoustic imaging (OAI/PAI) is a cutting-edge imaging technique that produces high-resolution images, effectively overcoming the challenges of optical scattering in biological tissues. This chapter delves into the fundamental principles of optoacoustic signal generation and its significant role in studying blood properties. OAI leverages the photoacoustic effect to visualize anatomical structures and quantify physiological parameters such as blood oxygenation and hemoglobin (Hb) concentration. By utilizing the distinct absorption spectra of Hb and other blood components, OAI enables the non-invasive imaging of blood vessels and real-time monitoring of hemodynamics.

Technological advancements, such as photoacoustic microscopy (PAM) and photoacoustic tomography (PAT), offer imaging at varying depths and resolutions, from the capillary level to whole organs. PAM provides high-resolution images for shallow tissue layers, while PAT penetrates deeper tissues, making it ideal for clinical applications. The chapter highlights the versatility of OAI in diagnosing and monitoring diseases like anemia, sickle cell disease, and cardiovascular conditions. Additionally, optoacoustic techniques show great promise in glucose monitoring for diabetes management, offering a non-invasive alternative to traditional methods.

The chapter also explores the potential of OAI in detecting circulating tumor cells (CTCs), providing a promising tool for early cancer detection and metastasis monitoring. Challenges such as enhancing image resolution, improving light delivery to deeper tissues, and optimizing clinical applicability are addressed alongside future research directions.

OAI provides a powerful, non-invasive method for visualizing blood properties and diagnosing various diseases. As technology advances, OAI is poised to make significant contributions to preclinical research and clinical diagnostics, particularly in functional and molecular imaging of the circulatory system.

9.1 Introduction

OAI is an innovative hybrid biomedical imaging technology that blends optical and acoustic methods to generate high-resolution images of tissues [1, 2]. It has seen a

doi:10.1088/978-0-7503-4806-5ch9

surge in interest over the past twenty years, particularly for its applications in biomedical imaging. Traditional optical imaging methods struggle to provide high-resolution images in deep biological tissues because of optical scattering. However, OAI can produce high-resolution optical contrast images at depths of up to several centimeters, making it a promising option for various clinical imaging applications [3]. As a powerful modality for *in vivo* imaging of small animals and humans, OAI provides anatomical, functional, and molecular contrast, effectively overcoming challenges posed by light scattering in deep tissues. Through various implementations ranging from microscopy to tomography, OAI is precious for visualizing vasculature and physiological function and tracking the distribution of specific molecules within biological tissues, including tumors, across diverse length scales from cellular structures up to whole organs [4, 5].

9.1.1 Overview of optoacoustic imaging technology

OAI utilizes the photoacoustic effect, first described by Alexander Graham Bell in 1880 [6]. Initially, this effect was underutilized due to the weak light-to-sound conversion and inefficient acoustic detectors. Significant advancements with the development of highly sensitive piezoelectric sensors and the invention of the laser in 1960 provided efficient acoustic detection and high-intensity, short light pulses crucial for effective photoacoustic generation. These innovations spurred further developments in instruments, image processing, molecular imaging, and functional imaging. The application of the photoacoustic effect for optical imaging within biological tissues became prominent in the 1990s, driven by the need to surpass the resolution limitations of traditional optical-based medical imaging techniques [7].

OAI leverages the rapid pulsing of a nanosecond laser (typically pulse durations <10 ns) to irradiate biological tissues. The absorption of light energy by molecular components in the tissue results in a rise in temperature through non-radiative relaxation. This heat rise induces a thermoelastic expansion of the molecule of interest, generating detectable acoustic waves propagating outwards [8]. The waves are detected by an ultrasound transducer benefiting from their substantially lower scatter in biological tissues—about 1000 times less than light—enabling them to penetrate tissues deeply with minimal loss and reconstructed into an image that maps the original optical absorption. These optoacoustic waves can generated from both endogenous and exogenous contrast agents, such as Hb and nanoparticles, offering a broad range of imaging possibilities [9, 10]. Additionally, OAI provides the advantage of adjustable image contrast by choosing different excitation laser wavelengths, which permits the independent imaging of various molecules within the same system.

Researchers have developed a variety of OAI setups that cater to different scales, such as micro, meso, and macro-scale, targeting organelles, cells, tissues, and organs using diverse combinations of optical illumination and acoustic detection, as shown in figure 9.1 [11]. Advancements in light delivery technologies led to more mobile, tunable, compact, and affordable OAI systems. These systems can be broadly categorized into two configurations [12].

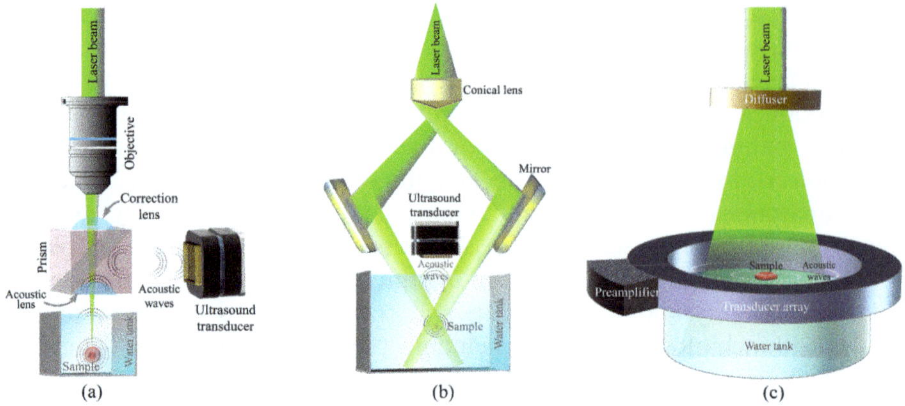

Figure 9.1. OAI configurations: (a) OR-PAM, (b) AR-PAM, (c) PAT.

1. PAM, utilizing a focused laser beam for high spatial resolution imaging at shallow depths.
2. PAT employs broader illumination schemes for deeper penetration, and the ultrasound transducer determines spatial resolution.

PAM and PAT can be carried out using optical or acoustic resolution configurations. In optical resolution, the spatial resolution is determined by the optical focal spot, while in acoustic resolution, it is determined by the transducer/array imaging characteristics.

In PAM, either optical illumination or ultrasonic detection is focused, capturing time-resolved photoacoustic signals at each lateral location to form a depth profile of tissue. Raster scanning the probe across the surface generates a two-dimensional (2D) cross-sectional or three-dimensional (3D) volumetric image. The axial resolution, inversely related to the acoustic detection bandwidth, is typically determined by a 100 MHz piezoelectric transducer with 100% receiving bandwidth, providing a theoretical axial resolution of 13.6 μm. PAM is further categorized as optical resolution PAM (OR-PAM) or acoustic resolution PAM (AR-PAM) based on whether optical or acoustic focus determines the lateral resolution.

PAM is a high-resolution OAI technique that can be further classified into optical resolution microscopy (OR-PAM) and acoustic resolution microscopy (AR-PAM), depending on the resolution type, as shown in figure 9.1(a) and (b). Additionally, PAT is differentiated by the configuration of its detectors, which include single, linear, ring, planar, cylindrical, and spherical array setups (figure 9.1(c)). Furthermore, integrating PAM and PAT technologies introduces the development of a photoacoustic endoscope (PAE) to facilitate intracavity imaging capabilities. In OAI, there is always a balance between resolution and detection depth, and each configuration is chosen based on the specific imaging requirements of the biological structures being studied, which are related to the number and arrangement of detectors [13].

OR-PAM provides the best imaging resolution and enhances optical microscopes by quantifying molecule-specific optical absorption contrast. It focuses light into a diffraction-limited spot within the tissue for confined photoacoustic excitation, resulting in the best lateral resolution (~1 μm). However, due to light scattering in tissues, effective optical focusing is limited to about 1 mm, restricting OR-PAM's imaging depth. Using sub-microjoule optical pulses, OR-PAM studies oxygen metabolism at capillary or red blood cell levels in the skin. Improvements in acoustic detection sensitivity could enhance OR-PAM in detecting single cells or organelles [14, 15].

AR-PAM utilizes wide-field optical excitation, enabling greater penetration depths but limiting resolution due to focused detection of high-frequency acoustic signals. Resolution in AR-PAM depends on the transducer's central frequency, bandwidth, and focusing geometry [16]. For instance, a 5 MHz transducer achieves 10.3 mm depth with 590 μm lateral resolution, while a 40 MHz transducer achieves 3.1 mm depth with 85 μm lateral resolution. Periyasamy *et al* [17] used a 30 MHz transducer and achieved a 57 μm axial resolution at a depth of 11 mm. In contrast, Moothanchery *et al* [18] used a 75 MHz transducer, producing an axial resolution of 53 μm at a depth of 1.8 mm [27, 32]. AR-PAM is utilized to diagnose human skin lesions and study brain function in small animal models.

PAT utilizes wide-field optical excitation, low-frequency array transducers, and inverse reconstruction algorithms for tomographic imaging and offers rapid 2D or 3D imaging at sub-millimeter resolutions [19]. It creates molecular-specific tomographic images at clinically relevant depths, prioritizing system sensitivity in its design by illuminating tissue over a broad surface area to ensure higher light doses reach deep targets (> 10 mJ). Various ultrasound transducer arrays, such as linear, ring, and 2D planar/hemispherical arrays, influence spatial resolution and imaging depths based on acoustic detection geometry and frequency. Unlike single-element PAM, PAT utilizes an array of unfocused acoustic detectors to capture a wider range of photoacoustic waves. A tomographic image is constructed by projecting individual measurements back to the object space along spherical surfaces, producing bright spots where optical absorbers are located. Spatial resolution in PAT depends on acoustic bandwidth and detection geometry, with moderate central frequency transducers (1–15 MHz) commonly used to resolve sub-millimeter details. The imaging depth in PAT is determined by light penetration into tissue, reaching up to 5 cm in the near-infrared (NIR) window. PAT shows early potential in whole-body imaging of small animals and breast cancer detection in clinical trials [20].

9.1.2 Importance of studying blood properties using optoacoustic methods

Recent research has evidenced that studying blood properties using optoacoustic methods is increasingly important due to several key advantages in biomedical imaging. Optoacoustic techniques, including OAI and spectroscopy, offer non-invasive, high-contrast, and high-resolution insights into blood's physiological and morphological characteristics (temperature, blood oxygenation, Hb concentration, and real-time monitoring of hemodynamic changes), which are crucial for diagnosing and treating various diseases various medical conditions, including cancer and cardiovascular diseases [21].

One of the critical benefits of optoacoustic methods is their ability to measure the temperature within vascularized tissues accurately, which is crucial for the safe and efficient treatment of lesions during thermal therapies [22]. The normalized temperature-dependent optoacoustic response in blood, which remains invariant with respect to hematocrit (HCT) at the isosbestic point of Hb, underscores the technique's potential for non-invasive thermometry. Additionally, the application of spectral analysis of photoacoustic signals further enhances the understanding of tissue microstructures and the concentration of different Hb types, facilitating the accurate estimation of Hb content [23].

Another primary advantage of optoacoustic methods is their ability to measure blood oxygenation and Hb concentration with high specificity and accuracy. This capability is vital for assessing the oxygenation status of tissues, which is essential in conditions like traumatic brain injury and neonatal care [24]. Moreover, these techniques can detect changes in blood viscosity and the aggregation level of red blood cells (RBCs), which are indicators of potential clot formation and are associated with cardiovascular diseases, infections, and inflammation [25].

Optoacoustic methods also excel in evaluating the morphological changes in RBCs, such as those caused by hematological disorders like sickle cell anemia and thalassemia. By analyzing the amplitude of photoacoustic signals, these techniques can detect variations in RBC concentration and morphology, offering a diagnostic signature for such conditions [26]. Furthermore, the ability to measure RBC count and physical properties simultaneously provides a comprehensive overview of blood's health status, which is not possible with conventional diagnostic methods [27].

The sensitivity of optoacoustic techniques to the spectral properties of blood enables the differentiation between oxygenated and deoxygenated RBCs, allowing for the assessment of blood oxygen saturation levels. This sensitivity is crucial for monitoring physiological processes and diagnosing diseases that alter blood's rheological properties [28, 29].

The advancement of contrast agents in OAI enhances its capabilities by improving the visibility of specific tissues or cellular processes. These agents are engineered with high absorption and efficient light-to-heat conversion properties, leading to clear and more precise imaging results. This feature is especially advantageous for tracking stem cells and monitoring their integration into target tissues, which is crucial for successful regenerative treatments [30].

Lastly, photoacoustic ultrasound spectroscopy (PAUS) has been proposed for simultaneously assessing red blood cell aggregation and oxygenation levels, providing a comprehensive framework for monitoring these critical blood properties. In summary, using optoacoustic methods, the study of blood properties offers an extensive, non-invasive, and highly accurate diagnostic tool for assessing various blood (physiological and pathological) parameters. These capabilities are essential for the early detection, diagnosis, and monitoring of a wide range of diseases, highlighting the importance of further research and development in this field [31, 32].

9.1.3 Objectives and scope of the chapter

This chapter comprehensively explores the optoacoustic properties of blood, covering a spectrum of topics from the fundamental aspects of signal generation to potential clinical applications and future research directions. It begins by delving into the intricate mechanisms underlying optoacoustic signal generation within biological tissues, highlighting the interaction between laser light and blood components that leads to the emission of acoustic waves. The chapter also discusses the technological advancements utilized for signal detection in imaging systems, providing insights into the complexities of OAI.

Moving forward, the chapter transitions into an in-depth analysis of the optical absorption properties of blood, with a specific focus on significant constituents like Hb. It explores how variations in blood oxygenation impact optical absorption, a crucial aspect relevant to OAI techniques.

Furthermore, the discussion extends to quantitative analysis methods tailored for optoacoustic signals, emphasizing the importance of accurate measurements in determining blood volume, concentration, and various hemodynamic parameters.

The chapter then shifts its attention to the imaging capabilities of optoacoustic techniques, showcasing their effectiveness in visualizing blood oxygenation levels, monitoring hemodynamics, and assessing morphological characteristics of blood vessels. It also explores potential clinical applications, including disease diagnosis and treatment monitoring, leveraging the strengths of OAI. Addressing the challenges and limitations of OAI, the chapter proposes potential solutions and outlines future research directions to enhance its capabilities and clinical utility. Lastly, the chapter concludes by summarizing key findings, discussing implications for scientific and clinical advancements, and suggesting avenues for further research and application in the dynamic field of OAI and hemodynamics.

9.2 Fundamentals of optoacoustic signal generation

Optoacoustic signal generation is a fundamental process at the intersection of optics and acoustics, essential for various biomedical imaging and sensing applications. It involves converting absorbed optical energy into detectable acoustic signals within biological tissues. Understanding the principles of optoacoustic signal generation is crucial for optimizing imaging depth, resolution, and sensitivity in OAI systems.

9.2.1 Principles of optoacoustic imaging in biological tissues

When a laser beam transitions between two different mediums, it undergoes refraction at the boundary of the second medium. The angle of refraction can be determined using Snell's law, as expressed in equation (9.1).

$$\sin \sin \theta_2 = \frac{n_1}{n_2} \sin \sin \theta_1 \tag{9.1}$$

where θ_2 is the angle of incidence of the laser beam in the second medium (refraction angle), θ_1 is the original angle of incidence of the laser beam, n_1 is the refractive index of the first medium, and n_2 is the refractive index of the second medium. The transmission of optical energy from the first medium to the second medium (T) is calculated using the below equation when the angle of incidence from the first medium to the second is 90 degrees.

$$T = \frac{4n_1 n_2}{(n_1 + n_2)^2} \tag{9.2}$$

Furthermore, the amount of reflected optical energy (R) directed back to the first medium is determined as,

$$R = 1 - T = \frac{(n_1 - n_2)^2}{(n_1 + n_2)^2} \tag{9.3}$$

The amount of optical energy scattered in tissue is determined by the scattering coefficient, assuming a homogenous distribution of scattering points. The scattering direction is influenced by the anisotropy value, which ranges from -1 to 1. Positive anisotropy values result in forward scattering, while zero anisotropy leads to isotropic scattering. Negative anisotropy values cause backward scattering, and the anisotropy value impacts the scattering coefficient and can be calculated as follows:

$$\mu_s' = (1 - g)\mu_s \tag{9.4}$$

The reduced scattering coefficient is denoted as $\mu_s{}'$, the anisotropy value as g, and the scattering coefficient as μ_s. The absorption coefficient calculates the amount of light absorbed by tissue, assuming a homogeneous distribution of absorbing points. This coefficient is influenced by the tissue type and the wavelength of the laser beam, as illustrated in figure 9.2.

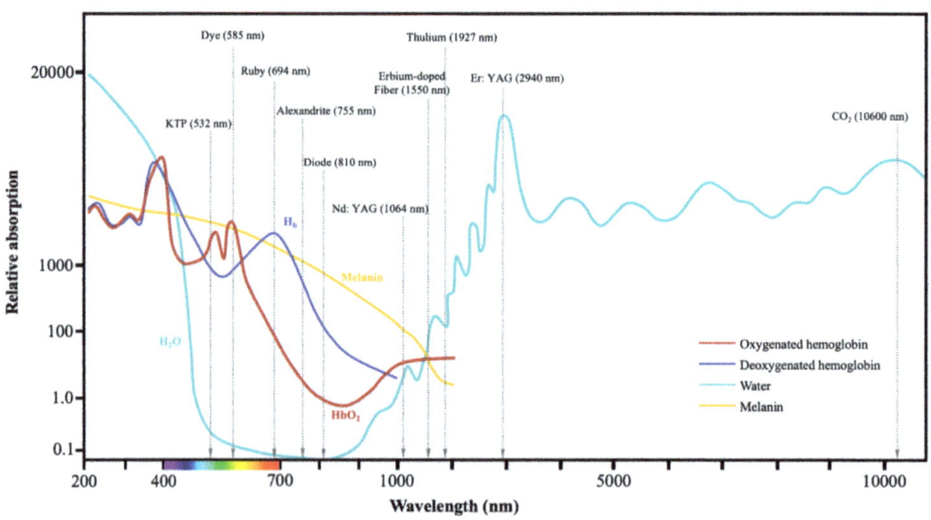

Figure 9.2. Absorption coefficients of different endogenous tissue constituents.

Optical imaging of tissues capitalizes on the spectroscopic interactions between light and tissue, including scattering, absorption, and polarization. These interactions are crucial because many tissue molecules exhibit distinct optical signatures, particularly in absorption, which can be effectively used to analyze tissues at functional and molecular levels. For instance, the absorption spectra for key tissue chromophores like Hb, melanin, lipids, and water can be distinctly identified, providing valuable diagnostic information [33].

This principle allows for detailed characterization of tissue properties, enhancing the understanding of biological processes at a cellular and subcellular level. Optical imaging leverages the distinct spectroscopic contrasts of biological molecules, which are pivotal in diagnosing various diseases. This imaging modality utilizes the unique light absorption properties of molecules such as Hb, melanin, and lipids, which have proven invaluable in medical diagnostics due to their specific interactions with light across different wavelengths [34–36]. However, the effectiveness of purely optical techniques diminishes at depths greater than a few millimeters because of the significant scattering of light within the tissue, which blurs images and reduces resolution at deeper levels [34].

On the other hand, ultrasound (US) imaging operates on a different principle, utilizing sound waves to insonify tissue and capture the returning echoes to construct acoustic reflectivity maps [37]. This modality remains highly favored in clinical settings due to its portability, cost-effectiveness, accessibility, and impressive spatial and temporal resolution. Despite these advantages, ultrasound imaging has its limitations, particularly when it comes to soft tissue contrast and the ability to distinguish between malignant and benign abnormalities in deep tissues, where it may lack the necessary sensitivity [38].

The interplay between optical and ultrasound imaging modalities suggests a complementary approach might be advantageous. By integrating these techniques, medical professionals could overcome the individual limitations of each system, offering a more comprehensive diagnostic tool that enhances disease detection and characterization in deeper tissues. This synergy could lead to advancements in diagnosing and monitoring conditions, paving the way for more targeted and effective treatments.

9.2.2 Interaction of laser light with blood components

Laser light propagation in tissues is a question of growing importance in many diagnostic and therapeutic applications in today's photomedicine. As suitable light sources for photo medical applications, Lasers provide highly monochromatic, temporally, and spatially coherent light with high radiation stability. The distribution of laser light in a tissue may considerably differ for various tissues depending on their structure and composition.

The interaction of laser light with blood components is a fundamental aspect of OAI and has significant implications in medical diagnostics and therapeutics [39]. It has been extensively studied, revealing a range of effects that vary depending on the type of laser used, its power, and the duration of exposure. Research has shown that laser light can influence the fundamental cellular and molecular components of blood, such as RBCs, platelets, and blood plasma proteins, affecting the micro-rheologic parameters of blood, and each absorbing light at specific wavelengths, which leads to distinct biological effects [40]. This interaction results in photo-chemical and photomechanical effects, depending on the energy and wavelength of the laser used.

- *Photothermal effects:* When absorbed light is converted into heat, it can be utilized for targeted destruction of abnormal blood vessels or tumors while minimizing damage to healthy tissues.
- *Photochemical effects:* Involve changes at the molecular level that can modify cell function or structure. They are beneficial in activating photosensitive drugs for the controlled treatment of diseases.
- *Photomechanical effects:* Rapid thermal expansion leading to mechanical disruption of tissues, applied in procedures like laser tattoo removal or treatment of skin conditions, ensuring targeted interventions with reduced side effects and improved efficacy.

Exposing human blood to helium–neon (He–Ne) and Nd:YAG lasers for 5 and 10 min increases RBC (erythrocyte) count, while white blood cells (WBCs) and platelets decrease (thrombocytopenia). Hb concentration, packed cell volume (PCV), and erythrocyte sedimentation rate (ESR) also increase after laser exposure, with varying effects based on laser power and exposure duration [41].

Moreover, laser-based methods have demonstrated potential in diagnosing blood-borne viruses like HIV (human immunodeficiency virus) and HCV (Hepatitis C virus) in human plasma, offering rapid, sensitive, and multiplex detection capabilities with minimal sample preparation. Laser sparks interact with blood components to differentiate HIV and HCV in plasma samples, enabling rapid virus identification with minimal sample preparation and providing results within minutes. Low-power helium–neon and diode lasers with wavelengths of 632.8 and 650 nm on some human blood samples alter their components, decreasing WBCs, RBCs, and blood viscosity (HCT) while increasing the number of neutrophils (NEUTs) and platelets (PLTs) and ESR. The laser may also affect intracellular calcium ions and plasma composition [42, 43].

Intravascular laser irradiation of blood (ILIB) has been explored for its stimulatory effects on blood cells. It has shown benefits for the immune system, microcirculation, and alleviation of pain and inflammation. Laser light at 450 and 520 nm affects RBCs' rheology, causing enhanced aggregation and shape changes at high levels of laser radiation (above 170.5 $J\,cm^{-2}$). Conversely, using lower levels of laser radiation (below 9.5 $J\,cm^{-2}$) improves RBC deformability, weakens cell–cell interactions during disaggregation, and revitalizes RBCs, especially in challenging conditions. [42, 44].

Research utilizing low-level laser radiation (LLLR) has indicated positive effects on the rheological properties of RBCs, such as flexibility and aggregability, which are crucial for healthy microcirculation [45]. Additionally, the interaction of He–Ne laser radiation with blood has been studied for its impact on the electrical conductivity of human blood, which is crucial for disease diagnosis and treatment. Factors like erythrocyte concentration, HCT volume, and blood plasma composition significantly influence blood's electrical conductivity. The laser-blood interaction causes light scattering and absorption, mainly influenced by erythrocytes due to their abundance and size, shaping blood's behavior under laser exposure [46].

Finally, Q-switched ultraviolet (355 nm) laser irradiation has been shown to cause RBC deformation and aggregation, affect Hb absorption spectra, and indicate structural changes in blood components. The reduced Hb absorbance and decreased RBC count with higher laser fluence indicated cell deformation and aggregation. This change in Hb absorption has implications for optical oximeters. Post-laser exposure, basophil-type WBCs increased significantly ($p \leqslant 0.05$), potentially activating the immune system against pathogens through mitochondrial changes and cell division. These findings collectively underscore laser light's complex and varied effects on blood, offering insights into potential diagnostic and therapeutic applications [47].

9.2.3 Generation of acoustic waves and their detection

9.2.3.1 Generation of photoacoustic signals

The optoacoustic effect revolves around the interaction of pulsed light with a material that absorbs part of this energy. This absorption triggers a temperature increase, leading to thermoelastic expansion, producing sound waves. These waves are detectable by ultrasound transducers, allowing the identification of the specific locations where light absorption occurs, thereby offering insights into the functional and molecular characteristics of the sample. This fundamental mechanism underpins PAI, which merges the molecular sensitivity of optical imaging with the penetrative power of ultrasound, providing a profound tool for deep tissue analysis [48]. The principle of OAI is illustrated in figure 9.3.

The essence of OAI lies in discerning the geometry and composition of a sample through the analysis of the spatial and temporal characteristics of optoacoustic signals. This technique hinges on a comprehensive understanding of how acoustic

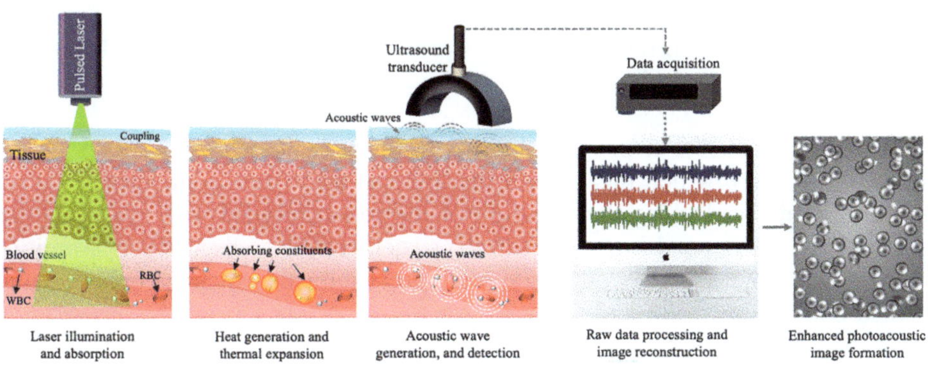

Figure 9.3. The photoacoustic principle.

waves are formed and propagated following the photoacoustic effect. In OAI, accurately describing these acoustic waves involves considering two critical temporal aspects, thermal confinement, and stress confinement, that influence how the waves are analyzed and interpreted, ensuring precise imaging results. These temporal conditions are crucial for effectively capturing and utilizing the acoustic data to reconstruct images that accurately reflect the physical properties of the targeted sample.

Thermal confinement: An optoacoustic signal from the sample is effectively generated and spatially distinguished in a sample when the pulse duration of the excitation laser is shorter than the thermal relaxation time of the targeted tissue. The thermal relaxation time, represented as τ_{th}, indicates the period required for the heat absorbed by a voxel, ideally a spherically symmetric volume excited through photon absorption, to disperse into the surrounding area. The thermal confinement, τ_{th}, *is* defined by.

$$\tau_{th} = \frac{d_v^2}{\alpha_{th}} \tag{9.5}$$

where *dv* is the characteristic dimension or voxel diameter, and α_{th} is the thermal diffusivity in the medium.

Stress confinement: If the pulse duration of the excitation laser is shorter than the stress relaxation time, denoted as τ_s, then the pressure increases during the excitation process across the medium are considered negligible. This condition ensures the medium remains relatively stable during the laser pulse.

$$\tau_s = \frac{d_v}{v_s} \tag{9.6}$$

where v_s is the speed of sound in the respective medium (in tissue ~1540 m s^{-1}). It is important to emphasize that to achieve high-resolution images in optoacoustic tomography, the detection bandwidth of the ultrasound probe must be sufficiently high. Optoacoustic tomography typically achieves resolutions of around 50 μ, corresponding to a stress relaxation time of approximately 30 nanoseconds. Consequently, τ_s is a critical determinant in selecting the excitation laser, with pulse durations commonly ranging from hundreds of picoseconds to a few nanoseconds to optimize optoacoustic signal generation effectively.

The wave equation for a propagating acoustic wave, where acoustic pressure is denoted as $p(\vec{r}, t)$, which meets both the thermal and stress confinement assumptions, can be derived using the equation of motion combined with the generalized Hooke's law. The resulting equation is structured to reflect these conditions, providing a framework for understanding how acoustic waves propagate under specified constraints:

$$\left(\nabla^2 - \frac{1}{c^2}\frac{\partial^2}{\partial t^2}\right) p(\vec{r}, t) = -\frac{\Gamma}{c^2}\frac{\partial}{\partial t}H(\vec{r}, t) \tag{9.7}$$

Here, the effect of heating on a material's volume is quantified by the dimensionless thermodynamic Gruneisen parameter.

$$\Gamma = \beta \frac{v_s^2}{C_p} \tag{9.8}$$

with β constituting the isobaric heat expansion coefficient and C_p the isobaric heat capacity of the absorber, respectively. A typical value for $\wp$ is 0.2 in soft tissue. Further, the heating function $H(\vec{r}, t)$ quantifies the rate and amount of energy absorption over time within a specific voxel, based on the energy of the absorbed photons or the general electromagnetic radiation. It is given by

$$H(\vec{r}, t) = \nu\mu(\vec{r})\Phi(\vec{r}, t) \tag{9.9}$$

In the equation, v represents the heat conversion efficiency, which is typically approximated to be close to 1, $\mu(\vec{r})$ is the absorption coefficient and $\Phi(\vec{r}, t)$ is the optical fluence rate. It is important to distinguish $\Phi(\vec{r}, t)$ from optical fluence and it corresponds to the temporal derivative of the laser excitation intensity,

$$\frac{\partial}{\partial t}\Phi(\vec{r}, t) = I(\vec{r}, t) \tag{9.10}$$

From equation (9.7), it is critical to note that the temporal derivative of $H(\vec{r}, t)$ on the right side indicates that optoacoustic excitation requires temporally differentiable illumination, such as that provided by pulsed or modulated lasers. This part of the equation generates optoacoustic signals, whereas the left side accounts for the propagation of acoustic waves through the medium.

To find a solution to equation (9.7), one would apply the corresponding Green's function, considering local stress confinement and localized energy absorption represented by a delta function, $H(t) = \delta\ (t)$. This approach allows the modeling of the pressure field in an infinite space, providing insights into how optoacoustic signals are generated and how they propagate and are detected through different media. The pressure field in infinite space can then be written as,

$$p(\vec{r}, t) = \frac{\Gamma}{4\pi v_s^2}\frac{\partial}{\partial t}\left[\frac{1}{v_s t}\iiint H(\vec{r}')\delta\left(t - \frac{\vec{r} - \vec{r}'}{v_s}\right)d\vec{r}'\right] \tag{9.11}$$

In this equation, the heating function encompasses integration over the volume illuminated by the light source, with $\vec{r}'$ located within this specific volume. The derived solution for a spherical absorber positioned at $\vec{r}_s$ with a radius a is described as.

$$p(\vec{r}, t) = p_I\left[U(a - v_s t - R) + \frac{R - v_s t}{2R}U(R - |a - v_s t|)\ U(a + v_s t + R)\right] \tag{9.12}$$

In this context, p_I represents the initial pressure amplitude, and U stands for the Heaviside function, which is defined as $H(x) = 0$ for $x < 0$ and $H(x) = 1$ for $x \geqslant 0$. Furthermore, R denotes the distance between the detector and the acoustic source, calculated as $R = |\vec{r} - \vec{r}'|$. Additionally, the absorber is described as having a finite volume and is assumed to maintain a homogeneous composition throughout its entire volume.

9.2.3.2 Ultrasound propagation and detection

When a laser pulse excites pressure within a medium, it acts as an acoustic source that triggers the propagation of acoustic waves throughout 3D space. In OAI, US waves in tissues generally maintain a constant speed of approximately 1540 m s^{-1}, with deviations typically less than 10%, which are often disregarded unless significant tissue heterogeneity exists. Acoustic scattering in tissues is substantially lower than optical scattering, contributing to OAI's enhanced imaging depth compared to other optical imaging methods that rely on focusing. This reduced scattering also highlights the importance of considering acoustic attenuation, which impacts wave propagation. The attenuation of all tissues is temperature and frequency-dependent. The frequency dependency of ultrasonic attenuation is described by,

$$\alpha = a_0 f^b \text{ (dB cm}^{-1}\text{)} \tag{9.13}$$

where a_0 is the tissue-dependent constant, b is a power law factor whose value usually ranges between 1 and 2 in the soft tissue, and f is the frequency ultrasound expressed in MHz.

The acoustic attenuation in tissues significantly impacts the imaging quality and resolution. For soft tissues, the attenuation coefficient, α, is generally about 1 dB cm^{-1} MHz^{-1}, but it can increase up to 20 dB cm^{-1} MHz^{-1} in denser tissues like bone, assuming a non-frequency-dependent ($b = 1$) attenuation model. This characteristic makes the frequency-dependent acoustic attenuation akin to a low-pass filter, where higher frequency signals are more attenuated, limiting the high-frequency content that reaches the detector and thus constraining the spatial resolution achievable.

The spatial resolution of an OAI system is influenced by several factors beyond acoustic attenuation, including the frequency bandwidth of the US detector, the detector's active surface area, the number of detector elements, the detector aperture, and the algorithms used for image reconstruction. Additionally, as the acoustic sensitivity of a US detector generally decreases with an increase in frequency, there is an inherent trade-off between imaging depth and spatial resolution. For instance, a study by Xia *et al* demonstrated that in an OAI system using a linear array US probe with a central frequency of 9 MHz, the axial resolution measured using targets immersed in water was 0.22 mm across a depth range of 13–36 mm. In contrast, the lateral resolution varied between 0.35 and 0.76 mm depending on the spatial location [49]. This complex interplay of factors underscores the need for careful consideration in designing and applying PAI systems to balance depth and resolution based on specific clinical or research requirements.

Linear array piezoelectric probes, commonly utilized in traditional ultrasound imaging, also serve as detectors in PAI, enabling simultaneous real-time US and photoacoustic imaging through a unified system [50]. This dual-modality approach provides supplementary contrast and facilitates clinical acceptance due to the prevalent utilization of US imaging. Progress in ultrasound probe technology, encompassing enhanced bandwidth and sensitivity, enhances the efficacy of PAI by accommodating the wide-ranging nature and diminished amplitude of photoacoustic signals. These advancements facilitate more accurate 2D or 3D imaging utilizing single-element transducers with mechanical scanning or multi-element arrays, amplifying diagnostic capabilities and seamlessly integrating PAI into clinical settings. Furthermore, incorporating alternative sensing technologies, like optical detection methods, is also feasible. These techniques present capabilities for contactless measurements and the potential for swift monitoring over extensive areas, albeit generally displaying reduced sensitivity and heightened noise levels at frequencies surpassing 1 MHz compared to piezoelectric detectors [51]. This classification of sensor categories emphasizes the compromises between distinct detection approaches concerning sensitivity, noise levels, and operational bandwidth, assisting in selecting technology based on specific application requirements.

9.3 Optical absorption properties of blood

9.3.1 Absorption spectra of major blood constituents (hemoglobin, oxyhemoglobin, deoxyhemoglobin)

In tissues, light propagation is influenced by absorption and scattering due to cells and molecules, quantified by the absorption coefficient (μ_a) and scattering coefficient (μ_s), respectively. When light energy is absorbed by biological tissue, it is converted into thermal energy, distributing heat within the absorber. The specific wavelengths at which absorption occurs are dictated by the molecular characteristics of the substances in the path of the light, highlighting how molecular structures influence light absorption [52].

Absorption primarily involves light-absorbing compounds in tissue called chromophores, such as Hb, myoglobin, and melanin, while scattering results from refractive index variations at structures like cellular membranes and collagen fibrils. These optical properties are essential for selecting diagnostic wavelengths that differentiate pathological tissues from healthy ones based on the distinct spectral signatures of tissue constituents such as Hb, lipids, and water. This differentiation is crucial for effective medical diagnostics [53]. Each chromophore has a unique absorption spectrum, where the specific extinction coefficient is expressed as a function of the wavelength. The typical spectral features of the main blood constituents, Hb, oxyhemoglobin (HbO_2), and deoxyhemoglobin, are shown in figure 9.4 [54].

In medical imaging, the absorption spectra of Hb and its oxygenated form, HbO_2, are pivotal. These blood constituents are major absorbers in the sub-1000 nm wavelength range, facilitating the imaging of vascular structures and the measurement of blood oxygen saturation (sO_2). The superior absorption properties of HbO_2 and HbR (reduced Hb) between 650 and 900 nm, compared to other chromophores such as lipids and water, enable high-contrast vascular imaging in PAT. This range

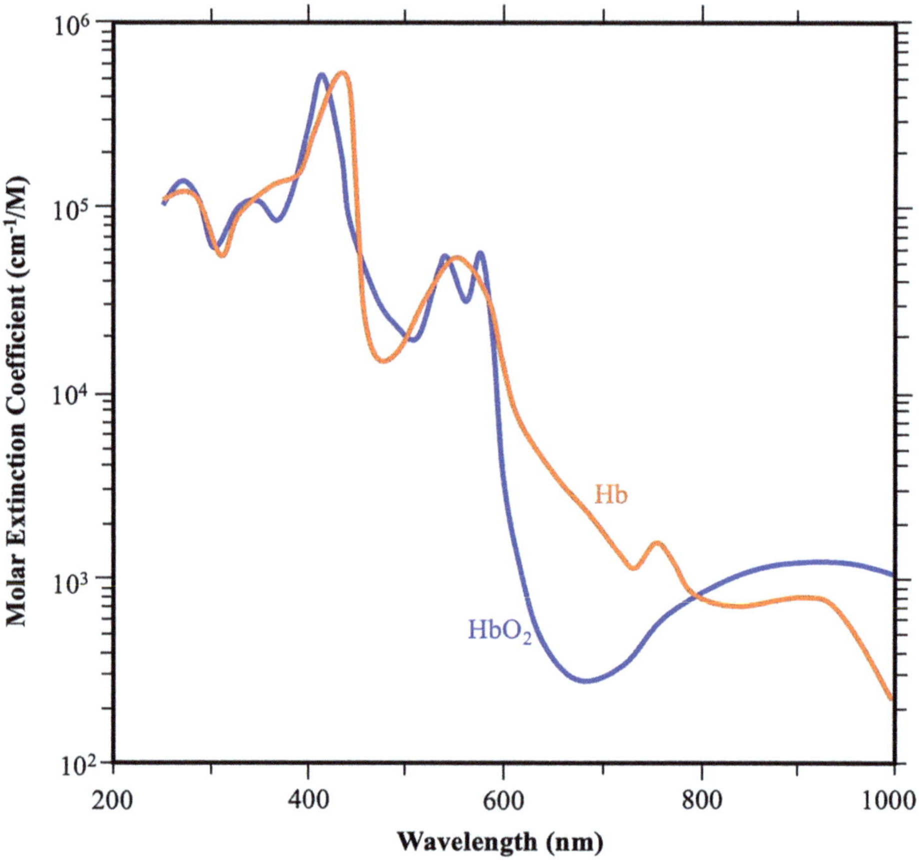

Figure 9.4. Absorption spectra for deoxyhemoglobin and oxyhemoglobin (HbO_2).

is specifically effective for vascular imaging without interference from melanin, which, despite its high absorption, is localized to areas like the skin and retina and does not affect blood oxygenation measurements. Understanding these spectral characteristics is crucial for enhancing the accuracy of non-invasive imaging diagnostics that monitor blood flow and tissue health [55].

9.3.2 Influence of blood oxygenation on optical absorption

The impact of blood oxygenation on optical absorption is a crucial element in various medical diagnostic and therapeutic contexts, as it directly impacts the optical characteristics of blood and thus affects the interaction of light with biological tissues. The absorption coefficient of blood, representing the amount of light absorbed by blood per unit length, exhibits notable variations based on the oxygenation status of Hb. This variability arises from the distinct absorption spectra of oxyhemoglobin and deoxyhemoglobin, which feature specific absorption bands in the visible and near-infrared spectral regions [31].

Studies have demonstrated that the absorption characteristics of human RBC suspensions are predominantly influenced by Hb absorption up to 1200 nm, with notable contributions from oxygen saturation levels [28]. Correspondingly, in interstitial photodynamic therapy, light-induced Hb deoxygenation triggers heightened light absorption, emphasizing the dynamic nature of blood's optical attributes under varying oxygenation conditions. This sensitivity to oxygen levels is leveraged in techniques for assessing blood oxygenation in the retina, where distinctions in the absorption coefficients of Hb and oxyhemoglobin are utilized to infer oxygenation levels [23, 25].

Moreover, the advancement of optical methodologies for detecting alterations in Hb oxygenation, such as two-dimensional absorption assessments, underscores the significance of precisely evaluating the oxygenation status for medical diagnostics, including screening tumors in breast tissue [29]. The influence of water absorption on signal baselines in *in vivo* measurements further highlights the intricacies involved in accurately determining the status of Hb in tissues [26].

Near-infrared spectroscopy (NIRS) and diffuse optical tomography (DOT) leverage the selective absorption of blood chromophores to measure concentrations of Hb and oxyhemoglobin, thereby offering insights into blood volume and oxygenation levels in tissues. These measurements play a critical role in the early detection of cancer through the characterization of tissue angiogenesis [24, 32].

Both *in vivo* and *in vitro* investigations have enhanced our comprehension of the impact of blood oxygenation on optical absorption, enabling the quantitative monitoring of changes in oxy-Hb content and total-Hb content in living tissues [56]. Additionally, the development of models to explore the influence of blood vessels on apparent absorption coefficients has enhanced algorithms for computing Hb saturation while considering background tissue absorption and the distribution of blood vessels [27]. Sensitivity analyses conducted in near-infrared spectral bands have pinpointed specific wavelengths where the effective absorption coefficient is most responsive to the concentration of oxygenated Hb, thereby facilitating precise saturation measurements in dense transmission samples like the forearm. This body of research collectively underscores the significant role of blood oxygenation in optical absorption, a fundamental aspect of advancing medical imaging and diagnostic methodologies.

9.3.3 Spectral characteristics and implications for optoacoustic imaging

OAI leverages the spectral characteristics of tissues to provide detailed insights into their physiological, cellular, and subcellular functions. The spectral dimension of OAI is crucial as it allows for the illumination of tissue at multiple wavelengths, enabling the differentiation of intrinsic chromophores and externally administered agents based on their unique absorption spectra. This multispectral approach facilitates the identification of physiological parameters such as blood oxygen saturation levels by employing spectral unmixing techniques to accurately sense intrinsic tissue chromophores like oxygenated and deoxygenated Hb, as well as extrinsically administered photo-absorbing agents and nanoparticles.

The spectral characteristics of blood, particularly the absorption spectra of oxygenated and deoxygenated Hb, play a crucial role in OAI. This technique offers a pathway to visualize and quantify sO_2 and monitor physiological states. OAI leverages the absorption of pulsed light by chromophores in the tissue, such as Hb, to generate ultrasound signals, which can be reconstructed to form images that reveal the morphological and functional characteristics of blood vessels [57, 58].

OAI can distinguish blood vessels by oxygen levels, with a discernment threshold of 4.6% in saturation at 15 mm depth. Using 1064 nm, OAI revealed oxygenated vessels up to 48 mm deep; with 757 nm, deoxygenated vessels were visible to 42 mm. It exploits the endogenous optical contrast of blood without needing external contrast agents or ionizing radiation [59].

A key aspect of OAI for blood analysis is the spectral unmixing techniques that differentiate intrinsic tissue chromophores and externally administered agents. This differentiation is vital for accurately sensing and quantifying blood parameters, such as sO_2 levels, by transforming the problem from the spatial to the spectral domain [22].

The quantitative photoacoustic assessment (QPA) further demonstrates the optical wavelength dependence in evaluating RBC aggregation and oxygen saturation, highlighting the dynamic interplay between absorber size, absorption coefficient, and the resulting photoacoustic signals during pulsatile blood flow [32].

Moreover, the wavelength-dependent light attenuation in tissue necessitates a spectral correction of optoacoustic signals to reliably estimate sO_2 levels, underscoring the importance of validating optical characterization and the spectral fitting process. Spectral analysis of photoacoustic signals in the ultrasound frequency domain also correlates changes in tissue microstructures with variations in the light distribution for different optical wavelengths, emphasizing the need for careful examination of spectral parameters [60, 61]

Recent advancements include the development of multi-wavelength high frame-rate light emittimg diode (LED) based photoacoustic/ultrasound imaging systems, which have demonstrated the capability to characterize the absorption spectrum of blood and other chromophores accurately. Dual-wavelength OAI systems have shown potential in visualizing arteriovenous anastomoses with high spatial resolution, employing structural and spectral information to distinguish between veins and arteries [59, 62].

Photoacoustic fluctuation imaging (PAFI) has been introduced to enhance image quality by exploiting absorption fluctuations due to blood flow, offering a new avenue for quantitative multispectral imaging for 3D blood oxygenation imaging [63]. This approach, along with OAI for generating diagnostic images of blood oxygen saturation without external contrast agents, illustrates the broad applicability of spectral characteristics in diagnosing conditions such as breast cancer [64]. Machine learning techniques, combined with Monte Carlo simulations and spectral optoacoustic data, are being explored to improve the reconstruction of the 3D distribution of blood oxygen saturation, highlighting the evolving landscape of OAI technology. Finally, the design of optoacoustic systems for clinical and preclinical applications emphasizes the importance of visualizing the distribution of optically absorbing molecules, such as Hb, for detecting and monitoring diseases.

9.4 Quantitative analysis of optoacoustic signals

9.4.1 Methods for quantifying blood volume and concentration

Optoacoustic technology is utilized for the absolute, accurate, continuous, and real-time measurement of various critical diagnostic variables. This includes non-invasive measurements of circulating blood volume (BV) and cardiac output (CO), cardiac index (CI), and systemic oxygen delivery (DO) from the measured variables. It also enables the measurement of concentrations of Hb derivatives (e.g., carboxyhemoglobin (HbCO), reduced Hb, oxygenated Hb (HbOxy), and methemoglobin (HbMet)), total Hb concentration tHb, and other substances such as lactate, myoglobin, cholesterol, body pigments, and exogenous dyes. Additionally, the invention can determine the content in tissues such as water, fat, protein, calcium, and blood and the density of hard and soft tissues. Furthermore, the optoacoustic technique can be used for accurate non-invasive measurement of blood pressure (or vascular pressure) in arteries, arterioles, veins, and capillaries using occlusion-induced changes in the optoacoustic signal induced in the circulating blood. The optoacoustic technique can be employed for single measurement, continuous measurement, or continuous monitoring of these variables [65].

PAM is used to achieve high-resolution imaging of optical absorption contrast in the optical diffusive regime. It quantifies optical absorption coefficients accurately at various optical wavelengths without needing information about optical fluence attenuation, acoustic pressure attenuation, or detection bandwidth.

The acoustic spectrum $S(\omega, \lambda)$ of the received PA signal from an absorbing target object of interest can be expressed, under the assumptions of linearity and shift invariance, as

$$S(\omega, \lambda) = F_I(\lambda)\ O(\omega, \lambda)\ a(\omega)H(\omega) \tag{9.14}$$

Here, λ denotes the optical wavelength, F_I represents the optical fluence received by the target object, $O(\omega, \lambda)$ is the original acoustic spectrum of the target object of interest (e.g., a blood vessel), $a\ (\omega)$ stands for the acoustic attenuation within the tissue situated between the target object and the ultrasonic transducer, and $H(\omega)$ defines the system transfer function of the ultrasonic detection system.

An absorption-fitting algorithm was developed to estimate optical absorption coefficients and relative incident fluence from acoustic spectra $\underline{S}(\omega, \lambda_i)$ at various wavelengths derived as:

$$\underline{S}(\omega, \lambda_i) = \frac{S(\omega, \lambda_i)}{S_{\mathrm{rms}}(\omega)} = \frac{F_I(\lambda_i)\ O(\omega, \lambda_i)}{\sqrt{\dfrac{\sum_{i=1}^{n} |\ F_I(\lambda_i)\ O(\omega, \lambda_i)\,|^2}{n}}} \tag{9.15}$$

Here, the acoustic spectrum $S(\omega, \lambda_i)$ (where $i = 1, 2, \ldots, n$) at each optical wavelength is normalized by the root-mean-square spectrum $S_{\mathrm{rms}}(\omega)$. The impacts of both the response $H(\omega)$ dependent on the system and the acoustic attenuation $a(\omega)$ related to the tissue are negated during the normalization procedure. The method was validated by quantifying the absorption coefficients of an oxygenated bovine blood phantom at 560, 565, 570, and 575 nm with errors less than 3%. Additionally, using AR-PAM, the study successfully quantified total Hb concentration [tHb] and Hb sO_2 in a live mouse using the acoustic spectral method, which demonstrated superior quantification accuracy compared to the conventional amplitude method in the optical diffusive regime [66].

Another study introduces a novel method for quantifying absolute particle concentrations in PAI without requiring laser fluence calibration. By analyzing photoacoustic signals statistically and leveraging Brownian motion-induced fluctuations governed by Poisson distribution, various particle concentrations, including RBCs, were accurately measured both *in vitro* and *in vivo*.

The power-based signal-to-noise ratio (SNR) of the photoacoustic signal is derived as,

$$\frac{1}{\mathrm{SNR_{PA}}} = (1 + {\alpha_p}^2)\frac{1}{E(N_P)} + \frac{1}{\mathrm{SNR_{th}}} + {\alpha_p}^2 \tag{9.16}$$

Where $E()$ denotes the mean, N_P is the particle count, α_P is the photon count fluctuation coefficient, the ratio between the mean squared PA amplitude (A_{PA}) and the variance of the electronic thermal noise of the ultrasonic transducer (n_{PA}) is $\mathrm{SNR_{th}} = \frac{E^2(A_{PA})}{Var(n_{PA})}$. When particles are sparse enough so that $\mathrm{E}(N_p) \gg {\alpha_p}^{-2}$, and if $E(N_p) \ll \mathrm{SNR_{th}}$, then the SNR becomes, $\mathrm{SNR_{PA}} \approx E(N_P)$. This fluence-independent approach offers a promising avenue for non-invasive particle concentration quantification of biological tissue in biomedical applications [67].

A planar Fabry–Pérot (FP) ultrasound scanner is used to acquire 3D photoacoustic images for quantitative PAT (qPAT) measurements to extract chromophore (blood, oxygen saturation) concentration ratios and validated by comparing the photoacoustic spectrum of copper (II) sulfate ($CuSO_4$) obtained with a spectrophotometer. The challenges include nonlinear tissue fluence distribution, a large-scale inverse problem, and the accuracy of experimental parameters. This study proposes a Monte Carlo-based inversion scheme with image segmentation to reduce variables. This inversion aimed to estimate relative concentration ratios R_k, with fixed background absorption and scattering. The objective function minimized as:

$$E(R_1, R_2, R_3) = \sum_{k=1}^{3}\sum_{i=1}^{N_\lambda} (\beta_k \cdot p_0^{\mathrm{exp}}(k, \lambda_i) - p_0^{\mathrm{sim}}(k, \lambda_i, R_k))^2 \tag{9.17}$$

The measured and modeled initial pressure distributions in tubes $k = 1,2,3$ denoted as $p_0^{\mathrm{exp}}(k, \lambda_i)$ and $p_0^{\mathrm{sim}}(k, \lambda_i, R_k)$ respectively, are determined at wavelength λ_i with concentration ratio R_k. These distributions are averaged over all pixels within the segmented volume corresponding to tube k. The scaling factor β_k is used to normalize both experimental and modeled data. Experimental validation in tissue-mimicking phantoms shows accurate parameter estimates within 5% of actual values for chromophore concentration ratios [68].

A photoacoustic-based blood glucose concentration (BGC) measurement setup was established using a Q-switched Nd: YAG-pumped optical parametric oscillator (OPO) pulsed laser. This setup employed a lateral detection model to capture photoacoustic signals from glucose. *In vitro* experiments with glucose solutions validated the real-time photoacoustic signal profile and identified characteristic wavelengths. Based on the least square fitting between photoacoustic peak-to-peak values and glucose concentrations, a prediction concentration model achieved a root mean square error (RMSE) of 0.77 $mmol\,l^{-1}$ [69].

PAI offers high-resolution blood Hb concentration and sO_2 detection. The correlation between photoacoustically determined total Hb and sO_2 with biochemical blood parameters across species was investigated using a commercial small animal imaging system (MSOT inVision 256-TF). *In vitro* experiments using blood from mice, rats, humans, and naked mole rats showed significant correlations between tHb and Hb, HCT, and RBC count. PAI accurately resolves inter-species differences in Hb, HCT, and oxygen dissociation curves, highlighting its sensitivity to species-specific variations [25].

Utilizing photoacoustic spectroscopy with near-infrared light, blood glucose concentrations were measured non-invasively. Results showed a clear correlation between glucose concentration and photoacoustic signal characteristics, with signal intensity and sound speed increasing with higher glucose concentrations, especially at wavelengths with high glucose absorbance. Quantitative estimation of glucose levels was achieved through signal intensity ratios at specific wavelengths, showing a linear relationship with glucose concentration [70].

9.4.2 Estimation of hemodynamic parameters (e.g., blood flow velocity, oxygen saturation)

Measuring multiple hemodynamic parameters simultaneously is crucial for understanding tissue function and disease progression. These responses occur in reaction to physical or organ activity, environmental shifts, and neural activity, ensuring adequate oxygen delivery to tissues.

Acoustic resolution photoacoustic flowmetry (AR-PAF) is a robust and accurate method for measuring microscale blood flow velocities, showcasing strong agreement with optical and photoacoustic flow measurements. It performs reliably even at higher RBC concentrations, demonstrating potential for diverse applications. AR-PAF is unaffected by physiological RBC aggregation, indicating its suitability for complex biological environments. Successful measurements using a clinical ultrasound scanner and whole blood pave the way for the clinical adoption of AR-PAF. The study underscores the need for further development of AR-PAF for real-time, non-invasive imaging of blood flow dynamics in clinical settings [71].

Thermal diffusion flowmetry (TDF) method based on photothermal excitation and photoacoustic measurement accurately measures blood velocity in a phantom vessel with minimal errors across a wide range of velocities. It utilizes a simplified lumped model to derive the velocity-PA signal relationship from heat and PA equations. The lumped temperature of the system for an impulse photothermal excitation is derived as,

$$\widetilde{T}(t) = \widetilde{T}(0)\exp\left(-\frac{t}{t_{\text{eff}}}\right) \tag{9.18}$$

Here, time constant is $t_{\text{eff}} = t_{\text{conduction}}^{-1} + t_{\text{convection}}^{-1}$, where $t_{\text{conduction}} = C_{\text{conduction}}\, R_{\text{conduction}}$, and $t_{\text{convection}} = C_{\text{convection}}\, R_{\text{convection}}$, C and R stand for capacitance and resistance. The estimated velocity of the fluid is determined as,

$$\widetilde{u}_{\text{est}} = \left(\frac{I_{\text{VUT}}}{t_{\text{eff}}}\right) \tag{9.19}$$

where, I_{VUT} is the optimal proportion parameter which is found by reducing errors between real (u) and estimated velocities. The method's reliance on light absorption suggests the potential for spectroscopic insights, allowing simultaneous measurement of blood velocity and sO_2 level with multispectral implementation [72].

Photoacoustic vector tomography (PAVT) breaks the optical diffusion limit, allowing deep hemodynamic imaging with quantification of blood flow speed and direction. The system setup included an ultrasonic probe, laser light delivery to blood vessels, and reconstruction using the universal back projection algorithm. By combining spatial blood heterogeneity and photoacoustic contrast, PAVT provides pixel-wise flow velocity estimation, surpassing typical limits to image deep blood vessels over five millimeters. The study emphasized the role of blood heterogeneity, particularly the spatial distribution of RBCs, in enhancing signal visibility for deep hemodynamic imaging [73].

The utility of carbogen-based functional imaging, combining PAI and blood oxygen level dependent (BOLD) magnetic resonance imaging (MRI), used to monitor early changes in tumor hemodynamics post-vascular targeted therapy. This approach reveals increased tumor Hb oxygen saturation levels and BOLD signal intensity in response to carbogen, while treatment with a vascular disrupting agent (VDA) reduces the tumor's hemodynamic response to carbogen as observed through PAI. Overall, this imaging technique effectively assesses and monitors tumor response to therapy, providing valuable insights into tumor oxygenation levels and hemodynamics and underlining the importance of non-invasive imaging modalities in evaluating treatment responses *in vivo* [74].

9.4.3 Techniques for enhancing signal-to-noise ratio and accuracy

Several factors limit the quality and resolution of optoacoustic images, thereby impeding this modality's potential for clinical application. These factors could stem from the components of the imaging hardware (noise from PA detection hardware, variations in laser pulse energy), the imprecise or approximate image reconstruction algorithms, the attenuating characteristics, and inhomogeneous light-tissue interaction phenomena or the specifics of the image acquisition process. These issues can materialize as image disturbances, artifacts, and suboptimal overall image accuracy [75, 76].

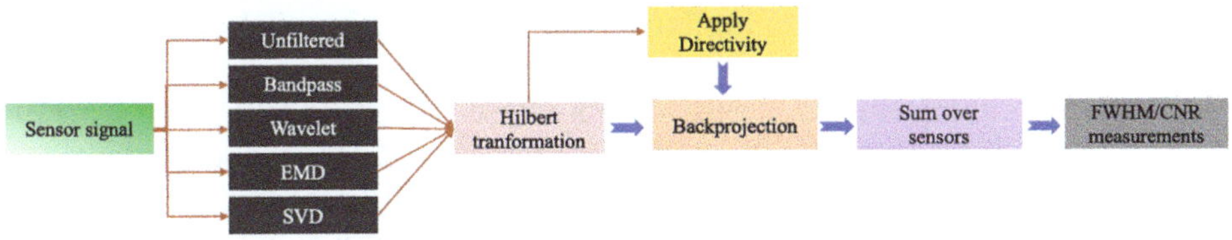

Figure 9.5. The workflow of the signal processing for various methods.

Enhancing the SNR and accuracy in OAI is crucial for improving image quality and resolution. Various techniques (figure 9.5) have been developed to address these challenges, each with unique approaches and benefits. Preprocessing methods such as band-pass filters, wavelet denoising, empirical mode decomposition (EMD), and singular value decomposition (SVD) have been compared, with band-pass filtering consistently yielding improvements in denoising performance and resolution when accounting for sensor directivity [77].

A combination of filters to reduce noise in PAM images, starting with an adaptive median filter, is particularly good at removing impulsive noise that appears as random bright or dark pixels. Following the adaptive median filter, an effective filter for background noise called a nonlocal means filter is used, which compares all parts of the image to reduce noise while preserving important details like edges and textures. This multistage approach aims to enhance the SNR significantly by as much as 16 dB in an *in vivo* study, demonstrating its effectiveness in improving image quality under noisy conditions without causing the blurring that often accompanies filtering techniques [78].

The researchers innovated a method merging light-induced sound with echoes, called the acoustic echo effect, which enhances image clarity and detail. The SNR of the combined signal, i.e., original 20 $(\frac{a}{b})$ and echo 20 $(\frac{\beta a}{b})$ signals, offers better SNR than the original when and expressed as,

$$\mathrm{SNR} = 20\,\frac{(1+\beta)a}{\sqrt{2}b} \tag{9.20}$$

where β is attenuation of the echo signal. This technique significantly improved PAI by enhancing axial positioning accuracy by 100% and increasing the SNR by ~2.8 dB experimentally. The echo signal properties using a multiwall carbon nanotube composite structure indicate practical implementation in PAI systems within a 3.9 mm working distance with water as the medium. Additionally, the method effectively enhanced photoacoustic images of RBCs, showcasing its versatility and effectiveness in improving image quality in biological samples [79].

Addressing pulse peak-power energy variations and timing jitter noise through a high-speed data acquisition (DAQ) system combined with a software-based approach has also been effective in enhancing photoacoustic signal accuracy. This method directly measures laser pulses' peak-power variation and temporal location using a fast photodetector and high-sampling-rate DAQ in an AR-PAM setup. To enhance processing efficiency and handle large data volumes effectively, an analysis platform using the C programming language, leveraging parallel and multi-thread processing for faster procedures [80].

Algorithmic enhancements, both learning-based and model-based, have been proposed to exceed the physical resolution limit of AR-PAM and achieve super-acoustic resolution imaging. The imaging enhancement problem from these two model-based algorithms is solved by utilizing the following equation,

$$I_{\mathrm{AR}} = W\ (\vec{r_t}) \otimes I_{GT} + N \tag{9.21}$$

where, $W\ (\vec{r_t})$ is point spread function kernel and N is the additive white Gaussian noise.

Using a mathematical degradation model, learning-based and model-based algorithms were applied to improve raw AR-PAM images. The results showed more than a 10-fold resolution enhancement, surpassing AR-PAM's physical limits and achieving super-acoustic resolution imaging in both synthetic and *in vivo* images [81].

Enhanced SNR and axial resolution of optoacoustic microscopy were achieved by correcting total impulse response (TIR) using spatially distributed optoacoustic point sources (SOAPs). To evaluate the SNR with or without TIR-spatial matched filter (SMF) correction, the following equation was used to determine the enhancement in image SNR, denoted as ΔSNR:

$$\Delta\mathrm{SNR} = 10\left[\frac{\sum_{x=0}^{n_x-1}\sum_{y=0}^{n_y-1}[a_r(x, y)]^2}{\sum_{x=0}^{n_x-1}\sum_{y=0}^{n_y-1}[a_r(x, y) - a_c(x, y)]^2}\right] \tag{9.22}$$

where a_r and a_c are the amplitude values for the raw and corrected images at the pixel positions x and y for all n_x and n_y pixels.

This technique improved the SNR by over 10 dB and axial resolution by about 30% by scanning a 250-nm thick gold layer with a focused laser to generate SOAPs across a 2D plane, enabling thorough signal mapping and validation against traditional methods [82].

Frequency-band model-based (fbMB) reconstruction in OAI enhances SNR and accuracy by separating frequency components, improving contrast, fidelity, and spectral unmixing for detailed anatomical structures. It uses a projected conjugate gradient as a non-negative least square (NNLS) to handle reconstruction equations in OAI. The formulation of the regularized inversion problem incorporating soft priors can be expressed as,

$$\begin{aligned}(x_1^*, \ldots\ldots, x_n^*) = \arg\arg\ &\| p - M(x_1 + \cdots + x_n)\|_2^2 \\ &(x_1, \cdots\cdots, x_n \geqslant 0) \\ &+ \lambda\ \| L(x_1 + x_2 + x_3 \cdots + x_n)\|_2^2 \\ &+ \eta\mu_1\ \| (id - F_1)\ Mx_1\ \|_2^2 \\ &+ \cdots + \eta\mu_n\ \| (id - F_n)\ Mx_n\ \|_2^2\end{aligned} \tag{9.23}$$

where $F1, \ldots, Fn$ are the n band-pass filters, and η, $\mu_1, \ldots, \mu_n$ the regularization parameters for the soft priors such that $\mu_1 + \cdots + \mu_n = 1$.

Machine learning accelerates fbMB for real-time clinical feedback, potentially improving multispectral optoacoustic tomography's (MSOT) clinical utility. Tuning the Tikhonov regularization parameter via the L-curve optimizes the balance between solution fidelity and regularization strength in standard model-based reconstruction [83].

A learning-based approach combining time-resolved signals, tomographic reconstructions, and artifact minimization enhances SNR and accuracy in OAI. The convolutional neural network (CNN)-based approach enhances optoacoustic image quality by training on both time-resolved signals and tomographic reconstructions, using reference human finger data from a full-ring array system for training. An algorithm was implemented to reduce acoustic reflection artifacts, which often occur due to structures with varying acoustic properties such as bones. Compared to other CNN-based methods focusing solely on image-domain data, this combined approach demonstrated superior performance in improving image quality [84].

Discriminative deep learning approaches have been developed to separate electrical noise from optoacoustic signals, demonstrating significant enhancements in morphological and spectral optoacoustic images. The researchers devised an intelligent computer program to distinguish between internal body signals and unwanted electrical noise in images captured through a unique camera technique. The obtained optoacoustic sinogram S can be partitioned into the original optoacoustic sinogram S_{OA} and the electrical noise contribution S_{noise}. The relationship is expressed as

$$S = S_{OA} + S_{noise} \tag{9.24}$$

They trained the program extensively on examples of noise and genuine signals to refine its ability to enhance image clarity. This strategy involved a systematic problem breakdown and employed a specialized framework to discern noise from useful camera signals [85]. Another method employs a deep learning algorithm, specifically an enhancement Unet (E-Unet), which improves SNR, structured similarity indexing (SSIM), RMSE, and Pearson correlation metrics by training on custom loss functions and evaluating performance on complicated phantoms in biological tissue [86]. Various loss functions and combinations listed below are utilized to obtain the enhanced reconstructed images.

$$\frac{1}{N}\sum(Y_{\text{true}} - Y_{\text{pred}})^2 \tag{9.25}$$

$$\frac{1}{N}\sum(Y_{\text{true}} - Y_{\text{pred}})^2 + PSNR\,(Y_{\text{true}}, Y_{\text{pred}}) \tag{9.26}$$

$$\frac{1}{N}\sum(Y_{\text{true}} - Y_{\text{pred}})^2 + CC\,(Y_{\text{true}}, Y_{\text{pred}}) \tag{9.27}$$

$$\frac{1}{N}\sum(Y_{\text{true}} - Y_{\text{pred}})^2 + PSNR\,(Y_{\text{true}}, Y_{\text{pred}}) + CC\,(Y_{\text{true}}, Y_{\text{pred}}) \tag{9.28}$$

where PSNR is the peak SNRo, *CC* denotes cross-correlation, and Y_{pred} is the predicted signal.

The methods discussed in this section encompass a variety of strategies aimed at improving the SNR and accuracy in OAI. This includes the utilization of advanced algorithms that are designed to process and analyze signals more effectively. Additionally, deep learning techniques are employed, allowing the system to learn and adapt based on a vast amount of data, leading to enhanced image quality and precision. Innovative signal processing techniques are also incorporated, enabling the system to differentiate between noise and relevant signals, resulting in clearer and more accurate imaging outcomes. Together, these approaches form a comprehensive and multifaceted strategy to optimize the performance of OAI systems.

9.5 Optoacoustic applications for blood diagnosis and imaging

The strong optical absorption characteristics of blood, specifically Hb, are effectively utilized by OAI. This allows for the differentiation between oxygenated and deoxygenated blood, which is crucial for assessing various physiological and pathological conditions such as hypoxia detection and monitoring tissue oxygenation levels. Moreover, the combination of optical and ultrasonic properties in OAI enables deeper tissue penetration compared to conventional optical imaging methods. As a result, it allows for detailed visualization of blood vessels and structures deep within the body without the need for invasive procedures.

Another significant advantage of OAI is its functional imaging capabilities, which enable real-time monitoring of dynamic biological processes. By utilizing multiple wavelengths of laser light, OAI can provide simultaneous information about blood volume, oxygen saturation, and flow dynamics. This makes it an invaluable tool for diagnosing and monitoring cardiovascular diseases, evaluating tumor angiogenesis, and assessing vascular health [87–89]. The non-invasive nature of OAI, combined with its ability to deliver quantitative functional data, positions it as a superior alternative to traditional imaging modalities. It enhances patient comfort and enables continuous monitoring in various clinical settings. In this section, we will provide a comprehensive overview of the primary applications of OAI in the field of blood-related diagnostics and imaging.

9.5.1 Optoacoustic as a diagnostic tool for anemia

Anemia is a medical condition where there is a lack of RBCs or Hb in the body, which leads to a decrease in the blood's ability to transport oxygen. This condition affects a large number of people worldwide and can be caused by various factors, including poor nutrition, chronic illnesses, and genetic disorders. It is important to diagnose anemia early and accurately in order to effectively treat and manage it. Traditional methods of diagnosis, such as complete blood count and Hb electrophoresis, often involve invasive procedures and laboratory testing. Recent advancements in OAI technology offer a promising non-invasive alternative for diagnosing and monitoring anemia.

OAI is a valuable tool in diagnosing anemia, as it utilizes the variations in optical absorption between oxyhemoglobin and deoxyhemoglobin in the visible and near-infrared spectral ranges. Multispectral optoacoustic tomography (MSOT) is an optoacoustic technique that employs several laser wavelengths to distinguish between HbO_2 and deoxyhemoglobin. By examining optoacoustic signals at various wavelengths, the total Hb concentration and sO_2 may be calculated.

MSOT has been shown to provide non-invasive assessment of Hb concentration in individuals with various degrees of anemia [90]. The research included 19 patients with moderate to severe anemia, as well as healthy controls. The MSOT signal intensity, especially the unmixed parameter for deoxyhemoglobin and the single wavelength of 700 nm, showed a substantial positive connection with the absolute Hb content as assessed by traditional blood tests. This link was especially strong for individuals with severe anemia who needed RBC transfusions. The study found a substantial positive association between MSOT signal intensity and Hb concentration, indicating that the approach is accurate and reliable for identifying and assessing anemia severity. MSOT, a non-invasive and functional imaging technique, provides a more convenient and informative alternative to established anemia diagnosis procedures.

9.5.2 Optoacoustic as a diagnostic tool for sickle cell

Sickle cell disease is a medical illness affecting RBCs caused by an Hb mutation. This mutation causes the cells to form a sickle shape, which has two significant consequences for the body. First, it lowers the quantity of oxygen that Hb can carry, resulting in a reduction in oxygen delivery to the tissues [91]. Second, irregularly formed cells tend to clump together, generating obstructions in blood flow and interfering with oxygen supply to tissues [92]. The clinical outcomes of sickle cell crises can vary widely, but early diagnosis is crucial for preventing and potentially reversing these adverse effects.

The differences between sickle cell hemoglobin (HbS) and normal adult hemoglobin (HbA) result in distinct characteristics in the photoacoustic signals of RBCs containing HbS compared to those containing HbA. The PA signal amplitudes of RBCs with HbS were found to be 2–4 times lower than those with HbA in linear mode imaging. PA imaging also revealed more variation in the distribution of Hb within sickle RBCs, possibly due to the presence of HbS polymer clusters with high optical absorption. Furthermore, PA signals differed between sickle RBCs that had undergone the sickling shape change and those containing HbS but had not yet sickled [93]. This suggests that the method could potentially detect changes in the ratio of irreversibly sickled cells to non-sickled cells in the circulation. However, further clinical studies are needed to determine if quantifying sickle cell ratios can predict or monitor vaso-occlusive crises (figure 9.6).

Monitoring the rheological behavior and movement of sickle RBCs in blood vessels using PAI may provide additional information for assessing vaso-occlusive

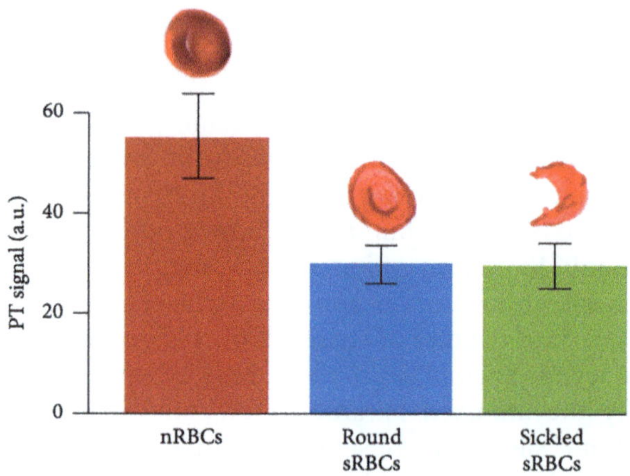

Figure 9.6. Photothermal (PT) signal amplitudes from individual nRBCs and sRBCs with round and deformed shapes. [93] John Wiley & Sons [reprinted with permission from Wiley] under the Creative Commons Attribution 4.0 International License (http://creativecommons.org/licenses/by/4.0/).

risk. The technique has shown the ability to identify RBC aggregations and quantify flow rates within the microvasculature [94]. Combining quantitative data on sickle cell ratios and microvascular rheology from photoacoustic techniques could offer valuable insights into the pathophysiology of vaso-occlusive events and acute pain crises in sickle cell patients.

9.5.3 Optoacoustic as a diagnostic tool for circulating cancer cells

Cancer is the second leading cause of death in the United States, with 90% of cancer-related deaths attributed to metastasis, which occurs when cells from the original tumor spread to distant parts of the body [95]. These CTCs are linked to higher rates of metastasis and worse patient outcomes [96]. Detecting CTCs early on could greatly improve cancer treatment by serving as an early warning sign of metastasis. Additionally, monitoring CTC levels can offer insights into tumor recurrence and the effectiveness of treatments. Ultimately, targeting CTCs to prevent metastasis could minimize the need for systemic therapies and improve patient outcomes.

There are various methods for detecting CTCs, each with its own advantages and limitations [97, 98]. One approach involves using cell surface markers that are specific to certain cell types. By targeting these markers with antibodies or other molecules, researchers can identify and isolate CTCs. Another method involves filtration, where a sample of blood or bodily fluid is passed through a filter that captures CTCs based on their size and shape.

Direct optical imaging systems are also utilized for CTC detection. These systems utilize light to visualize cells and can be classified into two main types: *ex vivo* and *in vivo* systems. *Ex vivo* systems, such as flow cytometry and Raman scattering, analyze cells that have been removed from the body and placed in a laboratory setting. While these systems allow for quick and efficient analysis of large cell numbers, they have limitations. Obtaining a large sample size can be challenging, especially for rare cell types like CTCs. Additionally, false negatives can occur due to the limited sample size or the presence of interfering cells [97, 98].

In contrast, *in vivo* optical imaging systems analyze cells within the body. These systems use light to visualize cells and can provide real-time monitoring of CTCs. Examples of *in vivo* optical imaging systems include wide-field fluorescence imaging and photo diagnostic infrared spectroscopy. These systems offer potential solutions to the limitations of *ex vivo* methods, as they do not require sample preparation and minimize the risk of false negatives. However, they are limited by scattering effects, which can hinder their ability to penetrate deep into the body and detect CTCs in deeper locations [97, 98].

PAI has shown promise as a potential alternative for detecting CTCs while overcoming the limitations of current detection methods. A recent study utilized high-frequency photoacoustic and ultrasound signals to identify cells in a blood sample [99]. The method leverages unique periodic features within the power spectrum that depend on cell size, structure, and morphology. By measuring the ultrasound and photoacoustic signals from individual cells using an acoustic microscope, the method can distinguish between RBCs, WBCs, and circulating melanoma cells. The signals from RBCs and melanoma cells show both ultrasound and photoacoustic components, while only an ultrasound signal is detected from WBCs. The method can estimate cell size from spectral periodicity and has potential applications in counting and identifying cells, including circulating melanoma cells (figure 9.7).

Another study that uses a two-phase microfluidic system in an *in vitro* setting has successfully detected CTCs derived from melanoma in bovine blood with a 100% detection rate at a concentration of 1 CTC μl^{-1} [100]. This high detection rate

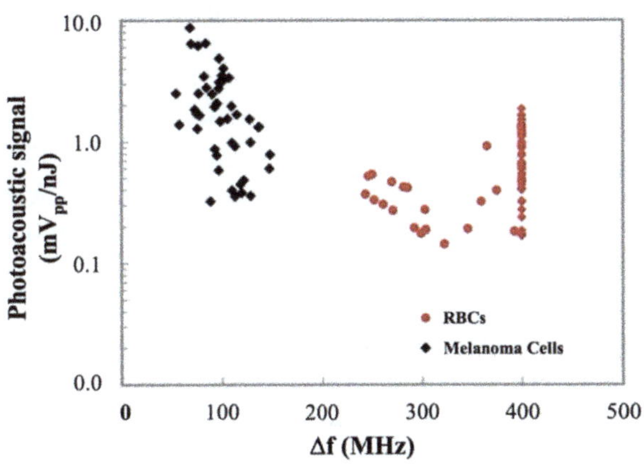

Figure 9.7. A graphical representation of the photoacoustic signal amplitude (log scale) and spectral spacing parameters. The peak–peak photoacoustic signal normalized to the laser energy versus spectral spacing for RBCs (red) and melanoma cells (black). [99] John Wiley & Sons [reprinted with permission from Wiley under the Creative Commons Attribution 4.0 International License (http://creativecommons.org/licenses/by/4.0/).

suggests that PAI may offer greater sensitivity compared to traditional methods like flow cytometry, especially when identifying rare cell populations like CTCs. Additionally, PAI offers a unique advantage over flow cytometry by enabling the imaging of multicellular cross-sections, providing a more comprehensive understanding of cellular structure and interactions within a sample. This capability of PAI holds the potential to offer valuable insights into the behavior and characteristics of CTCs.

9.5.4 Optoacoustic for blood glucose monitoring

Diabetes is a major concern in public health, affecting more than 38 million people in the United States [101]. The impact of high blood glucose levels goes beyond individual health, as it also poses a significant economic burden on the healthcare system, with costs estimated to be over $410 million annually and increasing [102]. To prevent complications, it is crucial to have a fast and reliable way to measure blood glucose levels. Therefore, the development of an accurate and non-invasive detection method is of utmost importance. Despite advancements in detection methods, there is still a need for innovative solutions to effectively address this urgent issue.

In the past, efforts to detect glucose levels without invasive methods, like urine glucose testing, faced challenges because the accuracy was affected by the patient's hydration levels, which tend to vary. To overcome these limitations, more sophisticated techniques like impedance spectroscopy and sonophoresis were introduced. However, these methods encountered problems such as skin irritation and other undesirable effects [103]. Despite these advancements, the search for a dependable and non-invasive glucose monitoring system continues, creating a notable void in the management of diabetes and other conditions related to glucose levels.

In 2015, photoacoustic spectroscopy (PAS) was used to measure glucose levels of varying degrees. The study's findings were presented in the form of a Clark error grid (CEG) plot, which visually represented the predicted glucose levels using PAS relative to the actual concentrations. The results demonstrated PAS as a safe and effective method for measuring glucose levels, with 100% of the measurements falling within the clinically acceptable range defined by the CEG criteria [104].

The CEG criteria, which define areas A and B as clinically acceptable variations, indicate that the PAS measurements were highly accurate and reliable. This high degree of accuracy is crucial for effective glucose monitoring, as it enables healthcare professionals to make informed decisions about patient care. The study's findings were further corroborated by another investigation that employed differential continuous-wave photoacoustic spectroscopy to measure glucose levels over a period of three hours [105]. This study using consensus error grid which also showed a similar response and variation, highlighting the consistency and reliability of the PAS method (see figure 9.8). The cumulative evidence from these studies underscores the potential of photoacoustic spectroscopy as a non-invasive and accurate tool for glucose detection.

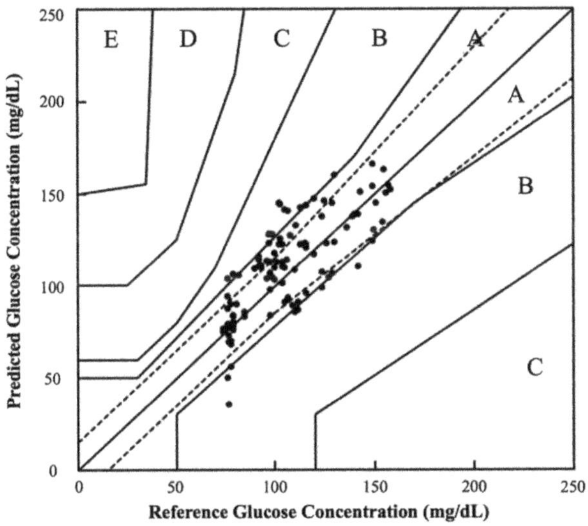

Figure 9.8. Consensus error grid. Comparison between reference glucose concentration from FGM (flash glucose monitoring) and predicted glucose concentration from DCW-PAS (Differential continuous-wave photoacoustic spectroscopy). [© [2019] IEEE. Reprinted, with permission, from [105] under the Creative Commons Attribution 4.0 International License (http://creativecommons.org/licenses/by/4.0/).]

9.6 Conclusion

In this chapter, we have explored the complex and diverse field of optoacoustics in relation to the properties of blood. Optoacoustic techniques combine optical absorption and acoustic detection to provide a valuable and non-invasive method for studying and diagnosing different blood-related conditions.

OAI/PAI imaging utilizes the unique characteristics of blood to facilitate a wide range of biomedical applications. Through the analysis of photoacoustic signals from RBCs, this method has proven to be highly effective in detecting and monitoring blood-related illnesses like anemia and sickle cell disease. The distinct acoustic patterns exhibited by these cells offer vital diagnostic insights, facilitating the early and accurate detection of diseases. In addition, photoacoustic imaging shows potential in detecting CTCs in the bloodstream, which can help with early cancer detection and monitoring for metastasis. Timely intervention and improved prognosis are dependent on early detection. Furthermore, photoacoustic spectroscopy provides a non-invasive approach for measuring blood glucose levels, representing a notable improvement compared to conventional glucose monitoring methods. The wide range of applications showcased the immense potential of PAI to improve diagnostic accuracy and elevate patient care.

Nevertheless, there are still obstacles to overcome in order to fully unlock the capabilities of photoacoustic blood imaging. These include the need to evaluate the dependability of quantitative findings and enhance the efficiency of delivering light to deeper tissues. Continuing research endeavors to tackle these challenges and advance photoacoustic techniques for use in clinical settings.

In summary, the unique optical and acoustic properties of blood, when combined with the strengths of PAI, open up exciting possibilities for non-invasive, functional, and molecular imaging of the circulatory system in health and disease. As the technology continues to advance, photoacoustic blood imaging is poised to make significant impacts in both preclinical research and clinical practice.

Abbreviations

2D	Two-dimensional
3D	Three-dimensional
AR-PAF	Acoustic resolution photoacoustic flowmetry
BGC	Blood glucose concentration
BOLD	Blood oxygen level dependent
BV	Blood volume
CC	Cross-correlation
CEG	Clark error grid
CI	Cardiac index
CNN	Convolutional neural network
CO	Cardiac output
CTCs	Circulating tumor cells
$CuSO_4$	Copper(II) sulfate
DAQ	Data acquisition
dB	Decibel
DCW-PAS	Differential continuous-wave photoacoustic spectroscopy
DO	Systemic oxygen delivery
DOT	Diffuse optical tomography
E-Unet	Enhancement Unet
EMD	Empirical mode decomposition
ESR	Erythrocyte sedimentation rate
fbMB	Frequency-band model-based
FGM	Flash glucose monitoring
FP	Fabry-Pérot
Hb	Hemoglobin
HbA	Adult hemoglobin
HbCO	Carboxyhemoglobin
HbMet	Oxygenated methemoglobin
HbO_2	Oxyhemoglobin
HbOxy	Oxygenated hemoglobin
HbR	Reduced hemoglobin
HbS	Sickle cell hemoglobin
HCT	Hematocrit
HCV	Hepatitis C virus
He-Ne	Helium–neon
HIV	Human immunodeficiency virus
ILIB	Intravascular laser irradiation of blood
LED	Light-emitting diode
LLLR	Low-level laser radiation
MHz	Megahertz
MRI	Magnetic resonance imaging

MSOT	Multispectral optoacoustic tomography
Nd: YAG	Neodymium: yttrium aluminum garnet
NEUT	Neutrophils
NIR	Near-infrared
NIRS	Near-infrared spectroscopy
NNLS	Non-negative least square
OAI	Optoacoustic imaging
OPO	Optical parametric oscillator
OR-PAM	Optical-resolution photoacoustic microscopy
PA	Photoacousctic
PAE	Photoacoustic endoscope
PAFI	Photoacoustic fluctuation imaging
PAI	Photoacoustic imaging
PAM	Photoacoustic microscopy
PAS	Photoacoustic spectroscopy
PAT	Photoacoustic tomography
PAUS	Photoacoustic ultrasound spectroscopy
PAVT	Photoacoustic vector tomography
PCV	Packed cell volume
PLT	Platelets
PSNR	Peak signal-to-noise ratio
PT	Photothermal
QPA	Quantitative photoacoustic assessment
qPAT	Quantitative photoacoustic tomography
RBC	Red blood cells
RMSE	Root mean square error
SMF	Spatial matched filter
SNR	Signal-to-noise ratio
sO_2	Blood oxygen saturation
SOAPs	Spatially distributed optoacoustic point sources
SSIM	Structured similarity indexing
SVD	Singular value decomposition
TDF	Thermal diffusion flowmetry
tHb	Total hemoglobin concentration
TIR	Total impulse response
US	Ultrasound
VDA	Vascular disrupting agent
WBC	White blood cells

Symbols

θ_1	Angle of incidence
θ_2	Angle of refraction
n_1	Refractive index of the first medium
n_2	Refractive index of the second medium
T	Transmission of optical energy
R	Reflected optical energy
g	Anisotropy value
μ_s'	Reduced scattering coefficient
μ_s	Scattering coefficient

τ_{th}	Thermal relaxation time (thermal confinement)
d_v	Characteristic dimension or voxel diameter
α_{th}	Thermal diffusivity in the medium
τ_s	Pulse duration (stress confinement)
v_s	Speed of sound (m s^{-1})
∇^2	Laplace operator
t	Time
Γ	Thermodynamic Gruneisen parameter
c	Speed of sound (m s^{-1})
$p(\vec{r}, t)$	Acoustic pressure
$H(\vec{r}, t)$	Heating function
β	Isobaric heat expansion coefficient
C_p	Isobaric heat capacity of the absorber
ν	Heat conversion efficiency
$\mu(\vec{r})$	Absorption coefficient
$\Phi(\vec{r}, t)$	Optical fluence rate
$I(\vec{r}, t)$	Laser intensity
$\delta(t)$	Delta function
$\vec{r}$	Observation point
$\vec{r}'$	Source point
p_I	Initial pressure amplitude
U	Heaviside function
a	Radius
R	Distance between the detector and the acoustic source
α	Attenuation coefficient (dB cm^{-1})
a_0	Tissue-dependent constant
b	Power law factor
f	Frequency (MHz)
$S(\omega, \lambda)$	Acoustic spectrum of the photoacoustic signal
λ	Optical wavelength
F_I	Optical fluence received by the target object
$O(\omega, \lambda)$	Original acoustic spectrum of the target object of interest
$a(\omega)$	Acoustic attenuation within the tissue situated between the target object and the ultrasonic transducer
$H(\omega)$	System transfer function of the ultrasonic detection system
$\underline{S}(\omega, \lambda_i)$	Normalized acoustic spectra
$S(\omega, \lambda_i)$	Raw acoustic spectra recorded at frequency ω and wavelength λ_i
$S_{rms}(\omega)$	Root-mean-square of the spectra across all wavelengths
n	Total number of different wavelengths
$E()$	Mean
N_P	Particle count
α_p	Photon count fluctuation coefficient
SNR	Signal-to-noise ratio
A_{PA}	Mean squared phpotoacoustic amplitude
n_{PA}	Electronic thermal noise of the ultrasonic transducer
R_k	Relative concentration ratio
$E(R_1, R_2, R_3)$	Objective function
N_λ	Number of different wavelengths
$p_0^{sim}(k, \lambda_i, R_k)$	Simulated initial pressure distribution
β_k	Scaling factor

$p_0^{\exp}(k, \lambda_i)$	Experimentally measured initial pressure distribution
$\widetilde{\tau}(t)$	Lumped temperature of the system
$\widetilde{\tau}(0)$	Initial lumped temperature ($t = 0$)
t_{eff}	Effective time constant
$t_{\mathrm{conduction}}$	Time constant for thermal conduction
$t_{\mathrm{convection}}$	Time constant for thermal convection
C	Capacitance
R	Resistance
$\widetilde{u}_{\mathrm{est}}$	Estimated velocity of the fluid
I_{VUT}	Photoacoustic signal related to the velocity of the fluid.
a	Variable for original signal
b	Variable for noise
β	Attenuation of the echo signal
I_{AR}	Acoustic resolution image in augmented reality
$W(\vec{r}_t)$	Point spread function kernel
I_{GT}	Ground truth image
N	Additive white Gaussian noise
ΔSNR	Change in signal-to-noise ratio
$a_r(x, y)$	Amplitude values for the raw image
$a_c(x, y)$	Amplitude values for the corrected image
n_x, n_y	Number of pixels
x	Signal components
p	Measured photoacoustic data or signal
M	System matrix or model that maps the reconstructed parameters
L	Regularization operator
η	Band-pass filter
	Regularization parameter
S	Obtained optoacoustic sinogram
S_{OA}	Original optoacoustic sinogram
S_{noise}	Electrical noise contribution
Y_{true}	Ground truth signal or image
Y_{pred}	Predicted signal or image
PSNR	Peak signal-to-noise ratio
CC	Cross-correlation

References

[1] Lutzweiler C and Razansky D 2013 Optoacoustic imaging and tomography: reconstruction approaches and outstanding challenges in image performance and quantification *Sensors* **13** 7345–84

[2] Wang L V and Hu S 2012 Photoacoustic tomography: *in vivo* imaging from organelles to organs *Science* **335** 1458–62

[3] Attia A B E, Balasundaram G, Moothanchery M, Dinish U S, Bi R, Ntziachristos V and Olivo M 2019 A review of clinical photoacoustic imaging: current and future trends *Photoacoustics* **16** 100144

[4] Razansky D 2014 Optoacoustic imaging *Comprehensive Biomedical Physics* **vol 4** ed F Alves and F Kiessling (Sweden: Elsevier) pp 281–300

[5] Shi X F, Ji B, Kong Y, Guan Y and Ni R 2021 Multimodal contrast agents for optoacoustic brain imaging in small animals *Front. Bioeng. Biotechnol.* **9** 746815

[6] Bell A G 1881 LXVIII. Upon the production of sound by radiant energy *Lond., Edinb., Dubl. Philos. Mag. J. Sci.* **11** 510–28

[7] Yao J, Xia J and Wang L V 2007 Photoacoustic tomography for biomedical applications *The Optics Encyclopedia* (Wiley) pp 1–34

[8] Lyamshev L M 1981 Optoacoustic sources of sound *Sov. Phys. Usp.* **24** 977

[9] Borg R E and Rochford J 2018 Molecular photoacoustic contrast agents: design principles & applications *Photochem. Photobiol.* **94** 1175–209

[10] Weber J, Beard P C and Bohndiek S E 2016 Contrast agents for molecular photoacoustic imaging *Nat. Methods* **13** 639–50

[11] Beard P 2011 Biomedical photoacoustic imaging *Interface Focus* **1** 602–31

[12] Hysi E, Moore M J, Strohm E M and Kolios M C 2021 A tutorial in photoacoustic microscopy and tomography signal processing methods *J. Appl. Phys.* **129** 141102

[13] Wang D, Wu Y and Xia J 2016 Review on photoacoustic imaging of the brain using nanoprobes *Neurophotonics* **3** 010901–1

[14] Li L 2014 Photoacoustic imaging *Pathobiology of Human Disease* ed L M McManus and R N Mitchell (New York: Elsevier) pp 3912–24

[15] Moothanchery M, Bi R, Kim J Y, Jeon S, Kim C and Olivo M 2018 Optical resolution photoacoustic microscopy based on multimode fibers *Biomed. Opt. Express* **9** 1190–7

[16] Park S, Lee C, Kim J and Kim C 2014 Acoustic resolution photoacoustic microscopy *Biomed. Eng. Lett.* **4** 213–22

[17] Periyasamy V, Das N, Sharma A and Pramanik M 2019 1064 nm acoustic resolution photoacoustic microscopy *J. Biophotonics* **12** e201800357

[18] Moothanchery M, Dev K, Balasundaram G, Bi R and Olivo M 2020 Acoustic resolution photoacoustic microscopy based on microelectromechanical systems scanner *J. Biophotonics* **13** e201960127

[19] Tian C, Zhang C, Zhang H, Xie D and Jin Y 2021 Spatial resolution in photoacoustic computed tomography *Rep. Prog. Phys.* **84** 036701

[20] Wang L V and Gao L 2014 Photoacoustic microscopy and computed tomography: from bench to bedside *Annu. Rev. Biomed. Eng.* **16** 155–85

[21] Majeed S H, Hasan J A and Khalil E G 2022 Photoacoustic technique for diagnosis of blood clotting *Int. J. Health Sci.* **6** 12195–205

[22] Ulrich L, Held K G, Jaeger M, Frenz M and Akarçay H G 2020 Reliability assessment for blood oxygen saturation levels measured with optoacoustic imaging *J. Biomed. Opt.* **25** 046005–5

[23] Bok T H, Hysi E and Kolios M C 2017 Preliminary photoacoustic imaging of the human radial artery for simultaneous assessment of red blood cell aggregation and oxygen saturation *in vivo 2017 IEEE Int. Ultrasonics Symp. (IUS)* (Piscataway, NJ: IEEE) pp 1–4

[24] Kravchuk D and Voronina K 2020 Studies of red blood cell aggregation and blood oxygenation on the basis of the optoacoustic effect in biological media *J. Biomed. Photon. Eng.* **6** 010307

[25] Hacker L, Brunker J, Smith E S J, Quiros-Gonzalez I and Bohndiek S E 2020 Photoacoustics resolves species-specific differences in hemoglobin concentration and oxygenation *J. Biomed. Opt.* **25** 095002–2

[26] Zhao W, Yu H, Wen Y, Luo H, Jia B, Wang X, Liu L and Li W J 2021 Real-time red blood cell counting and osmolarity analysis using a photoacoustic-based microfluidic system *Lab Chip* **21** 2586–93

[27] Hysi E, Saha R K and Kolios M C 2012 Photoacoustic ultrasound spectroscopy for assessing red blood cell aggregation and oxygenation *J. Biomed. Opt.* **17** 125006–6

[28] Esenaliev R O 2017 Optoacoustic monitoring of physiologic variables *Front. Physiol.* **8** 304070

[29] Gorey A, Biswas D, Kumari A, Gupta S, Sharma N, Chen G C and Vasudevan S 2019 Application of continuous-wave photoacoustic sensing to red blood cell morphology *Lasers Med. Sci.* **34** 487–94

[30] James S, Neuhaus K, Murphy M and Leahy M 2021 Contrast agents for photoacoustic imaging: a review of stem cell tracking *Stem Cell Res. Ther.* **12** 1–19

[31] Petrova E V, Oraevsky A A and Ermilov S A 2014 Red blood cell as a universal optoacoustic sensor for non-invasive temperature monitoring *Appl. Phys. Lett.* **105**

[32] Fadhel M N and Kolios M C 2017 Ultrasound spectral analysis of photoacoustic signals from red blood cell populations at different optical wavelengths *Photons Plus Ultrasound: Imaging and Sensing 2017* Vol. 10 064 (SPIE) pp 176–84

[33] Wang E B, Kaur R, Fierro M, Austin E, Jones L R and Jagdeo J 2019 Safety and penetration of light into the brain *Photobiomodulation in the Brain* (New York: Academic) pp 49–66

[34] Hamdy O, Abdel-Salam Z and Abdel-Harith M 2022 Optical characterization of biological tissues based on fluorescence, absorption, and scattering properties *Diagnostics* **12** 2846

[35] Waterhouse D J 2019 Translation of optical imaging techniques *Novel Optical Endoscopes for Early Cancer Diagnosis and Therapy* ed D J Waterhouse (Cham: Springer) pp 1–16

[36] Sanjay H S and Niranjanamurthy M 2023 Ultrasound imaging *Medical Imaging* (Scrivener Publishing) pp 121–49

[37] Morii T, Kishino T, Shimamori N, Motohashi M, Ohnishi H, Honya K, Aoyagi T, Tajima T and Ichimura S 2018 Differential diagnosis between benign and malignant soft tissue tumors utilizing ultrasound parameters *J. Med. Ultrason.* **45** 113–9

[38] Sanches J M, Laine A F and Sur J S 2012 *Ultrasound Imaging: Advances and Applications* (New York: Springer)

[39] Bosschaart N, Edelman G J, Aalders M C, van Leeuwen T G and Faber D J 2014 A literature review and novel theoretical approach on the optical properties of whole blood *Lasers Med. Sci.* **29** 453–79

[40] Priezzhev A V, Lugovtsov A E, Semenov A N, Ermolinskiy P B, Lee K, Shin S and Nikitin S Y 2020 Laser-optic methods for revealing molecular and microrheologic mechanisms of interaction of blood components and related impairment of metabolism at cardiovascular diseases *2020 Int. Conf. Laser Optics (ICLO)* (Piscataway, NJ: IEEE) p 1

[41] Obeed H H, Huzam M J, Ridha N J, Alosfur F K M, Tahir K J, Madlol R and Hussein B M 2022 Comprehensive study on the effect of laser on human blood *AIP Conf. Proc.* Vol. 2386 (AIP Publishing)

[42] Multari R A, Cremers D A, Nelson A, Fisher C, Karimi Z, Young S, Green V, Williamson P and Duncan R 2022 The use of laser-based diagnostics for the rapid identification of blood borne viruses in human plasma samples *J. Appl. Microbiol.* **132** 2431–40

[43] Slewa M Y, Bader B A, Hamam F M, Banoosh A M and Jarjees B W 2022 Laser therapy stimulation at red low-level on some human blood cells *NeuroQuantol.* **20** 166

[44] Zhu R, Avsievich T, Su X, Bykov A, Popov A and Meglinski I 2022 Hemorheological alterations of red blood cells induced by 450-nm and 520-nm laser radiation *J. Photochem. Photobiol., B* **230** 112438

[45] Meneguzzo D T, Ferreira L S, de Carvalho E M and Nakashima C F 2016 Intravascular laser irradiation of blood ed M R Hamblin, T Agrawal and M de Sousa *Handbook of Low-Level Laser Therapy* 1st edn (New York: Jenny Stanford Publishing)
[46] Rathore S and Ali B 2014 Effect of laser radiation on electrical conductivity of human blood *Int. J. Sci.* **3** 286–90
[47] Mohammed H H and Lafta M M A M J 2015 Q-switched UV laser interactions with the human blood *in vitro J. Natl. Sci. Res.* **5**
[48] Manwar R, Zafar M and Xu Q 2020 Signal and image processing in biomedical photoacoustic imaging: a review *Optics* **2** 1–24
[49] Xia W, Kuniyil Ajith Singh M, Maneas E, Sato N, Shigeta Y, Agano T, Ourselin S, West S J and Desjardins A E 2018 Handheld real-time LED-based photoacoustic and ultrasound imaging system for accurate visualization of clinical metal needles and superficial vasculature to guide minimally invasive procedures *Sensors* **18** 1394
[50] Pinheiro B R, Dinis H D, Catarino S O, Pinto V C, Sousa P J and Minas G 2023 Experimental characterization of a piezoelectric transducer for integration into a photoacoustic system *2023 IEEE 7th Portuguese Meeting on Bioengineering (ENBENG)* (Piscataway, NJ: IEEE) pp 84–7
[51] Linger C, Atlas Y, Winter R, Vandebrouck M, Faure M, Lucas T, Bridal S L and Gateau J 2023 Volumetric and simultaneous photoacoustic and ultrasound imaging with a conventional linear array in a multiview scanning scheme *IEEE Trans. Ultrason. Ferroelectr. Freq. Control* **70** 1607–20
[52] Bakker A, Smith B, Ainsli P and Smith K 2012 Near-infrared spectroscopy *Applied Aspects of Ultrasonography in Humans* ed P Ainslie (London: Intech Open)
[53] Sun C W and Chuang C C 2012 Hemodynamics study based on near-infrared optical assessment *Hemodynamics—New Diagnostic and Therapeutic Approaches* ed A S Artis (London: Intech Open)
[54] Prahl S 1999 https://omlc.org/spectra/hemoglobin/
[55] Li M, Tang Y and Yao J 2018 Photoacoustic tomography of blood oxygenation: a mini review *Photoacoustics* **10** 65–73
[56] Majeed S H, Hasan J A and Khalil E G 2022 Photoacoustic technique for diagnosis of blood clotting *Int. J. Health Sci.* **6** 12195–205
[57] Tzoumas S and Ntziachristos V 2107 2017. Spectral unmixing techniques for optoacoustic imaging of tissue pathophysiology *Philos. Trans. Royal Soc. A: Math., Phys. Eng. Sci.* **375** 20170262
[58] Bok T H, Hysi E and Kolios M C 2018 In vitro photoacoustic spectroscopy of pulsatile blood flow: probing the interrelationship between red blood cell aggregation and oxygen saturation *J. Biophotonics* **11** e201700300
[59] Zalev J *et al* 2019 Opto-acoustic imaging of relative blood oxygen saturation and total hemoglobin for breast cancer diagnosis *J. Biomed. Opt.* **24** 121915–5
[60] Shigeta Y, Sato N, Singh M K A and Agano T 2018 Multispectral photoacoustic characterization of ICG and porcine blood using an LED-based photoacoustic imaging system *Photons Plus Ultrasound: Imaging and Sensing 2018* Vol. 10494 (SPIE) pp 273–7
[61] Perekatova V, Nemirova S, Orlova A, Kirillin M, Kurnikov A, Pavlova K, Khilov A, Kovalchuk A and Subochev P 2021 Three-dimensional dual-wavelength optoacoustic angiography reveals arteriovenous anastomoses *Laser Phys. Lett.* **18** 045601

[62] Godefroy G, Arnal B and Bossy E 2022 Multispectral photoacoustic fluctuation imaging for full visibility SO_2 imaging *J. Acoust. Soc. Am.* **152** A225–5
[63] Valeriya P, Daria K, Aleksandr K and Mikhail K 2022 Combined Monte Carlo and k-Wave simulations for reconstruction of blood oxygen saturation in optoacoustics: a pilot study *J. Biomed. Photon. Eng.* **8** 40511
[64] Oraevsky A A 2009 Optoacoustic systems for functional and molecular imaging in clinical and preclinical research *2009 IEEE Int. Symp. on Biomedical Imaging: From Nano to Macro* (Piscataway, NJ: IEEE) pp 1199–200
[65] Prough D S, Esenaliev R O, Deyo D, Petrov Y Y and Petrova I YUniversity of Texas System 2008 Optoacoustic monitoring of multiple parameters *U.S. Patent Application* 12/101,891
[66] Guo Z, Favazza C, Garcia-Uribe A and Wang L V 2012 Quantitative photoacoustic microscopy of optical absorption coefficients from acoustic spectra in the optical diffusive regime *J. Biomed. Opt.* **17** 066011–1
[67] Zhou Y, Yao J, Maslov K I and Wang L V 2014 Calibration-free absolute quantification of particle concentration by statistical analyses of photoacoustic signals *in vivo J. Biomed. Opt.* **19** 037001–1
[68] Buchmann J, Kaplan B A, Prohaska S and Laufer J 2017 Experimental validation of a Monte-Carlo-based inversion scheme for 3D quantitative photoacoustic tomography *Photons Plus Ultrasound: Imaging and Sensing 2017* Vol. 10064 (SPIE) pp 168–75
[69] Ren Z, Liu G, Liu Y and Huang Z 2013 Exploration of noninvasive determination of blood glucose concentration by using photoacoustic technique *Int. Symp. on Photoelectronic Detection and Imaging 2013: Laser Sensing and Imaging and Applications* Vol. 8905 (SPIE) pp 250–6
[70] Namita T, Sato M, Kondo K, Yamakawa M and Shiina T 2017 Evaluation of blood glucose concentration measurement using photoacoustic spectroscopy in near-infrared region *Photons Plus Ultrasound: Imaging and Sensing 2017* Vol. 10064 (SPIE) pp 751–7
[71] Bücking T M 2019 Acoustic resolution photoacoustic flowmetry *PhD Dissertation* UCL (University College London)
[72] Sheinfeld A and Eyal A 2012 Photoacoustic thermal diffusion flowmetry *Biomed. Opt. Express* **3** 800–13
[73] Zhang Y, Olick-Gibson J, Khadria A and Wang L V 2024 Photoacoustic vector tomography for deep hemodynamic imaging *Nat. Biomed. Eng.* **8** 701–11
[74] Rich L J and Seshadri M 2015 Photoacoustic imaging of vascular hemodynamics: validation with blood oxygenation level–dependent MR imaging *Radiology* **275** 110–8
[75] Gröhl J, Schellenberg M, Dreher K and Maier-Hein L 2021 Deep learning for biomedical photoacoustic imaging: a review *Photoacoustics* **22** 100241
[76] Dimaridis I, Sridharan P, Ntziachristos V, Karlas A and Hadjileontiadis L 2022 Image quality improvement techniques and assessment adequacy in clinical optoacoustic imaging: a systematic review *Biosensors* **12** 901
[77] Huen I, Zhang R, Bi R, Li X, Moothanchery M and Olivo M 2023 An investigation of signal preprocessing for photoacoustic tomography *Sensors* **23** 510
[78] Guezzi N, Lee C, Le T D, Seong H, Choi K H, Min J J and Yu J 2022 Multistage adaptive noise reduction technique for optical resolution photoacoustic microscopy *J. Biophotonics* **15** e202200164

[79] Zhao W, Yu H, Wen Y, Li P, Wang X, Wang F, Yang Y, Liu L and Li W J 2021 Improving photoacoustic-imaging axial positioning accuracy and signal-to-noise ratio using acoustic echo effect *Sens. Actuators,* A **329** 112788
[80] Asadollahi A, Latifi H, Pramanik M, Qazvini H, Rezaei A, Nikbakht H and Abedi A 2021 Axial accuracy and signal enhancement in acoustic-resolution photoacoustic microscopy by laser jitter effect correction and pulse energy compensation *Biomed. Opt. Express* **12** 1834–45
[81] Zhang Z, Jin H, Zheng Z and Zheng Y 2022 Super acoustic resolution photoacoustic microscopy imaging enhancement *2022 IEEE Biomedical Circuits and Systems Conf. (BioCAS)* (Piscataway, NJ: IEEE) pp 208–12
[82] Seeger M, Soliman D, Aguirre J, Diot G, Wierzbowski J and Ntziachristos V 2020 Pushing the boundaries of optoacoustic microscopy by total impulse response characterization *Nat. Commun.* **11** 2910
[83] Longo A, Jüstel D and Ntziachristos V 2022 Disentangling the frequency content in optoacoustics *IEEE Trans. Med. Imaging* **41** 3373–84
[84] Davoudi N, Lafci B, Özbek A, Deán-Ben X L and Razansky D 2022 Learning-based enhancement of limited-view optoacoustic tomography based on image-and time-domain data *Photons Plus Ultrasound: Imaging and Sensing 2022* Vol. 11960 (SPIE) pp 7–13
[85] Dehner C, Olefir I, Chowdhury K B, Jüstel D and Ntziachristos V 2022 Deep-learning-based electrical noise removal enables high spectral optoacoustic contrast in deep tissue *IEEE Trans. Med. Imaging* **41** 3182–93
[86] Aggrawal D, Zafar M, Islam M T, Manwar R, Schonfeld D and Avanaki K 2023 E-Unet: a deep learning method for photoacoustic signal enhancement *Photons Plus Ultrasound: Imaging and Sensing* **vol 12379** (SPIE) pp 189–93
[87] Jin H *et al* 2023 A flexible optoacoustic blood 'stethoscope' for noninvasive multiparametric cardiovascular monitoring *Nat. Commun.* **14** 4692
[88] Oraevsky A A, Savateeva E V, Solomatin S V, Karabutov A A, Andreev V G, Gatalica Z, Khamapirad T and Henrichs P M 2002 Optoacoustic imaging of blood for visualization and diagnostics of breast cancer *Biomedical Optoacoustics III* Vol. 4618 (SPIE) pp 81–94
[89] Esenaliev R O 2017 Optoacoustic diagnostic modality: from idea to clinical studies with highly compact laser diode-based systems *J. Biomed. Opt.* **22** 091512–8
[90] Ganzleben I, Klett D, Hartz W, Götzfried L, Vitali F, Neurath M F and Waldner M J 2022 Multispectral optoacoustic tomography for the non-invasive identification of patients with severe anemia *in vivo Photoacoustics* **28** 100414
[91] Milner P F 1974 Oxygen transport in sickle cell anemia *Arch. Intern. Med.* **133** 565–72
[92] Manwani D and Frenette P S 2013 Vaso-occlusion in sickle cell disease: pathophysiology and novel targeted therapies *Blood* **122** 3892–8
[93] Cai C, Nedosekin D A, Menyaev Y A, Sarimollaoglu M, Proskurnin M A and Zharov V P 2016 Photoacoustic flow cytometry for single sickle cell detection *in vitro* and *in vivo Anal. Cell. Pathol.* **2016** 2642361
[94] Galanzha E I and Zharov V P 2011 *In vivo* photoacoustic and photothermal cytometry for monitoring multiple blood rheology parameters *Cytometry Part* A **79** 746–57
[95] Cl C 2011 A perspective on cancer cell metastasis *Science* **331** 1559–64
[96] Paterlini-Brechot P and Benali N L 2007 Circulating tumor cells (CTC) detection: clinical impact and future directions *Cancer Lett.* **253** 180–204

[97] Shen Z, Wu A and Chen X 2017 Current detection technologies for circulating tumor cells *Chem. Soc. Rev.* **46** 2038–56

[98] Habli Z, AlChamaa W, Saab R, Kadara H and Khraiche M L 2020 Circulating tumor cell detection technologies and clinical utility: challenges and opportunities *Cancers* **12** 1930

[99] Strohm E M and Kolios M C 2015 Classification of blood cells and tumor cells using label-free ultrasound and photoacoustics *Cytometry Part* A **87** 741–9

[100] O'Brien C M, Rood K D, Bhattacharyya K, DeSouza T, Sengupta S, Gupta S K, Mosley J D, Goldschmidt B S, Sharma N and Viator J A 2012 Capture of circulating tumor cells using photoacoustic flowmetry and two phase flow *J. Biomed. Opt.* **17** 061221–9

[101] National Diabetes Statistics Report, CDC 2024 https://cdc.gov/diabetes/php/data-research/index.html (accessed 15th May 2024)

[102] Parker E D, Lin J, Mahoney T, Ume N, Yang G, Gabbay R A, ElSayed N A and Bannuru R R 2024 Economic costs of diabetes in the US in 2022 *Diabetes Care* **47** 26–43

[103] Sim J Y, Ahn C G, Jeong E J and Kim B K 2018 *In vivo* microscopic photoacoustic spectroscopy for non-invasive glucose monitoring invulnerable to skin secretion products *Sci. Rep.* **8** 1059

[104] Pai P P, Sanki P K and Banerjee S 2015 A photoacoustics based continuous non-invasive blood glucose monitoring system *2015 IEEE Int. Symp. on Medical Measurements and Applications (MeMeA) Proc.* (Piscataway, NJ: IEEE) pp 106–11

[105] Tanaka Y, Tajima T, Seyama M and Waki K 2019 Differential continuous wave photo-acoustic spectroscopy for non-invasive glucose monitoring *IEEE Sens. J.* **20** 4453–8

Chapter 10

Optical coherence tomography and polarimetry of blood

Pauline John and Azhar Zam

This chapter explores the fundamental principles and clinical applications of optical coherence tomography (OCT) and polarimetry in blood analysis. It begins with a detailed explanation of OCT and discusses the various modalities of OCT, including time-domain, frequency-domain, spectral-domain, swept-source, Doppler, and spectroscopic OCT, highlighting their unique capabilities and limitations. The chapter also covers the theoretical foundation of polarimetry, which studies the polarization state of light and its interaction with matter, emphasizing the Stokes–Mueller formalism as a powerful tool for characterizing light polarization. The chapter then delves into the clinical applications of OCT and polarimetry, focusing on their potential to advance medical diagnosis and monitoring. Detailed examples are presented for various diseases and conditions, including leukemia, malaria, diabetes, and cardiovascular disease. The chapter highlights the advantages of OCT and polarimetry in providing real-time, non-invasive, and multi-faceted evaluations, enabling early disease detection, precise quantification of blood parameters, and improved therapeutic interventions. The impact of these technologies on clinical practice, underscoring their significant contributions to the fields of ophthalmology, cardiology, dermatology, and neurology, is also discussed. The chapter concludes with a discussion of the future directions and technological innovations that promise to further enhance the diagnostic and therapeutic capabilities of OCT and polarimetry in blood analysis.

10.1 Introduction

OCT, a medical imaging technique based on low-coherence interferometry, uses a broadband light source to obtain tomographic images of biological tissues non-invasively without using any contrast agents/labels [1]. Several advancements in OCT technology in terms of speed, resolution, and contrast have allowed OCT to take effectual strides in clinical research and medical applications since its invention

doi:10.1088/978-0-7503-4806-5ch10

[2]. Compared to other imaging techniques such as x-ray, computed tomography, magnetic resonance imaging, and ultrasound, the unique features of OCT, such as its non-invasive, non-contact, label-free, high-resolution (1–15 μm), cross-sectional and rapid real-time, *in vivo* imaging capabilities make it a favorable diagnostic tool for various medical applications such as ophthalmology, dermatology, cardiology, dentistry, gastroenterology, and neurology [1, 2]. Another important application of OCT is in oncology, as it is capable of performing 'optical biopsy' without the need for invasive tissue excision [3]. Besides imaging the superficial tissue layers, intravascular OCT is capable of imaging the inner layers of the lumen and vasculature with the help of catheters, thereby guiding in surgical intervention in endoscopy and locating atherosclerotic plaques in the blood vessel [3]. The cross-sectional OCT images or two-dimensional (2D) B-scans are obtained by measuring the time delay echo of backscattered light in the sample from multiple depth/axial or A-scans obtained transversely. Whereas the volumetric three-dimensional (3D) OCT images are obtained by raster scanning [4]. In addition to accessing morphological information of tissues, functional imaging and accessing of dynamic features such as flow velocity of particles in highly scattering media, visualization of changes in perfusion over time is also possible using Doppler OCT and OCT angiography (OCT-A), respectively [5–7]. Another modality of OCT is the spectroscopic OCT (S-OCT), which is capable of accessing the depth-resolved absorption properties of tissue [8]. Polarimetry has been used in the transparent medium for a long and successful period. Motivated by their biological potential, polarimetric methods have also lately drawn a lot of interest for biological tissue evaluation. More precisely, polarization can be a useful technique to improve contrast and tissue imaging resolution by discriminating against multiple dispersed light (which functions as a gating mechanism) [9]. Furthermore, a plethora of morphological and functional data of possible biological relevance is included in the intrinsic tissue polarimetry properties. However, various complications resulting from repeated scattering and simultaneous occurrences of several scattering and polarization events pose severe obstacles to precise measurements and tissue polarimetry signal interpretation in a complex random medium-like tissue.

This chapter provides an overview of OCT and polarimetry techniques for applications related to blood. The chapter includes the basic principle and theory of OCT, the different types of OCT systems, and the imaging modalities of OCT. The chapter also discusses polarized light basics, Stokes–Muller formalism, and methods of polarization measurements. In addition, the uses of OCT and polarimetry of blood for medical applications are discussed.

10.2 Optical coherence tomography (OCT)

10.2.1 Basic principles of optical coherence tomography

10.2.1.1 Michelson interferometry

Low-coherence interferometry measures the echo time delay and intensity of backscattered light by interfering with light that has traveled a known reference pathlength and time delay [4]. Measurements are performed using a Michelson

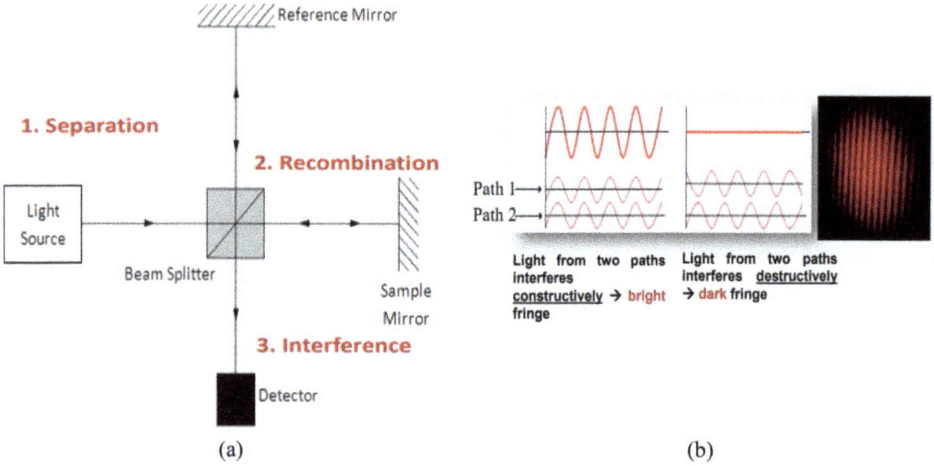

Figure 10.1. (a) Michelson interferometry. (b) Schematic representation of constructive and destructive interference.

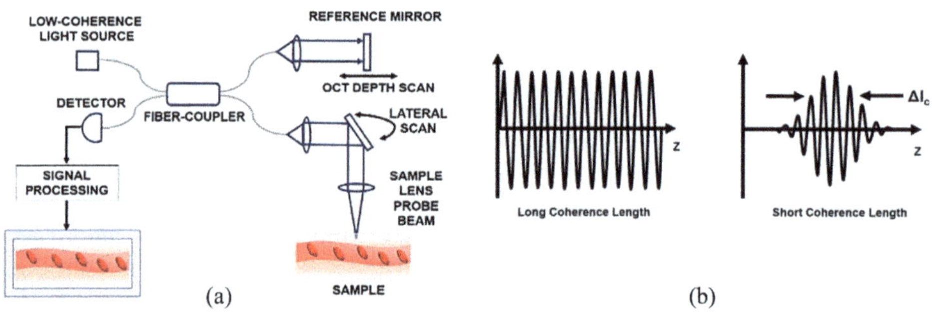

Figure 10.2. (a) Schematic of a typical time-domain OCT system. (b) Schematic representation of long and short coherence length.

interferometer, as shown in figure 10.1(a). Figure 10.1(b) illustrates the occurrence of constructive and destructive interference.

10.2.1.2 Theory of OCT

Light from a source is directed onto a beam splitter/fiber coupler, and one of the beams is incident onto the sample to be imaged, while the second beam travels a reference path with a variable pathlength, as shown in figure 10.2(a) [4]. The backscattered light from the sample is interfered with reflected light from the reference arm and detected with a photodetector at the interferometer output. If the light source is coherent, then interference fringes will be observed as the relative pathlengths are varied. However, if low-coherence light or short pulses are used, then interference occurs only when the two pathlengths match to within the coherence length of the light, as shown in figure 10.2(b). The echo time delay and intensity of backscattered light from sites within the sample can be measured by detecting and demodulating the interference output of the interferometer while scanning the reference pathlength.

Coherence length: The coherence length (l_c) of a source helps in defining the axial resolution (δz) of imaging in OCT systems. Considering a source with a Gaussian shaped spectrum with center wavelength λ_c, spectral bandwidth $\Delta\lambda$, and a medium with refractive index n, the axial resolution δz can be estimated as follows [4],

$$\text{Coherence length} = l_c = \delta z = \frac{2\ln 2}{n\pi}\left(\frac{\lambda_c^2}{\Delta\lambda}\right) \tag{10.1}$$

The principle of OCT can be understood by examining the interactions of the electromagnetic waves returning from the sample and the reference arms. For simplicity, first the approximation can be made that the source is monochromatic and emits plane waves [4]. Thus, the incident wave E_{source} from the source propagating in the z-direction is written as,

$$E_{\text{source}} = E_0 \exp\left[i(kz - \omega t)\right] \tag{10.2}$$

where $k = 2\pi/\lambda$ with λ being the wavelength of the source, ω is the angular frequency of the electric field, and the E_0 is the amplitude of the wave with the subscript '0' indicating that a monochromatic source is used. After this wave passes through the optical coupler the returning wave from the reference arm and sample arm are provided in equations (10.3) and (10.4), respectively

$$E_r = E_{r0} \exp\left[i(kz_r - \omega t)\right] \tag{10.3}$$

$$E_s = E_{s0} \exp\left[i(kz_s - \omega t)\right] \tag{10.4}$$

Here, z_r and z_s are the pathlengths from the optical coupler to the reference mirror and to a specific depth in the sample, respectively. The monochromatic wave amplitudes E_{r0} from the mirror and E_{s0} from the sample are quite different because only a small amount of light returns from the sample, whereas the mirror reflects most of the light incident on it. The total electric field E_{total} at the detector is given by the sum of the two returning waves as,

$$E_{\text{total}} = E_{r0} \exp\left[i(kz_r - \omega t)\right] + E_{s0} \exp\left[i(kz_s - \omega t)\right] \tag{10.5}$$

The intensity I_D at the detector of the light beams coming from the two arms of the interferometer is given by the square of the electric field amplitude,

$$I_D = \frac{n}{2\mu_o c} E_{\text{total}}\, E^*{}_{\text{total}} = \frac{n}{2\mu_o c}\left[E^2{}_{s0} + E^2{}_{r0} + 2E_{s0}E_{r0}\cos 2(kz_r - kz_s)\right] \tag{10.6}$$

where n is the refractive index of the transmission medium, μ_o is the permeability, and the asterisk (*) denotes the complex conjugate. Letting the intensity from the sample be,

$$I_{s0} = \frac{n}{2\mu_o c} E^2{}_{s0} \tag{10.7}$$

and the intensity from the reference mirror be,

$$I_{r0} = \frac{n}{2\mu_o c} E^2{}_{r0} \tag{10.8}$$

then the intensity at the detector can be expressed as

$$I_D = I_{s0} + I_{r0} + 2\sqrt{I_{s0}\, I_{r0}} \cos 2\left[\frac{2\pi}{\lambda}(z_r - z_s)\right] \tag{10.9}$$

where $\lambda = 2\pi/k$ is the wavelength of the optical source. The factor $z_r - z_s$ is the pathlength difference between the reference and the sample arms.

10.2.2 Different types of OCT systems

The two main types of OCT systems are the time-domain OCT (TD-OCT) and frequency-domain OCT, classified based on the configuration (source, detector, and scanning mechanism). Frequency-domain OCT is classified into spectral-domain OCT (SD-OCT) and swept-source OCT (SS-OCT). These modalities are further extended into polarization-sensitive OCT (PS-OCT), Doppler OCT, OCT angiography, full-field OCT, and spectroscopic OCT [5–8]. Apart from the above-mentioned modalities, multimodality systems, fluorescence combined with OCT, photoacoustic combined with OCT, and differential absorption-based OCT are also described [4].

10.2.2.1 Time-domain OCT system

The configuration of the time-domain OCT system is described in figure 10.3. The system consists of a scanning reference mirror, with a scanning mechanism

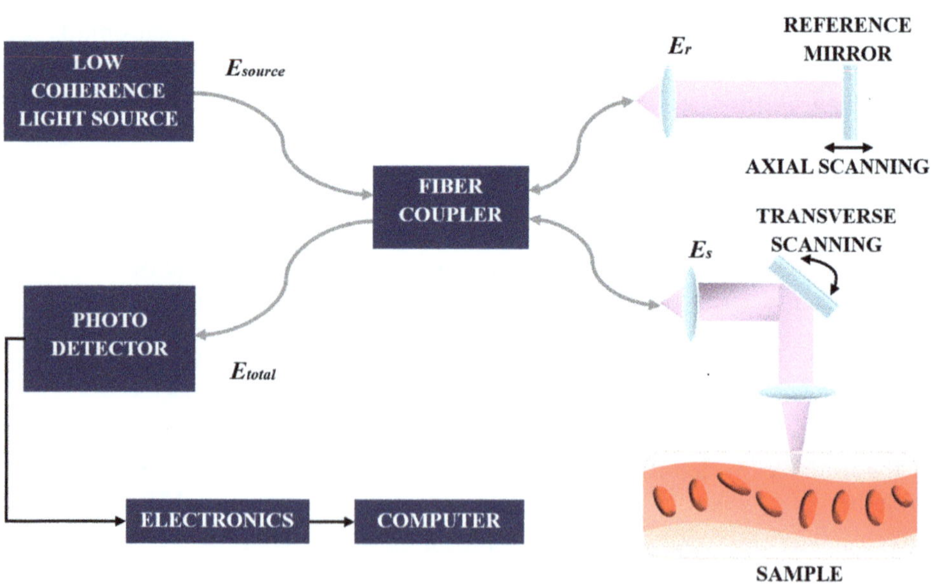

Figure 10.3. Schematic of a time-domain OCT system.

performed by different modes using piezoelectric or mechanical stepper motor to vary the reference arm length to match the delay in various layers of the sample for capturing the complete depth information. A photodetector or a camera records the interference pattern. The resulting interference signal is further processed to produce the axial scan or A-scan. Cross-sectional imaging in OCT is performed by measuring the magnitude and the delay in echo time of the backscattered light in the sample. The measurements along the depth provide axial or A-scans, whereas measurements performed multiple times along the depth axis transversely provide cross-sectional images or B-scans. Volumetric OCT images are obtained by scanning the incident light beam in a raster pattern. Although the TD-OCT system requires minimal post-processing procedures, the slow speed and motion artifacts caused by the mechanical movement of the reference mirror are its limitations [4].

10.2.2.2 Frequency-domain OCT system

Frequency-domain OCT (FD-OCT) allows high-speed imaging with a stationary reference arm, unlike the TD-OCT system. FD-OCT is further classified into spectral-domain OCT (SD-OCT), which uses a broadband light source, and a spectrometer, which records the interference pattern as a function of wavelength. Further post-processing using a Fourier transform provides cross-sectional information. Here, the resolution of the system depends on the resolution of the spectrometer, and the imaging speed depends on the readout time of the sensor in the spectrometer [10]. Swept-source OCT (SS-OCT) system incorporates a laser source sweeping across a band of wavelengths, and the spectral information is captured using a photodetector.

10.2.2.2.1 Spectral-domain OCT system

In SD-OCT, the mirror in the reference arm of the interferometer is kept stationary. The spectral interferogram acquired by the spectrometer consists of reflections from all the layers detected simultaneously. The schematic of SD-OCT is shown in figure 10.4. The spectral interferogram is Fourier transformed to obtain the axial or depth scan. The post-processing steps include the acquisition of reference, sample, and interferogram spectrum, background subtraction, mapping linear wavelength space to nonlinear k-space, mapping nonlinear k-space to linear k-space, interpolation, and inverse Fourier transform to obtain A-scan or the depth-resolved information from the sample.

10.2.2.2.2 Swept source OCT system

Swept-source OCT (SS-OCT) employs a fast wavelength scanning light source with a sweeping rate in the order of hundreds of kilohertz with ultrafast detection. The schematic of SS-OCT is shown in figure 10.5. Compared to the SD-OCT system, the SS-OCT system has a greater sensitivity and lower signal-to-noise ratio (SNR) at greater scanning depths. The speed of imaging depends on the sweep rate of the swept source. The source $k(t)$ is swept linearly in the rapidly tunable narrowband laser source,

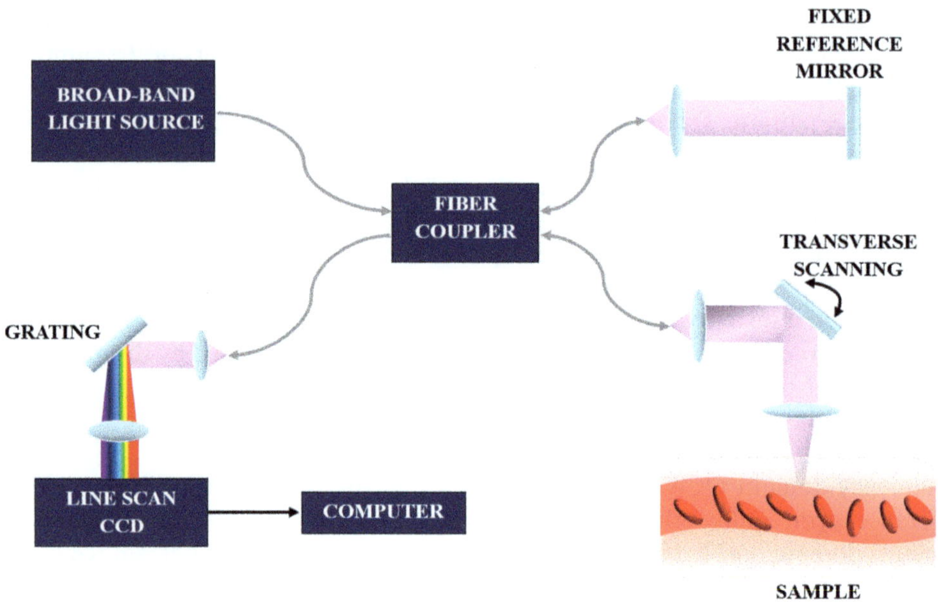

Figure 10.4. Schematic of a spectral-domain OCT system.

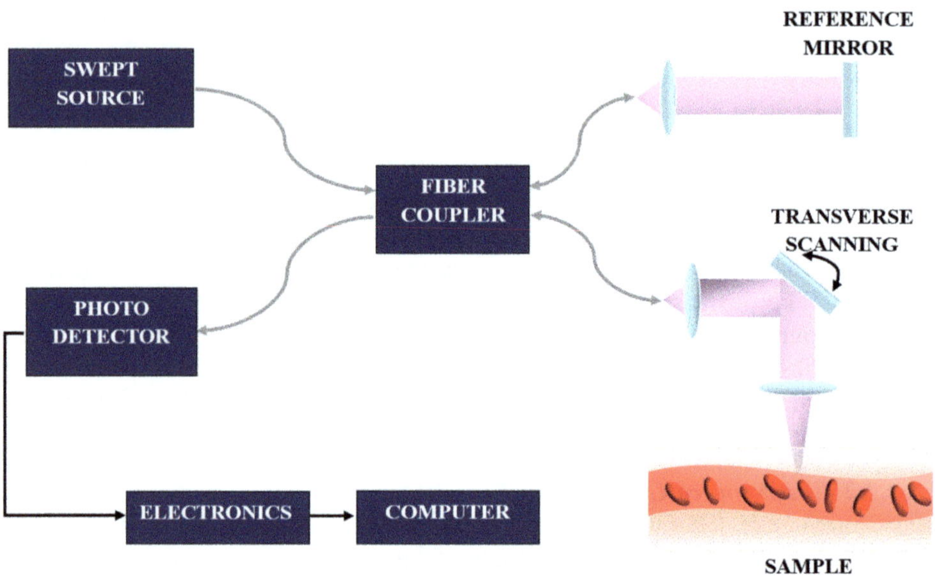

Figure 10.5. Schematic of a swept-source OCT system.

$$k(t) = k_o + \delta k \times t \tag{10.10}$$

$$\delta k = \Delta k / \Delta t \tag{10.11}$$

where Δk and Δt are the total bandwidth swept and sweep time, respectively. The depth scan range is provided by the following equation,

$$x_{\text{depth}} = \frac{M}{2} l_c \tag{10.12}$$

The signal is evenly spaced at M such that $M \times \delta k = \Delta k$ [11]. Discrete Fourier transform of the evenly spaced signal aids in deriving the depth scan of the sample.

10.2.3 Different modalities of OCT

10.2.3.1 Spectroscopic OCT

Spectroscopic OCT (S-OCT) provides morphological and spectroscopic information simultaneously from biological tissues. It is one of the functional OCT imaging techniques that enables quantitative measurement of wavelength-dependent and depth-resolved absorption or spectral backscattering of either native or foreign chromophores in the tissues. Figure 10.6 shows the concept of S-OCT compared to FD-OCT wherein time-frequency transformation (TFT) of OCT interferogram provides spectroscopic information of the sample compared to the limited diagnostic capability of stand-alone gray-scale OCT images.

S-OCT utilizes visible wavelength region and 800 nm region for obtaining enhanced image contrast, enabling the differentiation of tissue pathologies by their spectroscopic properties [8]. S-OCT can be performed either by a software- or hardware-based approach. In the hardware-based approach, a single broadband source like a supercontinuum laser source can be used, or two or multiple super-luminescent light-emitting diode (SLED) sources can be used with distinct bands of wavelengths, whereas software-based S-OCT is based on TFT of OCT interferograms. S-OCT/OCM (optical coherence microscopy) provides insights into the spectral properties of single cells without the requirement of exogenous contrasts, which may either reduce the viability of cells, especially in long-term cell cultures, or alter the function of the cells [8]. By using S-OCT/OCM, spectral-scattering information has been accessed from a 2D cell culture and cells seeded in a 3D agarose scaffold [4].

10.2.3.2 Doppler OCT

Doppler OCT is one of the functional imaging techniques of OCT, combining the Doppler and OCT principles to simultaneously image the cross-sectional structure of tissues and blood flow with a high resolution. Doppler OCT provides valuable information on blood flow in the vasculature, aiding in the diagnosis of various pathological conditions in dermatology, ophthalmology, dentistry, gastroenterology, and cardiology. The first one-dimensional coherent gated measurement of the localized flow velocity of water flowing in a duct was reported in 1991 using a moonbeam laser Doppler velocimeter [12]. Two-dimensional *in vivo* imaging of tissue structure and flow velocity using a short-time fast Fourier transformation (STFFT) and phase-resolved Doppler OCT to overcome the limited sensitivity of high-speed imaging of STFFT have been reported [13–15]. Imaging and quantifying blood flow

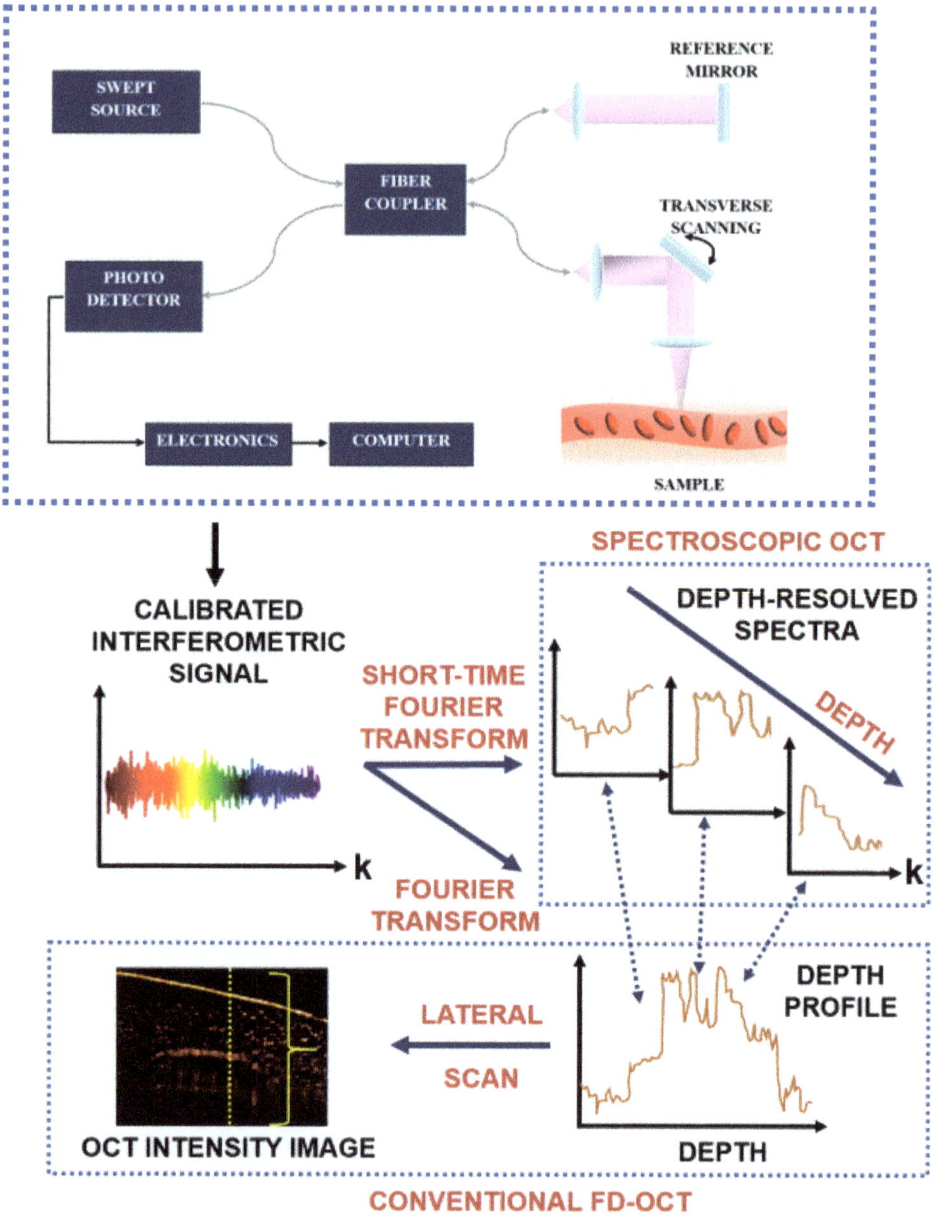

Figure 10.6. Schematic representation of FD-OCT and S-OCT.

based on phase-resolved Doppler OCT is performed by calculating the Doppler shift from the change observed in phase between the B-scans or C-scans [13]. Phase-resolved Doppler OCT is capable of imaging *in vivo* microcirculation in human tissues with a high speed by more than two orders of magnitude without any compromise in the spatial resolution and velocity sensitivity. Further, phase-resolved Doppler variance was developed to quantify transverse flow, unlike phase-resolved Doppler flow, wherein the flow direction is aligned with the probe beam, and also permits visualization of blood capillaries, making it useful for applications related to OCT angiography [13, 14].

10.2.3.2.1 Principle of doppler OCT

Doppler OCT has the potential to provide high-resolution tomographic images of both static and moving constituents in high-scattering media by integrating the Doppler principle with OCT. The Doppler principle is based on the Doppler frequency shift that occurs in the interference fringe when the light beam is backscattered from a moving particle and the reference beam interferes. Doppler frequency shift, Δf is provided as [4],

$$\Delta f = \frac{1}{2\pi}(k_s - k_i) \cdot V \tag{10.13}$$

where k_i is the incoming wave vector, k_s is the wave vector of scattered light and V is the velocity vector of the moving particle, V_T and V_L are the transverse and longitudinal flow velocities, respectively, as shown in figure 10.7.

Considering the angle between the flow and sample beam as θ, the Doppler frequency shift of the backscattered light in equation (10.13) is simplified to,

$$\Delta f = \frac{2 \times n \times V \times \cos(\theta)}{\lambda_0} \tag{10.14}$$

where n is the refractive index of the tissue, and λ_0 is the center wavelength of the light source.

The signal processing of Doppler OCT can be further realized by the following equations [4]. The field amplitude emitted by a low-coherence light source, $U(t)$, which is a complex-valued analytical signal of a stochastic process is represented by (10.15),

$$U(t) = \int_0^{\infty} \overline{U}(\nu)e^{2\pi i\nu t}dv \tag{10.15}$$

where $\overline{U}(\nu)$ is the corresponding spectral amplitude at optical frequency ν, the amplitude of low coherent light source coupled into the interferometer at time t, is represented as a harmonic superposition.

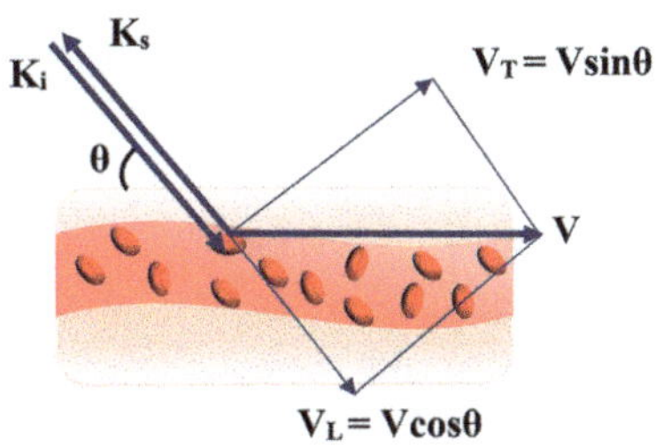

Figure 10.7. Schematic of flow direction and probe beam angle.

The cross spectral density of $\overline{U}(\nu)$ satisfies (10.16) as the stochastic process of the partially coherent light source is stationary.

$$\langle \overline{U}^*(\nu)\overline{U}^*(\nu')\rangle = S_0(\nu)\delta(\nu - \nu') \tag{10.16}$$

where $S_0(\nu)$ is the power spectral density of the source and $\delta(\nu - \nu')$ is the Dirac delta function. The light coupled back to the detector from the reference and sample is, $\overline{U}_r(\nu)$, and $\overline{U}_s(\nu)$, respectively, as provided below, assuming the light couples equally into the reference and sample arm with spectral amplitude of $\overline{U}_o(\nu)$.

$$\overline{U}_r(\nu) = e^{\frac{2\pi i\nu(2L_r+L_d)}{c}} K_r(\nu)\, e^{i\alpha_r(\nu)}\overline{U}_o(\nu) \tag{10.17}$$

$$\overline{U}_s(\nu) = e^{\frac{2\pi i\nu(2L_s+L_d)}{c}} K_s(\nu)\, e^{i\alpha_s(\nu)}\overline{U}_o(\nu) \tag{10.18}$$

where L_r and L_s are the optical pathlength of the reference arm and the sample arm, respectively, and L_d is the optical pathlength from the beam splitter to the detector, $K_r(\nu)\, e^{i\alpha_r(\nu)}$ and $K_s(\nu)\, e^{i\alpha_s(\nu)}$ are the amplitude reflection coefficients of light back-scattered from the reference mirror and the sample, respectively.

A time average of the squared light amplitude, $P_d(\tau)$, represents the total power detected at the output of the interferometer,

$$P_d(\tau) = \langle |U_s(\mathrm{t}) + U_r(\mathrm{t} + \tau)|^2\rangle \tag{10.19}$$

where τ represents the delay time between the light that traveled in the sample arm and reference arm.

The total power detected is the sum of sample, reference and interference fringe intensity,

$$P_d(\tau) = \int_0^{\infty} (P_r(\nu) + P_s(\nu) + P_{\mathrm{ODT}}(\nu))\, d\nu = I_r + I_s + \Gamma_{\mathrm{ODT}}(\tau) \tag{10.20}$$

where,

$$P_r(\nu) = S_0(\nu)|K_r(\nu)|^2 \tag{10.21}$$

$$P_r(\nu) = S_0(\nu)|K_s(\nu)|^2 \tag{10.22}$$

$$P_{\mathrm{ODT}}(\nu) = 2S_0(\nu)K_r(\nu)K_s(\nu)\cos\left[\left(2\pi\nu\left(\frac{\Delta_d}{c}\right) + \tau\right) + \alpha_s(\nu) - \alpha_r(\nu)\right] \tag{10.23}$$

$$I_r = \int_0^{\infty} P_r(\nu)d\nu \tag{10.24}$$

$$I_s = \int_0^{\infty} P_s(\nu)d\nu \tag{10.25}$$

$$\Gamma_{\mathrm{ODT}}(\tau) = \int_0^{\infty} P_{\mathrm{ODT}}(\nu)d\nu \tag{10.26}$$

The light scattered from a moving particle is equivalent to a moving phase front and hence (10.23) can be written as

$$\Delta_d = \Delta + 2\bar{n}V_z t \tag{10.27}$$

where Δ is the difference in the optical pathlength between the sample and reference arm, V_z is the velocity of the moving particle parallel to the probe beam, and $\bar{n}$ is the refractive index of the flow media.

The fringe signal in the spectral domain, $P_{\mathrm{ODT}}(\nu)$, neglecting the constants over the source and reference spectrum, α_s and α_r, and the corresponding time-domain signal, $\Gamma_{\mathrm{ODT}}(\tau)$, is given as follows.

$$P_{\mathrm{ODT}}(\nu) = 2S_0(\nu)K_r(\nu)K_s(\nu)\cos\left[\frac{(2\pi\nu(\Delta + 2\bar{n}V_z t)}{c} + \tau\right] \tag{10.28}$$

$$\Gamma_{\mathrm{ODT}}(\tau) = 2\int_0^{\infty} S_0(\nu)K_r(\nu)K_s(\nu)\cos\left[2\pi\nu\left(\frac{\Delta + 2\bar{n}V_z t}{c} + \tau\right)\right]d\nu \tag{10.29}$$

10.2.3.2.2 Phase-resolved doppler OCT

Phase-resolved Doppler OCT provides flow velocity images based on the phase change between sequential A-scans with an enhanced velocity sensitivity and imaging speed. The Doppler frequency shift Δf is derived through phase change using equation (10.14),

$$\Delta f = \frac{\Delta\varphi}{2 \times \pi \times \Delta T} \tag{10.30}$$

where $\Delta\varphi$ is the phase change, and ΔT is the time interval between sequential A-lines. $\Delta\varphi$ can be calculated using OCT complex data using equation (10.31),

$$\Delta\varphi = \tan^{-1}\left[\frac{Im\left(F_m \times F_{m+1}^*\right)}{\mathrm{Re}\left(F_m \times F_{m+1}^*\right)}\right] \tag{10.31}$$

where F_m and F_{m+1} are the OCT complex data acquired from the same location at a different time. By measuring the phase change of OCT signals as a function of time, combining equations (10.2), (10.14) and (10.15), the longitudinal flow velocity can be determined through equation (10.32),

$$V \times \cos(\theta) = \frac{\lambda \times \Delta\varphi}{4 \times \pi \times n \times \Delta T} = \frac{\lambda}{4 \times \pi \times n \times \Delta T} \times \tan^{-1}\left[\frac{Im\left(F_m \times F_{m+1}^*\right)}{\mathrm{Re}\left(F_m \times F_{m+1}^*\right)}\right] \tag{10.32}$$

Phase-resolved Doppler OCT method is capable of real-time visualization and quantification of blood flow with high-velocity sensitivity, high imaging speed and high spatial resolution simultaneously. However, this method cannot be used for ocular blood flow imaging when the Doppler angle is near 90°.

10.2.3.2.3 Doppler variance OCT

Doppler variance OCT overcomes the limitation of phase-resolved Doppler OCT by enabling imaging of transverse flow based on the bandwidth of Doppler frequency shift, B, which is the difference between the Doppler shifts generated by the two beams in figure 10.8 [14, 15].

$$B = f_1 - f_2 = \frac{4V \sin \theta NA_{\text{eff}}}{\lambda} \tag{10.33}$$

where $f_1 = \frac{2V\cos(\theta-\gamma)}{\lambda}$, $f_2 = \frac{2V\cos(\theta+\gamma)}{\lambda}$ and $\sigma = \frac{\pi V \sin\theta NA_{\text{eff}}}{8\lambda}$

The transverse flow velocity, V_T can be quantified by equation (10.34),

$$V \times \sin(\theta) = \frac{8 \times \lambda \times \sigma}{\pi \times n \times NA_{\text{eff}}} \tag{10.34}$$

where NA_{eff} is the effective numerical aperture of the scan lens. The standard deviation of the Doppler bandwidth can be determined by equation (10.35),

$$\sigma^2 = \frac{\int g(f)(f-\bar{f})^2 df}{\int g(f)(f)^2 df} = \frac{1}{(2\pi\Delta T)^2}\left(1 - \frac{2 \times \left|\left(F_m \times F^*_{(m+1)}\right)\right|}{|F_m|^2 + |F_{|m+1|}|^2}\right) \tag{10.35}$$

where f is the Doppler shift, $\bar{f}$ is the averaged Doppler shift, and $g(f)$ is the Doppler power spectrum.

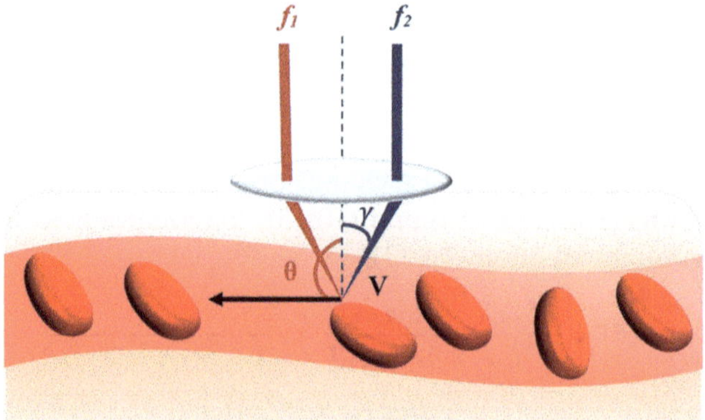

Figure 10.8. Schematic of phase-resolved variance Doppler OCT.

10.2.3.3 OCT angiography (OCT-A)

OCT angiography (OCT-A) based on both SD-OCT and SS-OCT is used in ophthalmology applications. The first commercial OCT-A system was the RTVue XR Avanti (Optovue), capable of providing images with a wide field of view of 6 × 6 mm, an axial resolution of 5 μm, lateral resolution of 15 μm, and an imaging speed of 70 000 A-scans per second [16]. SD-OCT-based Topcon's 3D OCT-1 system provides images with an axial resolution of 6 μm, lateral resolution of 20 μm, and a scanning speed of 50 000 A-scans per second, and Zeiss's Cirrus 6000 system provides images of axial and lateral resolution of 5 and 15 μm, respectively, with a high scanning speed of 100 000 A-scans per second [17]. SS-OCT provides faster scanning of images to improve the image resolution. SS-OCT-based SPECTRALIS from Heidelberg Engineering enables OCT-A imaging with an axial and lateral resolution of 3.9 and 5.7 μm, respectively. Topcon DRI Triton, AngioPlex OCT-A and, Zeiss PLEX Elite 9000, Xephilio OCT-S1 are the other SS-OCT-based OCT-A systems [17–20]. Advancements in AI-based OCT-A have also been reported [21].

The microvasculature consists of red blood cells (RBCs), the main oxygen carriers in blood. The hemodynamics and optical properties of blood in capillaries less than 10 μm in diameter, with RBCs flowing in a line, in macrovasculature with RBCs slowing side-by-side, and in microvasculature with a diameter ranging from 10 to 100 μm, are discussed in detail [22]. In microcapillaries, speed, flux, and linear density of RBCs, and macrovasculature, velocity or speed, flow rate, and hematocrit, are the primary hemodynamic parameters [23, 24]. The optical properties of RBCs, scattering, and absorption properties are attributed to the presence of hemoglobin and its complex refractive index [25]. The absorption of hemoglobin is found to be predominant at the visible and shorter wavelengths and is negligible at the near-infrared wavelength region, which is dominated by scattering. RBCs are considered to be the main scattering constituents in blood. The scattering of whole blood with an ensemble of RBCs with different orientations is characterized by parameters such as scattering coefficient, scattering phase function, scattering anisotropy, and the average of $\cos(\theta)$ over a solid angle. The whole blood is highly forward scattering compared to tissue, which is backscattering. The dynamics of the scatterer are accompanied by Doppler shift (which is the linear phase shift over time) and decorrelation (results in random change in both the OCT signal intensity and phase) [26]. Accurate quantification of OCT-A signals relies on understanding the interplay between hemodynamics, rheology, and RBC light scattering. Improvements in theoretical models, validated in microvasculature, could enhance this understanding. Exploring alternative measurements may mitigate challenges, improving the clinical impact of OCT-A [21].

10.2.3.3.1 Principle of OCT-A

Angiograms are created in OCT-A by separating the flowing scatterers from the blood vessel that is static by either Doppler shift or speckle variance [27]. It performs repeated detection of OCT signal over time at the exact location, with respect to the RBCs which move constantly, subsequently aiding in the visualization of microvasculature [28]. The volumetric OCT-A image is obtained by the steps described in figure 10.9 and the illustration in figure 10.10.

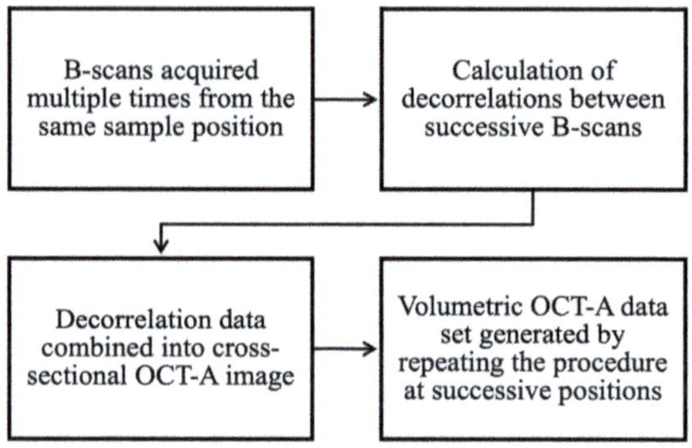

Figure 10.9. Flow chart representation for obtaining volumetric OCT-A.

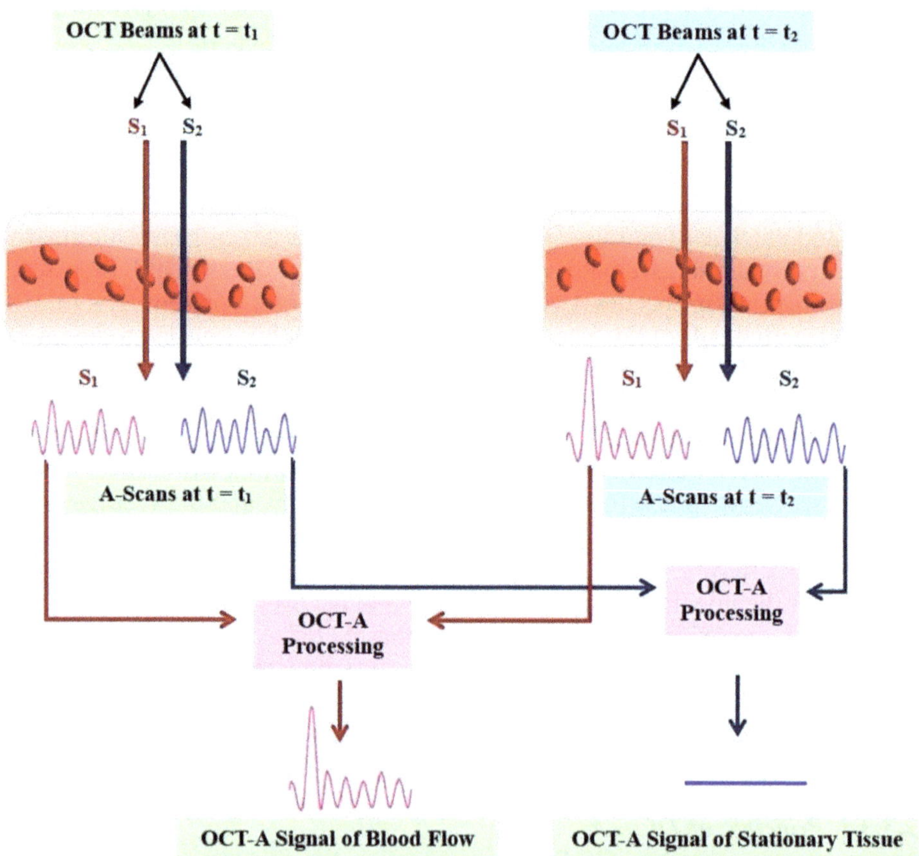

Figure 10.10. Schematic representing the principle of OCT-A: light beams striking the tissue interacting with flowing RBC (S_1—red arrow) and the stationary tissue (S_2—blue arrow) at time $t = t_1$ and $t = t_2$, and the A-scans of OCT obtained from the backscattered light signals from the flowing RBC and the stationary tissue represented as pink (S_1) and blue (S_2) traces at time t_1 and t_2. The averaged signals after processing form composite signals representing increased variability of the OCT signal from beam S_1 due to the movement of RBCs (pink) compared to the signal obtained from stationary tissue (blue).

Figure 10.9 illustrates the flow chart of OCT-A principle, representing the averaged OCT-A signals generated after processing the OCT signals backscattered from the RBC (S_1) and stationary tissue (S_2) at time t_1 and t_2, respectively.

10.2.3.3.2 OCT-A algorithms

The following are the various algorithms based on the intensity, phase, and a combination of both to overcome artifacts caused by moving blood cells.

(a) ***Split-spectrum amplitude-decorrelation angiography (SSADA)***

By using the split-spectrum amplitude-decorrelation angiography (SSADA) algorithm, the final flow signal is obtained by splitting into sub-bands the decorrelation in the consecutive B-scan intensity from the full OCT spectrum and averaging as shown in equation (10.36) [29]

$$\mathrm{Flow}_{\mathrm{SSADA}}(x, z) = 1 - \frac{1}{N-1}\frac{1}{M}\sum_{i=1}^{N-1} \times \sum_{m=1}^{M} \frac{I_{im}(x, z)I_{(i+1)m}(x, z)}{\left[\frac{1}{2}I_{im}(x, z)^2 + \frac{1}{2}I_{(i+1)m}(x, z)^2\right]} \tag{10.36}$$

where M is the number of split-spectrums, N is the number of B-scans acquired at the same location, $I_{im}(x, z)$ is the value of intensity measured in the ith B-scans of mth split-spectrum at the lateral location and depth position represented as x and z, respectively. The SNR is increased by splitting the spectrum into sub-bands without increasing the acquisition time.

(b) ***Optical microangiography (OMAG) algorithm***

The OMAG algorithm is based on both intensity and phase information, wherein the flow signal is calculated as shown in equation (10.37), with an increased sensitivity, by subtracting the consecutive complex signals after phase compensation is performed [29]

$$\mathrm{Flow}_{\mathrm{OMAG}}(x, z) = \frac{1}{N-1}\sum_{i=0}^{N-1} |C_{i+1}(x, z) - C_i(x, z)| \tag{10.37}$$

where N is the number of B-scans acquired at the same location, $C_i(x, z)$ is the complex signal consisting of both intensity and phase values in the ith B-scans at lateral location and depth position, x and z, respectively.

(c) ***Slab subtraction (SS) algorithm***

The SS algorithm removes projection artifacts caused by superficial layers, which is achieved by subtracting the superficial slab with maximum projected flow from the current slab as shown in equation (10.38) [30].

$$C_{\mathrm{slab2}} = \begin{cases} D_{\mathrm{slab2}} - D_{\mathrm{slab1}}, & \text{if } D_{\mathrm{slab2}} > D_{\mathrm{slab1}} \\ 0, & \text{otherwise} \end{cases} \tag{10.38}$$

where, D_{slab2} denotes the decorrelation value within the slab of interest from maximum flow projection, while D_{slab1} denotes the maximum flow projection of all layers above D_{slab2}.

(d) ***Projection resolved OCT-A (PR-OCT-A) algorithm***

The PR-OCT-A algorithm removes both the projection artifact and tail artifact from the vessels of the retina. The normalized flow signal F, is provided in equation (10.39) [30]

$$F = \frac{D}{S} \tag{10.39}$$

where D denotes the decorrelation and S denotes the log amplitude OCT signal. The PR-corrected values of decorrelation C_n, is expressed as,

$$C_n = \begin{cases} D_n, \text{ if } F_n > (1 + \alpha)\max(F_i),\ 1 \leqslant i \leqslant n - 1 \\ 0, \text{ otherwise} \end{cases} \tag{10.40}$$

where, i and n represent the index of a voxel in an A-line from the shallow inner and proximal end, respectively, and α denotes noise.

While OCT-A could be valuable for understanding pathogenesis by directly linking observables to key hemodynamic parameters, the lack of a well-established model poses a challenge. The current empirical models for OCT-A are limited, necessitating a more robust theoretical foundation that considers factors like multiple scattering and orientation effects for accurate interpretation. The simplicity of existing theoretical models for OCT-A, focusing only on single scattering, calls for advancements to include complexities like multiple scattering and orientation effects. Although empirical models for flow phantoms exist, uncertainties persist about their *in vivo* applicability. Rigorous *in vivo* validation, particularly in stable animal preparations, is crucial for assessing their reliability. Unique models for capillaries and macro vessels are essential due to variations in light scattering and hemodynamics, emphasizing the need for independent models for accurate interpretation. Quantification challenges arise from the irregular shape of RBCs, the orientation-dependent nature of RBC backscattering, and the substantial anisotropy in the RBC scattering phase function, resulting in multiple scattering within large vessels.

10.3 The nature of polarization and foundational formalisms

Polarization is an intrinsic property of electromagnetic radiation stemming from its vector and transverse nature. Classically, light is considered polarized if the extremity of the electric field vector (E) traces a stationary curve over a period of observation. Conversely, an electromagnetic wave is classified as unpolarized if the vector E exhibits random and varying orientations. The underlying quantum mechanical explanation is mutually consistent with this classical view; polarization is used to describe individual energy quanta (photons), which are presumed to be fully polarized and defined by a specific state vector. The observable polarization of the classical wave arises from the combined states of many individual photons [31, 32].

The classical propagation of polarized light through an optical system can be described using two main mathematical formalisms: Jones calculus [32, 33] and Stokes–Mueller calculus [34, 35]. Jones calculus provides a field-based representation that relies on the coherent addition of wave amplitudes and phases. However, the use of Jones formalism in tissue polarimetry is highly restricted because it is limited to describing only pure polarization states. It cannot account for partial polarization or the common phenomenon of depolarizing interactions found ubiquitously in biological tissues. Stokes–Mueller calculus, introduced by Stokes in 1852, is preferred in general scenarios, particularly those involving polarization loss, because it is an intensity-based representation that accommodates the incoherent addition of wave intensities.

10.3.1 The Stokes vector and polarization metrics

The polarization state of a light beam is represented by the Stokes vector (S), a 4 × 1 vector containing four quantifiable intensity values (*I, Q, U, V*) [33–35]. These parameters are defined relative to six specific intensity measurements (*I*) obtained using ideal polarizers:

- I_H: Horizontal linear polarizer (0 degrees)
- I_V: Vertical linear polarizer (90 degrees)
- I_P: 45 degrees linear polarizer
- I_M: 135 degrees (–45 degrees) linear polarizer
- I_R: Right circular polarizer
- I_L: Left circular polarizer

The Stokes vector (*S*) is defined by equation (10.41):

$$\mathrm{S} = \begin{bmatrix} I \\ Q \\ U \\ V \end{bmatrix} = \begin{bmatrix} I_H + I_V \\ I_H - I_V \\ I_P - I_M \\ I_R - I_L \end{bmatrix} \tag{10.41}$$

The element *I* represents the total detected light intensity, derived from the sum of two orthogonal component intensities. *Q* represents the intensity difference between horizontal and vertical polarization states. *U* denotes the intensity portion corresponding to the difference between linear + 45 degrees and –45 degrees polarization states. Finally, *V* quantifies the intensity difference between right circular and left circular polarization states.

The Stokes formalism allows for the calculation of polarization characteristics for any light beam [33–35]:

Net degree of polarization

$$\mathrm{DOP} = \frac{\sqrt{Q^2 + U^2 + V^2}}{I} \tag{10.42}$$

Degree of linear polarization

$$\mathrm{DOLP} = \frac{\sqrt{Q^2 + U^2}}{I} \tag{10.43}$$

Degree of circular polarization

$$\mathrm{DOCP} = \frac{V}{I} \tag{10.44}$$

For fully polarized light, the net degree of polarization is equal to one. When depolarization occurs, the DOP drops below one, reaching zero when the light is entirely depolarized.

10.3.2 The Mueller matrix: defining medium interaction

While the Stokes vector describes the polarization state of light, the transfer function of any medium during its interaction with polarized light is described by the Mueller matrix (M). Named after Hans Mueller (1940s), this 4 × 4 matrix relates the output Stokes vector (S_0) to the input Stokes vector (S_i) via simple matrix multiplication, as shown in equation (10.45) [33–35]:

$$S_o = \mathrm{M}\, S_i \tag{10.45}$$

The resulting output Stokes vector components are determined by the 16 elements (m_{ij}) of the Mueller matrix, demonstrating the inclusion of depolarization information:

$$\begin{bmatrix} I_o \\ Q_o \\ U_o \\ V_o \end{bmatrix} = \begin{bmatrix} m_{11} & m_{12} & m_{13} & m_{14} \\ m_{21} & m_{22} & m_{23} & m_{24} \\ m_{31} & m_{32} & m_{33} & m_{34} \\ m_{41} & m_{42} & m_{43} & m_{44} \end{bmatrix} \begin{bmatrix} I_i \\ Q_i \\ U_i \\ V_i \end{bmatrix} = \begin{bmatrix} m_{11}I_i + m_{12}Q_i + m_{13}U_i + m_{14}U_i \\ m_{21}I_i + m_{22}Q_i + m_{23}U_i + m_{24}U_i \\ m_{31}I_i + m_{32}Q_i + m_{33}U_i + m_{34}U_i \\ m_{41}I_i + m_{42}Q_i + m_{43}U_i + m_{44}U_i \end{bmatrix} \tag{10.46}$$

The real 4 × 4 Mueller matrix M can contain a maximum of 16 independent parameters (or 15 if absolute intensity is disregarded). Because its various components encode all the medium's polarization characteristics, the Mueller matrix is often conceptualized as the sample's complete 'optical polarization fingerprint'.

The Stokes–Mueller formalism holds particular utility in tissue polarimetry because it can describe all types of light polarization (natural, total, or partial), making it applicable to both polarizing and depolarizing optical systems. Furthermore, Stokes vectors and Mueller matrices can be measured easily using conventional intensity-measuring instruments suchating as polarimeters, radiometers, and spectrometers.

10.3.3 Medium polarization characteristics determined by the Mueller formalism

The Mueller matrix framework is employed to define the fundamental polarization properties of the interacting medium.

10.3.3.1 Depolarization

Depolarization is the property a system exhibits when a completely polarized incident state results in an exiting state where the degree of polarization is less than one. This effect is commonly caused by photon scattering. One factor contributing to depolarization is the presence of randomly oriented uniaxial birefringent domains. When the amplitudes and phases of the scattered fields are added incoherently, the resulting output polarization state is 'scrambled' [34, 36]. The general form of a pure depolarization Mueller matrix is given by equation (10.47):

$$\mathrm{M}_{\Delta} = \begin{pmatrix} 1 & 0 & 0 & 0 \\ 0 & a & 0 & 0 \\ 0 & 0 & b & 0 \\ 0 & 0 & 0 & 0 \end{pmatrix}, \ |a|, |b|, |c| \leqslant 1 \tag{10.47}$$

The depolarization factors for linear polarization are defined as $1 - |a|$ and $1 - |b|$ (for horizontal/vertical and +45 degrees/–45 degrees linear polarization, respectively), and $1 - |c|$ is the factor for circular polarization. The net depolarization factor is often calculated as:

$$\Delta = 1 - \frac{|a| + |b| + |b|}{3} = \frac{|(\mathrm{M}_{\Delta})^{T} - 1|}{3}, \ 0 \leqslant \Delta \leqslant 1 \tag{10.48}$$

It's important to note that the depolarization factor of the medium is defined differently than the conventional definition of degree of polarization of the light in section 3.1. The latter represents the level of polarization caused by various depolarization effects experienced by the beam and is also influenced by the initial Stokes vector. On the other hand, the depolarization factors discussed here reflect the pure depolarizing transfer function of the medium. In general, there is a rough relationship between the two, with $\mathrm{DOP}_{\mathrm{light}} \sim 1 - \Delta_{\mathrm{medium}}$ (the same applies to linear and circular states). However, it is important to note that this equality only holds true in specific scenarios. Generally speaking, a medium with a high value Δ will greatly reduce polarization, resulting in a low degree of polarization in the light after interaction.

10.3.3.2 Retardance

Retardance and diattenuation result from differences in refractive indices between various polarization states. Retardance specifically involves differences in the real parts of the refractive index, resulting in linear birefringence or circular birefringence. Retardance is defined as the phase shift that arises between two orthogonal polarizations of light. Linear retardance δ, or birefringence, is the phase difference that develops between orthogonal linear polarization states (such as vertical and horizontal, or 45 degrees and –45 degrees). Circular retardance (Ψ), also known as optical rotation, is the phase difference between right circularly polarized (RCP) and left circularly polarized (LCP) states. The Mueller matrix for a pure linear retarder, characterized by retardance δ and a fast axis oriented at angle θ relative to the horizontal, is given by equation (10.49) [34, 36]:

$$\begin{pmatrix} 1 & 0 & 0 & 0 \\ 0 & \cos^2 2\theta{+}\sin^2 2\theta \cos\delta & \sin 2\theta \cos 2\theta(1{-}\cos\delta) & -\sin 2\theta \cos\delta \\ 0 & \sin 2\theta \cos 2\theta(1{-}\cos\delta) & \sin^2 2\theta{+}\sin^2 2\theta \cos\delta & \cos 2\theta \sin\delta \\ 0 & \sin 2\theta \cos\delta & -\cos 2\theta \sin\delta & \cos\delta \end{pmatrix} \tag{10.49}$$

The Mueller matrix for a pure circular retarder, defined by an optical rotation value ψ is expressed by equation (10.50) [34, 36]:

$$\begin{pmatrix} 1 & 0 & 0 & 0 \\ 0 & \cos 2\psi & -\sin 2\psi & 0 \\ 0 & \sin 2\psi & \cos 2\psi & 0 \\ 0 & 0 & 0 & 1 \end{pmatrix} \tag{10.50}$$

10.3.3.3 Diattenuation

Diattenuation (d) refers to the differential (unequal) attenuation of orthogonal polarization states. This differential attenuation can be linear or circular. It is analogous to dichroism, which describes the unequal absorption of perpendicular polarization states (linear or circular). Diattenuation is a more comprehensive term, as it encompasses differential attenuation resulting from either scattering or absorption. Diattenuation is caused by differences in the imaginary parts of the refractive index (dichroism). The Mueller matrix for an ideal linear diattenuator is defined using intensity transmittance (or reflectance) parameters q and r for the two incident orthogonal polarization states, along with the orientation angle (θ) of the principal axis (equation (10.51)) [34, 36]:

$$\begin{pmatrix} q+r & (q-r)\cos 2\theta & (q-r)\sin 2\theta & 0 \\ (q-r)\cos 2\theta & (q+r)\cos^2 2\theta{+}2\sqrt{(qr)}\sin^2 2\theta & (q+r-2\sqrt{(qr)})\sin 2\theta\cos 2\theta & 0 \\ (q-r)\sin 2\theta & (q+r-2\sqrt{(qr)})\sin 2\theta\cos 2\theta & (q+r)\cos^2 2\theta{+}2\sqrt{(qr)}\sin^2 2\theta & 0 \\ 0 & 0 & 0 & 2\sqrt{(qr)} \end{pmatrix} \tag{10.51}$$

For circular diattenuation, the Mueller matrix takes the form of equation (10.52) [34, 36]:

$$\begin{pmatrix} q+r & 0 & 0 & q-r \\ 0 & 2\sqrt{(qr)} & 0 & 0 \\ 0 & 0 & 2\sqrt{(qr)} & 0 \\ q-r & 0 & 0 & q+r \end{pmatrix} \tag{10.52}$$

An example of a diattenuator is the ideal polarizer, which converts unpolarized light into fully polarized light, typically accompanied by a noticeable decrease in overall light intensity.

10.3.4 Measurement techniques in tissue polarimetry

Biomedical polarimetry seeks to enhance tissue imaging resolution by discriminating against multiply scattered light, and to provide detailed morphological, biochemical, and functional information through tissue characterization [37–39]. Accurate measurement of the polarization-retaining signal is vital for both objectives. However, traditional polarimetry systems (e.g., crossed linear polarizers used for thin *ex vivo* tissue slices) are unsuitable for thick biological tissues because multiple scattering induces depolarization noise, making the desired small polarization signal difficult to detect. Specialized experimental tools have been developed to enhance measurement sensitivity.

10.3.4.1 Stokes polarimetry measurement

The four Stokes parameters can be determined by either performing six intensity measurements (I_H, I_V, I_P, I_M, I_R, and I_L) involving linear and circular polarization states [35], or more efficiently, by using only four measurements, exploiting the property that ($I_H + I_V = I_P + I_M = I_L + I_R$) [40]. The four-measurement method typically uses a circular polarizer built from a linear polarizer and a quarter wave-plate (QWP). The linear polarizer's transmission axis is set at + 45 deg relative to horizontal, and the QWP's fast axis is parallel to the horizontal. Four intensity measurements are taken: three sets of [I_{Cir} (α)] by adjusting the circular polarizer angle α to 0, 45, and 90 degrees, and a final intensity measurement [I_{Lin} (α)] taken after flipping the combined polarizer to the opposite side and setting $\alpha = 0$ degrees. Collett originally proposed this measurement scheme [40]. The Stokes parameters are derived from these measurements using equation (10.53):

$$\begin{bmatrix} I \\ Q \\ U \\ V \end{bmatrix} = \begin{bmatrix} I_{Cir}(0deg) + I_{Cir}(90deg) \\ I - 2I_{Cir}(45deg) \\ I_{Cir}(0deg) - I_{Cir}(90deg) \\ -I + 2I_{Lin}(0deg) \end{bmatrix}. \tag{10.53}$$

Although this approach is used in depolarization studies for turbid media [41–43], applications requiring precise quantification of inherent tissue properties necessitate a more sensitive method, often involving polarization modulation combined with synchronous detection [38, 39]. These techniques manipulate polarization either incident on the sample or exiting the sample (via a modulator placed between the sample and the detector) [44–46].

10.3.4.2 Mueller matrix polarimetry measuremen

Mueller matrix polarimetry aims to determine the sample's polarization transfer function. Both modulation-based and static measurement procedures are employed. The static method requires cycling the input polarization through four distinct states (linear polarization at 0 degrees, 45 degrees, 90 degrees, and right circular polarization) and recording the complete output Stokes vector for each. The resulting four Stokes vectors (16 total values) are algebraically manipulated to solve for the Mueller matrix elements [47]. Equation (10.54) presents the algebraic solution for the Mueller matrix elements M(*i, j*), where the input states are designated by subscripts *H* (0 degrees), *P* (45 degrees), *V* (90 degrees), and *R* (right circular polarization):

$$M(i,j) = \begin{pmatrix} \frac{1}{2}(I_H + I_V) & \frac{1}{2}(I_H - I_V) & I_P - M(1,1) & I_R - M(1,1) \\ \frac{1}{2}(Q_H + Q_V) & \frac{1}{2}(Q_H - Q_V) & Q_P - M(2,1) & Q_R - M(2,1) \\ \frac{1}{2}(U_H + U_V) & \frac{1}{2}(U_H - U_V) & U_P - M(3,1) & U_R - M(3,1) \\ \frac{1}{2}(V_H + V_V) & \frac{1}{2}(V_H - V_V) & V_P - M(4,1) & V_R - M(4,1) \end{pmatrix}. \quad (10.54)$$

The indices $i, j = 1, 2, 3$, and 4 represent rows and columns, respectively.

The polarization modulation/synchronous detection approach is highly effective for Mueller matrix measurements in complex turbid media and actual biological tissues [47, 48]. The dual rotating retarder technique is a widely used modulation-based Mueller matrix polarimeter. In this technique, the incident polarization state is modulated by passing light through a fixed linear polarizer and then a rotating linear retarder (retardation δ_1, angular speed ω_1). The analyzing optics consist of a second rotating retarder (retardation δ_2, angular speed ω_2) and a fixed linear polarizer. A typical setup configuration uses equal retardation values ($\delta_1 = \boldsymbol{\delta}_2 = \pi/2$) and a 5:1 ratio for the angular speeds ($\omega_1 = \omega$ and $\omega_2 = 5\omega$). The resultant detected intensity signal is modulated due to the harmonic fluctuation in the orientation angle of the two retarders. This specific 5:1 ratio of rotation speeds is known to encode all 16 Mueller matrix components onto the amplitude and phases of 12 distinct frequencies within the observed intensity signal. These elements are then constructed via Fourier analysis using the Fourier coefficients. This framework can be generalized to use unrestricted values for linear retardations, rotation speed ratios, and polarizer axes, allowing optimization for improved determination precision or SNR for specific Mueller matrix elements. [49–51].

10.4 Clinical applications of OCT for blood

There are several research works on OCT-A, discussing about the advancements of OCT-A in terms of its use as a quantitative measurement tool [22], and the applications of deep learning in OCT-A imaging [21]. There exists an enormous interest in the application of OCT-A in ophthalmology, dermatology, gastroenterology, cardiology, neuroscience, and cancer biology, in studying the morphology of microvasculature and changes in perfusion over time using different modalities of OCT [52–62].

10.4.1 Ophthalmology

Fundus fluorescein angiography (FA) and indocyanine green angiography (ICGA) are the conventional modalities used in imaging the chorioretinal vasculature. These invasive procedures require intravenous injection of the dye, which might cause allergic reactions and are unsuitable during pregnancy [6]. OCT angiography (OCT-A) serves as an advanced alternative to conventional dye-based imaging techniques by providing real-time, non-invasive, high-resolution, and rapid visualization of deep and superficial capillary networks without the need for contrast agents [6]. OCT-A is widely used in ophthalmology, aiding in the identification of moving patterns of red blood cells (RBCs) in the retinal blood vessels to detect various pathologies of the eye, including diabetic retinopathy, age-related macular degeneration, diabetic macular ischemia, diabetic macular edema, and retinal vein occlusion [29]. FA is the gold standard for detecting macular capillary networks and macular ischemia. However, distinguishing superficial and deep capillary plexi using this method is not possible. Moreover, the acquisition speed and the label-free imaging are the advantages of OCT-A over FA. OCT-A helps in detecting various pathologies such as intraretinal microvascular abnormalities, microaneurysms, neovascularization, retinal non-perfusion regions and other structural changes caused by diabetic retinopathy which are subtle to be imaged using FA and color fundus photography [62–66]. The progression of diabetic retinopathy is determined by the quantitative measurements of several features such as the spacing, area density, length density, total length, diameter index and fractal dimension of the vessel, and the area of avascular zone in the fovea [61–72].

Advanced OCT-A imaging with a larger field of view provides insights into peripheral vascular abnormalities, aiding in the diagnosis and monitoring of diseases such as diabetic retinopathy (DR) and retinal vascular occlusions (RVO) [73]. In addition, it improves disease understanding, leading to earlier detection rates and more effective treatment planning and also helps in the detection of non-perfusion areas and vascular changes in retinal artery occlusion (RAO) and retinal vein occlusion (RVO), providing valuable information for predicting visual outcomes [74]. Further, it characterizes macular oedema, capillary dropout, and neovascularization, aiding in the diagnosis and management of RAO and RVO [75]. Computational approaches, including image binarization and choroidal vascularity index (CVI) derivation, enhance the precision of OCT-A in quantifying neovascular networks and evaluating choroidal alterations [76]. OCT-A further facilitates objective assessment, improves diagnostic accuracy, and guides treatment decisions for conditions such as neovascular AMD [77]. OCT-A assesses ischemia in limbal stem cells, guiding the identification of patients suitable for revascularization therapies [78]. OCT-A aids in diagnosing uveitis by revealing inflammation and vascular changes not visible through other imaging techniques. OCT-A proves valuable in detecting microvascular changes in glaucoma patients, including reductions in capillary density and altered blood flow [79–81].

Figure 10.11 shows the intraretinal microvascular abnormalities imaged using FA and OCT-A for a patient diagnosed with proliferative diabetic retinopathy, a condition characterized by the growth of abnormal new blood on the retinal surface, which may break and bleed leaking into the vitreous, leading to vision loss. Figures 10.11(a) and 10.11(b) show the fundus photograph and the FA, respectively [17]. Figures 10.11(c) and 10.11(d) are the 3 × 3 mm FA and OCT-A images, respectively, where the superficial collaterals and adjacent non-perfusion areas are indicated by the white and orange arrowheads, respectively. Figure 10.11(e) shows the corresponding SD-OCT B-scan. Figure 10.12 shows the OCT-A images of a normal eye, showing superficial and deep inner retina, non-vascularized outer retina, and choriocapillaris, obtained using RTVue XR Avanti (Optovue) with the software AgioVue used for processing [16]. OCT-A is capable of imaging the choroidal vessels and choriocapillaris, which are difficult to image using standard imaging techniques, including intensity-based OCT [5]. Key issues impacting flow analysis, especially in the choriocapillaris layer, include segmentation errors, projection artifacts, and shadowing artifacts [16].

Ocular diseases such as diabetic retinopathy, glaucoma and age-related macular degeneration may alter the retinal blood flow [5]. Quantification of blood flow using laser Doppler flowmetry (LDF), laser Doppler velocimetry (LDV), speckle fluctuations, and ultrasound-based approaches are reported. However, there is a need for rapid, label-free and non-contact imaging with a high-resolution [5]. Doppler OCT provides quantitative volumetric information on the retinal blood flow along with the vasculature and morphological anatomy.

Clinical limitations of OCT-A include difficulty in detecting vascular leakage, susceptibility to motion artifacts, and potential false-positive or false-negative results [82]. Evaluation of alterations in quantitative metrics of OCT-A in amblyopic eyes and investigation of their correlation with visual acuity in pediatric patients is reported [82–88]. Figure 10.13(a) shows the OCT fundus image in gray scale. The bright blood vessel structure attributes to the strong optical attenuation in blood. As a comparison, the 3D OCT volume from a depth range of 160–250 μm (corresponding to the inner/outer segment (IS/OS) junction to the retinal pigment epithelium (RPE) layer) and projected the mean intensity. An enhanced contrast from the microvasculature is seen in figure 10.13(b). Figure 10.13(b) shows the quantified mean sO_2 values in major vessels. A circular scanning pattern was used around the optic disk, as shown in figure 10.13(a), with 4096 A-lines, so that all the major vessels could be sampled. The circular scan was further expanded into a B-scan image, as shown in figure 10.13(c), where the vessel index corresponds to the numbers in figure 10.13(a). Figure 10.13(d) displays the values of sO_2 in individual vessels with

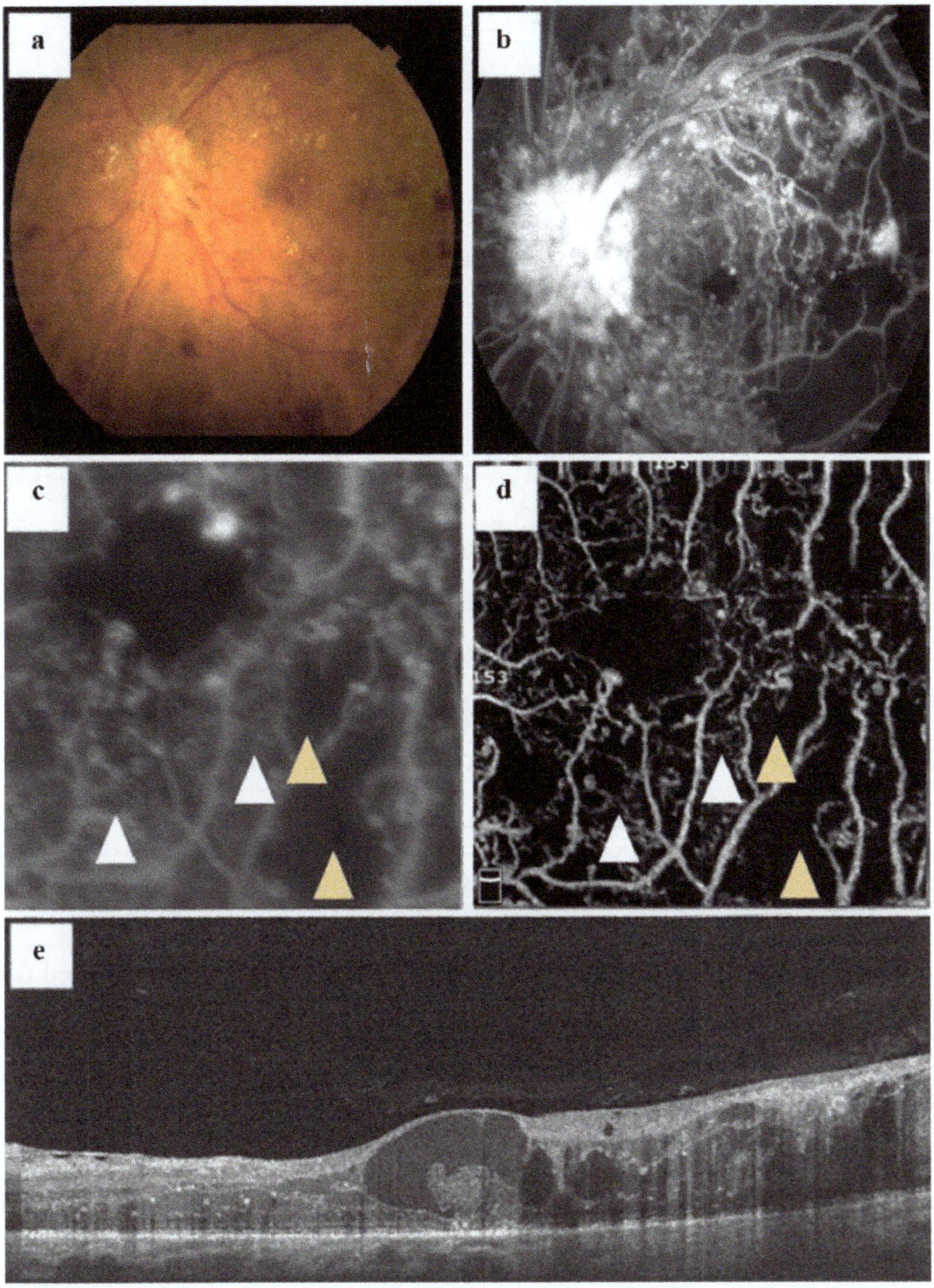

Figure 10.11. The intraretinal microvascular abnormalities imaged using FA and OCT-A for a patient diagnosed with proliferative diabetic retinopathy. (a) the fundus photograph and (b) FA, (c) the 3 × 3 mm FA and (d) OCT-A images (white arrowheads indicate the superficial collaterals and orange arrowheads indicate the adjacent non-perfusion areas), (e) shows the corresponding SD-OCT B-scan. Reproduced from [17], copyright 2017, Springer Nature Limited under the Creative Commons Attribution 4.0 International License (http://creativecommons.org/licenses/by/4.0/).

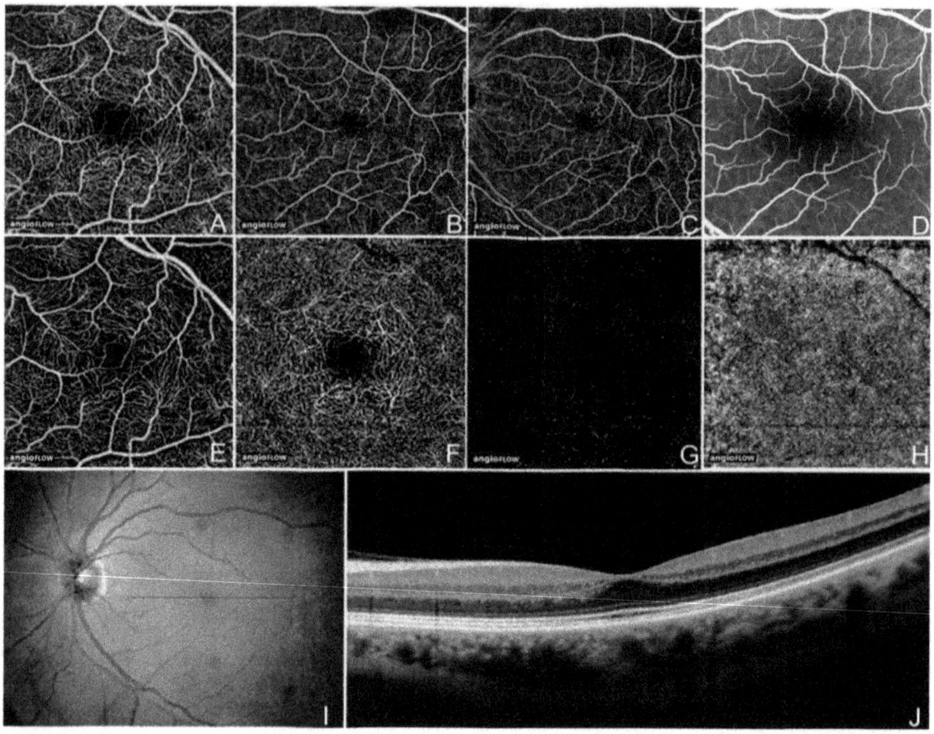

Figure 10.12. Normal eye image obtained using RTVue XR Avanti (Optovue) and AngioVue software (A) 3 × 3 mm, (B) 6 × 6 mm, and (C) 8 × 8 mm, OCT-A image, (D) 8 × 8 mm Fluorescein angiography image, 3 × 3 mm OCT-A image of the (E) 'Superficial' inner retina, and (F) 'Deep' inner retina, (G) non-vascularized outer retina, and (H) choriocapillaris, (I) En face intensity OCT image. (J) Highly sampled OCT B-scan image. Reproduced from [16], Copyright 2015, Springer Nature Limited under the Creative Commons Attribution 4.0 International License (http://creativecommons.org/licenses/by/4.0/).

red and blue colors labeling the arteries and veins. The sO_2 values estimated from arteries and veins were 95% ± 3% and 72% ± 7%, respectively. Qualitative visualization of lipid and artery distribution using a tri-band swept-source S-OCT at wavelengths 1315, 1509 and 1605 nm, based on the difference in the attenuation coefficients at these wavelength bands was reported [89].

S-OCT is capable of quantitative measurement of hemoglobin concentration and blood oxygen saturation levels from the spectroscopic information [90–102]. However, because of the challenge involved in quantitative analysis of the entire axial range, color map-based qualitative visualization of spectroscopic information is performed. S-OCT in the visible range was used for *in vivo* retinal oximetry application on pigmented rats (Long Evans rat, 500 g, Harlan Laboratories), wherein an analytical model was established to describe the optical scattering, absorption and packing factor of blood cells in whole blood. Using the visible OCT oximetry approach, the averaged sO_2 values of 95% and 72% were detected in arterial and venous blood, respectively [99]. The experimental setup based on a free-space SD-OCT system comprises a supercontinuum source (SiperK, NKT

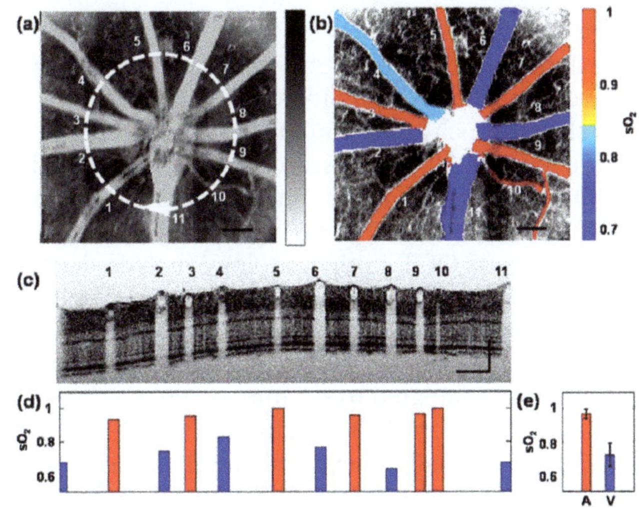

Figure 10.13. *In vivo* experimental results. (a) vis-OCT fundus image. The white circle highlights a circular scanning trajectory for the B-scan image shown in panel (c). (b) Fused vasculature image and sO_2 map in major vessels, (d) individual quantification of sO_2 in every vessel shown in panel (c), and (e) the average arterial and venous sO_2 values. Error bar = standard deviation. Bar = 200 μm. Reprinted with permission from [99] © Optical Society of America.

photonics), with a center wavelength of 585 nm and a FWHM bandwidth of 85 nm. The reflected light spectrum, I, is extracted by a series of short-time Fourier transforms (STFT) as,

$$I^2 = I_0^2 R_0 r \exp\left[-2nd\ \mu_{HbO_2}(sO_2) - 2nd\ \mu_{Hb}(1 - sO_2)\right] \tag{10.55}$$

where, I_0 is the incident intensity on the retina, which is the source spectrum, ignoring the optical attenuation of ocular lens and vitreous chamber, R_0 is the reflectance from reference arm, n denotes the mean refractive index of the blood (~1.35), d is the vessel diameter, and r (dimensionless) denotes the reflectance at the vessel wall. The attenuation coefficient of oxygenated and deoxygenated blood is denoted as μ_{HbO_2} and μ_{Hb}, respectively. The scattering spectrum is modeled as a power law under the first-order Born approximation $r(\lambda) = A\lambda - \alpha$, where A is a constant. The optical attenuation coefficient μ, denotes the attenuation coefficient which combines the absorption and scattering coefficients of whole blood which are dependent on both wavelength and oxygenation. By taking natural log and using the above expression, equation (10.13) becomes,

$$\ln\left(\frac{I(\lambda)}{I_0(\lambda)}\right) = -nd\ \left[(sO_2)\cdot\mu_{HbO_2}(\lambda) + (1 - sO_2)\cdot\mu_{Hb}\right] - \frac{1}{2}\alpha\ \ln(\lambda) + \frac{1}{2}\ln(AR_0) \tag{10.56}$$

The O_2, α and $\ln(AR_0)$ can be obtained by a least-squares fit to fit the spectrum. The blood cell packing factor W, weighs the scattering spectrum as, $\mu = \mu_a + W\mu_{s.}$

10.4.2 Dermatology

In skin tissue, scattering is the dominant phenomenon, making 1300 nm the preferred center wavelength due to its ability to penetrate deeper (1.2 mm) compared to sources with wavelengths such as 800 nm (0.7 mm) [2]. OCT has been increasingly utilized in dermatology and clinical research, with commercial OCT scanners, SkinDex300, ISIS Optronics GmbH, Mannheim, Germany Imalux Niris Imaging system, IMALUX, Cleveland, OH, USA and Sirius, 4optics, Lubeck, Germany [55, 103]. Various applications of OCT in dermatology include dermatological assessments, identifying skin layers, appendages, blood vessels, and distinguish intra-epidermal and subepidermal blisters, inflammatory skin condition such as dermatitis and psoriasis [104–106]. Dominant scattering and deeper penetration of 1.2 mm at 1300 nm centre wavelength compared to 0.7 mm at 800 nm, makes it preferable for skin tissue applications. Doppler OCT is a powerful imaging modality used for obtaining velocity profiles in small lumens and vessel at real-time acquisition rates, with a sensitivity 100 times more than Doppler ultrasound. Optical Doppler tomography combining OCT and Doppler velocimetry aids in measuring blood flow velocity in turbid tissue. The maximum imaging depth in skin tissue is limited to the blood vessel in the superficial skin surface. Besides Doppler OCT, spectroscopic OCT serves in the enhancement of image contrast, to differentiate skin tissue pathologies, as well as in obtaining functional and biochemical tissue information [107, 108].

A spectroscopic OCT for molecular imaging, capable of imaging endogenous and exogenous chromophores, has been demonstrated [98]. This approach utilizes a wide spectral bandwidth laser source of center wavelength 575 nm and bandwidth 240 nm, enabling the assessment of hemoglobin oxygen levels, contrast from available absorbers, and true-colour representation of samples. Figure 10.14(a) shows two major vessels, vein and artery on the right and left side, along with several branching vessels and capillary plexus. Figure 10.14(b), (c), (d), and (e) are the spectral profiles corresponding to the locations (b), (c), (d), and (e) marked in figure 10.14(a), where, the measured spectral profile (black trace) superposed with the theoretical hemoglobin molar extinction coefficient (red trace).

Molecular imaging true-colour spectroscopic OCT (METRiCS OCT) provides high spectral fidelity while imaging at a micrometer scale in three dimensions. This has significant implications for biomedical applications like ophthalmology, early cancer detection, and understanding diseases like hypoxia and angiogenesis.

In vitro, intralipid-based skin phantoms and *in vivo* animal and human subjects' measurement of changes in tissue scattering caused by variation in the glucose levels have been reported using the OCT technique at 1300 nm [109–111]. The ability of OCT to detect blood glucose-induced changes in tissue optical properties, shows a clear, linear decrease in signal slope [111]. Changes in OCT signal slope closely follow variations in blood glucose concentration, providing real-time feedback on glucose levels and allowing for potential non-invasive glucose monitoring [108]. Glucose measurement from blood, based on the changes in the attenuation coefficient of light was performed using an OCT system incorporating an SLED

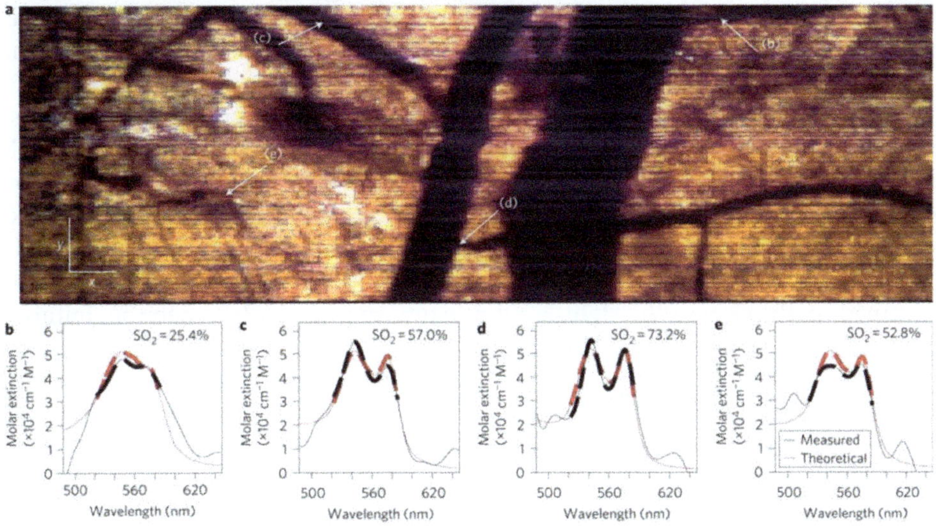

Figure 10.14. (a) En face molecular imaging true-colour spectroscopic optical coherence tomography (METRiCS OCT) image with arrows denoting locations where the spectra are quantified. (Scale bar 100 μm). (b–e) Spectral profiles attributing to the locations (b)–(e) marked in figure 10.14(a). The black trace denotes the measured spectral profile superposed with the red trace denoting the theoretical hemoglobin molar extinction coefficient. The region used to estimate the sO_2 levels is denoted with dashed lines on. Reprinted by permission from Springer Nature: *Nat. Photon.* [98] Copyright © 2011, Springer Nature Limited under the Creative Commons Attribution 4.0 International License (http://creativecommons.org/licenses/by/4.0/).

source of 930 nm and a glucose resolution of 65 mg dl^{-1} was reported in the whole blood and 133 mg dl^{-1} in saline diluted whole blood [112]. However, the attenuation of hemoglobin and water in the same wavelength region causes constraints in the selective measurement of glucose. Quantification of glucose in water, blood plasma and whole blood phantom using FD-OCT system using SLED source of center wavelength 1310 nm, based on the change in the refractive index that occurs with an increase in the concentration of glucose has been reported [113]. The main issues related to this approach of scattering induced by refractive index change are the effect of temperature change and the presence of other constituents such as fat, protein, and water that could affect the selective detection of glucose [114]. Hence, the selective detection of glucose using differential absorption low-coherence interferometry (LCI) is essential as it provides the selective detection of the analyte of interest [115, 116]. The concept of differential absorption OCT (DAOCT) was introduced by Schmitt *et al* for measuring water concentrations in tissue phantoms at 1310 and 1460 nm [117]. Differential absorption LCI used for detecting glucose selectively from phantoms and *ex vivo* gingival tissue has also been demonstrated in the first overtone and combination bands [118, 119]. However, further *in vivo* studies are required to validate the feasibility of this approach with standard blood glucometers.

The assessment of microvasculature of healthy and subjects with type 2 diabetes mellitus diabetic, based on OCT-A is also reported [120]. This pilot study explores

OCT-A application in dermatology, using multibeam VivoSight Dx-20 kHz line-scan rate with an axial resolution of 7.5 μm and a lateral resolution of 5.5 μm, aiming to establish reference values for skin microvascular parameters in the hands and feet. It provides age-dependent reference values for various microvascular metrics in healthy individuals and those with well-controlled type 2 diabetes mellitus (T2DM). Certain metrics, such as branchpoint density and changes in vessel diameter in response to post-occlusive reactive hyperemia, emerge as potential biomarkers distinguishing between healthy and T2DM groups, advancing the standardization of OCT-A in clinical practice and research [120]. All participants had imaging performed on the skin of the right-hand dorsum, specifically between the thumb and forefinger, as well as on the dorsum of the right hallux (big toe). Studies were conducted on 52 healthy individuals and 11 individuals with well-controlled T2DM. The study mentions individuals with well-controlled T2DM as one of the groups being investigated, highlighting potential differences in microvascular metrics compared to healthy participants. The investigation shows variations in microvascular metrics, shedding light on their dynamic behavior across distinct age groups. It uncovers notable disparities in microvascular characteristics between healthy participants and those with T2DM, contributing valuable insights into the potential implications of the disease on skin microvasculature. Additionally, the study delves into the influence of external stimuli on OCT-A measurements, showing the responsive nature of microvascular structures to specific stimuli and emphasizing the importance of considering these factors in clinical assessments. The study discusses the advantages of using OCT-A for assessing microvascular structure, including its sensitivity to small changes, potential as a diagnostic biomarker for diabetes, and its applicability for longitudinal monitoring. The study acknowledges several limitations, including the variability in metrics reported in the literature due to different imaging sites, OCT-A instrument variations, and image processing protocols. Additionally, the study recognizes the need for larger sample sizes, challenges in categorizing reference values based on age, and the impact of external factors on OCT-A measurements.

10.4.3 Cardiology

Intracoronary OCT plays a crucial role in cardiology in investigating the development of individual coronary lesions [121]. This serves the cardiology community in identifying and treating the vulnerable plaque. Various other intravascular OCT applications include follow-up measurements of the thickness of tissue growing inside the stents and characterization of lesions, which includes assessment of stenosed vessels and calcification before therapeutic intervention. The two main limitations of OCT in cardiology are the highly scattering blood, which needs to be cleared to maintain above 90 dB of SNRs, and the limited penetration depth, which is challenging to image through thick atherosclerotic plaque. Low-cost SLED light sources are suitable for cardiology applications. A high source power of ~20 mW for high scanning speeds and a resolution of greater than 50 μm is suitable to image large atherosclerotic lesions, unlike oncology applications which requires a high-resolution of 5 μm or better, with low powers [121]. LightLab OCT system based on polarization-insensitive design using an optical circulator is efficient in maximizing the overall efficiency, compared to Michelson interferometry and the rotating mirror for generating a linear scan [122, 123]. This system allows the implementation of spectroscopic, polarization and Doppler imaging modes in software by digitizing the raw signal early in the process. Another significant feature is its compatibility with different probes used in cardiology (rotary probes), microscopy (raster-scanning probes), and oncology (push-pull probes).

The importance of intracoronary imaging within the realm of interventional cardiology, with a specific focus on two primary modalities: intravascular ultrasound (IVUS) and OCT has been discussed [124]. Both IVUS and OCT play a pivotal role in guiding percutaneous coronary intervention (PCI) and furnishing detailed insights into coronary plaque characteristics, thus contributing to the comprehension of causes behind acute coronary syndrome (ACS) and enhancing clinical outcomes. Despite the valuable perspectives offered by both IVUS and OCT, there exists a dearth of conclusive clinical proof favoring one modality over the other, a trend reflected in existing guidelines. The functions of IVUS and OCT in diverse facets of coronary artery disease (CAD) by leveraging contemporary scientific evidence while also exploring future outlooks such as the emergence of hybrid OCT-IVUS catheters have been described. Hybrid systems that amalgamate IVUS and OCT technologies have been devised to overcome limitations and afford a more comprehensive depiction of plaque characteristics, demonstrating potential through trials conducted on both animal and human subjects.

Intravascular ultrasound (IVUS) and OCT play crucial roles in guiding percutaneous coronary intervention (PCI) and provide detailed information on coronary plaque characteristics, aiding in understanding acute coronary syndrome (ACS) causes and improving clinical outcomes. Hybrid OCT-IVUS catheters are being developed to combine the strengths of both imaging modalities, offering a more comprehensive approach to visualize plaque characteristics and potentially improve outcomes. Studies comparing IVUS and OCT have shown differences in detecting stent malapposition, tissue prolapse, and edge dissection, with OCT being more sensitive in detecting these issues post-PCI. Post-procedural fractional flow reserve (FFR) was greater in the OCT group compared to intravascular coronary angiography (ICA), leading to additional interventions in some cases.

OCT is a valuable tool for studying hemodynamic changes and developmental physiology in the embryonic chick model, offering high-resolution imaging capabilities. OCT can be used to non-invasively monitor blood flow and pressure alterations induced by experimental interventions such as surgical or chemical manipulations during cardiac development in chick embryos. While traditional techniques like Doppler echocardiography and catheter-based pressure measurements are commonly used, OCT presents a promising alternative with its ability to provide detailed imaging of cardiovascular structures and dynamics in a less invasive manner [125]. It also offers superior spatial and temporal resolution compared to Doppler echocardiography, generating tomographic images with 12–15 μm axial resolution [126, 127]. It provides detailed features of the vascular walls for detecting

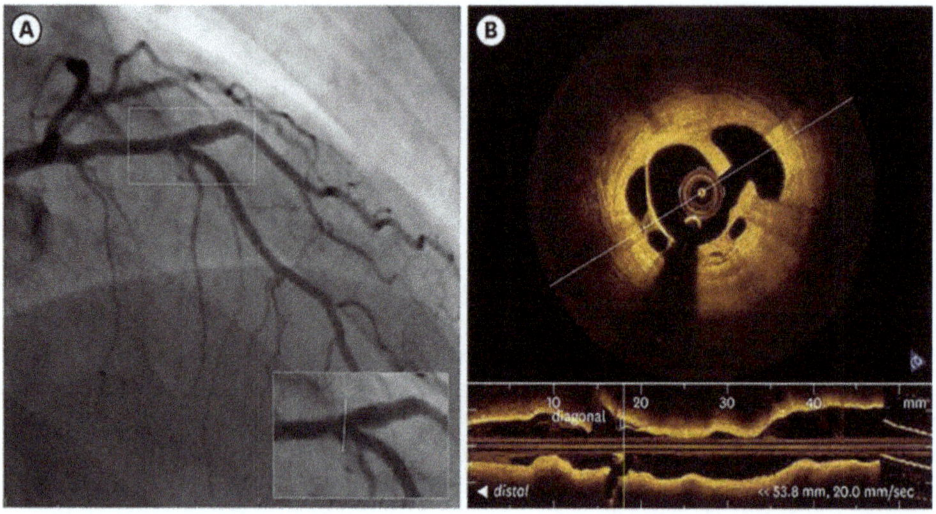

Figure 10.15. A representation showing the discrepancy between coronary angiography and OCT. A mild stenosis at the left anterior descending bifurcation lesion. B OCT image showing lotus root-like lesion consisting of multiple cavities with septation, not visible in coronary angiography. Reprinted with permission and modified from [127]. Copyright 2016 The Korean Association of Internal Medicine.

vulnerable plaque, faster pullback speed and automated analysis of diameters and lumen, and accurate assessment of stent interaction due to superior resolution. OCT is more accurate for assessing coronary lesions than IVUS or CAG, as shown in figure 10.15. However, the depth of OCT is limited to 1–2 mm compared to IVUS of 8–10 mm.

Besides cardiovascular diseases, intravascular OCT helps in imaging cerebrovascular diseases, specifically intracranial vessel wall abnormalities with luminal narrowing. A case of a 48-year-old man with exertional chest pain, where angiography showed minimal lesions but functional significance was revealed by FFR and intravascular OCT highlights the risk of underestimating lesion severity based solely on angiography. Figure 10.15(a) shows a minimal coronary stenosis in the left anterior descending artery (LAD). Figure 10.15(b) reveals a lotus root-like lesion in the mid-left anterior descending artery, consisting of multiple cavities within the fibrous plaque, suggesting a recanalized intracoronary thrombus. Patients with multi-vessel coronary disease may have challenging decisions for revascularization based on angiography alone, especially with intermediate or ambiguous lesions. Functional and physiological considerations are crucial for selecting the target vessel in such cases. The study emphasizes the importance of invasive imaging techniques to compensate for potential underestimation of lesion severity using angiography. The use of advanced imaging modalities like OCT can provide detailed insights into lesion characteristics, such as the presence of recanalized intracoronary thrombus, aiding in appropriate revascularization decisions and symptom relief.

Functional imaging of *ex vivo* lipid and artery was also demonstrated with porcine and mouse artery models [89]. This study is based on differential absorption LCI, where the attenuation coefficients of a sample at two different wavelength bands are expressed as,

$$\alpha_i(z) - \alpha_j(z) = \frac{1}{2}\frac{d}{dz}\ln\left[\frac{I_j(z)}{I_i(z)}\right] = \frac{1}{2(z - z_0)}\ln\left[\frac{I_j(z)}{I_i(z)}\right] \tag{10.57}$$

where α_i is the attenuation coefficient at the wavelength band i, z is the corresponding depth (difference in the light pathlength between the reference and sample arms), z_0 is the reference depth with normalized signal intensities, and $I_i(z)$ is the light intensity at the depth z.

By substituting $\Delta\alpha(z) = \alpha_i(z) - \alpha_j(z)$, equation (10.57) becomes,

$$\frac{I_i(z)}{I_j(z)} = e^{-i2\Delta\alpha(z-z_0)} \tag{10.58}$$

The negative-correlated attenuation coefficient difference between the two wavelength bands could be obtained with relative depth, by dividing the normalized intensity of sample images obtained from different wavelengths pixel-by-pixel. The differentiation of lipid and artery qualitatively using the tri-band S-OCT approach by the difference in the contrasting attenuation coefficient between 1.3/1.5 and 1.5/1.6 μm, has been reported.

10.4.4 Neurology

Longitudinal monitoring of recovery after conditions like experimental ischemic stroke can be conducted using OCT-A to observe vascular remodeling. The utility of OCT-A for studying brain microvasculature dynamics and potential applications in neurological research has been discussed [22]. A comparison between Doppler OCT and OCT-A of the microvasculature of mouse brain is shown in figure 10.16, where Doppler OCT detects phase changes caused by translational axial motion. Figure 10.16(a) and (b) shows the enhanced angiogram and OCT-A vascular graph of the mouse brain *in vivo*. Figure 10.16(c) shows the presence of vascular

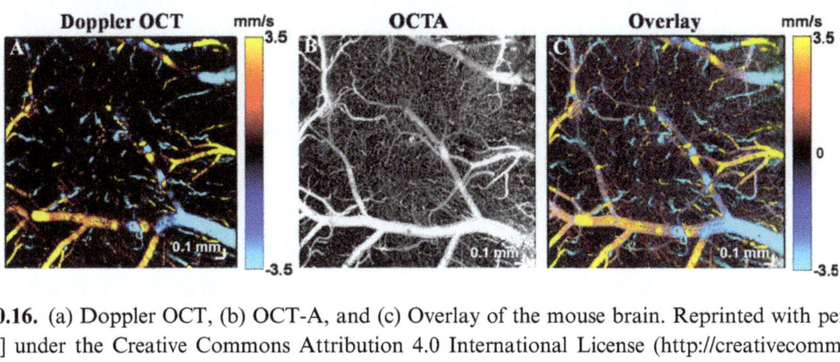

Figure 10.16. (a) Doppler OCT, (b) OCT-A, and (c) Overlay of the mouse brain. Reprinted with permission from [22] under the Creative Commons Attribution 4.0 International License (http://creativecommons.org/licenses/by/4.0/).

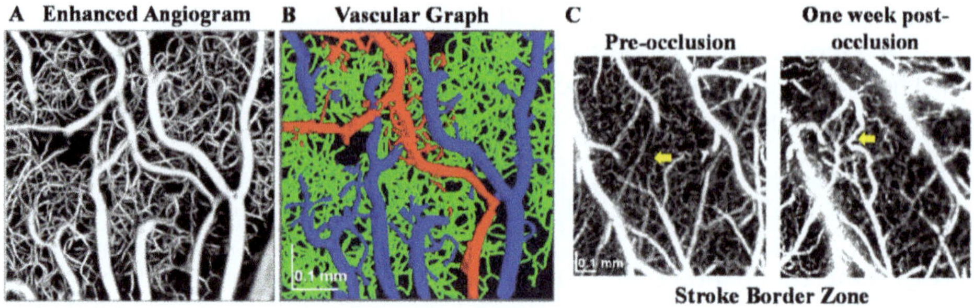

Figure 10.17. OCT-A microscopy of the mouse brain showing (A) Enhanced angiogram, (B) vascular graph, (C) longitudinal monitoring of microvasculature remodeling one week after occlusion of the distal middle cerebral artery. Reprinted with permission from [22] under the Creative Commons Attribution 4.0 International License (http://creativecommons.org/licenses/by/4.0/).

remodeling in the mouse brain, denoted by yellow arrows during longitudinal monitoring of the recovery phase one week after experimental ischemic stroke.

The predominate Doppler shift in macrovasculature is observed in figure 10.17(a), whereas, flow based on decorrelation (via intensity and/or phase) detected by OCT-A showing vasculature, which includes regions predominantly transverse flow and overlay, is shown in figure 10.17(b) and (c), respectively. The intricate details of blood flow patterns in the mouse brain showcase the potential of OCT-A for *in vivo* imaging of vascular structures.

The transit time distribution of blood in the cerebral microvasculature plays a crucial role in oxygen delivery and influences neuroimaging signals like blood-oxygen-level-dependent functional magnetic resonance imaging (BOLD fMRI) [128]. Quantifying capillary transit time distribution at a microscopic level has been challenging, limiting comprehensive understanding. A method called dynamic contrast OCT (DyC-OCT) for quantifying transit time metrics by imaging an intravascular tracer passing through the field of view is discussed. DyC-OCT provides accurate results even in highly scattering brain tissue without the need for optical focus calibration. The method was validated against dilution curves using a fluorescent plasma label in surface pial vessels. The study used DyC-OCT to investigate the transit time distribution in the microvasculature of the mouse somatosensory cortex, revealing laminar trends with earlier transit times and less heterogeneity in the middle cortical layers. The findings suggest that the early transit times in the middle cortical layers may contribute to the early onset times observed in BOLD fMRI, and the layer-dependencies in heterogeneity could explain how oxygen is delivered to different cortical layers with varying metabolic needs.

10.5 Clinical applications of polarimetry for blood analysis

There have been substantial advancements achieved in the use of polarimetry within the field of medicine. In particular, it has been shown to be an effective instrument for blood analysis, providing essential insights into the structural and functional features of blood components. In this sub-chapter, we will review the use of polarimetry in blood analysis. We will also emphasize the ways in which this method may significantly enhance our diagnostic and monitoring capacities for a variety of medical disorders.

10.5.1 Leukemia

Leukemia, a form of blood cancer, is typically diagnosed through histo-pathological examination of peripheral blood and bone marrow smears. This process involves a detailed microscopic examination of blood cells to identify any abnormal shapes and patterns that may indicate the presence of cancer. In addition, a comprehensive blood count (CBC) is performed to provide numerical data on the various types of blood cells found, assisting in the identification and classification of leukemia. While these traditional methods can be relied upon, they often require invasive procedures and extensive lab work.

Recent studies propose that polarimetric assessment of blood could serve as a valuable alternative for diagnosing and confirming leukemia [129, 130]. This method revolves around measuring alterations in the polarization state of light when it interacts with blood samples, providing insights into the optical characteristics of blood cells. RBCs play a significant role in light absorption and scattering due to their concentration and shape [131]. However, in cases of leukemia, where cancerous cells cause anemia, blood samples depolarize light to a lesser degree than healthy blood. This diminished depolarization is a consequence of the modified cellular structure and composition linked to leukemia, offering a unique optical signature that can be non-invasively detected through polarimetric analysis.

Forward scattered light from peripheral blood smears (PBS) was analyzed using a broadband wavelength source spanning 400–800 nm [129]. The transmitted light intensities were captured by a detector and stored on a computer, allowing a reconstruction of Mueller matrices for multiple samples. The detailed polarimetric data were extracted from these matrices. This analysis yielded transmission, diattenuation, and retardation spectra for both normal and samples of leukemia patients. The depolarization and transmission spectra of the samples revealed a drop in hemoglobin concentration, indicating acute lymphoblastic leukemia. The presence of a considerable number of leukocytes, especially lymphocytes such as T-cells or B-cells, was indicated by prominent peaks in the diattenuation and retardation spectra between 400–500 nm. Using the Mueller matrix to assess these polarization-altering characteristics provides a diagnostic tool for identifying tissue malignancies. The polarimetry approach offers a feasible option for *in vitro* leukemia blood analysis, possibly improving the accuracy and reliability of the current method of detection.

10.5.2 Malaria

Malaria continues to be a major parasitic illness, resulting in approximately 600 000 deaths annually [132]. Accurate detection and identification of malaria parasites are crucial for successful clinical diagnosis. In this process, one must differentiate between the asexual and sexual forms of the parasite, recognize various stages of maturation, and accurately quantify parasite density by measuring the number of parasites per unit volume of blood or the percentage of infected RBCs. In addition, understanding the development of antimalarial medications and assessing drug resistance involves examining the metabolic conditions and viability of the parasites. This thorough examination is crucial for advancing treatment approaches and improving patient outcomes in the fight against malaria.

Malaria parasites attack RBCs and catabolize hemoglobin, resulting in the creation of hemozoin (Hz), a pigment with strong absorption and birefringence characteristics. As the parasite grows within the RBC, it eventually releases Hz after its development cycle is complete. The presence and distinctive features of Hz in RBCs aid in the identification of diverse malaria species and stages of development. Observing Hz provides a reliable method for distinguishing between species and understanding the progression of the infection, making it a valuable marker in malaria diagnostics and research.

The bench-top flow cytometer (Cyflow SL, Partec/Sysmex) was utilized to conduct depolarized scatter measurement, enabling comprehensive comparisons between the cytometric detection of Hz-containing leukocytes and the Cell-Dyn microscope [133]. This investigation successfully demonstrated the accurate detection of Hz within infected erythrocytes (iRBCs) using flow cytometry, thus affirming its effectiveness as a diagnostic tool. This significant finding has initiated further research into the precise quantification and characterization of malaria-infected cells, potentially leading to improved diagnostic methods and a deeper understanding of malaria pathophysiology [134, 135].

Light depolarization measurements have become an important tool in the field of malaria research and diagnostics. This method enables the identification of Hz, whether it is found in the blood or inside infected RBCs (iRBCs) and leukocytes. Light depolarization measurements in malaria have a wide range of applications, offering valuable insights into different aspects of the disease. In addition, measuring Hz levels provides valuable data for diagnosing malaria infections and assessing the efficacy of treatments. By integrating Hz detection with additional parameters such as DNA or RNA content, researchers have the potential to enhance the precision and sensitivity of parasite detection. This, in turn, can contribute to advancements in the field of malaria diagnosis and research.

10.5.3 Diabetes

Diabetes remains a pressing health issue worldwide, impacting various countries with significant consequences. In the United States, diabetes is a major medical concern, affecting over 9% of the population and presenting significant challenges for individuals and the healthcare system [136]. Similarly, Germany is dealing with its own battle against this persistent condition, with statistics showing that at least about 7.2% of Germans between the ages of 18 and 79 are living with diabetes [137]. These statistics emphasize the widespread occurrence of diabetes and highlight the pressing need for global efforts in prevention, management, and research to address this growing public health crisis.

One of the main challenges faced by the various non-invasive techniques proposed for glucose monitoring is the limited and indirect relationship between the observed signal changes and the actual variations in glucose levels. However, polarimetry stands out among these methods as it holds great potential due to its dependence on the optical activity of glucose molecules, which possess chirality. This unique characteristic of glucose enables polarimetry to potentially deliver a more precise and reliable measurement of glucose levels, as it directly interacts with the distinctive optical properties of glucose. Consequently, polarimetry offers a promising solution for non-invasive monitoring of glucose.

Previous studies on non-invasive glucose monitoring techniques have demonstrated significant advancements in the field of polarimetry. The Stokes–Mueller matrix polarimetry system has shown its ability to measure glucose concentrations with a sensitivity of 20 mg dl^{-1}, representing an advancement in the accuracy of these measurements [138]. Expanding on this, a Mueller matrix polarimeter with dual photoelastic modulators was utilized, successfully attaining a sensitivity of 20 mg dl^{-1} [139]. This further strengthens the promise of polarimetric methods in glucose detection. Additional advancements were made through the implementation of multireflection polarimetry, which incorporates micro-mirrors to extend the optical pathlength [140]. This results in improved accuracy and reliability when measuring glucose levels. These studies demonstrate the changing landscape of polarimetric techniques, emphasizing their potential to enhance non-invasive glucose monitoring.

10.6 Conclusion

OCT and polarimetry have both established themselves as technologies that play a crucial role in the study and comprehension of blood. Significant improvements in medical diagnosis and research have been made possible as a result of these approaches, which provide precise and non-invasive insights into the structural and optical features of blood.

10.6.1 The contributions of OCT to blood analysis

OCT has transformed the study of blood by allowing for high-resolution, cross-sectional imaging of blood vessels and flow dynamics. This ability is critical for detecting vascular anomalies, monitoring hemodynamics, and evaluating the vascular system's integrity. In therapeutic settings, OCT's real-time imaging enables accurate visualization of blood artery architecture, helping the early diagnosis and treatment of disorders such as atherosclerosis, thrombosis, and microvascular illness. Furthermore, OCT's applications include the imaging of capillary networks and the assessment of blood flow velocity. These characteristics are especially useful in understanding microcirculation and its function in different disease conditions. OCT may help diagnose and monitor a variety of cardiovascular and hematological problems by offering a thorough image of blood flow patterns and arterial anatomy.

10.6.2 The contributions of polarimetry to blood analysis

Polarimetry enhances OCT by offering further insights into the optical characteristics of blood. Polarimetry is capable of uncovering structural and compositional features that OCT alone cannot detect by examining changes in the polarization state of light caused by blood and/or its components. This method is very efficient in identifying deviations in blood birefringence, which may signify alterations in blood cell shape, orientation, and clumping. The capability of polarimetry to evaluate the optical anisotropy of blood makes it a desirable instrument for investigating the behavior of erythrocytes and the orientation of hemoglobin. These insights are essential for comprehending illnesses such as leukemia, malaria, diabetes, and other blood-related disorders. Polarimetry improves the diagnostic capacities and facilitates a more profound knowledge of hematological health by offering a thorough investigation of blood characteristics.

10.6.3 Future directions and technological innovations

The ongoing development of OCT and polarimetry will have a significant influence on clinical practice. Enabling precise and non-intrusive imaging of blood characteristics can expedite the detection of various hematological and cardiovascular diseases, leading to early diagnosis and customized treatment regimens. These technologies will assist doctors by offering immediate and comprehensive analysis, enabling them to make better-informed choices. This will result in enhanced patient outcomes and increased quality of care. Moreover, the incorporation of OCT and polarimetry into regular clinical practice will stimulate additional investigation and advancement, revealing novel applications and augmenting our comprehension of blood-related illnesses. The ongoing cycle of feedback between technical advancement and clinical implementation will guarantee that these imaging techniques continue to be at the forefront of medical diagnosis.

10.6.4 Summary

To summarize, the use of OCT and polarimetry to analyze blood constitutes a major leap in medical imaging and diagnosis. These technologies give deep, non-invasive insights into the structural and optical features of blood, allowing us to better diagnose and monitor a variety of hematological and cardiovascular disorders. As research and technical developments advance, OCT and polarimetry promise to provide even more insights into blood health and illness, eventually changing the face of medical diagnostics and enhancing patient care. The future offers enormous promise for these technologies to progress, driven by continued innovation and the inclusion of AI, ushering in a new age of precision medicine and individualized healthcare solutions.

Abbreviations

2D	Two-dimensional
3D	Three-dimensional
ACS	Acute coronary syndrome
AMD	Age related macular degeneration
A-scan	Axial scan

BOLD fMRI	Blood-oxygen-level-dependent functional magnetic resonance imaging
CAD	Coronary artery disease
CBC	Comprehensive blood count
CVI	Choriodal vascular index
DAOCT	Differential absorption OCT
DOCP	Degree of circular polarization
DOLP	Degree of linear polarization
DOP	Net degree of polarization
DR	Diabetic retinopathy
DyC-OCT	Dynamic contrast optical coherence tomography
FA	Fluorescein angiography
FD-OCT	Frequency-domain optical coherence tomography
FFR	Fractional flow reserve
Hz	Hemozoin
ICA	Intravascular coronary angiography
ICGA	Indocyanine green angiography
iRBCs	Infected erythrocytes
IS/OS	Inner and outer segment
IVUS	Intravascular ultrasound
LAD	Left anterior descending artery
LCI	Low coherence interferometry
LCP	Left circularly polarized
LDF	Laser Doppler flowmetry
LDV	Laser Doppler velocimetry
METRiCS OCT	Molecular imaging true-colour spectroscopic optical coherence tomography
OCM	Optical coherence microscopy
OCT	Optical coherence tomography
OCT-A	Optical coherence tomography angiography
OMAG	Optical microangiography algorithm
PBS	Peripheral blood smears
PCI	Percutaneous coronary intervention
PR-OCT-A	Projection resolved OCT-A algorithm
PS-OCT	Polarization-sensitive optical coherence tomography
RAO	Retinal atery occlusions
RBCs	Red blood cells
RCP	Right circularly polarized
RPE	Retinal pigment epithelium
RVO	Retinal vascular occlusions
SD-OCT	Spectral-domain optical coherence tomography
SLED	Superluminescent light-emitting diode
SNR	Signal-to-noise ratio
S-OCT	Spectroscopic optical coherence tomography
SSADA	Split-spectrum amplitude-decorrelation angiography
SS-algorithm	Slab subtraction algorithm
SS-OCT	Swept-source optical coherence tomography
STFFT	Short-time fast Fourier transformation
T2DM	Type 2 diabetes mellitus
TD-OCT	Time-domain optical coherence tomography
TFT	Time-frequency transformation

Symbols

l_c	Coherence length
δz	Axial resolution
λ_c	Center wavelength of the source
$\Delta\lambda$	Spectral bandwidth
n	Refractive index
E_{source}	Incident wave from the source propagating in the z-direction
E_o	Amplitude of the wave with the subscript '0' indicating that a monochromatic source is used
z_r	Pathlengths from the optical coupler to the reference mirror
z_s	Pathlengths from the optical coupler to a specific depth in the sample
E_{r0}	Monochromatic wave amplitudes from the reference mirror
E_{s0}	Monochromatic wave amplitudes from the sample
E_{total}	Total electric field at the detector
ω	Angular frequency of the electric field
I_D	Intensity at the detector
μ_o	Permeability
$*$	Complex conjugate
Δk	Total bandwidth swept
Δt	Sweep time
Δf	Doppler frequency shift
k_i	Incoming wave vector
k_s	Wave vector of scattered light
V	Velocity vector of the moving particle
V_T	Transverse flow velocities
V_L	Longitudinal flow velocities
θ	Angle between the flow and sample beam
$U(t)$	Complex-valued analytical signal of a stochastic process
$\overline{U}(\nu)$	Spectral amplitude at optical frequency
$\underline{S_0}(\nu)$	Power spectral density of the source
$\overline{U}_r(\nu)$	Light coupled back to the detector from the reference
$\overline{U}_s(\nu)$	Light coupled back to the detector from the sample
$\overline{U}_o(\nu)$	Spectral amplitude
L_r	Optical pathlength of the reference arm
L_s	Optical pathlength of the sample arm
L_d	Optical pathlength from the beam splitter to the detector
$K_r(\nu)\,e^{i\alpha_r(\nu)}$	Amplitude reflection coefficients of light backscattered from the reference mirror
$K_s(\nu)\,e^{i\alpha_s(\nu)}$	Amplitude reflection coefficients of light backscattered from the sample
$P_d(\tau)$	Time average of the squared light amplitude
τ	Delay time between the light traveled in the sample arm and reference arm
Δ	Difference in the optical pathlength between the sample and reference arm
V_z	Velocity of the moving particle parallel to the probe beam
$\overline{n}$	Refractive index of the flow media
$P_{ODT}(\nu)$	The fringe signal in the spectral domain
$\Gamma_{ODT}(\tau)$	Time-domain signal
$\Delta\varphi$	Phase change
ΔT	Time interval between sequential A-lines
F_m and F_{m+1}	OCT complex data acquired from the same location at a different time

B	Bandwidth of Doppler frequency shift
NA_{eff}	Effective numerical aperture of the scan lens
$\underline{f}$	Doppler shift
$\bar{f}$	Averaged Doppler shift
$g(f)$	Doppler power spectrum
M	Number of split-spectrums
N	Number of B-scans acquired at the same location
$I_{im}(x, z)$	Value of intensity measured in the ith B-scans of mth split-spectrum at the lateral location and depth position represented as x and z, respectively
$C_i(x, z)$	Complex signal consisting of both intensity and phase values in the ith B-scans at lateral location and depth position, x and z, respectively
D_{slab2}	Decorrelation value within the slab of interest from maximum flow projection
D_{slab1}	Maximum flow projection of all layers above D_{slab2}
F	Normalized flow signal
D	Decorrelation
S	Log amplitude OCT signal
C_n	PR-corrected values of decorrelation
I_H	Horizontal linear polarizer (0 degrees)
I_V	Vertical linear polarizer (90 degrees)
I_P	45 degrees linear polarizer
I_M	135 degrees (-45 degrees) linear polarizer
I_R	Right circular polarizer
I_L	Left circular polarizer
S	The Stokes vector
Q	Difference in intensity between horizontal and vertical polarization states
U	Difference between intensities of linear + 45 deg and −45 deg polarization states
V	Difference between intensities of right circular and left circular polarization states
M	Transfer function of any medium in its interaction with polarized light
S_i	Stokes vector of the input light
$\mathrm{S_o}$	Stokes vector of the output light
M_Δ	Mueller matrix
ψ	Circular retardance/optical rotation
I	Reflected light spectrum extracted by a series of short-time Fourier transforms (STFT)
I_0	Incident intensity on the retina
R_0	Reflectance from reference arm
n	Mean refractive index of the blood
d	Vessel diameter
r	Reflectance at the vessel wall
$\mu_{\mathrm{HbO_2}}$	Attenuation coefficient of oxygenated
μ_{Hb}	Attenuation coefficient of deoxygenated blood
$r(\lambda)$	First-order Born approximation
μ	Optical attenuation coefficient
α_i	Attenuation coefficient at the wavelength band i
z	Depth
z_0	Reference depth with normalized signal intensities
$I_i(z)$	Light intensity at the depth z

References

[1] Swanson E A and Fujimoto J G 2017 The ecosystem that powered the translation of OCT from fundamental research to clinical and commercial impact *Biomed. Opt. Express* **8** 1638–64

[2] Fujimoto J and Swanson E 2016 The development, commercialization, and impact of optical coherence tomography *Invest. Ophthalmol. Vis. Sci.* **57** OCT1–13

[3] Leitgeb R *et al* 2021 Enhanced medical diagnosis for doctors: a perspective of optical coherence tomography *J. Biomed. Opt.* **26** 100601–1

[4] Drexler W and Fujimoto J G (ed) 2008 *Optical Coherence Tomography: Technology and Applications* (Berlin: Springer Science & Business Media)

[5] Leitgeb R A, Werkmeister R M, Blatter C and Schmetterer L 2014 Doppler optical coherence tomography *Prog. Retinal Eye Res.* **41** 26–43

[6] Javed A, Khanna A, Palmer E, Wilde C, Zaman A, Orr G, Kumudhan D, Lakshmanan A and Panos G D 2023 Optical coherence tomography angiography: a review of the current literature *J. Int. Med. Res.* **51** 03000605231187933

[7] Li Y, Chen J and Chen Z 2019 Advances in Doppler optical coherence tomography and angiography *Transl. Biophoton.* **1** e201900005

[8] Nam H S and Yoo H 2018 Spectroscopic optical coherence tomography: a review of concepts and biomedical applications *Appl. Spectrosc. Rev.* **53** 91–111

[9] Wang L V, Coté G L and Jacques S L 2002 Special section guest editorial: tissue polarimetry *J. Biomed. Opt.* **7** 278

[10] Drexler W, Liu M, Kumar A, Kamali T, Unterhuber A and Leitgeb R A 2014 Optical coherence tomography today: speed, contrast, and multimodality *J. Biomed. Opt.* **19** 071412–2

[11] Yaqoob Z, Wu J and Yang C 2005 Spectral-domainoptical coherence tomography: a better OCT imaging strategy *Biotechniques* **39** S6–S13

[12] Gusmeroli V and Martinelli M 1991 Distributed laser Doppler velocimeter *Opt. Lett.* **16** 1358–60

[13] Xie C, Gao W, Zhang Y and Shi W 2023 Quantitative parameter analysis of effects of particle density on the imaging signals in OCT *Opt. Commun.* **536** 129368

[14] Zhao Y, Chen Z, Saxer C, Xiang S, de Boer J F and Nelson J S 2000 Phase-resolved optical coherence tomography and optical Doppler tomography for imaging blood flow in human skin with fast scanning speed and high velocity sensitivity *Opt. Lett.* **25** 114–6

[15] Ren H, Brecke K M, Ding Z, Zhao Y, Nelson J S and Chen Z 2002 Imaging and quantifying transverse flow velocity with the Doppler bandwidth in a phase-resolved functional optical coherence tomography *Opt. Lett.* **27** 409–11

[16] De Carlo T E, Romano A, Waheed N K and Duker J S 2015 A review of optical coherence tomography angiography (OCTA) *Int. J. Retina Vitr.* **1** 1–15

[17] de Barros Garcia J M B, Isaac D L C and Avila M 2017 Diabetic retinopathy and OCT angiography: clinical findings and future perspectives *Int J Retina Vitr.* **3** 14

[18] Abdelsalam M M 2020 Effective blood vessels reconstruction methodology for early detection and classification of diabetic retinopathy using OCTA images by artificial neural network *Inform. Med. Unlocked* **20** 100390

[19] Pellegrini M, Cozzi M, Staurenghi G and Corvi F 2019 Comparison of wide field optical coherence tomography angiography with extended field imaging and fluorescein angiography in retinal vascular disorders *PLoS One* **14** e0214892

[20] Gendelman I *et al* 2020 Topographic analysis of macular choriocapillaris flow deficits in diabetic retinopathy using swept–source optical coherence tomography angiography *Int. J. Retina Vitr.* **6** 1–8

[21] John P, Damodaran V, Sujatha N and Vasa N J 2023 Recent developments in optical coherence tomography angiography imaging for the diagnosis and assessment of diabetic retinopathy *Photo Acoustic and Optical Coherence Tomography Imaging, Volume 1: Diabetic Retinopathy* (IOP Publishing) pp 1–2

[22] Zhu J, Merkle C W, Bernucci M T, Chong S P and Srinivasan V J 2017 Can OCT angiography be made a quantitative blood measurement tool? *Appl. Sci.* **7** 687

[23] Kamoun W S, Chae S S, Lacorre D A, Tyrrell J A, Mitre M, Gillissen M A, Fukumura D, Jain R K and Munn L L 2010 Simultaneous measurement of RBC velocity, flux, hematocrit and shear rate in vascular networks *Nat. Methods* **7** 655–60

[24] Schafer R T, Doerschuk P C, Olbricht W L and Chris B 2012 *In vivo* two-photon excited fluorescence microscopy *Am. J. Physiol. Heart Circ. Physiol.* **302** H1367–77

[25] Faber D J, Aalders M C, Mik E G, Hooper B A, van Gemert F M J and Van Leeuwen T G 2004 Oxygen saturation-dependent absorption and scattering of blood *Phys. Rev. Lett.* **93** 028102

[26] Srinivasan V J, Chan A C and Lam E Y 2012 Doppler OCT and OCT angiography for *in vivo* imaging of vascular physiology *Selected Topics in Optical Coherence Tomography* (Books on Demand) p 21

[27] Gao S S, Jia Y, Zhang M, Su J P, Liu G, Hwang T S, Bailey S T and Huang D 2016 Optical coherence tomography angiography *Invest. Ophthalmol. Vis. Sci.* **57** OCT27–36

[28] Matsunaga D R, Yi J J, De Koo L O, Ameri H, Puliafito C A and Kashani A H 2015 Optical coherence tomography angiography of diabetic retinopathy in human subjects *Ophthal. Surg., Lasers Imag. Retina* **46** 796–805

[29] Wang J, Hormel T T, Gao L, Zang P, Guo Y, Wang X, Bailey S T and Jia Y 2020 Automated diagnosis and segmentation of choroidal neovascularization in OCT angiography using deep learning *Biomed. Opt. Express* **11** 927–44

[30] Jia Y *et al* 2014 Quantitative optical coherence tomography angiography of choroidal neovascularization in age-related macular degeneration *Ophthalmology* **121** 1435–44

[31] Ronchi V and Barocas V 1970 *The Nature of Light: An Historical Survey* (Heinemann)

[32] Kliger D S and Lewis J W 2012 *Polarized Light in Optics and Spectroscopy* (Amsterdam: Elsevier)

[33] Collett E 1992 *Polarized Light. Fundamentals and Applications* (Marcel Dekker)

[34] Gross H, Dörband B and Müller H 2012 Polarimetry *Handbook of Optical Systems: Volume 5: Metrology of Optical Components and Systems* (Wiley) pp 559–642

[35] Bickel W S and Bailey W M 1985 Stokes vectors, Mueller matrices, and polarized scattered light *Am. J. Phys.* **53** 468–78

[36] Lu S Y and Chipman R A 1996 Interpretation of Mueller matrices based on polar decomposition *JOSA* A **13** 1106–13

[37] Jacques S L, Ramella-Roman J C and Lee K 2002 Imaging skin pathology with polarized light *J. Biomed. Opt.* **7** 329–40

[38] Ghosh N, Wood M and Vitkin A 2010 Polarized light assessment of complex turbid media such as biological tissues us-ing mueller matrix decomposition *Handbook of Photonics for Biomedical Science* (Boca Raton, FL: CRC Press) pp 289–318

[39] Wood M F, Ghosh N, Guo X and Vitkin I A 2008 Towards noninvasive glucose sensing using polarization analysis of multiply scattered light *Handbook of Optical Sensing of Glucose in Biological Fluids and Tissues* (CRC Press) p 12
[40] Collett E 1984 Measurement of the four Stokes polarization parameters with a single circular polarizer *Opt. Commun.* **52** 77–80
[41] Sankaran V, Schönenberger K, Walsh J T and Maitland D J 1999 Polarization discrimination of coherently propagating light in turbid media *Appl. Opt.* **38** 4252–61
[42] Sankaran V, Walsh J T Jr. and Maitland D J 2002 Comparative study of polarized light propagation in biologic tissues *J. Biomed. Opt.* **7** 300–6
[43] Ghosh N, Patel H S and Gupta P K 2003 Depolarization of light in tissue phantoms-effect of a distribution in the size of scatterers *Opt. Express* **11** 2198–205
[44] Côté D and Vitkin I A 2004 Balanced detection for low-noise precision polarimetric measurements of optically active, multiply scattering tissue phantoms *J. Biomed. Opt.* **9** 213–20
[45] Studinski R C and Vitkin I A 2000 Methodology for examining polarized light interactions with tissues and tissue-like media in the exact backscattering direction *J. Biomed. Opt.* **5** 330–7
[46] Silverman M P, Ritchie N, Cushman G M and Fisher B 1988 Experimental configurations using optical phase modulation to measure chiral asymmetries in light specularly reflected from a naturally gyrotropic medium *JOSA* A **5** 1852–62
[47] Ghosh N, Wood M F and Vitkin I A 2008 Mueller matrix decomposition for extraction of individual polarization parameters from complex turbid media exhibiting multiple scattering, optical activity, and linear birefringence *J. Biomed. Opt.* **13** 044036–6
[48] Ghosh N, Wood M F, Li S H, Weisel R D, Wilson B C, Li R K and Vitkin I A 2009 Mueller matrix decomposition for polarized light assessment of biological tissues *J. Biophoton.* **2** 145–56
[49] Azzam R M A 1978 Photopolarimetric measurement of the Mueller matrix by Fourier analysis of a single detected signal *Opt. Lett.* **2** 148–50
[50] Goldstein D H 1992 Mueller matrix dual-rotating retarder polarimeter *Appl. Opt.* **31** 6676–83
[51] Smith M H 2002 Optimization of a dual-rotating-retarder Mueller matrix polarimeter *Appl. Opt.* **41** 2488–93
[52] Ishibazawa A, Nagaoka T, Takahashi A, Omae T, Tani T, Sogawa K, Yokota H and Yoshida A 2015 Optical coherence tomography angiography in diabetic retinopathy: a prospective pilot study *Am. J. Ophthalmol.* **160** 35–44
[53] de Carlo T E, Bonini Filho M A, Chin A T, Adhi M, Ferrara D, Baumal C R, Witkin A J, Reichel E, Duker J S and Waheed N K 2015 Spectral-domain optical coherence tomography angiography of choroidal neovascularization *Ophthalmology* **122** 1228–38
[54] Gambichler T *et al* 2005 Applications of optical coherence tomography in dermatology *J. Dermatol. Sci.* **40** 85–94
[55] Tsai T H *et al* 2014 Endoscopic optical coherence angiography enables 3-dimensional visualization of subsurface microvasculature *Gastroenterology* **147** 1219–21
[56] Lee H C *et al* 2016 Circumferential optical coherence tomography angiography imaging of the swine esophagus using a micromotor balloon catheter *Biomed. Opt. Express* **7** 2927–42
[57] Srinivasan V J, Jiang J Y, Yaseen M A, Radhakrishnan H, Wu W, Barry S, Cable A E and Boas D A 2010 Rapid volumetric angiography of cortical microvasculature with optical coherence tomography *Opt. Lett.* **35** 43–5

[58] Srinivasan V J *et al* 2011 Optical coherence tomography for the quantitative study of cerebrovascular physiology *J. Cereb. Blood Flow Metab.* **31** 1339–45

[59] Jung Y, Zhi Z and Wang R K 2010 Three-dimensional optical imaging of microvascular networks within intact lymph node *in vivo J. Biomed. Opt.* **15** 050501–1

[60] Vakoc B J *et al* 2009 Three-dimensional microscopy of the tumor microenvironment *in vivo* using optical frequency-domainimaging *Nat. Med.* **15** 1219–23

[61] Tey K Y, Teo K, Tan A C, Devarajan K, Tan B, Tan J, Schmetterer L and Ang M 2019 Optical coherence tomography angiography in diabetic retinopathy: a review of current applications *Eye Vision* **6** 1–10

[62] Couturier A, Mané V, Bonnin S, Erginay A, Massin P, Gaudric A and Tadayoni R 2015 Capillary plexus anomalies in diabetic retinopathy on optical coherence tomography angiography *Retina* **35** 2384–91

[63] Khadamy J, Aghdam K A and Falavarjani K G 2018 An update on optical coherence tomography angiography in diabetic retinopathy *J. Ophthal. Vision Res.* **13** 487

[64] Sim D A *et al* 2013 The effects of macular ischemia on visual acuity in diabetic retinopathy *Invest. Ophthalmol. Vis. Sci.* **54** 2353–60

[65] Early Treatment Diabetic Retinopathy Study Research Group 1991 Early photocoagulation for diabetic retinopathy: ETDRS report number 9 *Ophthalmology* **98** 766–85

[66] Nesper P L, Roberts P K, Onishi A C, Chai H, Liu L, Jampol L M and Fawzi A A 2017 Quantifying microvascular abnormalities with increasing severity of diabetic retinopathy using optical coherence tomography angiography *Invest. Ophthalmol. Vis. Sci.* **58** BIO307–15

[67] Kim A Y, Chu Z, Shahidzadeh A, Wang R K, Puliafito C A and Kashani A H 2016 Quantifying microvascular density and morphology in diabetic retinopathy using spectral-domain optical coherence tomography angiography *Invest. Ophthalmol. Vis. Sci.* **57** OCT362–70

[68] Durbin M K, An L, Shemonski N D, Soares M, Santos T, Lopes M, Neves C and Cunha-Vaz J 2017 Quantification of retinal microvascular density in optical coherence tomographic angiography images in diabetic retinopathy *JAMA Ophthalmol.* **135** 370–6

[69] Toto L, D'Aloisio R, Di Nicola M, Di Martino G, Di Staso S, Ciancaglini M, Tognetto D and Mastropasqua L 2017 Qualitative and quantitative assessment of vascular changes in diabetic macular edema after dexamethasone implant using optical coherence tomography angiography *Int. J. Mol. Sci.* **18** 1181

[70] Freiberg F J, Pfau M, Wons J, Wirth M A, Becker M D and Michels S 2016 Optical coherence tomography angiography of the foveal avascular zone in diabetic retinopathy *Graefe's Arch. Clin. Exp. Ophthalmol.* **254** 1051–8

[71] Bhanushali D, Anegondi N, Gadde S G, Srinivasan P, Chidambara L, Yadav N K and Roy A S 2016 Linking retinal microvasculature features with severity of diabetic retinopathy using optical coherence tomography angiography *Invest. Ophthalmol. Vis. Sci.* **57** OCT519–25

[72] Alam M, Zhang Y, Lim J I, Chan R V, Yang M and Yao X 2020 Quantitative optical coherence tomography angiography features for objective classification and staging of diabetic retinopathy *Retina* **40** 322–32

[73] Grewal D S, Agarwal M and Munk M R 2024 Wide field optical coherence tomography and optical coherence tomography angiography in uveitis *Ocular Immunol. Inflam.* **32** 105–15

[74] Fraser-Bell S, Symes R and Vaze A 2017 Hypertensive eye disease: a review *Clin. Exp. Ophthal.* **45** 45–53

[75] Haddar S, Mahjoub A, Ghorbel M, Mahjoub H, Knani L and Krifa F 2021 Retinal vein occlusions: an OCT-angiography analysis *La Tunisie Med.* **99** 538–43

[76] Agrawal R, Gupta P, Tan K A, Cheung C M G, Wong T Y and Cheng C Y 2016 Choroidal vascularity index as a measure of vascular status of the choroid: measurements in healthy eyes from a population-based study *Sci. Rep.* **6** 21090

[77] Malamos P, Tsolkas G, Kanakis M, Mylonas G, Karatzenis D, Oikonomopoulos N, Lakoumentas J and Georgalas I 2017 OCT-angiography for monitoring and managing neovascular age-related macular degeneration *Curr. Eye Res.* **42** 1689–97

[78] Kate A and Basu S 2022 Role of anterior segment-optical coherence tomography angiography in acute ocular burns *Diagnostics* **12** 607

[79] Yarmohammadi A, Zangwill L M, Diniz-Filho A, Saunders L J, Suh M H, Wu Z, Manalastas P I C, Akagi T, Medeiros F A and Weinreb R N 2017 Peripapillary and macular vessel density in patients with glaucoma and single-hemifield visual field defect *Ophthalmology* **124** 709–19

[80] Miguel A, Silva A, Barbosa-Breda J, Azevedo L, Abdulrahman A, Hereth E, Pinto L A, Lachkar Y and Stalmans I 2022 OCT-angiography detects longitudinal microvascular changes in glaucoma: a systematic review *Br. J. Ophthalmol.* **106** 667–75

[81] Iovino C, Iodice C M, Pisani D, Damiano L, Di Iorio V, Testa F and Simonelli F 2023 Clinical applications of optical coherence tomography angiography in inherited retinal diseases: an up-to-date review of the literature *J. Clin. Med.* **12** 3170

[82] Wong E S, Zhang X J, Yuan N, Li J, Pang C P, Chen L, Tham C C, Cheung C Y and Yam J C 2020 Association of optical coherence tomography angiography metrics with detection of impaired macular microvasculature and decreased vision in amblyopic eyes: the Hong Kong children eye study *JAMA Ophthalmol.* **138** 858–65

[83] Yilmaz I, Ocak O B, Yilmaz B S, Inal A, Gokyigit B and Taskapili M 2017 Comparison of quantitative measurement of foveal avascular zone and macular vessel density in eyes of children with amblyopia and healthy controls: an optical coherence tomography angiography study *J. Am. Assoc. Pediatr. Ophthalmol. Strabismus* **21** 224–8

[84] Lonngi M, Velez F G, Tsui I, Davila J P, Rahimi M, Chan C, Sarraf D, Demer J L and Pineles S L 2017 Spectral-domain optical coherence tomographic angiography in children with amblyopia *JAMA Ophthalmol.* **135** 1086–91

[85] Sobral I, Rodrigues T M, Soares M, Seara M, Monteiro M, Paiva C and Castela R 2018 OCT angiography findings in children with amblyopia *J. Am. Assoc. Pediatr. Ophthalmol. Strabismus* **22** 286–9

[86] Borrelli E, Lonngi M, Balasubramanian S, Tepelus T C, Baghdasaryan E, Pineles S L, Velez F G, Sarraf D, Sadda S R and Tsui I 2018 Increased choriocapillaris vessel density in amblyopic children: a case-control study *J. Am. Assoc. Pediatr. Ophthalmol. Strabismus* **22** 366–70

[87] Demirayak B, Vural A, Onur I U, Kaya F S and Yigit F U 2019 Analysis of macular vessel density and foveal avascular zone using spectral-domain optical coherence tomography angiography in children with amblyopia *J. Pediatr. Ophthalmol. Strabismus* **56** 55–9

[88] Chen W, Lou J, Thorn F, Wang Y, Mao J, Wang Q and Yu X 2019 Retinal microvasculature in amblyopic children and the quantitative relationship between retinal perfusion and thickness *Invest. Ophthalmol. Vis. Sci.* **60** 1185–91

[89] Yu L, Kang J, Jinata C, Wang X, Wei X, Chan K T, Lee N P and Wong K K 2015 Tri-band spectroscopic optical coherence tomography based on optical parametric amplification for lipid and vessel visualization *J. Biomed. Opt.* **20** 126006–6

[90] Faber D J, Mik E G, Aalders M C and van Leeuwen T G 2003 Light absorption of (oxy-) hemoglobin assessed by spectroscopic optical coherence tomography *Opt. Lett.* **28** 1436–8
[91] Faber D J, Mik E G, Aalders M C and van Leeuwen T G 2005 Toward assessment of blood oxygen saturation by spectroscopic optical coherence tomography *Opt. Lett.* **30** 1015–7
[92] Kagemann L, Wollstein G, Wojtkowski M, Ishikawa H, Townsend K A, Gabriele M L, Srinivasan V J, Fujimoto J G and Schuman J S 2007 Spectral oximetry assessed with high-speed ultra-high-resolution optical coherence tomography *J. Biomed. Opt.* **12** 041212–2
[93] Lu C W, Lee C K, Tsai M T, Wang Y M and Yang C C 2008 Measurement of the hemoglobin oxygen saturation level with spectroscopic spectral-domain optical coherence tomography *Opt. Lett.* **33** 416–8
[94] Liu X and Kang J U 2010 Depth-resolved blood oxygen saturation assessment using spectroscopic common-path Fourier domain optical coherence tomography *IEEE Trans. Biomed. Eng.* **57** 2572–5
[95] Robles F E, Chowdhury S and Wax A 2010 Assessing hemoglobin concentration using spectroscopic optical coherence tomography for feasibility of tissue diagnostics *Biomed. Opt. Express* **1** 310–7
[96] Yi J and Li X 2010 Estimation of oxygen saturation from erythrocytes by high-resolution spectroscopic optical coherence tomography *Opt. Lett.* **35** 2094–6
[97] Bosschaart N, Faber D J, Van Leeuwen T G and Aalders M C 2011 *In vivo* low-coherence spectroscopic measurements of local hemoglobin absorption spectra in human skin *J. Biomed. Opt.* **16** 100504–4
[98] Robles F E, Wilson C, Grant G and Wax A 2011 Molecular imaging true-colour spectroscopic optical coherence tomography *Nat. Photonics* **5** 744–7
[99] Yi J, Wei Q, Liu W, Backman V and Zhang H F 2013 Visible-light optical coherence tomography for retinal oximetry *Opt. Lett.* **38** 1796–8
[100] Yi J, Chen S, Backman V and Zhang H F 2014 *In vivo* functional microangiography by visible-light optical coherence tomography *Biomed. Opt. Express* **5** 3603–12
[101] Chen S, Yi J and Zhang H F 2015 Measuring oxygen saturation in retinal and choroidal circulations in rats using visible light optical coherence tomography angiography *Biomed. Opt. Express* **6** 2840–53
[102] Chong S P, Merkle C W, Leahy C, Radhakrishnan H and Srinivasan V J 2015 Quantitative microvascular hemoglobin mapping using visible light spectroscopic optical coherence tomography *Biomed. Opt. Express* **6** 1429–50
[103] Huang D *et al* 1991 Optical coherence tomography *Science* **254** 1178–81
[104] Welzel J, Lankenau E, Birngruber R and Engelhardt R 1997 Optical coherence tomography of the human skin *J. Am. Acad. Dermatol.* **37** 958–63
[105] Welzel J, Bruhns M and Wolff H H 2003 Optical coherence tomography in contact dermatitis and psoriasis *Arch. Dermatol. Res.* **295** 50–5
[106] Welzel J 2001 Optical coherence tomography in dermatology: a review *Skin Res. Technol.* **7** 1–9
[107] Schmitt J M 1999 Optical coherence tomography (OCT): a review *IEEE J. Sel. Top. Quantum Electron.* **5** 1205–15
[108] Xu C, Marks D L, Do M N and Boppart S A 2004 Separation of absorption and scattering profiles in spectroscopic optical coherence tomography using a least-squares algorithm *Opt. Express* **12** 4790–802

[109] Larin K V, Eledrisi M S, Ashitkov T V, Motamedi M and Esenaliev R O 2002 Monitoring of tissue optical properties using OCT: application for blood glucose analysis *Saratov Fall Meeting 2001: Optical Technologies in Biophysics and Medicine III* Vol. 4707 (SPIE) pp 181–8

[110] Feng S, Yuan K and Ye D 2008 Precision of glucose measurement in Intralipid suspensions with optical coherence tomography *2008 Int. Conf. on Information Technology and Applications in Biomedicine* (Piscataway, NJ: IEEE) pp 510–3

[111] Feng S, Yuan K and Ye D 2010 Effect of multiple scattering on measured signal losses using optical coherence tomography studied by Monte Carlo simulation *Int. J. Innov. Comput. Inf. Control* **6** 4249–62

[112] De Pretto L R, Yoshimura T M, Ribeiro M S and Zanardi de Freitas A 2016 Optical coherence tomography for blood glucose monitoring *in vitro* through spatial and temporal approaches *J. Biomed. Opt.* **21** 086007–7

[113] Ullah H, Gilanie G, Hussain F and Ahmad E 2015 Autocorrelation optical coherence tomography for glucose quantification in blood *Laser Phys. Lett.* **12** 125602

[114] Potts R O, A. Tamada J and J. Tierney M 2002 Glucose monitoring by reverse iontophoresis *Diabetes/Metab. Res. Rev.* **18** S49–53

[115] Pircher M, Götzinger E, Leitgeb R, Fercher A F and Hitzenberger C K 2003 Measurement and imaging of water concentration in human cornea with differential absorption optical coherence tomography *Opt. Express* **11** 2190–7

[116] Zhou Y, Zeng N, Ji Y, Li Y, Dai X, Li P, Duan L, Ma H and He Y 2011 Iris as a reflector for differential absorption low-coherence interferometry to measure glucose level in the anterior chamber *J. Biomed. Opt.* **16** 015004–4

[117] Schmitt J M, Xiang S H and Yung K M 1998 Differential absorption imaging with optical coherence tomography *J. Opt. Soc. Am.* A **15** 2288–96

[118] John P, Vasa N J, Sujatha N and Rao S R 2019 Glucose sensing in ex-vivo human gingival tissue with enhanced sensitivity in combination band *IEEE Sens. J.* **19** 7347–54

[119] John P, Vasa N J, Sujatha N and Rao S R 2017 Glucose sensing in oral tissue mimicking phantoms using supercontinuum laser source *Conf. on Lasers and Electro-Optics/Pacific Rim* (Optica Publishing Group) p s1781

[120] Untracht G R, Dikaios N, Durrani A K, Bapir M, Sarunic M V, Sampson D D, Heiss C and Sampson D M 2023 Pilot study of optical coherence tomography angiography-derived microvascular metrics in hands and feet of healthy and diabetic people *Sci. Rep.* **13** 1122

[121] Tearney G J, Jang I K and Bouma B E 2008 Imaging coronary atherosclerosis and vulnerable plaques with optical coherence tomography *Optical Coherence Tomography: Technology and Applications* (Berlin: Springer) pp 1083–101

[122] Rollins A M and Izatt J A 1999 Optimal interferometer designs for optical coherence tomography *Opt. Lett.* **24** 1484–6

[123] Petersen C L and Schmitt J M 2007 Design of an OCT imaging system for intravascular applications *Optical Coherence Tomography in Cardiovascular Research* (Boca Raton, FL: CRC Press) pp 51–8

[124] Tsigkas G, Spyropoulou P, Bousoula E, Apostolos A, Vasilagkos G, Karamasis G, Dimitriadis K, Moulias A and Davlouros P 2023 Intracoronary imaging: current practice and future perspectives *Rev. Cardiovasc. Med.* **24** 39

[125] Sukumaran V, Mutlu O, Murtaza M, Alhalbouni R, Dubansky B and Yalcin H C 2023 Experimental assessment of cardiovascular physiology in the chick embryo *Dev. Dyn.* **252** 1247–68
[126] Lee C H and Hur S H 2019 Optimization of percutaneous coronary intervention using optical coherence tomography *Korean Circ. J.* **49** 771–93
[127] Yoon H J, Cho Y K, Nam C W, Kim K B and Hur S H 2016 Angiographically minimal but functionally significant coronary lesion confirmed by optical coherence tomography *Korean J. Int. Med.* **31** 807
[128] Merkle C W and Srinivasan V J 2016 Laminar microvascular transit time distribution in the mouse somatosensory cortex revealed by dynamic contrast optical coherence tomography *Neuroimage* **125** 350–62
[129] Aziz T, Firdous S, Khan M A, Ikram M and Rahman T U 2013 Polarimetric study of leukemia human peripheral blood smears in 400–800 nm spectral range *Optik-Int. J. Light Electron Opt.* **124** 2936–42
[130] Wang W, Min L, Tian P, Wu C, Liu J and Hu X H 2022 Analysis of polarized diffraction images of human red blood cells: a numerical study *Biomed. Opt. Express* **13** 1161–72
[131] Tuchin V V 1997 Light scattering study of tissues *Phys. Usp.* **40** 495
[132] World Health Organization 2023 *WHO Malaria Policy Advisory Group (MPAG) Meeting Report* (World Health Organization) 18–20 April 2023
[133] Hänscheid T, Romão R, Grobusch M P, Amaral T and Melo-Cristino J 2011 Limitation of malaria diagnosis with the Cell-Dyn® analyser: not all haemozoin-containing monocytes are detected or shown *Int. J. Lab. Hematol.* **33** e14–6
[134] Frita R, Rebelo M, Pamplona A, Vigario A M, Mota M M, Grobusch M P and Hänscheid T 2011 Simple flow cytometric detection of haemozoin containing leukocytes and erythrocytes for research on diagnosis, immunology and drug sensitivity testing *Malar. J.* **10** 1–14
[135] Rebelo M, Shapiro H M, Amaral T, Melo-Cristino J and Hänscheid T 2012 Haemozoin detection in infected erythrocytes for *Plasmodium falciparum* malaria diagnosis—prospects and limitations *Acta Trop.* **123** 58–61
[136] Diabetes Statistics 2019 https://diabetesresearch.org/diabetes-statistics
[137] Heidemann C and Scheidt-Nave C 2017 Prevalence, incidence and mortality of diabetes mellitus in adults in Germany—a review in the framework of the diabetes surveillance *J. Health Monitor.* **2** 98
[138] Phan Q H and Lo Y L 2017 Stokes–Mueller matrix polarimetry system for glucose sensing *Opt. Lasers Eng.* **92** 120–8
[139] Mukherjee P, Hagen N and Otani Y 2019 Glucose sensing in the presence of scattering by analyzing a partial Mueller matrix *Optik* **180** 775–81
[140] Al-Hafidh M H, Glidle A, Wilson R, Kelly A E, Reboud J and Cooper J M 2019 Multireflection polarimetry in microfluidics *IEEE Sens. Lett.* **3** 1–4

IOP Publishing

The Optics of Blood
A Handbook
Alexandre Douplik

Chapter 11

Blood and Photodynamic Therapy: two-directional interactions

Lothar Lilge

11.1 Introduction

Photodynamic therapy (PDT) exploits the use of light-sensitive, non-toxic drugs called photosensitizers (PSs), administered topically or systemically. These drugs are preferentially accumulated and retained in highly proliferating tissues, such as malignancies, skin, and other tissues. Upon absorption of a photon matching the PS's absorption spectrum to reach the singlet excited state, the photon's quantum energy is utilized through photophysical and photochemical mechanisms to generate cytotoxic reactive oxygen species (ROS), predominantly singlet oxygen ($^1O_2$). PSs also generate fluorescence and thus permit the visualization of malignant tissues [1, 2].

PDT is extensively used in precursors, potentially leading to malignancies, such as Barrett's esophagus [3] and actinic keratosis [4], as well as a range of malignancies on organ surfaces, including basal cell carcinoma [5], bladder [6, 7], cervical [8], esophageal [9] and lung cancer [10] among others. Additionally, deep-seated malignancies such as gliomas in the brain [11, 12], prostate [13–15], and head and neck tumors [16, 17] are also accessible via interstitial placement of optical fibers with distal diffusing tips [18].

The association between blood and PDT dates back to the inception of the therapy, as the original PS initially developed for oncology, hematoporphyrin derivative or HpD, was synthesized from dried blood [19]. Today, the associations between blood, its components, and vascular structure, and PDT are much more complex, given that blood can be the primary target causing subsequent apoptosis and necrosis in the illuminated volume or, conversely, blood and the vasculature can modify the secondary response to the therapy.

The cardiovascular system and blood are critical elements for effective PDT throughout the clinical target volume (CTV), starting with the systematic delivery of two of PDT's efficacy-determining parameters, the PS and molecular oxygen ($^3O_2$), particularly in the case of solid tumor treatment. Conversely, the light absorption by

doi:10.1088/978-0-7503-4806-5ch11

hemoglobins restricts the effective treatment volume a single light source can target. The cytotoxins generated by PDT can directly affect the cardiovascular system, including the endothelial and internal elastic lamina, thereby indirectly impacting the vessel's barrier function and all components of the blood, particularly leukocytes and platelets. Rapid vasoconstriction during PDT delivery disrupts the supply of $^3O_2$ to the target tissue, stalling the production of the cytotoxic ROS, thus limiting or abrogating a further increase in the local PDT dose.

Some indications include macular degeneration and port wine stains [20], prostate cancer [15, 21], and spider veins [22]. The vasculature is the primary target of PDT, and permanent vascular stasis is a required endpoint.

PDT's interactions with leukocytes can export local PDT treatment effects systemically, primarily through the activation or deactivation of signaling pathways associated with the immune system, post-PDT inflammatory processes, and tissue healing.

Through the complex interaction of PDT with blood and the vascular system, local modifications to blood flow, blood viscosity, and blood leakage into the surrounding tissue change blood properties. These can hinder treatment dosimetry or be exploited as potential monitoring mechanisms for assessing PDT efficacy. Thus, the interactions between delivering a curative PDT dose to tissue and the blood within the clinical target volume are bidirectional. PDT affects the blood, and the blood, in turn, affects the efficacy of PDT.

11.2 Principles of photodynamic therapy

PDT was first observed at the beginning of the 20th century during microbial inactivation and coined shortly after that. It was revived for oncological indications in the 1970s due to the efforts of Thomas Dougherty at Roswell Park in Buffalo, NY [23–25].

PDT describes the conversion of a light photon through absorption by the PS into oxygen radicals, predominantly singlet oxygen. Approved PSs or those under investigation are mostly organic molecules of small molecular weight and can be synthesized [26], metal-based [27], nanoparticles [28, 29], or from natural sources [30]. Toxic moieties are produced either by Type I (oxygen-independent) or Type II (oxygen-dependent) pathways, so Type II, with the production of ROS, is dominant. The biochemical reactions for Type I reactions include tryptophan, phenol coupling, phenylalanine hydroxylation, protein cross-linking, and carbonylation. In contrast, Type II reactions lead to lipid hydroperoxides and radical chain reactions, cholesterol, 5, 6-hydroperoxides, and nucleic acids 5-carboxamide or 5 formamide production, and histidine and tryptophan oxygen addition, cysteine disulfide and methionine sulfoxide formation, and proteolysis among others [31].

Upon absorption of a light quantum, the PS is raised to the first electronic excited singlet state, $^1PS^*$, into its lowest triplet excited state, ^3PS. This enables it to interact with ground-state oxygen present in a triplet state, $^3O_2$, to exchange spin and energy, generating singlet oxygen, $^1O_2$, and returning to its ground state. Thus, the PS acts as a catalyst, generating 10^3–10^5 ROS [32]. The term $^1O_2$ refers to the lowest energy excited species $^1\Delta_g$ of molecular oxygen.

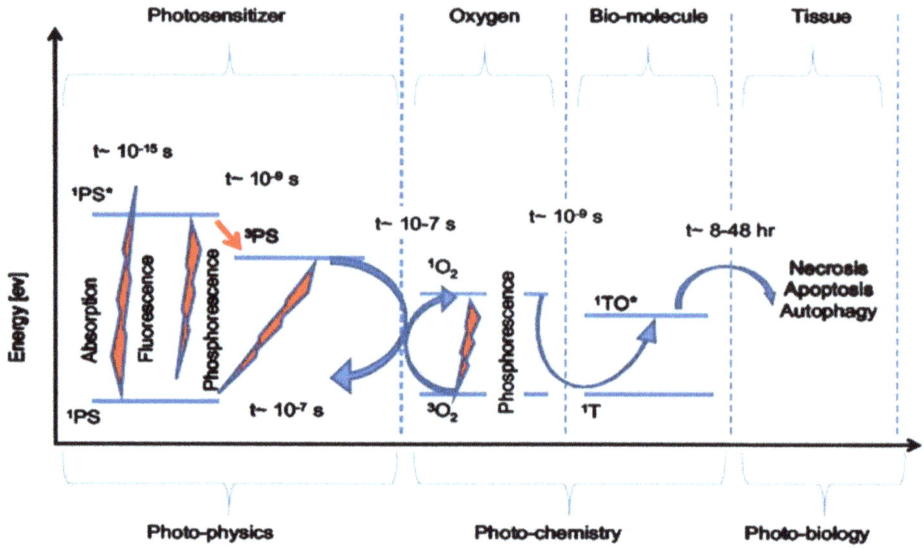

Figure 11.1. Energy transfer from photon absorption to tissue necrosis is done through a sequence of photophysical, photochemical, and photo-biological processes.

For effective PDT, there needs to be a spatial-temporal overlap between the photon, PS, and oxygen to allow the efficient spin and energy transfer between $^1O_2$ and the oxidation target, lipids, or proteins within the short $^1O_2$ lifetime ($<10^{-8}$ s) and thus restricted diffusion distance (<200 nm) [33] figure 11.1 illustrates the energy transfer from the photon's quantum energy to the oxidation of the biomolecules.

In PDT, one differentiates between cellular and vascular action. In the former, cellular structures throughout the CTV are targeted, whereas in the latter, only the vasculature is targeted [34].

For surface irradiation and interstitial applications, the power density is typically maintained below 200 mW cm^{-2} to prevent hyperthermia, which has been shown to modulate the tissue response. While some enhancement of the PDT efficacy is possible [35, 36], excessive heat due to high power densities during interstitial delivery close to minor arteries or veins will exacerbate vascular stasis and block further PDT dose delivery to tissue volumes serviced by that artery or vein.

The PS's activation wavelength is selected to provide the largest penetration depths inside the tissue. These are typically flanked by 630 nm at the low end and generally less than 750 nm. The former minimizes absorption by the hemoglobins, which increases by several orders of magnitude between 630 and 520 nm [37] and at the long wavelength end by the minimum quantum energy required for the efficient population of the PS's triplet state and energy and spin transfer to generate $^1O_2$. As most PSs are administered i.v. they must be water-soluble or utilize a drug delivery carrier, such as dextran or micelles [38, 39]. Other approaches to augment cellular uptake involve usurping surface receptors upregulated in target tissues, such as the transferrin receptor [40].

Given that the PS and $^3O_2$ concentrations as well as the photon density rates govern the ROS generation and, hence, the photodynamic dose and PDT efficacy, most PDT dosimetry concepts are built on one or more of these three efficacy-determining parameters.

The clinical dosing of PDT is determined by the drug dose given in [mg kg^{-1}] and the light intensity given either as power density call irradiance, φ, [mW cm^{-2}] for surface irradiation or as fluence rate [mW cm^{-2}] for interstitially placed cylindrical diffusing tip optical fiber and the treatment time, T, determining the energy density, called radiant exposure and fluence, for surface illumination and interstitial light delivery, respectively, denoted by H [J cm^{-2}]. To quantify the spatially resolved dose of ROS and $^1O_2$ in particular, the PS's concentration, [PS] [mM], throughout the clinical target volume (CTV), multiplied by its molar extinction coefficient, $\varepsilon(\lambda)$ [L mol^{-2} cm^{-2}], at the excitation wavelength, λ, the fluence rate, φ given in units of photons per area and time [$h\nu$ cm^{-2} s^{-1}] and the partial oxygen pressure in the tissue pO_2 [%] must be known.

Assuming molecular oxygen is not the rate-limiting educt for the PDT reaction, which is satisfied for vascular application as long as the $pO_2 > 2\%$ throughout the treatment time, the dose is given by.

$$D_{\mathrm{PDT}} = \int_0^T \phi(t)\varepsilon(\lambda)[PS](t)dt \tag{11.1}$$

as used, for example, in the photodynamic threshold model [41]. The associate threshold values, which represent the number of photons absorbed by the PS per unit volume, have been published for various tissues and PSs [42–47] and employed in PDT treatment planning software [48]. PDT dose models have also been published with the inclusion of the local molecular oxygen concentration [$^3O_2$],

$$D_{\mathrm{PDT}} = \int_0^T \xi\frac{[3O_2](t)}{[3O_2](t) + \beta}\phi(t)\varepsilon(\lambda)[PS](t)dt \tag{11.2}$$

For photofrin-mediated PDT using 630 nm excitation light, the photophysical parameter $\xi = 3.7\ 10^{-3}\ cm^2\ s^{-1}\ mW^{-1}$, representing the specific oxygen consumption rate, and $\beta = 11.9\ \mu M$, the oxygen quenching threshold concentration, which has been previously determined. This model is also currently being investigated for PDT treatment planning purposes [49–51].

The latter model implicitly acknowledges the well-established fact that if the oxygen saturation drops during PDT, as expressed in the oxygen consumption model by Foster *et al* [52], in the interstitial space and the cells throughout the irradiated clinical target volume. In the case of vascular PDT, the effect becomes important if stasis in the vascular flow occurs as a biological response during light delivery therapy.

The reactive oxygen species, including hydroxy anion, hydrogen peroxide, and singlet oxygen [53–55], will interact indiscriminately with the cell's lipids and proteins, exceeding the cell's ability to replenish the damaged structures and leading to apoptosis and necrosis as dominant cell death mechanisms. The efficacy of the PS is commonly expressed by its singlet oxygen quantum yield or the number of cytotoxic oxygen molecules generated per photon absorbed. Given the longer lifetimes of H_2O_2 and OH^{2-}, cells have developed defense mechanisms in the form of scavengers; however, due to the short lifetime of $^1O_2$, cellular defenses against this cytotoxin are very limited [33].

Due to the extremely short lifetime of singlet oxygen, approximately 200 ns, its diffusion distance is limited to much less than μm in mammalian cells. Thus, the subcellular localization of the PS determines the primary organelles damaged by the photodynamic action. Most current PSs include porphyrins, chlorines, purpurins, and phthalocyanines, hence cations, and localize them at the inner mitochondrial membrane. One pathway for cell death is severe inner mitochondrial membrane damage leading to the release of cytochrome C into the cytoplasm, activating the caspase cascade and causing apoptosis. Direct damage to the nucleus is rarely observed but can be demonstrated in *in vitro* or liquid models using comet assays when phagocytosis is absent [56, 57]. Targeting the DNA is generally avoided in PDT so as not to cause single or double-strand breaks at sub-lethal PDT doses, possibly giving rise to future disease. For more detailed mechanistic information, see reviews by Agostinis *et al* [58] and Castano *et al* [59].

Besides the tetrapyrrole-based PSs listed above, recent developments are ongoing with BOPIDY derivatives as PSs, given their high absorption coefficient; however, they are hampered by low triplet quantum yields in their basic form. Adding heavy atoms to the structures can increase the triplet and singlet oxygen quantum yields. Most BODIDY derivatives are excited with green and orange wavelengths (540–580 nm), limiting their indications to those with shallow CTV in oncology and antimicrobial settings. Transition metals, such as TLD1433 [60, 61], and other ruthenium [42], osmium [62], and rhenium-based coordination complexes have comparably short excitation wavelengths, and the majority of their efficacy still needs to be demonstrated in pre-clinical studies.

There has been a solid effort to develop nanoparticles (NPs) as PSs. These nanoparticles can be categorized as constructs with conjugated σ-π-orbitals, as in the case of fullerenes, semiconducting polymers, and other polymer-based structures, nanostructures comprised of photoactive materials, such as titanium dioxide, and core–shell upconversion NPs. The latter permits the absorption of near-infrared (NIR) photons and generates visible light to excite the PS [54]. Particular self-assembly NPs combine the PS and the structure themselves, as in the case of porphysomes [63, 64]. These porphysomes are currently in the first clinical trial in humans [65, 66].

As the PS is delivered by intravenous administration, the distribution of the PS in the tumor parenchyma and the vascular system per se is essential for the PDT efficacy of all PSs. Hence, two principal approaches for PDT targeting in oncology exist, called cellular or vascular PDT. In the first, the PS targets the tumor cells directly, which necessitates its leakage from the vasculature into the tumor parenchymal, whereas, in the second, the PS remains in the vasculature, whereby the vascular epithelial cells and the blood are direct targets of the PDT generated ROS, see the examples mentioned above. Targeting the tumor's vascular supply requires the PS to remain at high concentrations in the vasculature without leaking into the parenchymal or being cleared from the blood by the hepatic or renal systems [67]. Targeting the tumor vasculature requires tighter timing between PS administration and the onset of light delivery.

Monitoring the effects of blood and the vasculature in response to PDT requires *in vivo* model systems that enable direct imaging of the vasculature and blood during and after PDT, preferably in a longitudinal manner. The two most common model systems are the chick chorioallantoic membrane (CAM) model [68] or one of the various window chamber models [69]. For some indications, such as PDT for port wine stain [70] and the retina for macular degeneration [71], direct imaging access is also provided during clinical studies, given the transparent nature of the eye's overlaying cornea, lens, and vitreous humor.

The remainder of this chapter discusses how blood affects PDT efficacy, how PDT targets blood and blood components and the vascular system to mediate tumour destruction, how these PDT-induced changes could be utilized for treatment progress monitoring, and how they impact the immune system. PDT can also be used as an antimicrobial treatment effort to sterilize blood products, as reported at this chapter's end.

11.3 Impact of blood on the efficacy of photodynamic therapy

11.3.1 Optical attenuation by blood

Given the need for delivery of the PS and $^3O_2$ by a well-developed vascular system, including a high capillary density [72], absorption by blood and thus limiting the light propagation in the tissue is always of concern throughout the CTV [73].

The impact of blood absorption can be mitigated by either switching to a less absorbent wavelength in the 780–830 nm range, currently available only to Tookad as a PS or alternatively by replacing the blood with non-hemoglobin-containing liquids, as demonstrated using STEEN fluid during pre-clinical *ex vivo* and *in vivo* lung perfusion experiments [43].

11.3.2 Photosensitizer transport in the cardiovascular system

Cellular-acting PSs have longer blood circulation times and clearance rates, such as protoporphyrin IX, which has a plasma half-life of $\sim$3.6 ± 1.8 h following oral administration of its pro-drug aminolaevulinic acid (ALA) [74–76]. PSs with long circulation times include Photofrin and Foscan [77].

At short drug light intervals, all PSs can be found predominantly in the blood plasma, causing damage to the vascular wall upon photon activation which can sometimes be exploited, albeit with limited selectivity between malignant and normal tissues. For vascular-acting PSs such as WST09, also known as Tookad, and Benzoporphyrin derivative monoacid (BPD-MA), also known as Visudyne, the blood clearance half-lives are rapid, at >0.05 h [78] and 0.1 h [79, 80], respectively. To achieve the required PDT dose according to equations (11.1) or (11.2) and the limited PS circulation time, the fluence rate needs to be increased, causing only mild hyperthermia, reaching >200–300 mW cm^{-2}. If longer irradiation times are necessary, the PS must be administered continuously via a syringe pump.

From a PDT dosimetry viewpoint, the PS's blood plasma concentration at the time of light delivery is of interest as it is a primary determinant of intentional or unintentional vascular damage. The former relates to the efficacy of vascular PDT, and the latter relates to therapy-associated morbidity. Table 11.1 lists the blood plasma concentration of various PSs in absolute concentration and as a specific uptake ratio (SUR), calculated from the administered sensitizer dose and the concentration.

The data indicate that no PSs have a non-negligible presence in the blood plasma at the time of clinical light delivery. While for low PS concentration or for fast mean transfer times (MTTs), this temporal generation of ROS may not be high enough to damage the vessel's endothelial cell and intima; however, at high plasma PS concentration, [PS], or slow MTT, damage to the vasculature within the illuminated tissue volume may not be preventable.

11.3.3 Molecular oxygen transport during PDT

The loss in blood oxygen saturation, pO_2, was experimentally demonstrated to be dependent on the [PS] and the photon fluence rate, φ and the photon fluence, H. Higher PS, φ, or H all results in a monotonous faster drop in the blood's oxygen saturation, pO_2, which can reach 0% during *ex vivo* studies, and as low as 25% *in vivo* given reperfusion. However, in either case, PDT is rendered ineffective. *Ex vivo* experiments showed an 80% loss in blood pO_2 after exposure to clinical doses of sulfonated aluminum phthalocyanine PS to 20 J cm^{-2} [79]. Hence, reperfusion and recovery of high pO_2 throughout the CTV can be achieved through moderation of, φ, thus maintaining a well-developed capillary system for effective PDT. The need to maintain reperfusion of the CTV led to the development of online monitoring systems, such as blood-flow-informed PDT [80], further discussed below, and diffuse correlation spectroscopy (DCS) [79].

11.4 Effects of PDT on blood and the blood's vascular structure

11.4.1 Blood flow and blood volume

Blood flow and pO_2 are two of the major aspects of monitoring the vascular aspects of PDT during and after PDT, independent of the mode of action, cellular or vascular. Optical techniques permitting flow measurements either on an interval or categorical scale include, for the former, laser Doppler (LD) [67], Diffuse correlation spectroscopy (DCS) [81] or laser speckle contrast imaging (LSCI) [82, 83] and for the latter, speckle optical coherence tomography (sOCT) [135]. While Doppler-based methods only quantify blood flow along the optical observation axis, speckle-based techniques are independent of the blood flow direction relative to the observation axis. Doppler-based methods offer better flow speed resolution, whereas speckle-based methods exhibit poor flow speed resolution. DCS is more sensitive to microvascular flow than Doppler-based methods, which are generally sensitive to and hence dominated by the higher flow rates in arteries and veins; however, DCS-determined flow is qualitative

Table 11.1. PS concentration in blood plasma.

Photo-sensitizer	Administered dose [mg kg^{-1}]	Species	Time of light illumination [h]	Plasma concentration [μg ml^{-1}]	SUR	References
Photofrin	1	Human	48	~10	10	[136]
Photofrin	2	Human	48	7.65	3.82	[137]
Photofrin	5	Mice	24	100	20	[138]
Photofrin	20	Rat	24	2	0.1	[139]
HPPH	3–6	Human	0.45	0.4–0.8	0.13	[140]
BPD-MA	4	Mice	1	3.44	0.86	[141]
BPD-MA	4	Human	1	6.49 ± 0.94	1.62	[142]
Hypericin	5	Mice	3	3.04 ± 0.32	0.61	[143]
m-THPC	0.3	Rat	24	2.34	7.8	[144]
AlPcS4	20	Rat	24	2	0.1	[145]
Motexafin Lutetium	10	Mice	2	5.7	0.57	[146]

rather than quantitative. The temporal evolution of blood flow, as measured by DCS in transmission mode, during and following ALA-induced PpIX mediated PDT, delivering 100 J cm^{-2} of 514 nm light over 2000 s, revealed an initial increase in flow due to the PDT-related consumption of oxygen followed at the 1200 s timepoint with a sudden loss of flow in the artery supplying the tumor as well as in the tumor microvasculature.

DCS, LSCI, and sOCT provide inherent information about the blood volume as long as no thrombus is formed. Photoacoustic imaging (PAI) and microscopy (PAM) provide a flow-independent assessment of the blood volume [84], and if combined with multiwavelength excitation [85], oxygen saturation can also be quantified.

A recent study by Saeidi *et al* [86] aimed to determine if knowledge of MRI-derived blood flow and blood volume can become a predictor of local PS uptake in the brain; however, the variability in the leakiness of the blood vessels between an intact blood-brain-barrier and leaky tumor vasculature did not permit to establish a direct correlation in this immune privileged organ.

11.4.2 PDT effects on blood components

The interactions of platelets and PDT are also bidirectional. Platelets were loaded with nanochemotherapeutics, in particular chemotherapeutics linked to chlorin e6 composites, whereby the release of the chemotherapeutic drug was activated by light irradiation in the CTV. When associated with doxorubicin, leading to DNA damage, as in the case of iron oxide-polyglycerol linked [87], or targeting particular cancers for breast cancer [88] and glioma [89].

Conversely, PDT effects on platelets have also been investigated. One complication is that UV and short-wavelength blue light alone have been shown to cause platelet aggregation [90]. Upon irradiation with irradiances associated with low-level laser therapy, now referred to as photobiomodulation (see chapter 12), it has also been demonstrated to modify platelet function, including alterations in their biochemistry [91].

While UV light exposure enhanced platelet self-aggregation, photofin-mediated PDT lowered their binding potential and adhesion to the extracellular matrix and other known coagulation factors. However, aggregation to collagen was shown to increase. This renders large vessels less thrombogenic, whereas veins and arterioles are at an increased risk for thrombus formation. The former has a low collagen content versus a high collagen content in the latter [92].

11.4.3 Immediate effects on erythrocytes due to photodynamic therapy

Applying ALA topically to rat skin followed after 2 h with $H = 30$ J cm^{-2} delivered at $\varphi = 50$ mW cm^{-2} of 635 nm irradiation caused a significant increase in the met-hemoglobin concentrations to ~50 mM in the blood even after 24 h, compared to <2 mM in non-PDT treated animals, indicating blood erythrocyte breakdown with potential systemic effects. Due to its higher molar extinction coefficient than oxy-hemoglobin throughout the red and NIR spectrum, significant amounts of met-hemoglobin will significantly under report the pO_2 [%] [93].

11.4.4 Immediate effects on leukocytes due to photodynamic therapy

Uptake differences between stimulated and resting peripheral blood mononuclear cells, including lymphocytes and monocytes, have been noted for different phthalocyanines, whereby stimulated leukocytes demonstrated a stronger uptake of the phthalocyanine, indicating that some activated immune cells can be targeted selectively [94]. A difference in the uptake of cyclosporine A by normal leukocytes and human myeloid leukemia cell lines was noted by Ignatova *et al* [95], whereby the latter uptake was more than twice that of normal leukocytes. The team noted that this also translated into normal leukocytes and erythrocytes being less sensitive to PDT compared to the leukemia cell lines *in vitro* in a PS concentration-dependent manner. Additional effects mediated by leukocytes are listed in the paragraph relating to the immune responses to PDT.

11.4.5 Changes to the blood vessel structures during photodynamic therapy

Vascular targeting PDT aims to achieve a complete cessation of blood flow long enough to deprive the tissue of oxygen or nutrition, resulting in its death. For Verteporfin, mediated PDT initiated within 15 min of drug administration caused complete flow arrest at 6 h, whereas longer time delays reduced only blood flow. During *in vivo* experiments, the former resulted in a 10-day growth delay, and the latter only in a 4-day delay [67]. Fingar noted similar responses for Verteporfin [96]. Similar effects were demonstrated for various PSs, including pyropbeophorbide acid [97], talaporfin sodium [98], and hypericin [99], when light illumination follows shortly after i.v. PS delivery.

Vascular stasis following PDT is the goal in the treatment of port wine stain [100], glaucoma [101], optical disc and retinal vessel [72], atherosclerosis [102], and oral cancer [103]. Laser speckle monitoring is often employed to monitor cessation of blood flow in these situations [97, 104].

11.5 Systemic effects of photodynamic therapy mediated by blood or blood cells

PDT can directly or indirectly affect the blood via damage to blood components such as red blood cells (RBCs), leucocytes, and neutrophils, or via the release of signaling molecules from the damaged cells in the CTV [105], resulting in a systemic therapeutic effect [106]. It was shown that post-photofrin or tetra(m-tetrahydroxyphenyl) chlorin (m-THPC), -mediated PDT, a significant increase in infiltration of activated neutrophils was noted in the peripheral blood of mice, possibly due to an efflux of these cells from the bone marrow [107]. This is commonly initiated via a nuclear factor κB (NFκB) mediated inflammatory response by the release of damage-associated molecular patterns (DAMPs), in particular, the heat shock proteins and inflammatory cytokines [108]. This effect was observed for multiple

PSs [109]. However, the original intracellular location of the PDT-induced damage can result in different DAMPs being released into the bloodstream [110]. The DAMPs released into the bloodstream can be lipid fragments or metabolites, ATP [111] or endoplasmatic reticulum-associated proteins [112]. These DAMPs recruit macrophages, dendritic cells, and other neutrophils. The latter have a pivotal effect on PDT outcome, given that their availability within the bloodstream appears to determine the overall therapeutic efficacy [113]. While this signaling and activation of the innate and adaptive immune response in furthering anti-tumour effects is desirable locally and systematically to achieve a complete local response and suppress and eliminate potential distant metastasis, general immunosuppression following PDT has attracted less curiosity in the research community. Some of the cytokines released, including IL-10 and transforming growth factor β (TGF-β), can stimulate $CD4^+$ T cells to differentiate into regulatory T cells (Tregs), leading to the generation of anergic or tolerogenic $CD8^+$ T cells [114]. Significantly elevated Tregs have been demonstrated in the spleens and lymph nodes of mice post-PDT [115], indicating the potential for systemic effects mediated by leukocytes in the blood.

11.5.1 PDT effects related to leucocytes

D Mono-L-aspartyl chlorine 6 (NPe6) mediated PDT using 664 nm and delivery, $H = 10\ \mathrm{J\,cm^{-2}}$ increased the expression of Mac-1 by 3-fold in polymorphonuclear leukocytes, which may play a cytocidal role in the treatment of oral cancer [116].

11.6 Using blood to monitor the photodynamic therapy progress

11.6.1 Monitoring of photodynamic therapy

The cytotoxic load generated with photodynamic therapy often exceeds mM concentrations of oxygen radicals, affecting the blood cells' integrity and blood vessels. While low doses of PDT can result in an increase in blood flow and inflammation, high doses of photonic therapy, particularly for vascular-acting PSs, can result in rapid flow stasis and thrombus formation.

As indicated above, laser speckle imaging is the preferred method to monitor blood flow in superficial applications, such as the window chamber models or the chick embryo chorioallantoic membrane model [97, 104]. DCS was used to quantify the blood flow in subcutaneous mouse tumors treated with low and high irradiances post-photofrin injection. The onset and slope of blood perfusion loss were positively correlated with irradiance, resulting in a reduction of blood flow by up to 50% [85]. Using DCS, it was shown that modulating the PDT irradiance based on the rate of blood flow loss could not only minimize the total irradiation time and improve the overall clonogenic tumor cell kill by PDT.

Laser Doppler imaging is another method for monitoring blood perfusion intraoperatively, as applied in port wine stain therapy during vascular-targeted photodynamic therapy [117].

11.7 PDT and blood outside of the human body

11.7.1 Improving safety for blood and blood products

The use of PDT to inactivate blood-borne pathogens, including bacteria and viruses, had been previously demonstrated [118–120]. Given the substantial changes in the absorption coefficient between oxygenated and deoxygenated blood in the 500–650 nm spectral range, PDT dosimetry depends strongly on the blood's oxygen saturation, simulated by Monte Carlo for merocyanine-540-mediated PDT [121]. These simulations are desired or required to calculate the maximum permissible cuvette flow speed that achieves high mammalian or microbial kill in the flow cell volume distal to the light source, while not damaging or causing necrosis in normal blood cells in the flow volume proximal to the light source.

11.7.2 Extracorporeal PDT treatment of blood

Extracorporeal PDT was developed for two different indications as extracorporeal photopheresis (ECP) for the treatment of cutaneous T-cell lymphoma and, building on the ability to inactivate microbes, extracorporeal PDT was tested *in vivo* in a process coined photodynamic bBlood purification (PBP) therapy. In both indications, blood is harvested from the patient, exposed to the PS and light outside the body, and then re-infused into the patient.

ECP using 8-methoxy psoralen (8-MOP) followed by ultraviolet A (UV-A) radiation was approved in the 1990s and is used, among others, to mediate graft-versus-host disease and organ transplant rejection [122]. High-quantum energy UV-A light is used to eliminate the potential for DNA damage. Recent studies evaluated ALA-induced PpIX blue light-mediated PDT for ECP. It was shown that activated $CD3^{+}$, $CD4^{+}$ $CD25^{+}$, and $CD8^{+}$ T cells showed a high synthesis and accumulation of PpIX with lower cell survival than for the standard 8-MOP UV-A protocol. Conversely, resting T cells show less damage than the 8-MOP UV-A protocol. During the co-culture of activated and resting cells reflecting clinically relevant conditions, activated cells were destroyed more selectively while sparing dendritic cells, demonstrating the high potential of ALA-induced PpIX for various ECP applications [123].

Extracorporeal PBP treatment of circulatory blood with hematoporphyrin-monomethyl-ether mediated PDT resulted in a transient increase in WBCs (lasting 1–3 days but returning to normal on 7 days). For repeat PBP, a monotonous decrease in RBCs is noted. Even three PDT exposures over 1 week did not significantly decrease the functionality of the analyzed blood at doses sufficient to reduce the bacterial or viral loads significantly [124]. The biochemical analysis of other blood components, including platelets alanine aminotransferase, aspartate aminotransferase, alkaline phosphatase, γ-glutamyl transpeptidase, uric acid, blood urea nitrogen, and creatinine showed no differences to a control non-PDT exposed group, or only transient changes of maximal 30% even after 3 PDT treatments.

11.7.3 Treatment of blood products

Antimicrobial PDT (aPDT) has also been investigated for inactivating pathogens in whole blood, plasma, and platelets. While a rare occurrence, hundreds of transfusion-transmitted infections occur each year, primarily bacterial (2/3) and viral (~1/3), and seldom parasitic.

To date, three PSs have been approved for blood and blood product sterilization: a psoralen derivative called amotosalen, riboflavin, and methylene blue (MB), the first two requiring UV excitation and the latter blue light activation. All three PS are targeting predominantly viruses. The current efforts are to expand aPDT for blood product sterilization beyond viruses to include bacteria, fungi, and protozoa. *Candida albicans* typically colonize the gastrointestinal tract and other mucosal surfaces and can affect the host immune system and bacterial flora. Once it enters the bloodstream, the mortality rate approximates 40%; hence, elimination from blood products is critical [125]. *C. albicans* was successfully treated with aPDT mediated by hematoporphyrin, photofrin, chlorins, and ALA-induced PpIX in planktonic solutions.

11.8 Vasculature as the entry point for PDT light delivery

The vasculature is used as a common access point for a wide range of medical interventions. Transvascular access is used for a range of clinical indications, such as reducing restenosis following femoral angioplasty [126] or coronary-stent placement [127, 128], for atherosclerotic plaque [129–132] and as a preventive method to inhibit intimal hyperplasia [133–135], using a range of PSs. These studies demonstrated that endovascular PDT, with laser irradiation from within the vessel, is well tolerated by large vessels without inducing stenosis, thrombosis, aneurysms, and vessel rupture, providing no prior damage or biological modifications to the vessel wall.

Glossary of terms

Antimicrobial photodynamic therapy	aPDT
Chick chorioallantoic membrane	CAM
Clinical target volume	CTV
Damage-associated molecular patterns	DAMPs
Diffuse correlation spectroscopy	DCS
Diffuse correlation spectroscopy	DCS
Electronic excited singlet state	$^{1}PS^{*}$
Fluence	J cm^{-2} or hν cm^{-2}
Fluence-rate	mW cm^{-2} or hν cm^{-2} s^{-1}
Irradiance	φ mW cm^{-2} or hν cm^{-2} s^{-1}
Laser Doppler	LD
Laser speckle contrast imaging	LSCI
Molar extinction coefficient	$\varepsilon(\lambda)$, L mol^{-2} cm^{-2}
Molecular oxygen	$^{3}O_2$
Near-infrared	NIR
Oxygen consumption rate	β, μM s^{-1}
Photoacoustic imaging	PAI

Photoacoustic microscopy	PAM
Photodynamic blood purification	PBP
Photophysical parameter	ξ, $cm^2\ s^{-1}\ mW^{-1}$
Photosensitizer	PS
Photosensitizer concentration	[PS]
Radiant exposure	H, J cm^{-2} or hν cm^{-2}
Reactive oxygen species	ROS
Red blood cells	RBC
Regulatory T cells	Tregs
Singlet oxygen	$^1O_2$
Specific uptake ratio	SUR
Speckle optical coherence tomography	sOCT
Time	T, s
Transforming growth factor β	TGF-β
Triplet excited state	^3PS
Wavelength	λ, nm
White blood cells	WBC

References

[1] Casas A 2020 Clinical uses of 5-aminolaevulinic acid in photodynamic treatment and photodetection of cancer: a review *Cancer Lett.* **490** 165–73

[2] Rink M *et al* 2013 Hexyl aminolevulinate-guided fluorescence cystoscopy in the diagnosis and follow-up of patients with non-muscle-invasive bladder cancer: a critical review of the current literature *Eur. Urol.* **64** 624–38

[3] Wu H, Minamide T and Yano T 2019 Role of photodynamic therapy in the treatment of esophageal cancer *Dig. Endosc.* **31** 508–16

[4] Szeimiesa R M *et al* 2002 Photodynamic therapy using topical methyl 5-aminolevulinate compared with cryotherapy for actinic keratosis: a prospective, randomized study *J. Am. Acad. Dermatol.* **47** 258–62

[5] Braathen L R *et al* 2007 Guidelines on the use of photodynamic therapy for nonmelanoma skin cancer: an international consensus *J. Am. Acad. Dermatol.* **56** 125–43

[6] Li H, Long G and Tian J 2023 Efficacy and safety of photodynamic therapy for non-muscle-invasive bladder cancer: a systematic review and meta-analysis *Front. Oncol.* **13**

[7] Kulkarni G S *et al* 2022 A phase 1b clinical study of intravesical photodynamic therapy in patients with bacillus Calmette–Guérin-unresponsive non-muscle-invasive bladder cancer *Eur. Urol. Open Sci.* **41** 105–11

[8] Hillemanns P *et al* 1999 Photodynamic therapy in women with cervical intraepithelial neoplasia using topically applied 5-aminolevulinic acid *Int. J. Cancer* **81** 34–8

[9] Bartusik-Aebisher D *et al* 2022 Advancements in photodynamic therapy of esophageal cancer *Front. Oncol.* **12** 1024576

[10] Usuda J *et al* 2006 Photodynamic therapy (PDT) for lung cancers *J. Thorac. Oncol.* **1** 489–93

[11] Lietke S *et al* 2021 Interstitial photodynamic therapy using 5-ALA for malignant glioma recurrences *Cancers (Basel)* **13** 1767

[12] Stepp H *et al* 2007 ALA and malignant glioma: fluorescence-guided resection and photodynamic treatment *J. Environ. Pathol. Toxicol. Oncol.* **26** 157–64

[13] Koudinova N V *et al* 2003 Photodynamic therapy with Pd-bacteriopheophorbide (TOOKAD): successful *in vivo* treatment of human prostatic small cell carcinoma xenografts *Int. J. Cancer* **104** 782–9
[14] Selman S H 2007 Photodynamic therapy for prostate cancer: one urologist's perspective *Photodiagnosis Photodyn. Ther.* **4** 26–30
[15] Azzouzi A-R *et al* 2017 Padeliporfin vascular-targeted photodynamic therapy versus active surveillance in men with low-risk prostate cancer (CLIN1001 PCM301): an open-label, phase 3, randomised controlled trial *Lancet Oncol.* **18** 181–91
[16] Jerjes W *et al* 2010 Clinicopathological parameters, recurrence, locoregional and distant metastasis in 115 T1-T2 oral squamous cell carcinoma patients *Head Neck Oncol.* **2** 9
[17] Lou P-J *et al* 2004 Interstitial photodynamic therapy as salvage treatment for recurrent head and neck cancer *Br. J. Cancer* **91** 441–6
[18] Brown S B, Brown E A and Walker I 2004 The present and future role of photodynamic therapy in cancer treatment *Lancet Oncol.* **5** 497–508
[19] Moan J, Sandberg S, Christensen T and Elander S 1983 Hematoporphyrin derivative: chemical composition, photochemical and photosensitizing properties *Porphyrin Photosensitization* (Springer) pp 165–79
[20] Jasim Z F and Handley J M 2007 Treatment of pulsed dye laser-resistant port wine stain birthmarks *J. Am. Acad. Dermatol.* **57** 677–82
[21] Weersink R A *et al* 2005 Techniques for delivery and monitoring of TOOKAD (WST09)-mediated photodynamic therapy of the prostate: clinical experience and practicalities *J. Photochem. Photobiol.,* B **79** 211–22
[22] Buzzá H H *et al* 2019 Photodynamic therapy versus glucose for the treatment of telangiectasia: a randomised controlled study in a rabbit ear model *Eur. J. Vasc. Endovasc. Surg.* **58** 583–91
[23] Dougherty T J 1984 Photodynamic therapy (PDT) of malignant tumors *Crit. Rev. Oncol. Hematol.* **2** 83–116
[24] Waldow S M, Henderson B W and Dougherty T J 1984 Enhanced tumor control following sequential treatments of photodynamic therapy (PDT) and localized microwave hyperthermia *in vivo Lasers Surg. Med.* **4** 79–85
[25] Dougherty T J *et al* 1998 Photodynamic Therapy *JNCI J. Natl. Cancer Inst.* **90** 889–905
[26] Savelyeva I O, Zhdanova K A, Gradova M A, Gradov O V and Bragina N A 2023 Cationic porphyrins as antimicrobial and antiviral agents in photodynamic therapy *Curr. Issues Mol. Biol.* **45** 9793–822
[27] Frei A, Verderosa A D, Elliott A G, Zuegg J and Blaskovich M A T 2023 Metals to combat antimicrobial resistance *Nat. Rev. Chem.* **7** 202–24
[28] Chen X *et al* 2023 Current and promising applications of Hf(iv)-based MOFs in clinical cancer therapy *J. Mater. Chem.* B **11** 5693–714
[29] Overchuk M, Weersink R A, Wilson B C and Zheng G 2023 Photodynamic and photothermal therapies: synergy opportunities for nanomedicine *ACS Nano* **17** 7979–8003
[30] Aziz B *et al* 2023 An overview of potential natural photosensitizers in cancer photodynamic therapy *Biomedicines* **11** 224
[31] Alvarez N and Sevilla A 2024 Current advances in photodynamic therapy (PDT) and the future potential of PDT-combinatorial cancer therapies *Int. J. Mol. Sci.* **25** 1023
[32] Ochsner M 1997 Photophysical and photobiological processes in the photodynamic therapy of tumours *J. Photochem. Photobiol.,* B **39** 1–18

[33] Moan J and Berg K 1991 The photodegradation of porphyrins in cells can be used to estimate the lifetime of singlet oxygen *Photochem. Photobiol.* **53** 549–53

[34] Chen B, Pogue B W, Hoopes P J and Hasan T 2006 Vascular and cellular targeting for photodynamic therapy *Crit. Rev. Eukaryot Gene Expr.* **16** 279–306

[35] Zhu Y *et al* 2022 Oxygen self-supply engineering-ferritin for the relief of hypoxia in tumors and the enhancement of photodynamic therapy efficacy *Small* **18** e2200116

[36] Udrea A M *et al* 2023 Photosensitizers-loaded nanocarriers for enhancement of photodynamic therapy in melanoma treatment *Pharmaceutics* **15** 2124

[37] Veenstra C *et al* 2019 Quantification of total haemoglobin concentrations in human whole blood by spectroscopic visible-light optical coherence tomography *Sci. Rep.* **9** 15115

[38] Kwon S, Ko H, You D G, Kataoka K and Park J H 2019 Nanomedicines for reactive oxygen species mediated approach: an emerging paradigm for cancer treatment *Acc. Chem. Res.* **52** 1771–82

[39] Ziental D *et al* 2020 Titanium dioxide nanoparticles: prospects and applications in medicine *Nanomaterials* **10** 387

[40] Kaspler P *et al* 2016 A ruthenium(II) based photosensitizer and transferrin complexes enhance photo-physical properties, cell uptake, and photodynamic therapy safety and efficacy *Photochem. Photobiol. Sci.* **15** 481–95

[41] Patterson M S, Wilson B C and Graff R 1990 *In vivo* tests of the concept of photodynamic threshold dose in normal rat liver photosensitized by aluminum chlorosulphonated phthalocyanine *Photochem. Photobiol.* **51** 343–9

[42] Ankathatti Munegowda M, Manalac A, Weersink M, McFarland S A and Lilge L 2022 Ru (II) containing photosensitizers for photodynamic therapy: a critique on reporting and an attempt to compare efficacy *Coord. Chem. Rev.* **470** 214712

[43] Ramadan K T *et al* 2021 Determination of optical properties and photodynamic threshold of lung tissue for treatment planning of *in vivo* lung perfusion assisted photodynamic therapy *Photodiagnosis Photodyn. Ther.* **35** 102353

[44] de Faria C M G, Inada N M, Kurachi C and Bagnato V S 2016 Determination of the threshold dose distribution in photodynamic action from *in vitro* experiments *J. Photochem. Photobiol.,* B **162** 168–75

[45] Lilge L *et al* 1996 The sensitivity of normal brain and intracranially implanted VX2 tumour to interstitial photodynamic therapy *Br. J. Cancer* **73** 332–43

[46] Lilge L D *et al* 1997 Preclinical Studies of Photodynamic Therapy of Intracranial Tissues *Proc. SPIE 2972, Optical Methods for Tumor Treatment and Detection: Mechanisms and Techniques in Photodynamic Therapy VI* T J Dougherty (SPIE) pp 64–73

[47] Chen Q, Chopp M, Madigan L, Dereski M O and Hetzel F W 1996 Damage threshold of normal rat brain in photodynamic therapy *Photochem. Photobiol.* **64** 163–7

[48] Yassine A-A *et al* 2018 Automatic interstitial photodynamic therapy planning via convex optimization *Biomed. Opt. Express* **9** 898

[49] Kareliotis G, Liossi S and Makropoulou M 2018 Assessment of singlet oxygen dosimetry concepts in photodynamic therapy through computational modeling *Photodiagn. Photodyn. Ther.* **21** 224–33

[50] Beeson K *et al* 2022 Photodynamic therapy in a pleural cavity using monte carlo simulations with 2D/3D graphical visualization *Global J. Cancer Ther.* **8** 21–33

[51] Sheng T, Ong Y, Busch T M and Zhu T C 2020 Reactive oxygen species explicit dosimetry to predict local tumor growth for photofrin-mediated photodynamic therapy *Biomed. Opt. Express* **11** 4586
[52] Foster T H *et al* 1991 Oxygen consumption and diffusion effects in photodynamic therapy *Radiat. Res.* **126** 296
[53] Baptista M S, Cadet J, Greer A and Thomas A H 2021 Photosensitization reactions of biomolecules: definition, targets and mechanisms *Photochem. Photobiol.* **97** 1456–83
[54] Escudero A *et al* 2021 Photodynamic therapy: photosensitizers and nanostructures *Mater. Chem. Front.* **5** 3788–812
[55] Baptista M S *et al* 2017 Type I and Type II photosensitized oxidation reactions: guidelines and mechanistic pathways *Photochem. Photobiol.* **93** 912–9
[56] Rousset N *et al* 2000 Use of alkaline comet assay to assess DNA repair after m-THPC-PDT *J. Photochem. Photobiol.,* B **56** 118–31
[57] Yoo J-O and Ha K-S 2012 New insights into the mechanisms for photodynamic therapy-induced cancer cell death *Int. Rev. Cell Mol. Biol.* **295** 139–74
[58] Agostinis P *et al* 2011 Photodynamic therapy of cancer: an update *CA Cancer J. Clin.* **61** 250–81
[59] Castano A P, Demidova T N and Hamblin M R 2005 Mechanisms in photodynamic therapy: part three—photosensitizer pharmacokinetics, biodistribution, tumor localization and modes of tumor destruction *Photodiagnosis Photodyn. Ther.* **2** 91–106
[60] Kaspler P *et al* 2016 Ru(II) complex mediated PDT for bladder cancer, Biology and dosimetry *2016 Int. Conf. Laser Optics (LO)* (Piscataway, NJ: IEEE) p S2–51
[61] Monro S *et al* 2019 Transition metal complexes and photodynamic therapy from a tumor-centered approach: challenges, opportunities, and highlights from the development of TLD1433 *Chem. Rev.* **119** 797–828
[62] Lazic S *et al* 2017 Novel osmium-based coordination complexes as photosensitizers for panchromatic photodynamic therapy *Photochem. Photobiol.* **93** 1248–58
[63] Lovell J F, Jin C, Huynh E *et al* 2011 Porphysome nanovesicles generated by porphyrin bilayers for use as multimodal biophotonic contrast agents *Nat. Mater.* **10** 324–32
[64] Huynh E and Zheng G 2014 Porphysome nanotechnology: a paradigm shift in lipid-based supramolecular structures *Nano Today* **9** 212–22
[65] Valic M S, Fisher C J, Zheng M *et al* 2025 Radiopharmaceutical kit to prepare Copper-64 labelled porphyrin-lipid nanoparticles for radiotracer imaging studies in cancer patients *Eur. J. Nucl. Med. Mol. Imaging*
[66] Sahovaler A, Valic M S, Townson J L *et al* 2024 Nanoparticle-mediated photodynamic therapy as a method to ablate oral cavity squamous cell carcinoma in preclinical models *Cancer Res. Comm.* **4** 796–810
[67] Chen B *et al* 2003 Effect of photodynamic therapy with verteporfin on tumor blood flow *Proc. SPIE 4952, Optical Methods for Tumor Treatment and Detection: Mechanisms and Techniques in Photodynamic Therapy XII* D Kessel (SPIE) p 48
[68] Samkoe K S, Clancy A A, Karotki A, Wilson B C and Cramb D T 2007 Complete blood vessel occlusion in the chick chorioallantoic membrane using two-photon excitation photodynamic therapy: implications for treatment of wet age-related macular degeneration *J. Biomed. Opt.* **12** 034025
[69] Khurana M *et al* 2009 Drug and light dose responses to focal photodynamic therapy of single blood vessels *in vivo J. Biomed. Opt.* **14** 064006

[70] Chen B, Cheng L, Li D, Wu T and Zeng W 2022 Experimental study of combined photodynamic and photothermal therapy in the treatment of port wine stain *Lasers Med. Sci.* **38** 26

[71] Schmidt-Erfurth U *et al* 1996 Benzoporphyrin-lipoprotein-mediated photodestruction of intraocular tumors *Exp. Eye Res.* **62** 1–10

[72] Dogan B *et al* 2023 Optic disc and retinal vessel densities assessment by optical coherence tomography angiography in patients with keratoconus *Photodiagnosis Photodyn. Ther.* **41** 103218

[73] Foster T H and Gao L 1992 Dosimetry in photodynamic therapy: oxygen and the critical importance of capillary density *Radiat. Res.* **130** 379

[74] Webber J, Kessel D and Fromm D 1997 Plasma levels of protoporphyrin IX in humans after oral administration of 5-aminolevulinic acid *J. Photochem. Photobiol.,* B **37** 151–3

[75] O'Connor A E, Gallagher W M and Byrne A T 2009 Porphyrin and nonporphyrin photosensitizers in oncology: preclinical and clinical advances in photodynamic therapy *Photochem. Photobiol.* **85** 1053–74

[76] Baskaran R, Lee J and Yang S-G 2018 Clinical development of photodynamic agents and therapeutic applications *Biomater. Res.* **22** s40824-018-0140-z

[77] Aveline B, Hasan T and Redmond R W 1994 Photophysical and photosensitizing properties of benzoporphyrin derivative monoacid ring a (BPD-MA) *Photochem. Photobiol.* **59** 328–35

[78] Richter A M *et al* 1993 Liposomal delivery of a photosensitizer, benzoporphyrin derivative monoacid ring a (BPD), to tumor tissue in a mouse tumor model *Photochem. Photobiol.* **57** 1000–6

[79] Stratonnikov A A, Douplik A Y, Klimov D V, Loschenov V B and Mizin S V 1998 Influence of light irradiation on blood oxygen saturation level *in vitro* and *in vivo* during photodynamic therapy *Proc. SPIE* **3247** 128–36

[80] Ong Y, Miller J, Zhu T C, Yodh A G and Busch T M 2018 Blood-flow-informed photodynamic therapy (PDT) improves therapeutic efficacy *Biophotonics Congress: Biomedical Optics Congress* (Microscopy/Translational/Brain/OTS) OSA Technical Digest CF2B.6

[81] Ong Y H *et al* 2020 Blood flow measurements enable optimization of light delivery for personalized photodynamic therapy *Cancers (Basel)* **12** 1584

[82] Liu Q, Zhou S, Zhang Z and Luo Q 2005 Laser speckle contrast imaging: monitoring blood flow dynamics and vascular structure of photodynamic therapy *Proc. SPIE* **5630** 26

[83] Kruijt B, de Bruijn H S, van der Ploeg -, van den Heuvel A, Sterenborg H J C M and Robinson D J 2006 Laser speckle imaging of dynamic changes in flow during photodynamic therapy *Lasers Med. Sci.* **21** 208–12

[84] Shao P, Chapman D W, Moore R B and Zemp R J 2015 Monitoring photodynamic therapy with photoacoustic microscopy *J. Biomed. Opt.* **20** 106012

[85] Merdasa A *et al* 2021 Photoacoustic imaging of the spatial distribution of oxygen saturation in an ischemia-reperfusion model in humans *Biomed. Opt. Express* **12** 2484

[86] Saeidi , Foltz T, Zabel W D *et al* 2025 Are blood flow and blood volume predictors of localized photosensitizer accumulation in the brain? *Photodiag. Photody. Ther.* **54** 104689

[87] Li Q-R *et al* 2023 Laser-triggered intelligent drug delivery and anti-cancer photodynamic therapy using platelets as the vehicle *Platelets* **34**

[88] Song Y, Tan X and Gao Y 2022 Platelet-biomimetic nanoparticles for *in vivo* targeted photodynamic therapy of breast cancer *J. Biomater. Sci. Polym. Ed.* **33** 1383–97
[89] Xu H-Z *et al* 2022 Targeted photodynamic therapy of glioblastoma mediated by platelets with photo-controlled release property *Biomaterials* **290** 121833
[90] Povlishock J T, Rosenblum W I, Sholley M M and Wei E P 1983 An ultrastructural analysis of endothelial change paralleling platelet aggregation in a light/dye model of microvascular insult *Am. J. Pathol.* **110** 148–60
[91] Maurer H M, Haggins J C and Still W J S 1976 Platelet injury during phototherapy *Am. J. Hematol.* **1** 89–96
[92] Fungaloi P *et al* 2002 Platelet adhesion to photodynamic therapy-treated extracellular matrix proteins *Photochem. Photobiol.* **75** 412
[93] Teles de Andrade C *et al* 2016 Optical spectroscopy of radiotherapy and photodynamic therapy responses in normal rat skin shows vascular breakdown products *Proc. SPIE* **9694** 10
[94] Frackowiak D *et al* 2001 The interactions of phthalocyanines with stimulated and resting human peripheral blood mononuclear cells *Acta Biochim. Pol.* **48** 257–69
[95] Ignatova A A, Maslova A S, Kirpichnikov M P and Feofanov A V 2009 Interaction of the photosensitizer 13,15-N-(3′-hydroxypropyl)cycloimide chlorin p6 with normal and cancerous blood cells *Russ. J. Bioorg. Chem.* **35** 746–51
[96] Fingar V H *et al* 1999 Analysis of acute vascular damage after photodynamic therapy using benzoporphyrin derivative (BPD) *Br. J. Cancer* **79** 1702–8
[97] Liu Q, Zhou S, Zhang Z and Luo Q 2005 Laser speckle contrast imaging: monitoring blood flow dynamics and vascular structure of photodynamic therapy *Proc. SPIE* **5630** 26
[98] Suzuki T *et al* 2020 Vascular shutdown by photodynamic therapy using talaporfin sodium *Cancers (Basel)* **12** 2369
[99] Chen B, Zupkó I and de Witte P A 2001 Photodynamic therapy with hypericin in a mouse P388 tumor model: vascular effects determine the efficacy *Int. J. Oncol.* **18** 737–42
[100] Wang L, Li L and Huang C 2023 Efficacy of photodynamic therapy in the treatment of port wine stains: a systematic review and meta-analysis *Front. Med.* **10** 1111234
[101] Köse H C and Tekeli O 2022 Comparison of microvascular parameters and diagnostic ability of optical coherence tomography angiography between eyes with primary angle closure glaucoma and primary open angle glaucoma *Photodiagnosis Photodyn. Ther.* **40** 103114
[102] Zou L *et al* 2023 Chlorin e6 (Ce6)-loaded plaque-specific liposome with enhanced photodynamic therapy effect for atherosclerosis treatment *Talanta* **265** 124772
[103] Yang T-S, Hsiao Y-C, Chiang Y-F and Chang C-J 2023 Imaging and histopathological analysis of microvascular angiogenesis in photodynamic therapy for oral cancer *Cancers (Basel)* **15** 1110
[104] Goldschmidt R, Vyacheslav K and Scherz A 2017 Real time laser speckle imaging monitoring vascular targeted photodynamic therapy *Proc. SPIE* **10047** 0M
[105] Cecic I and Korbelik M 2002 Mediators of peripheral blood neutrophilia induced by photodynamic therapy of solid tumors *Cancer Lett.* **183** 43–51
[106] van Straten D, Mashayekhi V, de Bruijn H, Oliveira S and Robinson D 2017 Oncologic photodynamic therapy: basic principles, current clinical status and future directions *Cancers (Basel)* **9** 19

[107] Cecic I, Parkins C S and Korbelik M 2001 Induction of systemic neutrophil response in mice by photodynamic therapy of solid tumors *Photochem. Photobiol.* **74** 712
[108] Korbelik M, Sun J and Cecic I 2005 Photodynamic therapy-induced cell surface expression and release of heat shock proteins: relevance for tumor response *Cancer Res.* **65** 1018–26
[109] Castano A P, Mroz P and Hamblin M R 2006 Photodynamic therapy and anti-tumour immunity *Nat. Rev. Cancer* **6** 535–45
[110] Reginato E 2014 Immune response after photodynamic therapy increases anti-cancer and anti-bacterial effects *World J. Immunol.* **4** 1–11
[111] Garg A D, Nowis D, Golab J and Agostinis P 2010 Photodynamic therapy: illuminating the road from cell death towards anti-tumour immunity *Apoptosis* **15** 1050–71
[112] Garg A D *et al* 2010 Immunogenic cell death, DAMPs and anticancer therapeutics: an emerging amalgamation *Biochim. Biophys. Acta (BBA)—Rev. Cancer* **1805** 53–71
[113] de Vree W J *et al* 1996 Evidence for an important role of neutrophils in the efficacy of photodynamic therapy *in vivo Cancer Res.* **56** 2908–11
[114] Griffith T S *et al* 2007 Apoptotic cells induce tolerance by generating helpless CD8 + T cells that produce TRAIL *J. Immunol.* **178** 2679–87
[115] Reginato E *et al* 2013 Photodynamic therapy plus regulatory T-cell depletion produces immunity against a mouse tumour that expresses a self-antigen *Br. J. Cancer* **109** 2167–74
[116] Kobayashi W *et al* 2004 Photodynamic therapy upregulates expression of Mac-1 and generation of leukotriene B4 by human polymorphonuclear leukocytes *Oral Oncol.* **40** 506–10
[117] Chen D, Ren J, Wang Y, Li B and Gu Y 2016 Intraoperative monitoring of blood perfusion in port wine stains by laser Doppler imaging during vascular targeted photodynamic therapy: A preliminary study *Photodiagnosis Photodyn. Ther.* **14** 142–51
[118] Abe H *et al* 2000 Elimination of both cell-free and cell-associated HIV infectivity in plasma by a filtration/methylene blue photoinactivation system *Transfusion (Paris)* **40** 1081–7
[119] Wagner S J *et al* 2000 The use of dimethylmethylene blue for virus photoinactivation of red cell suspensions *Dev. Biol. (Basel)* **102** 125–9
[120] Floyd R A, Schneider J E and Dittmer D P 2004 Methylene blue photoinactivation of RNA viruses *Antiviral. Res.* **61** 141–51
[121] Alanazi R S and Laref A 2022 Monte Carlo simulations of photodynamic therapy in human blood model *Lasers Med. Sci.* **37** 1515–29
[122] Alfred A *et al* 2017 The role of extracorporeal photopheresis in the management of cutaneous T-cell lymphoma, graft-versus-host disease and organ transplant rejection: a consensus statement update from the UK Photopheresis Society *Br. J. Haematol.* **177** 287–310
[123] Darvekar S *et al* 2020 Selective killing of activated T cells by 5-aminolevulinic acid mediated photodynamic effect: potential improvement of extracorporeal photopheresis *Cancers (Basel)* **12** 377
[124] Yin H *et al* 2014 Preliminary safety evaluation of photodynamic therapy for blood purification: an animal study *Artif. Organs* **38** 510–5
[125] Spampinato C and Leonardi D 2013 Candida infections, causes, targets, and resistance mechanisms: traditional and alternative antifungal agents *BioMed. Res. Int.* **2013** 204237
[126] Jenkins M P *et al* 2002 Clinical study of adjuvant photodynamic therapy to reduce restenosis following femoral angioplasty *BR. J. Surg.* **86** 1258–63
[127] Usui M *et al* 2004 A first trial in the clinical application of photodynamic therapy for the prevention of restenosis after coronary-stent placement *Lasers Surg. Med.* **34** 235–41

[128] Kereiakes D J *et al* 2003 Phase I drug and light dose-escalation trial of motexafin lutetium and far red light activation (phototherapy) in subjects with coronary artery disease undergoing percutaneous coronary intervention and stent deployment *Circulation* **108** 1310–5
[129] Allison B A *et al* 1997 Delivery of benzoporphyrin derivative, a photosensitizer, into atherosclerotic plaque of watanabe heritable hyperlipidemic rabbits and balloon-injured New Zealand rabbits *Photochem. Photobiol.* **65** 877–83
[130] Hsiang Y N *et al* 1993 *In vitro* AND *in vivo* uptake of benzoporphyrin derivative into human and miniswine atherosclerotic plaque *Photochem. Photobiol.* **57** 670–4
[131] Jain M *et al* 2016 Intra-arterial drug and light delivery for photodynamic therapy using visudyne®: implication for atherosclerotic plaque treatment *Front. Physiol.* **7**
[132] Waksman R *et al* 2008 Photopoint photodynamic therapy promotes stabilization of atherosclerotic plaques and inhibits plaque progression *J. Am. Coll. Cardiol.* **52** 1024–32
[133] LaMuraglia G M *et al* 1994 Photodynamic therapy inhibition of experimental intimal hyperplasia: acute and chronic effects *J. Vasc. Surg.* **19** 321–31
[134] Nyamekye I *et al* 1996 Inhibition of intimal hyperplasia in balloon injured arteries with adjunctive phthalocyanine sensitised photodynamic therapy *Eur. J. Vasc. Endovasc. Surg.* **11** 19–28
[135] Nagae T *et al* 2001 Endovascular photodynamic therapy using mono-L-aspartyl-chlorin e6 to inhibit Intimal hyperplasia in balloon-injured rabbit arteries *Lasers Surg. Med.* **28** 381–8
[136] Qureshi M M *et al* 2023 Advances in laser speckle imaging: from qualitative to quantitative hemodynamic assessment *J. Biophotonics* **17** e202300126
[137] Vogeser M *et al* 2005 Development of an HPLC method for monitoring of Photofrin II therapy *Clin. Biochem.* **38** 73–8
[138] Igbaseimokumo U 2004 Quantification of *in vivo* Photofrin uptake by human pituitary adenoma tissue *J. Neurosurg.* **101** 272–7
[139] Yumita N *et al* 2004 Sonodynamic therapy on chemically induced mammary tumor: pharmacokinetics, tissue distribution and sonodynamically induced antitumor effect of porfimer sodium *Cancer Sci.* **95** 765–9
[140] Peng Q *et al* 1991 Sensitizer for photodynamic therapy of cancer: a comparison of the tissue distribution of Photofrin II and aluminum phthalocyanine tetrasulfonate in nude mice bearing a human malignant tumor *Int. J. Cancer* **48** 258–64
[141] Bellnier D A *et al* 2006 Clinical pharmacokinetics of the PDT photosensitizers porfimer sodium (photofrin), 2-[1-hexyloxyethyl]-2-devinyl pyropheophorbide-a (photochlor) and 5-ALA-induced protoporphyrin IX *Lasers Surg. Med.* **38** 439–44
[142] Richter A M *et al* 1990 Biodistribution of tritiated benzoporphyrin derivative (3H-BPD-MA), a new potent photosensitizer, in normal and tumor-bearing mice *J. Photochem. Photobiol. B, Biol.* **5** 231–44
[143] Busetti A *et al* 1999 High efficiency of benzoporphyrin derivative in the photodynamic therapy of pigmented malignant melanoma *Br. J. Cancer* **79** 821–4
[144] Chen B and de Witte P A 2000 Photodynamic therapy efficacy and tissue distribution of hypericin in a mouse P388 lymphoma tumor model *Cancer Lett.* **150** 111–7
[145] Jones H J, Vernon D I and Brown S B 2003 Photodynamic therapy effect of m-THPC (foscan) *in vivo*: correlation with pharmacokinetics *Br. J. Cancer* **89** 398–404
[146] Busch T M *et al* 2010 Increasing damage to tumor blood vessels during motexafin lutetium-PDT through use of low fluence rate *Radiat. Res.* **174** 331–40

IOP Publishing

The Optics of Blood
A Handbook
Alexandre Douplik

Chapter 12

Photobiomodulation exposure of blood and its components: from local to systemic effects

Lothar Lilge

12.1 Introduction

Photobiomodulation (PBM), formerly also referred to as low-level laser therapy (LLLT), low-intensity laser therapy (LILT), and other terms, is part of phototherapy therapies that have been employed for medical indications such as vitiligo and psoriasis over several millennia. PBM refers to light-driven endogenous photochemical reactions that impact overall cell metabolism, ranging from increased ATP production to the induction of DNA strand breaks, which can result in cell death. Given the currently available photon sources, PBM encompasses the optical wavelength spectrum from 222 to 1064 nm. PBM should not cause a thermal elevation of the tissue target, and thus, a common upper limit is given by the solar irradiance at sea level, generally around $0.2\ \mathrm{W \cdot cm^{-2}}$. Thermal effects can occur at irradiances as low as $50\ \mathrm{mW \cdot cm^{-2}}$, albeit it is not known if these are direct thermal effects or are subsequent to improved microcirculatory flow [1].

Across the optical spectrum, the photon's quantum energy determines the photochemistry that can be executed by the biomolecule acting as the absorber.

The use of UV light for sterilization is now well-established [2, 3]. Cutaneous synthesis of previtamin D3 from 7-dehydrocholesterol by exposure to ultraviolet photons with λ 290–320 nm, whereby the exposure levels required present approximately 25% of the minimum erythematic dose (MED) covering a quarter of a person's skin surface to produce the equivalent of 1000 IU of vitamin D [4].

Biologically active chromophores susceptible to activation or inhibition by visible and NIR photons have been identified. Cryptochromes and flavoproteins absorb blue wavelengths. Type II cryptochromes found in vertebrates are known to couple the circadian clock to metabolism via glucocorticoid receptors and thus are considered clock proteins. While their circadian functions can occur independently of light, their clock speed can be influenced by the absorption of photons.

doi:10.1088/978-0-7503-4806-5ch12

Photoexcitation of flavoproteins [5], the flavin cofactors, leads to changes in redox and protonation states that remodel protein conformation and molecular interactions across a diverse family of proteins.

Green wavelengths, λ = 510–565 nm, play a crucial role in the trans-cis isomerization of opsins. These are G-protein-coupled receptors that become light-sensitive through A Retinal. Opsins are found in the retina's photoreceptor cells and are instrumental in vision, facilitating the conversion of photons into electrochemical signals. Melanopsin, a type of opsin, is involved in circadian rhythms and pupillary reflexes. Opsins have been engineered to absorb different wavelengths and are the foundation of optogenetics, a key tool in neurobiology [6].

Red/NIR wavelengths overlap with the absorption spectrum of complex IV, cytochrome c oxidase (CCO), [7, 8] of the mitochondrial respiratory chain across the 620–930 nm range. CCO transfers an electron from cytochrome c to oxygen as part of the respiratory redox cycle. The chromophore's color centers are generated through the presence of two heme groups (heme a and heme b) and two copper centers (Cu_A and Cu_B) in the enzyme. Heme, a metalloprotein, has an extremely short, excited-state lifetime of <230 ps, as measured by two-photon fluorescence spectroscopy. It is photochemically inert but involves other metabolic pathways, such as oxidative phosphorylation.

Heme exists in both reduced and oxidized forms, with absorption in their Soret bands at 430 and 415 nm, and in their Q-bands at 555 and 542/576 nm, respectively. Heme is metabolically active and involved in oxygen transport beyond the CCO, as it integrates into hemoglobins, and is of central importance to oxidative phosphorylation and metabolic regulation. The additional color centers of CCO are two copper metal centers, both absorbing in their reduced and oxidized forms, for CuA at 620 and 820 nm, and Cu_B at 760 and 680 nm, respectively [9]. CCO is a strong, biologically active absorber given its high molar extinction coefficient, ε, and its high *in vivo* concentrations ranging from 6.5 mM (rat brains) to 70 mg g^{-1} dry weight in human skeletal muscle [10], resulting in an absorption probability of $\sim$1500 cm^{-1}. Augmentation of the respiratory redox efficacy by the added photon quantum energy results in the generation of ATP, reactive oxygen species (ROS), and release of NO, a known vasodilator that leads to increased tissue perfusion and additionally impacts the lymphatics by dilating the vessels and reducing their porosity. The generation of Ca^{2+} as an intracellular messenger leads to the activation of transcription factors such as NF-κB and AP-1, which in turn result in the up- or downregulation of gene expression via the AMPK and Akt pathways [11]. The release of Ca^{2+} can also result from photon absorption by ion channels, albeit at shorter wavelengths.

Absorption of NIR photons resulting in thermal activation of heat-gated ion channels has also been demonstrated, whereby bound water in the immediate vicinity of the ion channels is the primary absorber. These photothermal effects can occur at irradiances below 0.2 W $\cdot$ cm^{-2}, so the literature is somewhat fluent regarding these limits.

A red and NIR photon's quantum energy is insufficient for electronic excitation of the primary chromophore and, hence, cis-trans isomerization, as in the case of the opsins, and activation of higher vibrational states, as in the case of NIR absorption by bound water, remains feasible. The conformational changes following cis-trans isomerization are sensed by a secondary protein, such as retinal in the case of the opsins, which augments the electronic excitation and converts it for further biological activities. In the case of thermal activation, the ion channel function is strongly temperature-dependent.

As PBM is most often delivered via the skin, looking at other essential chromophores and their potential biological activity is advisable. Eumelanin and pheomelanin, responsible for the brown and reddish/yellow skin color, respectively, are now considered as composed of stacked oligomeric 'proto-molecules' with overlapping π/π^* orbitals, resulting in a rapid non-radiative energy-transfer between proto-molecules and ultimate thermal conversion of the photon's quantum energy [12]. This is also reflected by the extremely low fluorescence quantum yield $\Phi_{fl} < 7 \times 10^{-4}$ following UV excitation [13].

While hemoglobins deoxy (Hb_{deox}) and oxy (Hb_{ox}) are the dominant absorbers in the skin, other potential absorbers are still under investigation, including proteins undergoing conformational changes, forming dimers, tetramers, or larger aggregates, and are involved in transcription, such as the glucocorticoid receptor and others.

12.2 Delivery of photobiomodulation

There are no limitations on the light sources used in PBM, with respect to wavelength, pulsed versus continuous wave emission, power P [W] emitted, or exposure time t [s], resulting in energy E [J] and frequency of the light illumination sessions. However, there are limits on the irradiance, Φ [mW $\cdot$ cm^{-2}], or power density at the tissue surface, and thus the attainable radiant exposure, $\boldsymbol{H}$, or energy density delivered to the tissue surface. Φ needs to be low enough to prevent a macroscopic, biologically significant temperature increase. For Φ exceeding the solar irradiance constant, $\sim$200 mW $\cdot$ cm^{-2}, the skin's intrinsic cooling mechanisms, diffusion, and convection can no longer maintain normal organ temperature, and thermal effects must be considered when evaluating tissue responses.

Light illumination is typically performed via small points, such as at known acupuncture points, or over larger areas when targeting muscle groups, or in pain management. Multiple illumination points are targeted simultaneously or sequentially for skeletal joints or larger organs. Irradiances of less than 10 mW $\cdot$ cm^{-2} to an excess of 500 mW $\cdot$ cm^{-2} and radiant exposures between 0.1 and >80 J $\cdot$ cm^{-2} can be found in the literature. Depending on the indication, PBM is delivered only once or repeatedly, ranging from once daily to 2–3 times per week for several weeks for indications such as wound healing or neurodegenerative preventive therapy [26].

Reports of a biphasic tissue response indicate that, for a range of low irradiance and radiance exposure, PBM can result in favorable outcomes versus unfavorable or detrimental outcomes at higher irradiances or radiant exposures, providing a biological response limit to the PBM treatment parameters [14, 15]. Hence, when developing PBM protocols, the irradiance and radiant exposure must be matched for a given indication and the employed wavelength.

12.3 Current indications

The current indications can be found predominantly in pain management, wound healing, traumatic brain injury, stroke, and neurodegenerative diseases, accelerating exercise muscle recovery, and the management of treatment-related morbidities, particularly in oncology, as well as in some cosmetic indications.

12.3.1 Pain management

PBM pain relief is one of the most common uses of PBM. The patient reports modification of pain sensation subjectively using the visual analog scale [16]. However, biomarkers from serum levels, such as reductions in TNF- and IL-8, are also reported [17].

Randomized clinical studies related to pain relief have been performed for low back pain [18], in women post-cesarean section [19], simple tooth extraction [20], hip replacement [17], migraine relief [17], and now oncological indications [21], among others [22, 23]. Visual light exposure to reduce pain conditions, including migraines and fibromyalgia, was demonstrated only with green light (wavelengths of 520–550 nm). Cutaneous photon delivery is generally limited to 10–30 s, or at most a couple of minutes per point, whereas visual application requires hours of exposure. Pain management is ultimately achieved by modifying signal transduction centrally in the brainstem and spinal cord, as well as peripherally at the root ganglia and nociceptor levels [24].

12.3.2 Wound healing

The most frequently investigated wounds are acute skin incisions, which typically show an initial accelerated wound closure rate. However, at later times in the healing process, the difference in wound area is no longer statistically significant, suggesting a saturation of the PBM effect for repeat irradiation sessions [25]. Wounds in bone, muscle, burns, and skin grafts are repeatedly investigated, employing a variety of wavelengths and irradiation protocols. The effect of PBM in infected wounds was recently reviewed for a range of treatment wavelengths [26].

Blood serum and tissue biopsies are collected for analysis to quantify the PBM effect. Upregulation of the adenosine, GH, and FGF levels has been reported [27]. PBM in diabetic murine wounds reduced the expression of MMP-2 and MMP-9, resulting in a redistribution of collagen types I and III [28–30]. In burn wounds, PBM demonstrated equal efficacy in healing compared to sodium alginate/chitosan-based films, as evaluated by epithelialization, blood vessel formation, and collagenization processes [31]. Angiogenesis is often among the biological effects reported; see below for the effects of PBM on vascularity and angiogenesis.

12.3.3 Traumatic brain injury, stroke, and neurodegenerative diseases

The use of PBM in the brain is motivated by the knowledge that mitochondrial dysfunction plays a key role in neurodegeneration. Given the localization of CCO on the inner mitochondrial membrane, PBM presents a logical option for mitigating retinal and brain damage subsequent to mitochondrial failure [32–35]. PBM stimulates anti-inflammatory, anti-apoptotic, and antioxidant responses by enhancing the metabolic capacity of neurons and astrocytes. It is also said to initiate neurogenesis and synaptogenesis. PBM has been shown to increase regional blood flow [36] and cerebral tissue oxygenation, as well as improve memory and cognitive function [37] in young volunteers and the elderly with aged brains [37]. However, detailed studies of the sequence of events are not available. Is the increased regional cerebral blood flow a cause or an effect of improved cognitive function, neurogenesis, and synaptogenesis?

Clinical studies in stroke patients and patients with traumatic brain injury have been performed, whereby murine studies with focal ischemic damage suggest that PBM can protect the blood–brain barrier (BBB) and thus reduce neuroinflammation by limiting leukocyte infiltration [38].

By now, it is well-documented that seasonal affective disorder can be mitigated by exposing the patient to a bright, diffuse light source for more than 1 h per day [39]. Here, PBM acts via the visual stimulation pathway. Similarly, clinical PBM pilot studies in patients suffering from major depression and anxiety [40] showed that irradiation of the forehead resulted for $\sim$60% of the participants in an immediate psychological improvement, accompanied by an increase in frontal lobe regional cerebral blood flow [41]. A review by Semyachkina-Glushkovskaya *et al* [42] suggests a range of potential mechanisms beyond those listed above, some of which are strongly interrelated, including increased angiogenesis and lymphatic drainage, as well as improved neuroprotection through increases in the antioxidants SOD, survivin, and BCL2. PBM-induced reduction of glutamate caused excitotoxicity. Additionally, activation of brain repair pathways via neurotrophins, including BDNF, NGF, and NT-3, as well as neuroprogenitor cells, was observed [36].

Not all neurodegenerative diseases or their symptoms have been successfully treated with PBM at this time. One example is fatigue in patients with relapsing-remitting multiple sclerosis, where no clinical or quality-of-life beneficial effects could be demonstrated [32].

12.3.4 Muscle recovery

Delivering PBM prior to or after exercise demonstrated an increase in the number of repetitions at 80% of max load, or for a fixed number of contractions, an increase in the mean work performed was noted. Simultaneously, blood lactate levels were significantly reduced, allowing for shorter recovery periods between workouts. For some protocols, the post-exercise creatine kinase level was also reduced [43, 96].

12.3.5 Cancer therapy-related morbidities

Clinical application of PBM in oncology is currently dominated as an adjuvant to prevent or mitigate therapy-induced morbidity following radiation therapy, chemotherapy, or hematopoietic stem cell transplantation [44]. The most researched indications are acute oral mucositis [45, 46] and epithelitis. For the latter, the randomized phase III TRANSDERMIS showed that PBM is an effective supportive care method to prevent acute radiodermatitis in adjuvant breast cancer radiotherapy [47]. Dysphagia may be diagnosed in two-thirds of head and neck cancer patients and can persist for the mid- and long-term, commonly causing or promoting severe complications such as mucositis [48] or pneumonitis in up to 20% of patients [49]. PBM decreased the incidence of acute dysphagia and opioid use for pain management. Xerostomia or abnormal dryness of the mouth occurs in over 75% of patients after radiotherapy for head and neck cancer, reduced to 30% in intensity-modulated conformal radiation therapy [50].

12.3.6 Cosmetic indications

Cosmetic indications present the next frontier for PBM, mainly related to body contouring, where areas with excess subcutaneous adipose tissue are targeted with large areas emitting photon sources or scanning devices. Some clinical studies have shown that a radiant exposure of 10 J cm^{-2} at 635 nm, three times per week, reduced the waist, hip, and upper thigh circumference within two weeks. The proposed mechanism pertains to achieving leakiness of the adipocyte's plasma membrane [50].

12.4 Short critical comments on the state of PBM

Research into PBM has primarily evolved into an industry-led effort, which presents several challenges. First, the companies involved generally cannot afford large-scale, double-blinded studies. Hence, most published clinical trials comprise only a moderate number of participants, with some exceptions, including the NEST-1, NEST-2, and NEST-3 clinical trials in stroke patients [51–54]. The two smaller clinical trials, NEST-1 and NEST-2, showed a PBM benefit. In contrast, the last and largest trial had to be terminated early, based on the recommendation of the data monitoring board, because the effect size could not be demonstrated with high significance.

Given the ANSI Z136.3 Standards [55] or the safe exposure of skin, which now also includes bright photon sources such as LEDs, too many *ex vivo* and *in vivo* publications are still listed under the PBM header when the irradiances significantly exceed the prescribed limits, thus also inducing photothermal effects. These studies do not allow for the separation of photonic and thermal effects following exposure to blood or blood products. This happens when Class IV lasers are employed as photon sources. Studies quoting irradiances above the solar irradiance constant, $\sim$200 mW $\cdot$ cm^{-2}, should be considered cautiously. Claims that lasers are essential for PBM are also not supported, as spatial and temporal coherence are rapidly lost. The coherence length, L, is given by $L = \frac{c}{\pi \Delta v}$ with v being the optical bandwidth typically defined through the cavity length. A HeNe laser with a bandwidth of 1 MHz can have a coherence length of up to 1000 m, whereas the bandwidth of most diode lasers is in the high GHz or THz, and a coherence length of $\ll$ 1 cm.

Loss of coherence in biological tissue is due to a rapid increase in beam divergence induced by light scattering and, more importantly, due to motion and flow, predominantly by blood, within the treatment tissue volume [56]. This added randomization of the photon direction results in a rapid loss of spatial and temporal coherence after a path length of a couple of 100 μm in biological tissue. In highly perfused tissues, the loss of coherence after the tissue surface is the strongest. Hence, beyond a depth of 100–200 μm, the potential benefit of a laser's coherence is lost, and LEDs can provide similar efficacy.

The two effects that could cause efficacy differences between LEDs and Lasers are the angle of incidence and monochromatic versus polychromatic illumination.

For the former, it was demonstrated that exploiting the spatial coherence of a laser prior to entering the biological tissue and aligning the beam with the normal relative to the tissue's surface provides a slightly deeper depth distribution of the fluence rate. As LEDs inherently have a diverging beam, fewer photons enter the tissue surface normally and therefore cannot achieve the same depth distribution.

The difference for the latter stems from the fact that PBM is based on quantum effects. That is, photons need to be absorbed by the target chromophore to initiate a photochemical or photothermal-mediated downstream biological effect. Hence, the absorption probability of the sum of all LED polychromatic photons needs to be equal to that of the monochromatic photons from a laser. In particular, for high-power LEDs, having a wider spectral bandwidth, this is often not the case.

12.5 Light propagation in turbid media and biological tissue primer

The photon scattering and absorption probabilities govern light propagation in turbid media, the former being given by the scattering coefficient, μ_s, and the absorption coefficient, μ_a, both with units of inverse distance, commonly expressed in [cm^{-1}] or the probability to undergo a scattering or absorption event, respectively. At its core is the radiative transport equation,

$$\begin{aligned}\frac{1}{c}\frac{\partial L(\vec{r}, \hat{s}, t)}{\partial t} = &- \nabla \cdot L(\vec{r}, \hat{s}, t)\hat{s} - \mu_t L(\vec{r}, \hat{s}, t) \\ &+ \mu_s \int_{4\pi} L(\vec{r}, \hat{s}', t) f(\hat{s}, \hat{s}')\mathrm{d}\Omega' + S(\vec{r}, \hat{s}, t),\end{aligned} \tag{12.1}$$

where $\hat{s}$ is the direction of the light irradiance L, $\vec{r}$ is the spatial location, t is the time, f is the scattering function from direction $\hat{s}'$ into direction $\hat{s}$, Ω is the solid angle, $\mu_t = \mu_s + \mu_a$ is the total attenuation coefficient. No easily workable solutions to the transport equation are available; hence, to calculate the power and energy densities below the surface, approximate analytical and numerical methods are employed. Analytical methods are derivatives of the transport equation; in particular, the diffusion solution and numerical methods are based either on finite element implementation of the diffusion solution or Monte Carlo methods. Nevertheless, studies are ongoing to find solutions for the radiative transport equation for certain tissue geometries [57, 58].

In its simplest form, the one-dimensional steady-state diffusion equation for a point source in an infinite medium,

$$\phi(\vec{r}) = \frac{\Phi_o}{4 \cdot \pi \cdot D \cdot \vec{r}} \cdot e^{-\mu_{\text{eff}} \cdot \vec{r}} \tag{12.2}$$

or the general solution of the diffusion equation to calculate the temporal and spatial evolution of the photon density or fluence rate

$$\phi(\vec{r}, t; \vec{r}', t') = \frac{c}{[4\pi Dc(t - t')]^{3/2}} e^{\left[-\frac{|\vec{r}-\vec{r}'|^2}{4Dc(t-t')}\right]} e^{[-\mu_a c(t-t')]} \tag{12.3}$$

with $D = \frac{1}{3\mu_{tr}} = \frac{1}{3(\mu_a + \mu_{s'})} = \frac{1}{3(\mu_a + (\mu_s(1-g)))}$ wherein g represents the average cosine of the light scattering angle and $\mu_{\text{eff}} = \sqrt{3\mu_a(\mu_a + \mu_{s'})}$ denotes the effective attenuation coefficient of the tissue, whereby the inverse of μ_{eff} is defined as the light penetration depth into a tissue or the distance at which the fluence rate has dropped to 37% of the initial value.

Numerical solutions of the photon transport are widely available and require an *in silico* model of the tissues involved in the planning treatment volume, absorption and scattering coefficients for these tissues, in conjunction with one of the open source or online Monte Carlo simulators [59] including MCX [60, 61], FullMonte [62, 63] and Cloud Monte Carlo [64, 65].

Knowing the light propagation in biological tissues is important because the depth of the clinical target under the skin depends on the body shape, that is, BMI, muscle mass, and water lipid ratios in the tissues. Hence, the fluence and fluence rate at the clinical target can vary widely between patients. However, the empirically derived PBM treatment protocols consider body shapes and other confounders, such as age and skin type [66], only in the broadest of categories, varying the radiant exposure by a factor of less than a factor 5, despite the skin-to-target depth can vary easily over 4 or more optical penetration depth.

Another unsolved issue in PBM is the lack of knowledge regarding the required number of photons to be absorbed and the rate of photon absorption at the clinical target, which is necessary to elucidate the desired biological response. While the required fluence rate or photon density could be determined using 3D imaging of the planning treatment volume and simulations of the photon propagation within this volume, it needs to be correlated with a reported clinical outcome.

If the clinical response is mediated by photon absorption in the blood, one needs to additionally consider the mean and range of the blood's transit time through the planning treatment volume. The issue with blood transition through the treatment volume is that it depends on the ratio of capillaries and major vessels therein. Hence, determining the required photon density of fluence for blood-mediated PBM requires not only anatomical imaging but also functional imaging that provides blood flow and volume information.

12.6 Blood as an impediment to local PBM therapy

PBM is reported to have both local and systemic effects on biological processes. When talking about locally induced modification to biological processes, the effective depth-dependent PBM dose is given by the absorber concentration, its molar extinction coefficient, and the photon density according to equation (12.2). The effective attenuation over the commonly used PBM spectral range from 600 to 900 nm, $\mu_{\text{eff}}(\lambda) = \sqrt{3\mu_a(\lambda)(\mu_a(\lambda) + \mu_{s'}(\lambda))}$ is weakly modified by $\mu_{s'}(\lambda) = a(\frac{\lambda}{500\text{ nm}})^{-b}$ [67], with a and b in muscle reported by Jacques to be 13.0 cm^{-1} and 0.926, respectively; equivalent to only a ~30% reduction in $\mu_{s'}$. The absorption coefficient $\mu_a(\lambda) = \sum \mu_{a,\,x}(\lambda)$, whereby x represents all major absorber, including the hemoglobins, CCO, and other tissue chromophores, can span close to three orders of magnitude across the same wavelength range.

Considering CCO as the primary absorber, which causes modulation of the post-exercise muscle recovery time, only the fraction of photons absorbed by it can initiate the desired effect. The molar absorption coefficient of CCO in both its oxidized and reduced forms exceeds that of the hemoglobins significantly across this wavelength range. Using 800 nm at the isosbestic point for oxy and deoxyhemoglobin, the reduced form of CCO is about seven times higher, and the oxidized CCO is close to 1000 times higher. However, given its limited concentration (for example, ~45 ng ml^{-1} in skeletal muscle and ~35 ng ml^{-1} in heart muscle equivalent to 2.25 and 1.75 μM, respectively) versus the higher hemoglobin concentration (~0.2 mM) indicates that a considerable fraction of the photons is lost due to blood, particular when a high fraction of reduced CCO is present in mitochondria. The high concentration of hemoglobin in blood and its contribution to the tissue's μ_a across the PBM wavelength range results in a higher μ_{eff} and consequently steeper $\phi(\vec{r})$ gradient limiting the effective PBM target depth.

To reach deep-seated targets, PBM can exploit longer wavelengths as long as the absorber's extinction coefficient is not too low, resulting in long exposure times or the need for higher irradiances. The potential thermal effects caused by high irradiances are, in turn, partially mitigated by convective cooling provided by the blood flow across the light irradiation volume. The maximum permissible exposure of skin, according to the ANSI z136.3 standard [55], should not be exceeded as thermal effects will become evident, and separation of photophysical/photochemical from photothermal effects will become difficult.

12.7 Blood and blood components following PBM

In most cases, it is very difficult to assess if changes observed in blood cells, plasma, or platelets are due to direct photobiological effects on these blood components or if the modifications are a response to changes in the surrounding tissue's metabolism and signaling. *In vivo*, it is impossible to expose only the vasculature to light, as the penetration depth, even of blue light, is larger than the majority of arteries and veins proximal to the skin surface. Conversely, exposing harvested blood to external stressors prior to re-administration immune modulation (i.m.) is a well-documented i.m. therapy, whereby the stressor can also include UV and NIR light. Applying multiple stressors, UVC, NIR, and ozone *ex vivo* and re-administration i.m. was shown to cause downregulation of proinflammatory cytokines and upregulation of anti-inflammatory cytokines [68].

Various studies investigated the effects of PBM on erythrocytes, leukocytes, and platelets *in vitro*. If the biological findings of these studies are also relevant to *in vitro* PBM of whole blood or *in vivo*, it is unclear at present.

12.7.1 Erythrocytes

PBM of whole blood can result in both increased proliferation and resistance to oxidative stress, as indicated by reduced hemolysis. Reduction of hemolysis was noticed throughout the NIR spectral range and exposures for a few minutes; however, longer exposure reversed the beneficial effects, and lysis increased beyond that of control samples. Of note is that these effects would be observed for exposure limited to individual wavelengths in the 750–900 nm range or broadband illumination, suggesting that a particular chromophore responsible for the observed effects could be identified [69]. The observation that pulsed light delivery permits increased fluence delivery compared to continuous wave delivery suggests that internal conversion of photon energy is the dominant photophysical, rather than photochemical, effect driving PBM. While both the oxidized and reduced forms of heme absorb throughout the 750–1000 nm range (molar extinction coefficients are in the 200–2000 cm^{-1} M^{-1} range), heme has a very short singlet excited-state lifetime in the sub-nanosecond domain, suggesting internal conversion and local thermal effects as a driving mechanism.

Increases in the erythrocyte and hemoglobin concentration were also noted following the illumination of arteries and veins transcutaneously. Dos Santos Malavazzi *et al* [69] achieved their observation by delivering 80 J $\cdot$ cm^{-2}, 780 nm radiation to the base of a rat tail following a cryoinjury-induced acute muscle damage. The non-PBM treated animals did not show the same erythrocyte concentration increase. The differential in erythrocyte and hemoglobin concentration is credited for reduced inflammation at the muscle damage site and accelerated repair, as the PBM irradiation location was not within the muscle damage site, the effects mediated by blood act systemically.

A similar systemic effect of PBM was noted by Pereira *et al* [70] in pneumonia patients whose thorax is illuminated by 300 LEDs emitting 5400 J at 940 nm. Here, the increase in erythrocytes was accompanied by a statistically significant reduction of lymphocytes and leukocytes.

These observations of increased erythrocytes and hemoglobin could also contribute to the improved blood oxygen saturation in the brains of Alzheimer's disease mice following transcranial illumination of the brain with 1267 nm light, up to 32 J cm^{-2} each day, for up to 9 days [71]. The activation of the cerebral lymphatics also facilitated the clearance of the beta-amyloid from the mice's brains.

12.7.2 Platelets

While for erythrocytes the observation of independent groups are all pointing to an increased concentration post-PBM, the observations for platelets are more diverse.

Exposing platelet-rich plasma (PRP) derived from human blood sustained and controlled release of growth factors following exposure to a broadband light source (600–1200 nm) for 10 min. The observed effects were increased ATP secretion and calcium release, followed by lamellipodia extension, filopodia formation, and agglomeration, indicating platelet activation. The growth factor release was sustained for up to 28 days [72] to support accelerated healing of wounds.

Conversely, Jadah *et al* [73] investigated the effects of 650 nm radiation (130 mW · cm^{-2} for 30 s) irradiation of autologous PRP injected into the knee to mitigate osteoarthritis and noted an inhibition of PRP release growth factors. Here, the reduction of growth factors is seen as a contributing factor to the accelerated healing of osteoarthritis.

In vitro, whole blood irradiation with broadband visible and NIR light (400–1000 nm) at irradiances from 0.75–50 mW · cm^{-2} for up to 8 h noted a 35% drop in platelets at 2 h and also a significant platelet inhibition for irradiances >1.5 mW · cm^{-2}. This was accompanied by changes in discoid platelet shape and reduced aggregation. No change in hemolysis was noted for the first 5 h of 1.5 mW · cm^{-2} irradiation compared to the control group; however, hemolysis increased at later time points [67].

12.7.3 Oxygen saturation

An increase in blood oxygenation, as reported by Semyachkina-Glushkovskaya *et al* [71] was also noted by other groups [74–81]. This is potentially due to the body's autoregulation following increased oxygen consumption following light absorption by cytochrome c oxidase, causing nitric oxide dissociation from heme and copper binding sites, permitting the binding of oxygen [78]. Hence, oxygen saturation of the blood must be seen as a transient mechanism; however, it may also have systemic effects.

12.7.4 Nitric oxide signaling

904 nm mediated PBM delivering 130 J to the femur muscle prior to a workout can mediate post-exercise fatigue, which is thought to cause systemic NO release, a known signaling molecule related to blood pressure [35]. 660 nm mediated PBM was shown by Oishi *et al* [79] to prevent blood pressure increase in a murine obesity model delivering 5.6 J across six illumination spots three times per week. The blood nitric oxide concentration was restored to that of normal, non-obese mice, and the blood pressure increase stopped.

12.7.5 Blood flow

Improvement in blood flow post-PBM, delivered over large areas or in an acupuncture-style manner, has been demonstrated by multiple groups using photoplethysmography or laser Doppler flowmetry. Improved blood flow changes are commonly accompanied by variations in overall blood volume and improvements in the microcirculation. The direct causes are not clear and may be related to small temperature rises resulting from laser irradiation, even at levels below 200 mW · cm^{-2}. Gavish *et al* [80] noted a minimum 20% increase in the microcirculation's blood volume and blood flow only in patients who demonstrated at least a 0.5 °C temperature increase in the irradiated area while delivering either 633 or 830 nm light at 70 or 55 mW · cm^{-2}, respectively. While this could suggest only a temporal effect driven by the autoregulatory function due to the temperature increase, it was noted that the PBM-induced arteriolar vasodilatation was long-lasting.

12.7.6 Blood glucose

Improvements in the blood glucose levels through increased muscle glycogen were demonstrated repeatedly in diabetic mouse models. Gong *et al* [81] also demonstrated insulin resistance and the reversal of metabolic abnormalities in skeletal muscle following delivery of 43.3 J · c^{-2} m-635 nm radiation over 10 min daily for 10 weeks. Castro *et al* [82] obtained similar results using a cluster of 69 lEDs emitting at 630 or 850 nm while delivering up to 60 J · cm^{-2}. The greatest increase in muscle glycogen was observed for 10 J · cm^{-2}. They noted that the induction of greater muscle glycogen synthesis was independent of physical exercise.

12.8 Vasculature and associated structures

PBM is often employed to accelerate the healing process post-injury, including open skin wounds [83], burns [84, 85], skeletal-muscular damage [86–88], or dramatic brain injury [75, 91], to name but a few.

12.8.1 Angiogenesis

Angiogenesis is often a reported anatomical modification post-PBM. This was demonstrated across a wide range of experimental models, including co-cultured *in vitro* studies, chick egg chorioallantoic membrane (CAM) assays, and *in vivo* studies. Organs for which PBM-mediated angiogenesis was demonstrated include the skin, brain, heart, and others. As angiogenesis requires 24 h or more to become evident, it is difficult to determine *in vivo* whether angiogenesis is a primary stimulating effect post-injury or if it is initiated due to increased oxygen demand by the mitochondria in the irradiated zone and accelerated cell division.

Winter *et al* investigated the PBM effect directly on the proliferation of vascular endothelial cells and thus angiogenesis in two co-culture models, *in vitro* using human umbilical vein endothelial cells with additional stem cells, and *in vivo* in the CAM model augmented with stem cells. PBM consisted of 635 nm radiant exposure of 24 J · cm^{-2} delivered at 80 mW · cm^{-2}. The *in vitro* studies demonstrated a doubling of cell division, accompanied by significantly improved cellular network formation and reduced cellular compactness. The CAM model showed a significant increase in vessel junction density [90].

An upregulation of angiogenesis-related gene expression was observed for HIF-1 alpha, VEGF, and TGF-beta, both *in vivo* after irradiation of grafts and *in vitro* when co-culturing different cells, such as BMSCs and HUVECs [88].

Zhang *et al* exposed human umbilical vein endothelial cells to 1 J · cm^{-2} of 632.8 nm radiation and demonstrated that vascular endothelial growth was mediated via the VEGFA/VEGFR2/STAT3 pathways to promote angiogenesis in wound healing [91].

Whittaker *et al* claim that the 'optimal' range for laser on the ischemic heart is 5–15 mW · cm^{-2}, showing the best angiogenesis effect of PBM [92]. A long-lasting impact up to 45 days of PBM post-myocardial infarct in the rat model was demonstrated to be driven by inducible heat shock proteins dominated by HSP70i, resulting in more than doubling of the cell density, and a three-fold increase in newly formed blood vessels in the heart [93].

In a clinical study involving 48 patients with Alzheimer's disease and 37 patients with vascular Parkinsonism (VP), Maksimovich [94] demonstrated that all patients underwent angiogenesis stimulation, resulting in cerebral collateral capillary revascularization and closure of arteriovenous shunts. The cognitive improvements, often resulting in a reduction in the required medication, lasted for up to 15 years.

12.8.2 Blood–brain barrier

Disruption of the BBB has been suggested as a culprit of cognitive decline across a broad spectrum of disorders [95]. Restoring the barrier function is considered a crucial step in maintaining or regaining cognitive abilities.

Equally, preconditioning of MPTP mice as a model of Parkinson's disease daily with 4 J · cm^{-2} doses of 670 nm light via the dorsum and hindlimbs for at least 10 days showed modulation of the BBB along with loss simultaneously reduced loss of midbrain tyrosine hydroxylase-positive dopaminergic cells and mitigated the increase in FOS-positive neurons in the caudate-putamen complex [89]. These changes have been attributed to an improvement in the performance of the BBB [96]. Conversely, Zhou *et al* [97] investigated the ability of PBM to improve drug delivery and noted that 10 or 30 J · cm^{-2} of 808 nm radiation increases the permeability of an *in vitro* BBB model via an increase in the mitochondrial activity, the concentration of ROS, and a Ca^{2+} influx. Additionally, inhibition of proteins associated with matrix metalloproteinases and endothelial cells' tight junction proteins was found. Hence, the actual effects of PBM on the BBB remain a topic of study.

12.9 Summary

Given the high molar extinction coefficients of hemoglobin in its oxidized and reduced form, paired with the extremely short singlet excited state, blood is acting primarily photothermally. Effects on platelets, leucocytes, and lymphocytes can either be driven by direct photochemical effects or rely on some thermal activation energy provided by the RBC. Given the lack of immediately modified biomarkers indicating the chemical changes during PBM, new and clever experiments need to be conceived to determine if photothermal or photochemical mechanisms are dominant.

One point, however, is clear: blood is a very important medium to facilitate systemic responses to PBM. Here, blood and blood plasma serve as photon absorbers and the primary site of signaling molecule generation. Alternatively, irradiated cells release signaling molecules into the blood, which are then transported to distant sites.

Open questions remain, including the molecular basis for the frequently observed biphasic PBM response as a function of irradiance or radiant exposure. Is blood playing any role here, given the changes in blood volume or blood flow documented during PBM?

The picture for PBM molecular mechanisms must be further developed, including the identification of other biologically effective chromophores beyond heme and CCO, and, thus, other competing signaling pathways to explain the plethora of clinical observations post-PBM. In particular, the impact of dynamic changes in the blood transmission of PBM radiation needs to be considered in most future *in vivo* studies.

References

[1] Gavish L, Hoffer O, Rabin N *et al* 2020 Microcirculatory response to photobiomodulation-why some respond and others do not: a randomized controlled study *Lasers Surg. Med.* **52** 863–72

[2] Ramos R C C, Roque A, Sarmiento J L A, D B *et al* 2022 Use of ultraviolet-C in environmental sterilization in hospitals: a systematic review on efficacy and safety *Int. J. Health Sci.* **14** 52–65

[3] Pereira A R, Braga D F, Vassal M *et al* 2023 Ultraviolet C irradiation: a promising approach for the disinfection of public spaces? *Sci. Total Environ.* **879** 163007

[4] Dominguez L J, Farruggia M, Veronese N and Barbagallo M 2021 Vitamin D sources, metabolism, and deficiency: available compounds and guidelines for its treatment *Metabolites* **11** 255

[5] Conrad K, Manahan C and Crane B 2014 Photochemistry of flavoprotein light sensors *Nat. Chem. Biol.* **10** 801–9

[6] Chen W, Li C, Liang W *et al* 2022 The roles of optogenetics and technology in neurobiology: a review *Front. Aging Neurosci.* **4** 867863

[7] Karu T I 2008 Mitochondrial signaling in mammalian cells activated by red and near-IR radiation *Photochem. Photobiol.* **84** 1091–9

[8] Passarella S and Karu T 2014 Absorption of monochromatic and narrow band radiation in the visible and near IR by both mitochondrial and non-mitochondrial photoacceptors results in photobiomodulation *J. Photochem. Photobiol.,* B **140** 344–58

[9] Karu T 2010 Mitochondrial mechanisms of photobiomodulation in context of new data about multiple roles of ATP *Photomed. Laser Surg.* **28** 159–60

[10] Akeson A, Börck G and Simon R 1969 On the content of cytochrome c in human muscles *Acta Med. Scand.* **185** 287–92

[11] Karu T 1999 Primary and secondary mechanisms of action of visible to near-IR radiation on cells *J. Photochem. Photobiol. B: Biol.* **49** 1–17

[12] Meredith P and Sarna T 2006 The physical and chemical properties of eumelanin *Pigment Cell Res* **19** 572–94

[13] Meredith P and Riesz J 2004 Radiative relaxation quantum yields for synthetic eumelanin *Photochem. Photobiol.* **79** 211–6
[14] Hamblin M R 2017 Mechanisms and applications of the anti-inflammatory effects of photobiomodulation *AIMS Biophys.* **4** 337–61
[15] Nie F, Hao S, Ji Y, Zhang Y *et al* 2023 Biphasic dose response in the anti-inflammation experiment of PBM *Lasers Med. Sci.* **738** 66
[16] Hawker G A, Mian S, Kendzerska T and French M 2011 Measures of adult pain: Visual Analog Scale for Pain (VAS Pain), Numeric Rating Scale for Pain (NRS Pain), McGill Pain Questionnaire (MPQ), Short-Form McGill Pain Questionnaire (SF-MPQ), Chronic Pain Grade Scale (CPGS), Short Form-36 Bodily Pain Scale (SF-36 BPS), and Measure of Intermittent and Constant Osteoarthritis Pain (ICOAP) *Arthritis Care Res* **63** S240–52
[17] Langella L G, Casalechi H L, Tomazoni S S *et al* 2018 Photobiomodulation therapy (PBMT) on acute pain and inflammation in patients who underwent total hip arthroplasty-a randomized, triple-blind, placebo-controlled clinical trial *Lasers Med. Sci.* **33** 1933–40
[18] Ammar T 2015 Monochromatic infrared photo energy versus low level laser therapy in chronic low back pain *J. Lasers Med. Sci.* **6** 157–61
[19] de Holanda Araujo A M P, de Sena K R R, da Silva Filho E M *et al* 2020 Low-level laser therapy improves pain in postcesarean section: a randomized clinical trial *Lasers Med. Sci.* **35** 1095–102
[20] Momeni E, Kazemi F and Sanaei-Rad P 2022 Extraoral low-level laser therapy can decrease pain but not edema and trismus after surgical extraction of impacted mandibular third molars: a randomized, placebo-controlled clinical trial *BMC Oral Health* **22** 417
[21] Zecha J A, Raber-Durlacher J E and Nair R G 2016 Low level laser therapy/photobiomodulation in the management of side effects of chemoradiation therapy in head and neck cancer: part 1: mechanisms of action, dosimetric, and safety considerations *Support Care Cancer.* **24** 2781–92
[22] Kawakubo M, Ferraresi C, Kaippert B *et al* 2018 2018 Pain management using photobiomodulation: mechanisms, location, and repeatability quantified by pain threshold and neural biomarkers in mice *J. Biophotonics* **11** e201700370
[23] Kemper K J 2018 'Let there be light.' Research on phototherapy, light therapy, and photobiomodulation for healing—alternative therapy becomes mainstream *Complement. Ther. Med.* **41** A1–6
[24] Cheng K, Martin L F, Slepian M J *et al* 2021 Mechanisms and pathways of pain photobiomodulation: a narrative review *J. Pain.* **22** 763–77
[25] Shen Q, Guo H and Yan Y 2024 Photobiomodulation for neurodegenerative diseases: a scoping review *Int. J. Mol. Sci.* **25** 1625
[26] Singh N and Lilge L 2025 Light-based therapy of infected wounds: a review of dose considerations for photodynamic microbial inactivation and photobiomodulation *J. Biomed. Opt.* **30** 030901
[27] Mohammed Ihsan F R 2005 Low-level laser therapy accelerates collateral circulation and enhances microcirculation *Photomed. Laser Surg.* **23** 289
[28] Bayat M, Delbari A, Almaseyeh M A *et al* 2005 Low-level laser therapy improves early healing of medial collateral ligament injuries in rats *Photomed. Laser Surg.* **23** 556–60
[29] Aparecida Da Silva A, Leal-Junior E C, Alves A C *et al* 2013 Wound-healing effects of low-level laser therapy in diabetic rats involve the modulation of MMP-2 and MMP-9 and the redistribution of collagen types I and III *J. Cosmet. Laser Ther.* **15** 210–6

[30] Ayuk S M, Abrahamse H and Houreld N N 2016 The role of matrix metalloproteinases in diabetic wound healing in relation to photobiomodulation *J. Diabetes Res.* **2016** 2897656

[31] Dantas M D, Cavalcante D R, Araújo F E *et al* 2011 Improvement of dermal burn healing by combining sodium alginate/chitosan-based films and low level laser therapy *J. Photochem. Photobiol.,* B **105** 51–9

[32] Salehpour F, Mahmoudi J and Kamari F 2018 Brain photobiomodulation therapy: a narrative review *Mol. Neurobiol.* **55** 6601–36

[33] Chamkouri H, Liu Q, Zhang Y *et al* 2024 Brain photobiomodulation therapy on neurological and psychological diseases *J. Biophotonics* **17** e202300145

[34] Hennessy M and Hamblin M R 2016 Photobiomodulation and the brain: a new paradigm *J. Opt.* **19** 013003

[35] Toma R L, Oliveira M X, Renno A C M *et al* 2018 Photobiomodulation (PBM) therapy at 904 nm mitigates effects of exercise-induced skeletal muscle fatigue in young women *Lasers Med. Sci.* **33** 1197–205

[36] Hamblin M R 2017 Photobiomodulation for stroke *Translational Research in Stroke. Translational Medicine Research* ed P Lapchak and G Y Yang (Singapore: Springer)

[37] Cardoso F D S, Gonzalez-Lima F and Gomes da Silva S 2021 Photobiomodulation for the aging brain *Ageing Res. Rev.* **70** 101415

[38] Cunningham D A, Varnerin N, Machado A *et al* 2015 Stimulation targeting higher motor areas in stroke rehabilitation: a proof-of-concept, randomized, double-blinded placebo-controlled study of effectiveness and underlying mechanisms *Restor. Neurol. Neurosci.* **33** 911–26

[39] Golden R N, Gaynes B N, Ekstrom R D *et al* 2005 The efficacy of light therapy in the treatment of mood disorders: a review and meta-analysis of the evidence *Am. J. Psychiatry* **162** 656–62

[40] Cassano P, Petrie S R, Mischoulon D *et al* 2018 Transcranial photobiomodulation for the treatment of major depressive disorder. The ELATED-2 pilot trial *Photomed. Laser Surg.* **36** 634–46

[41] Schiffer F, Johnston A L, Ravichandran C *et al* 2009 Psychological benefits 2 and 4 weeks after a single treatment with near infrared light to the forehead: a pilot study of 10 patients with major depression and anxiety *Behav. Brain Funct.* **5** 46

[42] Semyachkina-Glushkovskaya O, Abdurashitov A, Dubrovsky A *et al* 2020 Photobiomodulation of lymphatic drainage and clearance: perspective strategy for augmentation of meningeal lymphatic functions *Biomed. Opt. Express* **11** 725–34

[43] De Marchi T, Schmitt V M, Machado G P *et al* 2017 Does photobiomodulation therapy is better than cryotherapy in muscle recovery after a high-intensity exercise? A randomized, double-blind, placebo-controlled clinical trial *Lasers Med. Sci.* **32** 429–37

[44] Robijns J, Nair R G, Lodewijckx J *et al* 2022 Photobiomodulation therapy in management of cancer therapy-induced side effects: WALT position paper *Front Oncol.* **12** 927685

[45] Antunes H S, Herchenhorn D, Small I A *et al* 2013 Phase III trial of low-level laser therapy to prevent oral mucositis in head and neck cancer patients treated with concurrent chemo-radiation *Radiother. Oncol.* **109** 297–302

[46] Gautam A P, Fernandes D J, Vidyasagar M S *et al* 2015 Low level laser therapy against radiation induced oral mucositis in elderly head and neck cancer patients-a randomized placebo controlled trial *J. Photochem. Photobiol.,* B **144** 51–6

[47] Robijns J, Censabella S, Claes S, Pannekoeke L, Bussé L, Colson D *et al* 2018 Prevention of acute radiodermatitis by photobiomodulation: a randomized, placebo-controlled trial in breast cancer patients (TRANSDERMIS trial) *Lasers Surg. Med.* **50** 763–71

[48] Gautam A P, Fernandes D J, Vidyasagar M S *et al* 2012 Low level laser therapy for concurrent chemoradiotherapy induced oral mucositis in head and neck cancer patients—a triple blinded randomized controlled trial *Radiother. Oncol.* **104** 349–54

[49] Russi E G, Corvò R, Merlotti A *et al* 2012 Swallowing dysfunction in head and neck cancer patients treated by radiotherapy: review and recommendations of the supportive task group of the Italian Association of Radiation Oncology *Cancer Treat. Rev.* **38** 1033–49

[50] Nutting C M, Morden J P, Harrington K J *et al* 2011 Parotid-sparing intensity modulated versus conventional radiotherapy in head and neck cancer (PARSPORT): a phase 3 multicentre randomised controlled trial *Lancet Oncol.* **12** 127–36

[51] Jackson R F, Dedo D D, Roche G C *et al* 2009 Low-level laser therapy as a non-invasive approach for body contouring: a randomized, controlled study *Lasers Surg. Med.* **41** 799–809

[52] Lampl Y, Zivin J A, Fisher M *et al* 2007 Infrared laser therapy for ischemic stroke: a new treatment strategy: results of the NeuroThera Effectiveness and Safety Trial-1 (NEST-1) *Stroke* **38** 1843–9

[53] Huisa B N, Stemer A B, Walker M G *et al* 2013 Transcranial laser therapy for acute ischemic stroke: a pooled analysis of NEST-1 and NEST-2 *Int. J. Stroke.* **8** 315–20

[54] Zivin J A, Sehra R, Shoshoo A *et al* 2014 NeuroThera(R) Efficacy and Safety Trial-3 (NEST-3): a double-blind, randomized, sham-controlled, parallel group, multicenter, pivotal study to assess the safety and efficacy of transcranial laser therapy with the NeuroThera(R) laser system for the treatment of acute ischemic stroke within 24 h of stroke onset *Int. J. Stroke.* **9** 950–5

[55] https://lia.org/resources/laser-safety-information/laser-safety-standards/ansi-z136-standards/z136-3

[56] Fixler D, Duadi H, Ankri R and Zalevsky Z 2011 Determination of coherence length in biological tissues *Lasers Surg. Med.* **43** 339–43

[57] Liemert A, Reitzle D and Kienle A 2017 Analytical solutions of the radiative transport equation for turbid and fluorescent layered media *Scient. Rep.* **7** 3819

[58] Liemert A, Martelli F, Binzoni T and Kienle A 2019 P3 solution for the total steady-state and time-resolved reflectance and transmittance from a turbid slab *J. Opt. Soc. Am.* A **58** 4143–8

[59] Jacques S L 2023 Tutorial on Monte Carlo simulation of photon transport in biological tissues *Biomed. Opt. Express* **14** 559–76

[60] Fang Q and Yan S 2022 MCX Cloud-a modern, scalable, high-performance and in-browser Monte Carlo simulation platform with cloud computing *J. Biomed. Opt.* **27** 083008

[61] Nina-Paravecino F, Yu L, Fang Q and Kaeli D 2017 High-performance Monte Carlo simulations for photon migration and applications in optical brain functional imaging *Handbook of Large-Scale Distributed Computing in Smart Healthcare. Scalable Computing and Communications* ed S Khan, A Zomaya and A Abbas (Cham: Springer)

[62] Cassidy J, Nouri A, Betz V and Lilge L 2018 High-performance, robustly verified Monte Carlo simulation with FullMonte *J. Biomed. Opt.* **23** 085001

[63] Young-Schultz T, Brown S, Lilge L and Betz V 2019 FullMonteCUDA: a fast, flexible, and accurate GPU-accelerated Monte Carlo simulator for light propagation in turbid media *Biomed. Opt. Express* **10** 4711–26

[64] Doronin A V and Meglinski I V 2012 Peer-to-Peer Monte Carlo simulation of photon migration in topical applications of biomedical optics *J. Biomed. Opt.* **17** 090504
[65] Meglinski I V and Doronin A V 2012 Monte Carlo modeling for the needs of biophotonics and biomedical optics *Advanced Biophotonics: Tissue Optical Sectioning* ed V V Tuchin and R K Wang (Taylor & Francis)
[66] Souza-Barros L, Dhaidan G, Maunula M *et al* 2018 Skin color and tissue thickness effects on transmittance, reflectance, and skin temperature when using 635 and 808nm lasers in low intensity therapeutics *Lasers Surg. Med.* **50** 291–301
[67] Jacques S L 2013 Optical properties of biological tissues: a review *Phys. Med. Biol.* **58** R37–61
[68] Nolan Y, Campbell V A, Bolton A E and Lynch M A 2005 Evidence of an anti-inflammatory role for vasogen's immune modulation therapy *Neuroimmunomodulation* **12** 113–6
[69] Dos Santos Malavazzi T C, Andreo L, Martinelli A *et al* 2024 Preventive and therapeutic vascular photobiomodulation decreases the inflammatory markers and enhances the muscle repair process in an animal model *J. Photochem. Photobiol.* B **256** 112921
[70] Pereira P C, de Lima C J, Fernandes A B *et al* 2022 Systemic effects of photobiomodulation on blood components in the treatment of community-acquired pneumonia *Photobiomodul. Photomed. Laser Surg.* **40** 51–8
[71] Semyachkina-Glushkovskaya O, Klimova M, Iskra T *et al* 2021 Transcranial photobiomodulation of clearance of beta-amyloid from the mouse brain: effects on the meningeal lymphatic drainage and blood oxygen saturation of the brain *Adv. Exp. Med. Biol.* **1269** 57–61
[72] Irmak G, Demirtaş T T and Gümüşderelioğlu M 2020 Sustained release of growth factors from photoactivated platelet rich plasma (PRP *Eur. J. Pharm. Biopharm.* **148** 67–76
[73] Jadah N A and Shamkhi I A 2021 A comparative study of low-level laser efficacy on autologous activity of PRP injected in knee arthritis, *in vivo* study *Lasers Med. Sci.* **36** 357–63
[74] Walski T, Grzeszczuk-Kuć K, Mehl J *et al* 2024 Biphasic dose-response and effects of near-infrared photobiomodulation on erythrocytes susceptibility to oxidative stress *in vitro J. Photochem. Photobiol.,* B **257** 112958
[75] Hamblin M R 2016 Shining light on the head: photobiomodulation for brain disorders *BBA Clin.* **6** 113–24
[76] Wang X, Tian F, Soni S S *et al* 2016 Interplay between up-regulation of cytochrome-c-oxidase and hemoglobin oxygenation induced by near-infrared laser *Sci. Rep.* **6** 30540
[77] Salehpour F, Khademi M, Bragin D E and DiDuro J O 2022 Photobiomodulation therapy and the glymphatic system: promising applications for augmenting the brain lymphatic drainage system *Int. J. Mol. Sci.* **23** 2975
[78] Mitrofanis J and Henderson L A 2020 How and why does photobiomodulation change brain activity? *Neural Regen. Res.* **15** 2243–4
[79] Oishi J C, de Moraes L H O, Filho J C C *et al* 2024 Long-term effects of photobiomodulation therapy on blood pressure in obese rats induced by a high-fat diet *Lasers Med. Sci.* **39** 20
[80] Gavish L, Hoffer O, Rabin N *et al* 2020 Microcirculatory response to photobiomodulation —why some respond and others do not: a randomized controlled study *Lasers Surg. Med.* **52** 863–72
[81] Gong L, Zou Z, Liu L *et al* 2021 Photobiomodulation therapy ameliorates hyperglycemia and insulin resistance by activating cytochrome c oxidase-mediated protein kinase B in muscle *Aging* **13** 10015–33

[82] Castro K M R, de Paiva Carvalho R L, Junior G M R *et al* 2020 Can photobiomodulation therapy (PBMT) control blood glucose levels and alter muscle glycogen synthesis? *J. Photochem. Photobiol.,* B **207** 111877
[83] Mosca R C, Ong A A, Albasha O, Bass K and Arany P 2019 Photobiomodulation therapy for wound care: a potent, noninvasive, photoceutical approach *Adv. Skin Wound Care* **32** 157–67
[84] Khan I, Rahman S U, Tang E *et al* 2021 Accelerated burn wound healing with photobiomodulation therapy involves activation of endogenous latent TGF-β1 *Sci. Rep.* **11** 13371
[85] Firouz B, Faihs L, Slezak P *et al* 2023 Testing the effects of photobiomodulation on angiogenesis in a newly established CAM burn wound model *Sci. Rep.* **13** 22985
[86] Ferraresi C, Huang Y Y and Hamblin M R 2016 Photobiomodulation in human muscle tissue: an advantage in sports performance? *J. Biophotonics* **9** 1273–99
[87] Gendron D J and Hamblin M R 2019 Applications of photobiomodulation therapy to musculoskeletal disorders and osteoarthritis with particular relevance to Canada *Photobiomodul. Photomed. Laser Surg.* **37** 408–20
[88] Bai J, Li L, Kou N *et al* 2021 Low level laser therapy promotes bone regeneration by coupling angiogenesis and osteogenesis *Stem Cell Res. Ther.* **12** 432
[89] Bathini M, Raghushaker C R and Mahato K K 2022 The molecular mechanisms of action of photobiomodulation against neurodegenerative diseases: a systematic review *Cell Mol. Neurobiol.* **42** 955–71
[90] Winter R, Dungel P, Reischies F M J *et al* 2018 Photobiomodulation (PBM) promotes angiogenesis *in vitro* and in chick embryo chorioallantoic membrane model *Sci. Rep.* **8** 17080
[91] Zhang G, Yi L, Wang C *et al* 2022 Photobiomodulation promotes angiogenesis in wound healing through stimulating the nuclear translocation of VEGFR2 and STAT3 *J. Photochem. Photobiol.,* B **237** 112573
[92] Whittaker P and Patterson M 2000 Ventricular remodeling after acute myocardial infarction: effect of low-intensity laser irradiation *Lasers Surg. Med.* **27** 29–38
[93] Yaakobi T, Shoshany Y, Levkovitz S, Rubin O, Ben Haim S A and Oron U 2001 Long-term effect of low energy laser irradiation on infarction and reperfusion injury in the rat heart *J. Appl. Physiol.* **90** 2411–9
[94] Maksimovich I V 2023 Stimulation of cerebral angiogenesis and neurogenesis with transcatheter intracerebral laser photobiomodulation therapy in Alzheimer's disease and vascular Parkinsonism aggravated by dementia *Alzheimer's Dement* **19** e073677
[95] Che J, Sun Y, Deng Y *et al* 2024 Blood-brain barrier disruption: a culprit of cognitive decline? *Fluids Barriers CNS* **21** 63
[96] Ganeshan V, Skladnev N V, Kim J Y, Mitrofanis J, Stone J and Johnstone D M 2019 Preconditioning with remote photobiomodulation modulates the brain transcriptome and protects against MPTP insult in mice *Neuroscience.* **21400** 85–97
[97] Zhou T, Ohulchanskyy T Y and Qu J 2021 Effect of NIR light on the permeability of the blood-brain barriers in *in vitro* models *Biomed. Opt. Express* **12** 7544–55
[98] Ferraresi C, Parizotto N A, Pires de Sousa M V *et al* 2015 Light-emitting diode therapy in exercise-trained mice increases muscle performance, cytochrome c oxidase activity, ATP and cell proliferation *J. Biophotonics* **8** 740–54

www.ingramcontent.com/pod-product-compliance
Ingram Content Group UK Ltd.
Pitfield, Milton Keynes, MK11 3LW, UK
UKHW051908100926
8556IPUK00005B/802

9 780750 34804